Seminars in Clinical Psychopharmacology

Third Edition

College Seminars Series

For details of available and forthcoming books in the College Seminars Series please visit www.cambridge.org/series/college-seminars-series/

Seminars in Clinical Psychopharmacology

Third Edition

Edited by

Peter M. Haddad

Senior Consultant Psychiatrist, Hamad Medical Corporation, Doha, Qatar; Clinical Professor of Psychiatry, Qatar University, Qatar; Honorary Consultant Psychiatrist, Greater Manchester Mental Health NHS Foundation Trust, Manchester, United Kingdom; Honorary Professor of Psychiatry, University of Manchester, United Kingdom

David J. Nutt

Edmond J. Safra Professor of Neuropsychopharmacology and Head of the Centre for Neuropsychopharmacology, Division of Psychiatry, Department of Brain Sciences, Imperial College London, United Kingdom

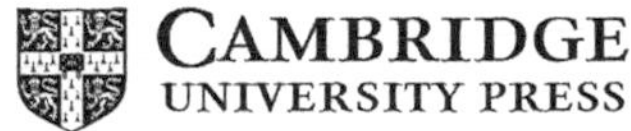

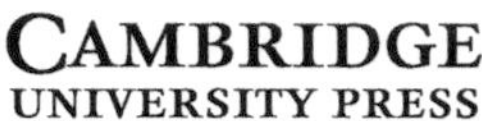

University Printing House, Cambridge CB2 8BS, United Kingdom

One Liberty Plaza, 20th Floor, New York, NY 10006, USA

477 Williamstown Road, Port Melbourne, VIC 3207, Australia

314–321, 3rd Floor, Plot 3, Splendor Forum, Jasola District Centre, New Delhi – 110025, India

79 Anson Road, #06–04/06, Singapore 079906

Cambridge University Press is part of the University of Cambridge.

It furthers the University's mission by disseminating knowledge in the pursuit of education, learning, and research at the highest international levels of excellence.

www.cambridge.org
Information on this title: www.cambridge.org/9781911623458
DOI: 10.1017/9781911623465

This book was previously published by The Royal College of Psychiatrists.

First published 1995, The Royal College of Psychiatrists
Second edition 2004, The Royal College of Psychiatrists
This third edition published by Cambridge University Press 2020

Printed in the United Kingdom by TJ International Ltd. Padstow Cornwall

A catalogue record for this publication is available from the British Library.

Library of Congress Cataloging-in-Publication Data
Names: Haddad, Peter M., editor. | Nutt, David J., 1951– editor.
Title: Seminars in clinical psychopharmacology / edited by Peter M. Haddad, David J. Nutt.
Other titles: College seminars series.
Description: Third edition. | New York, NY : Cambridge University Press, 2020. | Series: College seminars series | Includes bibliographical references and index.
Identifiers: LCCN 2019030912 (print) | ISBN 9781911623458 (paperback) | ISBN 9781911623465 (epub)
Subjects: MESH: Psychotropic Drugs | Psychopharmacology
Classification: LCC RM315 (print) | LCC RM315 (ebook) | NLM QV 77.2 | DDC 615.7/88–dc23
LC record available at https://lccn.loc.gov/2019030912
LC ebook record available at https://lccn.loc.gov/2019030913

ISBN 978-1-911-62345-8 Paperback

Contents

Contributors

Nicoletta Adamo
Visiting Research Fellow, Social, Genetic and Developmental Psychiatry Centre (PO80) Institute of Psychiatry, Psychology & Neuroscience, King's College London; Consultant Child and Adolescent Psychiatrist, South London and Maudsley (SLaM) National Services, NHS Foundation Trust, London, UK

Katherine J. Aitchison
Professor, Department of Psychiatry; Adjunct Professor, Department of Medical Genetics; Associate Director, Mental Health, Neuroscience and Mental Institute and Consulting Psychiatrist, Mood and Anxiety Disorders Program; University of Alberta, Edmonton, Canada

David S. Baldwin
Professor of Psychiatry, Clinical and Experimental Sciences, Faculty of Medicine, University of Southampton, United Kingdom; Honorary Professor of Psychiatry, University of Cape Town, South Africa; Visiting Professor, Shandong Mental Health Centre, China

Stuart Banham
Principal Pharmacist, South London and Maudsley (SLaM) NHS Foundation Trust, London, UK

Thomas R. E. Barnes
Emeritus Professor of Clinical Psychiatry, Imperial College London, UK

Alistair Burns
Professor of Old Age Psychiatry, University of Manchester, Jean McFarlane Building, University of Manchester, Oxford Road, Manchester, UK

David Christmas
Consultant Psychiatrist and Honorary Senior Lecturer, Advanced Interventions Service, Ninewells Hospital & Medical School, Dundee, UK

Anthony Cleare
Professor of Psychopharmacology & Affective Disorders, Institute of Psychiatry, Psychology and Neuroscience, King's College London, London, UK

David Coghill
Professor of Psychiatry, Financial Markets Foundation Chair of Developmental Mental Health, Departments of Paediatrics and Psychiatry, Faculty of Medicine, Dentistry and Health Sciences, University of Melbourne; Murdoch Children's Research Institute, Melbourne, Australia

Stephen J. Cooper
Professor Emeritus, Queen's University Belfast, United Kingdom; Clinical Lead for the National Clinical Audit of Psychosis, Centre for Quality Improvement, Royal College of Psychiatrists, London, UK

Simon J. C. Davies
Associate Professor, Geriatric Psychiatry Division, Centre for Addiction & Mental Health (CAMH), Toronto and Department of Psychiatry, University of Toronto, Canada

Richard Drake
Senior Lecturer, University of Manchester, United Kingdom; Honorary Consultant in Rehabilitation Psychiatry,

Greater Manchester Mental Health NHS Foundation Trust, Manchester, UK

Ross Dunne
Consultant Psychiatrist for Later Life, Greater Manchester Mental Health NHS Foundation Trust, Park House, North Manchester General Hospital, Manchester, UK

A. Richard Green
Honorary Professor of Neuropharmacology, School of Life Sciences, Queen's Medical Centre, University of Nottingham, Nottingham, UK

Peter M. Haddad
Senior Consultant Psychiatrist, Hamad Medical Corporation, Doha; Clinical Professor of Psychiatry, Qatar University, Qatar; Honorary Consultant Psychiatrist, Greater Manchester Mental Health NHS Foundation Trust; Honorary Professor of Psychiatry, University of Manchester, UK

Beatriz C. Henriques
Masters in Psychiatry student, Departments of Psychiatry and Medical Genetics, University of Alberta, Edmonton, Canada

Oliver D. Howes
Professor of Molecular Psychiatry, King's College London, Institute of Medical Sciences (Imperial College) and Honorary Consultant Psychiatrist, Maudsley Hospital, London, UK

Nathan T. M. Huneke
MRC Clinical Research Fellow, Clinical and Experimental Sciences, Faculty of Medicine, University of Southampton, and Honorary Registrar in General Adult Psychiatry, Southern Health NHS Foundation Trust, Southampton, UK

John Hutchison
Chief Medical Officer, Autifony Therapeutics Ltd, Stevenage Bioscience Catalyst, Stevenage, Hertfordshire, UK

Ian Jones
Professor of Psychiatry, Cardiff University; Honorary Consultant Psychiatrist in Cardiff and Vale NHS Trust, UK

Stephen J. Kaar
Clinical Research Worker, Institute of Psychiatry, Psychology and Neuroscience, King's College London and Specialty Trainee, South London and Maudsley NHS Trust, UK

Diego L. Lapetina
Postdoctoral Fellow, Departments of Psychiatry and Medical Genetics, University of Alberta, Edmonton, Canada

Brian E. Leonard
Emeritus Professor of Pharmacology, National University of Ireland, Galway, Ireland

Keith Matthews
Professor of Psychiatry and Honorary Consultant Psychiatrist, University of Dundee, Ninewells Hospital & Medical School, Dundee, UK

Robert McCutcheon
Wellcome Clinical Research Training Fellow, Institute of Psychiatry, Psychology and Neuroscience, King's College London and Specialty Trainee, South London and Maudsley NHS Trust, UK

Patrick McLaughlin
Specialist Registrar in Psychiatry, National Affective Disorders Service, South London and Maudsley NHS Foundation Trust, Maudsley Hospital, London, UK

Ulrich Müller-Sedgwick
Consultant Psychiatrist, Adult ADHD Service, Barnet Enfield Haringey Mental Health NHS Trust, Springwell Centre, Barnet Hospital, London; Honorary Visiting Fellow, Department of Psychiatry, University of Cambridge, Cambridge, UK

Joanna C. Neill
Professor of Psychopharmacology, Division of Pharmacy and Optometry, School of Health Sciences, University of Manchester, Manchester, United Kingdom

David J. Nutt
Edmond J. Safra Professor of Neuropsychopharmacology and Head of the Centre for Neuropsychopharmacology, Division of Psychiatry, Department of Brain Sciences, Imperial College London, UK

Aileen O'Brien
Reader in Psychiatry and Education, and Honorary Consultant Psychiatrist, St. George's, University of London, UK

Caroline Parker
Consultant Mental Health Pharmacist, St Charles Hospital, Central and North West London NHS Foundation Trust, London, United Kingdom

Maxine X. Patel
Consultant Psychiatrist, Oxleas NHS Foundation Trust, and Honorary Clinical Senior Lecturer, King's College London, London, UK

Lesley Peters
Consultant Addiction Psychiatrist, My Recovery Tameside, Change Grow Live, UK

Gavin P. Reynolds
Professor Emeritus, Queen's University Belfast; Honorary Professor, Biomolecular Sciences Research Centre, Sheffield Hallam University, UK

Jane A. Sedgwick-Müller
Senior Teaching Fellow, Programme Lead BSc Mental Health Nursing: Florence Nightingale Faculty of Nursing &, Midwifery & Palliative Care, Institute of Psychiatry, Psychology & Neuroscience, King's College London; ADHD/ASD Coach & Psychosocial Therapist, UK

Faisil Sethi
Consultant Psychiatrist, Maudsley Hospital, South London and Maudsley NHS Foundation Trust, London, UK

Mohammed Shahid
Senior Adviser in Translational Research, Orion Pharma, Nottingham, UK

Julia Sinclair
Professor of Addiction Psychiatry, and Honorary Consultant in Alcohol Liaison, University Hospital Southampton, UK

Dilveer S. Sually
Clinical Trial Coordinator, Department of Psychological Medicine, Institute of Psychiatry, Psychology and Neuroscience, King's College London, London, UK

Peter S. Talbot
Senior Lecturer, University of Manchester; Honorary Consultant Psychiatrist, Greater Manchester Mental Health NHS Foundation Trust, Manchester, UK

David Taylor
Professor of Psychopharmacology, Institute of Pharmaceutical Science, King's College London, London, UK

Esther H. Yang
Research Assistant, Departments of Psychiatry and Medical Genetics,

University of Alberta, Edmonton, Canada

Allan H. Young
Director, Centre for Affective Disorders, Department of Psychological Medicine, Institute of Psychiatry, Psychology and Neuroscience, King's College London, London, UK

Angelika Wieck
Honorary Senior Lecturer in Psychiatry, University of Manchester, Manchester, UK

Foreword

'Most psychiatric patients with anxiety, depression, and schizophrenia, and a good previous personality can now quickly be got well ... but one must be prepared to use every *physical* treatment now available (Sargant, 1966)(his italics). The clumsy quote from this lecture was written at the apogee of physical treatments in psychiatry and published a month before I took up the post of House Physician in Psychological Medicine under the tutelage of William Sargant. This post became a master-class of excess, and I learnt more about both the value and risks of psychopharmacology in the following six months than I would ever have done in a conventional post.

This post stimulated my interest and in 1982 I edited a book on psychopharmacology (Tyrer, 1982). In the introduction I offered a (pretty specious) excuse for error or omission by trumpeting that such was 'the pace of change that by the time this book is published it will be already out of date'. But the pace has slowed, dramatically, and I do not think I would write in the same way today, and even though we know so much more about drugs, we have not made the great advances achieved by the introduction of imipramine and chlorpromazine.

Drug treatment in psychiatry is now at the crossroads. On one side it is being buffeted by other mental health practitioners promoting psychological treatments as fundamentally superior in effecting change, while on the other it is assailed by a motley crowd of anti-psychiatry supporters, dissatisfied patients and worried observers who in different ways attack the prescriber more than the drug for the unthinking and industrialized marketing of pills. The drug prescriber is viewed as the idiot who does not have the competence to talk to patients, only the prescription pad.

So what is the way forward past the crossroads? As the Irish priest said, 'it is the straight and narrow path between right and wrong'. It is right to continue to develop new drugs, to test them independently without favour, and to have new horizons of understanding, but wrong to overstate the pharmacology of mechanism when understanding is low, to listen too closely to the claims made by representatives of pharmaceutical companies, or to minimize the importance of the adverse effects of drugs while promoting their benefits.

Correcting these errors is going to require hard work, and I am glad to say that this new edition of *Seminars in Psychopharmacology* has put this off to a good start. A lot of the former arrogance of the subject has been lost, so now we do not have chapters on 'antidepressants' and 'anxiolytics' but 'drugs for depression' and 'drugs for anxiety', so emphasizing that what Donald Klein called 'pharmacological dissection' (Klein, 1987) (the notion that a diagnosis such as panic disorder could be identified solely by drug response) is remarkably rare. The chapter format represents an excellent balance between science and practice, and, despite my interest in the subject, I am glad there is not a chapter on drug treatment in personality disorders, as it would be very difficult to write and would be remarkably unedifying.

It is also very good to have frequent guidance on the careful monitoring of drug treatment and the early recognition of adverse effects, subjects that have come to the fore with the excellent work of Thomas Barnes and Carol Paton who have just completed ten years of the Prescribing Observatory for Mental Health (POMH-UK); a title that reminded me of a telescope when I first came across it but now, with the careful analysis that has been central to their work, is more akin to a microscope. This work has also helped to bring pharmacists more closely into the arena of the subject, and their value as independent experts with key knowledge has doubtless improved the cost-effectiveness of drug treatment enormously.

The last, but probably the most important, need for psychopharmacology is for its practitioners to improve their image. I accept that they have been traduced unfairly, but they have not always defended themselves well in public fora. When there are powerful and eloquent voices on the other side of the fence such as Joanna Moncrieff (2007) and David Healy (2013) it is wrong to dismiss them as psychiatrists who are just beyond the pale.

In particular, you need to remove the perception that psychotherapists of all persuasions are warm and empathic while those who prescribe drugs are detached and impersonal and more interested in their wallets than patient welfare. In so doing, I think these words of Philip Cowen, a scientist and psychopharmacologist of distinction, but also a careful clinician, are worth keeping very close to your heart:

'Psychopharmacology is important to many patients, can be difficult to manage safely and effectively, and is controversial. The best way to secure the future of the discipline is to ensure that psychiatrists who prescribe have a deep understanding of the relevant clinical science as well as the ability to assess clinical trials of whatever provenance in a critical yet balanced way. In terms of individual treatment, initiation of medication with a follow-up appointment several weeks hence, perhaps with a different clinician, is not the way to use medicines successfully. Like psychotherapy, successful prescribing in psychiatry requires a collaborative and reflective clinical relationship characterised by continuity as well as warmth, kindness and hope' (Cowen, 2011).

As one of my Lancastrian teachers used to say, 'think on'.

Peter Tyrer
Centre for Psychiatry, Imperial College, London

References

Cowen PJ (2011). Has psychopharmacology got a future? *Br J Psychiatry*, 198, 333–335.

Healy D (2013). *Pharmageddon*. Berkeley: University of California Press.

Klein DF (1987). Anxiety reconceptualised: gleaning from pharmacological dissection – early experience with imipramine and anxiety. *Mod Probl Pharmacopsychiatry*, 22, 1–35.

Moncrieff J (2007). *The Myth of the Chemical Cure: A Critique of Psychiatric Drug Treatment*. London: Palgrave Macmillan.

Sargant W (1966). Psychiatric treatment in general hospitals: a plea for a mechanistic approach. *BMJ*, 2, 257–262.

Tyrer PJ (ed.) (1982). *Drugs in Psychiatric Practice*. London: Butterworth.

Preface

The second edition of this book was edited by David King and published in 2004. Since then there have been major advances in psychopharmacology in terms of new medications coming to the market, increased understanding of the mechanisms of drug action and new data on the efficacy, tolerability, safety and clinical effectiveness of a range of medications. Partly as a result, clinical guidelines for many psychiatric disorders have altered. As such, a new edition of this textbook was essential and we were delighted when the College approached us to edit the third edition. This was a major endeavour that was only possible with the commitment and expertise of the authors. We wish to thank them and also Professor Peter Tyrer for writing the foreword.

The book has been rewritten and greatly expanded since the second edition appeared. There are 21 chapters rather than 16 and the number of contributing authors has increased from 22 to 44. With one exception all the authors are new. We aimed to achieve a wider range of authors than in previous editions and are particularly pleased to have contributors from outside the UK including Australia, Canada and Ireland. Most authors are psychiatrists but preclinical scientists, pharmacists and the nursing profession are also represented. The lead authors of each chapter are all acknowledged experts and opinion leaders in their respective fields and many have contributed to national clinical guidelines. We are indebted to the editors and authors of the two earlier editions which provided a foundation for our work. In particular, we have retained the division of the book into three broad sections as in the second edition (i.e. Basic Science and General Principles, Psychopharmacology of the Main Psychotropic Drug Groups, Specific Therapeutic Areas) and ensured that the integration of basic sciences, pharmacology and clinical practice within each chapter, a strength of the earlier editions, remains.

A particular challenge in any book on psychopharmacology is nomenclature. We asked contributors where possible to incorporate the Neuroscience-based Nomenclature (NbN) in their chapters. In NbN each drug is named after the primary neurotransmitter system(s) that the drug acts on followed by its mode of action. This contrasts to 'traditional' terminology where drugs are named after one psychiatric disorder that they treat, for example antidepressants and antipsychotics. This ignores the fact that most psychiatric drugs are efficacious in several disorders and naming them after one disorder may cause confusion. In addition, traditional terminology does not help clinicians to make informed choices about next step pharmacological treatment. NbN overcomes these drawbacks. However, no nomenclature is ideal for all purposes and clinicians are likely to use a combination of NbN and traditional terminology in their work. As such, a pragmatic approach is adopted in this book and older generic terms, for example antidepressant, antipsychotic and anxiolytic, still appear. However, where a generic label is needed, we tend to prefer for example 'drugs for depression' rather than 'antidepressants' as the former seems less likely to imply a uniform domain and mechanism of action than the latter. An editor's note provides further information on NbN including a summary table showing the pharmacological target(s) and mode of action of a range of psychiatric drugs.

We hope that this book will be useful to psychiatrists from core trainees to consultants, non-medical prescribers, psychiatric pharmacists and basic science researchers. Most importantly we hope that this edition will contribute to evidence-based prescribing that is appropriate and safe and leads to better clinical outcomes for patients.

Peter M. Haddad and David J. Nutt

Editor's Note on Nomenclature

Neuroscience-Based Nomenclature (NbN): The Future Nomenclature for Psychiatry

David J. Nutt

For all my professional life I have been unhappy with the way in which the terms we use in psychiatry are imprecise and confusing, e.g. we use antidepressants to treat anxiety disorders, some antipsychotics to augment antidepressants in depression, etc. Such imprecision can lead to more stigma and also poor clinical practice. For example, other medical professionals may assume that someone once prescribed an antipsychotic must have been psychotic at some point or even suffer from schizophrenia.

Another major imprecision is with the acronyms used for psychiatric drugs which have zero coherence. Perhaps the most ridiculous are in the field of drugs for depression where we have TCAs (tricyclic antidepressants) named after a chemical structure that they share with chlorpromazine for instance. Then we have SSRIs (selective serotonin reuptake inhibitors) which might lead one to suppose that SNRI meant selective noradrenaline reuptake inhibitor but it does not – instead it means serotonin and noradrena line reuptake inhibitor. Mirtazapine was the original NASSA which has been expanded as either noradrenaline and selective serotonin antagonist or noradrenaline antihistamine and selective serotonin antagonist, neither of which communicate much in the way of mechanistic data. Noradrenaline reuptake inhibitors, even if very selective, for example reboxetine, are called NARIs not Selective NARIs.

A few years ago, I published a paper arguing for a new approach to nomenclature (Nutt, 2009) and this idea was taken up by the European College of Neuropsychopharmacology (ECNP) who formed a working group comprising experts from five international organizations: the ECNP, the American College of Neuropsychopharmacology (ACNP), the Asian College of Neuropsychopharmacology (AsCNP), the International College of Neuropsychopharmacology (CINP) and the International Union of Basic and Clinical Pharmacology (IUPHAR). The group tasked itself '*to examine ways of improving the current nomenclature in psychopharmacology*'. Specifically, the new nomenclature was to (i) be based on contemporary scientific knowledge; (ii) help clinicians to make informed choices when working out the next 'pharmacological step'; (iii) provide a system that does not conflict with the use of medications; and (iv) be future proof to accommodate new types of compounds. An initial proposal (Zohar et al., 2014) was discussed in the scientific community and accordingly revised (Zohar et al., 2015).

After several years work the current version, now called Neuroscience-based Nomenclature (NbN), is available as a fee app on both the Android and i-player platforms (http://nbnomenclature.org/) and the NbN terminology has been accepted by the majority of leading psychopharmacology journals. These include the *Journal of Psychopharmacology, European Neuropsychopharmacology, Biological Psychiatry, CNS Spectrums, European Psychiatry, International Journal of Neuropsychopharmacology, Journal of Clinical Psychopharmacology, Neuropsychopharmacology, Pharmacopsychiatry, World Journal of Biological Psychiatry.*

The editors of the current volume asked chapter authors to incorporate the NbN process and philosophy in this book as far as possible. Using NbN required authors to clarify their meaning when they use a term to describe a drug, for example when they use a term such as 'antidepressant' do they mean drugs for depression or for anxiety or even, in some cases, for pain or enuresis? A glossary of preferred terms is provided as an appendix to this chapter.

Despite the preference for NbN, readers will find that older generic terms (e.g. antidepressant, antipsychotic, anxiolytic) still appear. However, where a generic label is needed the editors prefer, for example 'drugs for depression' rather than 'antidepressants'; the former seems less likely to imply a uniform domain and mechanism of action than the latter.There are several reasons why a hybrid of NbN and traditional generic terms appear in this book. Firstly, most clinicians will not be familiar with NbN; in contrast, terms such as 'tricyclic antidepressant' and 'antipsychotic' are widely used in clinical discussions with other healthcare professionals and with patients. It will take time for the terminology used to alter and for a full appraisal of the benefits, and any potential limitations of NbN to become apparent. Secondly, the benefits of NbN are probably greatest for researchers and scientists and the subtilities of the system may be irrelevant or even confusing to many patients and so doctors are likely to continue to use some traditional terms in discussions with patients. Finally, NbN is a new system and is continuing to evolve.

NbN is a pharmacologically driven system in which each drug is named after its pharmacological domain (i.e. the primary neurotransmitter system(s) that the drug acts on) followed by its mode of action. In contrast, drugs have previously been named according to their indication, sometimes with a vague attempt to refer to their mechanism of action. This can be illustrated by an example. Previously a journal article may have referred to '*olanzapine, an atypical antipsychotic*'. In NbN this wording would become '*olanzapine, a dopamine, serotonin antagonist*'. '*Dopamine, serotonin*' refers to the drug's pharmacological domain and '*antagonist*' refers to its mode of action.

It is important to note that in NbN the underlying disorder that is being treated is not referred to. This makes sense as many psychiatric drugs have an evidence base supporting their efficacy in a range of disorders. For example, olanzapine is efficacious in the acute and maintenance treatment of schizophrenia and mania and also has supporting evidence as an augmenting agent when there has been a partial response to an 'antidepressant' in major depressive disorder. Of course, this example shows a potential problem with NbN; as here we refer to 'antidepressant' which is not consistent with NbN! As already highlighted, there are likely to be occasions when clinicians find older generic terms including 'antidepressants' and 'antipsychotics' a useful shorthand to refer to drug 'classes', albeit with their inherent drawbacks.

NbN is scientifically precise and extendable: new drug targets or modes of action can be easily added to the system once accepted by the scientific community. It is fairly comprehensive: at the present time it includes over 130 compounds which span the great majority of what is currently used in the practice of psychopharmacology. However, this very precision requires of authors and readers to adjust some well-worn habits: for example, use of the terms 'second-generation' or 'atypical antipsychotic', or even more so a group reference such as 'anxiolytics' referring to a group of substances with quite heterogeneous receptor targets and mode of action.

The editors realize that NbN posed some additional challenges for our authors and may also do for some readers. Nevertheless we believe that readers and ultimately the field will benefit greatly – first, by the self-imposed terminology precision itself, and second, by sometimes making it clear where gaps in our knowledge still exist, especially when the modes of action of drugs with relationship to our evolving understanding of the neurobiology of mental illness are concerned (Millan et al., 2015).How does NbN work in practice? To 'translate' between old and new nomenclature, the easiest and recommended way is to use the approved app, which is available on the project's website, as well as in the software repositories of the various platforms for which it is available.

The NbN effort is an organic process. For example, a child and adolescent version is now also available (NbNC&A) and neuropharmacology sections are still being completed and updated. Moreover, discussion with pharmaceutical companies on how to name their new compounds to make them NbN compliant is underway.

Overall and importantly, I believe that a clearer understanding of pharmacology will greatly benefit translational neuroscience and the discovery of new treatments for brain disorders.

References

Millan MJ, Goodwin GM, Meyer-Lindenberg A, Ögren SO (2015). 60 years of advances in neuropsychopharmacology for improving brain health, renewed hope for progress. *Eur Neuropsychopharmacol*, 25(5), 591–598. [Epub ahead of print 7 February 2015] doi:10.1016/j.euroneuro.2015.01.015. PubMed PMID: 25799919.

Nutt DJ (2009). Beyond psychoanaleptics – can we improve antidepressant drug nomenclature? *J Psychopharmacol*, 23(4), 343–345. doi:10.1177/0269881109105498. Erratum in: *J Psychopharmacol* 2009, 23(7), 861. PubMed PMID: 19433474.

Zohar J, Nutt DJ, Kupfer DJ, et al. (2014). A proposal for an updated neuropsychopharmacological nomenclature. *Eur Neuropsychopharmacol*, 24(7), 1005–1014. [Epub ahead of print 18 September 2013] doi:10.1016/j.euroneuro.2013.08.004. PubMed PMID: 24630385.

Zohar J, Stahl S, Moller HJ, et al. (2015). A review of the current nomenclature for psychotropic agents and an introduction to the Neuroscience-based Nomenclature. *Eur Neuropsychopharmacol*, 25(12), 2318–2325. [Epub ahead of print 7 September 2015] doi:10.1016/j.euroneuro.2015.08.019. PubMed PMID: 26527055.

Neuroscience-Based Nomenclature Glossary

Pharmacological target NbN3	Mode of action NbN3	Drug
acetylcholine	enzyme inhibitor	donepezil
		rivastigmine
	multimodal	galantamine
	partial agonist	varenicline
alcohol	enzyme inhibitor	disulfiram
dopamine	agonist	pramipexole
	antagonist	amisulpride
		fluphenazine
		haloperidol
		perphenazine
		pimozide
		sulpiride
		zuclopenthixol
	reuptake inhibitor	modafinil
dopamine, norepinephrine	multimodal	amphetamine (D) and (D,L)
		lisdexamfetamine
		methylphenidate (D) and (D,L)
dopamine, norepinephrine, serotonin	enzyme inhibitor	selegiline
dopamine, serotonin	antagonist	blonanserin
		chlorpromazine
		cyamemazine
		flupenthixol
		iloperidone
		loxapine
		lurasidone
		olanzapine
		perospirone
		pipotiazine
		sertindole
		thioridazine
		trifluoperazine
		ziprasidone
		zotepine
	partial agonist and antagonist	aripiprazole
		brexpiprazole
		cariprazine
dopamine, serotonin, norepinephrine	antagonist	asenapine
		clozapine
		paliperidone
		risperidone
	multimodal	quetiapine
GABA	agonist	baclofen
		sodium oxybate (GHB)
	antagonist	flumazenil
	positive allosteric modulator	alprazolam
		chloral hydrate, chloral betaine
		chlordiazepoxide
		clomethiazole
		clonazepam
		clorazepate
		diazepam
		estazolam
		eszopiclone
		flunitrazepam
		flurazepam
		lorazepam

Pharmacological target NbN3	Mode of action NbN3	Drug
		lormetazepam
		midazolam
		nitrazepam
		oxazepam
		quazepam
		temazepam
		triazolam
		zaleplon
		zolpidem
		zopiclone
GABA, glutamate	unclear	topiramate
glutamate	channel blocker	carbamazepine, oxcarbazepine
		gabapentin
		lamotrigine
		pregabalin
	NMDA antagonist	memantine
	unclear	acamprosate
		valproate
glutamate, opioid	unclear	tianeptine
histamine	antagonist	diphenhydramine
		hydroxyzine
		pitolisant
histamine, dopamine	antagonist	promethazine
lithium	enzyme modulator	lithium
melatonin	agonist	melatonin
		ramelteon
melatonin, serotonin	agonist and antagonist	agomelatine
norepinephrine	agonist	clonidine
		guanfacine
		lofexidine
	antagonist	prazosin
	multimodal	mianserin
	reuptake inhibitor	atomoxetine
		desipramine
		maprotiline
		nortriptyline
		protriptyline
		reboxetine
norepinephrine, dopamine	multimodal	bupropion
norepinephrine, serotonin	multimodal	doxepin
		mirtazapine
	reuptake inhibitor	amoxapine
		levomilnacipran
		lofepramine
		milnacipran
opioid	agonist	methadone
opioid	antagonist	nalmefene
opioid		naloxone
opioid		naltrexone
opioid	partial agonist	buprenorphine
orexin	antagonist	suvorexant
serotonin	agonist and antagonist	flibanserin
	antagonist	pimavanserin
	antagonist and agonist	nefazodone
	multimodal	trazodone
		vilazodone
		vortioxetine
	partial agonist	buspirone
		tandospirone

Pharmacological target NbN3	Mode of action NbN3	Drug
	reuptake inhibitor	citalopram
		escitalopram
		fluoxetine
		fluvoxamine
		paroxetine
		sertraline
serotonin, dopamine	antagonist	trimipramine
serotonin, norepinephrine	multimodal	amitriptyline
	reuptake inhibitor	clomipramine
		desvenlafaxine
		dosulepin
		duloxetine
		imipramine
		venlafaxine
serotonin, norepinephrine, dopamine	enzyme inhibitor	isocarboxazid
		moclobemide
		phenelzine
	multimodal	tranylcypromine

GHB: gamma-hydroxybutyrate

Abbreviations

ABC	ATP binding cassette
AChE	Acetylcholinesterase
AChEI	Acetylcholinesterase inhibitor
ACTH	Adrenocorticotrophic hormone
ADHD	Attention deficit hyperactivity disorder
ADR	Adverse drug reaction
ALDH	Acetaldehyde dehydrogenase
AMPA	α-Amino-3-hydroxy-5-methyl-4-isoxazolepropionic acid
ASD	Autism spectrum disorder
AT	Adenosine triphosphate
AUC	Area under the curve
AUD	Alcohol use disorder
AVP	Arginine vasopressin
AWS	Alcohol withdrawal syndrome
BAP	British Association for Psychopharmacology
BChE	Butyrylcholinesterase
BDNF	Brain-derived neurotrophic factor
BMI	Body mass index
BNF	*British National Formulary*
BPD	Borderline personality disorder
BPSD	Behavioural and psychological symptoms of dementia
cAMP	Cyclic 3,5-adenosine monophosphate
CAR	Constitutive androstane receptor
CATIE	Clinical Antipsychotic Trials of Intervention Effectiveness
CBT	Cognitive behavioural therapy
CCK	Cholecystokinin
cGMP	Cyclic guanosine monophosphate
CNS	Central nervous system
CO	Carbon monoxide
COMT	Catechol-*O*-methyltransferase
COX	Cyclo-oxygenase
CPIC	Clinical Pharmacogenetics Implementation Consortium
CRH	Corticotrophin-releasing hormone
CSF	Cerebrospinal fluid
CSM	Committee for Safety of Medicines
CUtLASS	Cost Utility of the Latest Antipsychotic Drugs in Schizophrenia Study
CVD	Cardiovascular disease
CYP	Cytochrome P450
DA	Dopamine

DALYs	Disability-adjusted life years
DBS	Deep brain stimulation
DHCR7	7-Dehydrocholesterol reductase
DLB	Dementia with Lewy bodies
DLPFC	Dorsolateral prefrontal cortex
DMPP	Dimethylphenylpipirazonium
DNA	Deoxyribonucleic acid
DVLA	Driver and Vehicle Licensing Agency
ECG	Electrocardiogram
ECS	Electroconvulsive stimulation
EEG	Electroencephalogram
EM	Extensive metabolizer
EMA	European Medicines Agency
EPSE	Extrapyramidal side effects
FDA	Food and Drug Administration
FGA	First-generation antipsychotic
FMO	Flavin-containing monooxygenases
GABA	Gamma-aminobutyric acid
GAD	Generalized anxiety disorder
GHB	Gamma-hydroxybutyrate
GlyT	Glycine transporter
GTP	Guanosine triphosphate
HDRS	Hamilton Depression Rating Scale
HIV	Human immunodeficiency virus
5-HT	5-Hydroxytryptamine
ICD-10	10th revision of the International Statistical Classification of Diseases and Related Health Problems
ID	Intellectual disability
IM	Intermediate metabolizer
iPSC	Induced pluripotent stem cells
Inter SePT	International Suicide Prevention Trial
Ki	Inhibition constant
LAI	Long-acting injectable
MADRS	Montgomery–Asberg Depression Rating Scale
MAO	Monoamine oxidase
MAOI	Monoamine oxidase inhibitor
MATRICS	Measurement and Treatment Research to Improve Cognition in Schizophrenia
MDD:	Major depressive disorder
M-ECT	Maintenance ECT
MHRA	Medicines and Healthcare products Regulatory Authority
MRI	Magnetic resonance imaging
MSM	Men who have sex with men

NA	Noradrenaline
NbN	Neuroscience-based Nomenclature
NICE	National Institute for Health and Care Excellence
NIMH	National Institute of Mental Health
NM	Normal metabolizer
NMDA	*N*-methyl-D-aspartate
NMS	Neuroleptic malignant syndrome
NPY	Neuropeptide Y
NRT	Nicotine replacement therapy
NSAID	Non-steroidal anti-inflammatory drug
OAP	Oral antipsychotic
OATP	Organic anion-transporting polypeptide
OCD	Obsessive-compulsive disorder
OST	Opioid substitution therapy
PANSS	Positive and Negative Syndrome Scale
PCE	Pharmacological cognitive enhancement
PCP	Phencyclidine
PD	Parkinson's disease
PDD	Parkinson's disease dementia
PET	Positron emission tomography
PFC	Prefrontal cortex
P-gp	P-glycoprotein
PGE_2	Prostaglandin E_2
PM	Poor metabolizer
PoC	Proof of concept
POMH	Prescribing Observatory for Mental Health
PXR	Pregnane X receptor
R&D	Research and development
RCPsych	Royal College of Psychiatrists
RCT	Randomized controlled trial
RDoC	Research Domain Criteria
RID	Relative infant dose
rTMS	Repetitive transcranial magnetic stimulation
scPCP	Subchronic phencyclidine
SDM	Shared decision making
SGA	Second-generation antipsychotic
SJS	Stevens–Johnson syndrome
SMD	Standardized mean difference
SNP	Single nucleotide polymorphism
SNRI	Serotonin and noradrenaline reuptake inhibitor
SPC	Summary of Product Characteristics
SSRI	Selective serotonin reuptake inhibitor
SXR	Steroid and xenobiotic receptor

STAR*D	Sequenced Treatment Alternatives for the Relief of Depression
TADS	Treatment for Adolescents with Depression Study
TCA	Tricyclic antidepressant
tDCS	Transcranial direct current stimulation
TDM	Therapeutic drug monitoring
TEN	Toxic epidermal necrolysis
tVNS	Transcutaneous vagus nerve stimulation
UGT	Uridine diphosphate (UDP)-glucuronosyltransferase
UM	Ultrarapid metabolizer
UTR	Untranslated region
VDR	Vitamin D receptor
VMAT-2	Vesicular amine transporter 2
VNS	Vagus nerve stimulation
WKS	Wernicke–Korsakoff syndrome
Y-BOCS	Yale-Brown Obsessive Compulsive Scale

Chapter 1 A Brief History of Psychopharmacology

Peter M. Haddad, David J. Nutt and A. Richard Green

1.1 Introduction

The Oxford English Dictionary defines psychopharmacology as '*the scientific study of the effect of drugs on the mind and behaviour*' (Oxford English Dictionary Online, 2018). The earliest reference to the term was in 1548 when Reinhard Lorichius published the prayer book *Psychopharmakon, hoc est Medicina Animae* (Lehmann, 1993; Wolman, 1977). Lorichius coined the term '*psychopharmakon*' to refer to spiritual medicine that could reduce human suffering. The word psychopharmacology was first used in a scientific paper in 1920 by a pharmacologist working at Johns Hopkins University who wrote a short paper entitled 'Contributions to psychopharmacology' (Macht, 1920).

The 1950s saw psychopharmacology emerge as a scientific discipline. The first textbook of psychopharmacology, *Pharmakopsycologie und Psychopathologie* by Wolfgang de Boor, was published in 1956 and the first journal dedicated to this research area, *Psychopharmacologia* (title subsequently changing to *Psychopharmacology*), appeared soon after in 1959. The term was first used in *Index Medicus* in 1960. *Psychopharmacology* published papers on both preclinical and clinical psychopharmacology, an approach followed by two subsequent major journals; *Journal of Psychopharmacology* and *Neuropsychopharmacology*. It was also in the 1950s that the first scientific society dedicated to psychopharmacology research was formed, the Collegium Internationale Neuro-Psychopharmacologicum (CINP), their first meeting being held in Rome in 1958 (Ban & Ray, 1996). The foundation of the American College of Neuropsychopharmacology (ACNP) followed in 1961 (Ray, 2007). The British Association for Psychopharmacology (BAP) was founded in 1974 (Green & Haddad, 2016) and the European College of Neuropsychopharmacology (ECNP) in 1985. All these societies hold regular meetings.

Many cultures have used naturally occurring psychoactive substances to alter mental functioning as part of religious ceremonies, for pleasurable effects or to alleviate mental distress. Psychedelic mushrooms and cacti were used in prehistoric times (Akers et al., 2011; El-Seedi et al., 2005). Alcohol has been fermented by many cultures for thousands of years, with the earliest documented use being in China in approximately 7000 BCE (McGovern et al., 2004). In the nineteenth century several physicians attempted to investigate the effect of naturally occurring drugs on human behaviour. They included Jacques-Joseph Moreau who studied the potential for hashish to treat mental illness (Moreau, 1845). It has only been in the last 200 years that knowledge of organic chemistry allowed scientists to synthesize non-naturally occurring drugs to alter human behaviour. A key milestone was the synthesis of barbital, the first barbiturate, in 1902 by Fischer and von Mering. The start of modern psychopharmacology is usually dated to 1949 when John Cade reported on the beneficial use of lithium in treating acute mania (Cade, 1949). This was followed by a decade of rapid drug development, the 1950s seeing the introduction of the first tricyclic antidepressants (TCAs), monoamine oxidase inhibitors (MAOIs) and antipsychotics, an era often referred to as the 'psychopharmacology revolution'. These developments had immense benefit for patients and their families and also spurred research into the biological causes of psychiatric illness.

Today psychopharmacology is a key part of the management of many psychiatric disorders. This does not in any way invalidate the importance of psychosocial factors in the aetiology of mental illness or of psychosocial interventions in their treatment. The optimum outcome for a person with a mental health disorder results from an individualized package of care and this will often incorporate psychopharmacological, social and psychological treatments. Furthermore, for many psychiatric disorders, especially those that are milder, the most appropriate treatment is to use psychosocial interventions alone.

The areas covered in this chapter fall into three main parts. The first part reviews the development of drugs to treat psychiatric illness from 1850 to the current time. Most attention is devoted to drug development since 1950. It is not possible, nor would it be of interest to most readers, to exhaustively review each new drug or drug class that has entered use since 1850. Rather, we have chartered some of the major developments that have occurred over this time. The middle part of the chapter reviews preclinical psychiatric drug development including the preclinical research that led to ideas about the mechanism of action of psychiatric drugs and several of the current pharmaceuticals available. The last part of the chapter examines the benefits that have stemmed from psychopharmacology, the controversies it has generated and the problems that the field currently faces.

1.2 Clinical Psychopharmacology 1850 to 1900

The second half of the nineteenth century saw the introduction of a range of sedative and hypnotic drugs that were widely used to treat behavioural symptoms of psychiatric disorders within the asylums. Some of these drugs were alkaloids and as a result psychopharmacology in the second half of the nineteenth century has been referred to as the '*alkaloids era*' (Shorter, 1997). However, the reality is that a wider range of drugs than alkaloids were used during this period.

Alkaloids are a group of naturally occurring nitrogenous bases. The earliest alkaloid used in psychiatry was morphine which was isolated from opium in 1805 by the German pharmacist Friedrich Sertürner. Wilhelm Griesinger (1861) highlighted the role of opium in treating various psychiatric symptoms, including anxiety and excitement, in the second edition of his textbook *Pathology and Treatment of Mental Diseases*. The alkaloids that were most widely used in psychiatry were those isolated from species of the Solanaceae family of flowering plants. This included hyoscyamine, isolated in 1839, and hyoscine (also called scopolamine), isolated in 1880. Hyoscyamine and hyoscine were often used as part of drug 'cocktails' administered in the asylums to control severe agitation. Norton (1979) refers to the 'Hyoscine Co A' cocktail, a mixture of hyoscine, morphine and atropine that was used in the 1930s to control agitation, aggression and excitement at the Bethlem Royal Hospital, London.

Chloral hydrate was synthesized in 1832. It started being used as a hypnotic in 1869 and was widely used for this indication throughout the remainder of the nineteenth century. Bromides were also widely used in the second half of the nineteenth century as sedatives and anticonvulsants. Indeed, until the introduction of phenobarbitone in 1912, potassium bromide was the only effective anticonvulsant drug (Pearce, 2002). The side-effects of bromides, plus their long half-life, meant that prolonged use could lead to their accumulation in the body. Symptoms of bromide toxicity (bromism) included neurological and psychiatric symptoms (restlessness, irritability, ataxia, confusion, hallucinations, psychosis and, in severe cases, coma), gastrointestinal effects (nausea, vomiting, anorexia, constipation) and rashes (Tillim, 1952). The bromides were replaced by the barbiturates in the early twentieth century. Much later it was discovered that all these drugs worked in one way or another on the $GABA_A$ receptor system in the brain.

The 1880s saw the introduction of paraldehyde, the cyclic trimer of acetaldehyde, into medicine. It became widely used as a sedative and anticonvulsant. Norton (1979), reflecting on his experience of working as a psychiatrist in the UK in the late 1930s, commented '*The smell of this last drug* [paraldehyde] *contributed – with that of the rubber chamber pots and the rubber lining of the padded room – to the characteristic odour of acute psychiatric wards all over Britain.*' Intramuscular paraldehyde continued to be used to treat severe agitation in psychiatric wards in the UK up to the 1980s (Holden & Cavanagh, 1987).

The nineteenth century witnessed several important discoveries by chemists in Germany that laid the foundation for the synthesis of new drugs in the twentieth century. In 1883 the structure of the phenothiazine ring was deduced by Heinrich Bernthsen, an industrialist chemist, who was trying to develop artificial dyes to replace more expensive natural dyes (Ohlow & Moosmann, 2011). The phenothiazine ring was used to synthesize chlorpromazine and other phenothiazine antipsychotics in the 1950s. In 1887 Lazăr Edeleano synthesized amphetamine, though its stimulant properties were not recognized until the 1930s. In 1899 Friedrich Thiele and Otto Holzinger deduced the structure of the iminodibenzyl nucleus, two benzene rings joined together by a nitrogen atom and an ethylene bridge. This structure was used by Geigy Pharmaceuticals to synthesize imipramine, the first TCA, in the 1950s.

1.3 Clinical Psychopharmacology and Physical Treatments 1900 to 1949

In 1903 two chemists at Bayer, Emil Fischer and Joseph von Mering, synthesized barbital, the first barbiturate. This was marketed as Veronal. It was followed by phenobarbital, marketed as Luminal, in 1912. By the 1950s over 2000 barbiturates had been synthesized of which approximately 50 were introduced into clinical practice as hypnotics, sedatives, anticonvulsants and general anaesthetics. The barbiturates replaced the bromides as drugs of choice as sedatives, hypnotics and anticonvulsants.

The first half of the twentieth century also saw the introduction of various new physical treatments for severe mental illness. In 1917 the Austrian psychiatrist Julius Wagner-Jauregg introduced malarial therapy for neurosyphilis, for which he was later awarded a Nobel Prize (Tsay, 2013). Malarial therapy was effective in arresting the course of neurosyphilis in some patients as the fever associated with malaria killed the bacteria *Treponema pallidum* that causes syphilis. The treatment was associated with significant mortality. Malarial therapy became obsolete in the 1940s after Stokes et al. (1944) reported the effectiveness of penicillin in treating neurosyphilis, including general paralysis of the insane (GPI). GPI was a common cause for admission to asylums in the first half of the twentieth century. Its symptoms included grandiose delusions, ataxia, asymmetrical pupils and dementia and prior to the introduction of effective treatments it was fatal. GPI virtually disappeared following the introduction of penicillin.

In the 1920s barbiturate-induced deep sleep was used to treat schizophrenia (Windholz & Witherspoon, 1993). In the 1930s, Manfred Sakel, a psychiatrist working in Vienna, introduced insulin-coma treatment, also known as insulin-shock treatment. The treatment was introduced to Britain in 1935 and became widely used, predominantly to treat schizophrenia. Insulin injections were given to induce a coma and, in some cases, a seizure. After approximately 20 minutes the coma would be reversed by administering glucose, either intravenously or via a nasal tube. Treatment was given most days for several weeks. Side effects included brain damage and it is estimated that there was a 1% mortality rate (Jones, 2000).

Another so-called 'shock treatment' was introduced in 1937 by Ladislas von Meduna, a Hungarian physician, who provoked seizures by the intravenous injection of pentylenetetrazole (also known as Metrazol and Cardiazol) primarily as a treatment for schizophrenia. The seizures were difficult to control and when severe could lead to spinal fractures. By the mid-1940s chemically induced seizures had been replaced by electroconvulsive therapy (ECT) as an electric shock was a more reliable and safer method for seizure induction (McCrae, 2006). Moreover, ECT did not suffer the adverse effect of anxiety generation that pentylenetetrazole did if a seizure was not produced and which could be profoundly distressing to the patient (Nutt, 1990).

A surgical approach to changing brain function called prefrontal leucotomy was developed by António Egas Moniz, a Portuguese neurologist, in the 1930s and led to him being a joint recipient of the 1949 Nobel Prize in Physiology or Medicine. Moniz was previously, and unsuccessfully, nominated on two occasions for a Nobel Prize for his work on cerebral angiography. Moniz's operation entailed cutting the pathways from the frontal cortex to the rest of the brain. He conducted the first prefrontal leucotomy in 1935. The first such operation was performed in the UK in 1940 (Hutton et al., 1941) and between 1942 and 1954 it is estimated that approximately 10 000 patients in England and Wales underwent this treatment (Tooth & Newton, 1961). Side effects included brain damage, marked personality change and epilepsy, and the mortality of the procedure was approximately 3% (Board of Control for England and Wales, 1947).

Over time, insulin-coma, barbiturate-induced deep sleep treatment and leucotomy were all recognized as having no benefit and became obsolete. The demise of insulin-coma partly reflected a trial that showed no difference in outcome between patients receiving insulin-coma treatment and those who had a period of unconsciousness produced by barbiturates (Ackner et al., 1957). Although both insulin-coma and leucotomy were on the wane by the early 1950s, the introduction of the first antipsychotic drugs in the mid-1950s contributed to their demise. The use of ineffective physical treatments during the first half of the twentieth century partly reflects the fact that at that time evidence-based medicine did not exist. In addition, the suffering caused to patients and their families by mental illness, the absence of any effective treatment and the poor conditions within asylums (overcrowding, underfunding and understaffing were commonplace) meant that clinicians were desperate for new therapies that offered hope. The only physical treatment introduced in that period that remains in use today is ECT. Today, ECT is largely used as a treatment option for severe depressive illness in urgent or emergency situations, such as depressive stupor, or where other treatments have failed (Cleare et al., 2015). There is a strong evidence base supporting the efficacy of ECT in severe depression (see Chapter 16). Current practice for ECT involves the patient being given a general anaesthetic and administered a muscle relaxant to attenuate the muscular activity in the seizure. This is in contrast to the use of unmodified ECT in the 1940s, when the electroshock was given without anaesthesia and a muscle relaxant, and the treatment was used in a much broader range of disorders, including schizophrenia.

In 1937 Charles Bradley, a psychiatrist working in Rhode Island, reported a small study that showed that Benzedrine (amphetamine sulphate) led to a marked improvement in the behaviour and school work of children with behavioural problems (Bradley, 1937). This was the first report that psychostimulants could treat certain behavioural problems in children. Bradley confirmed his findings with a second larger study published in 1940 (Bradley & Bowen, 1940). His work received little attention for the next 20 years and it has been suggested that this reflected the prevailing view that behavioural problems did not have an underlying biological cause and that psychological interventions alone were required (Lange et al., 2010). In the mid-1950s another stimulant drug, methylphenidate, started being used as a treatment for children with what would now be diagnosed as attention deficit hyperactivity disorder (ADHD). At that time methylphenidate was also used for various indications in adults including the treatment of chronic fatigue, depression and narcolepsy (Physicians' Desk Reference, 1956).

The first half of the twentieth century saw a variety of drugs being used to treat depression including amphetamine and tincture of morphine and various vitamins and hormones but none was successful. So, in summary, advances in drug treatments for psychiatric disorders in the first half of the twentieth century were limited. The major successes were penicillin as a treatment for neurosyphilis and the introduction of barbiturates to treat anxiety and sleep disturbance, though barbiturates were often fatal in overdose. A series of physical treatments were also introduced that were later shown to be ineffective, the exception being ECT, which remains an important treatment option primarily for severe depression. There were no effective drugs to treat depression or schizophrenia, but this situation changed dramatically in the 1950s.

1.4 The 1950s and the Psychopharmacology Revolution

The 1950s saw the introduction of the first antidepressant and antipsychotic drugs, the early development of randomized, placebo-controlled clinical trials to assess drug efficacy and the creation of psychopharmacology as a discipline. The importance of this decade is highlighted by the fact that it is often referred to as the 'psychopharmacology revolution'. The first breakthrough came in 1949 when the Australian physician John Cade reported the benefit of lithium in treating manic patients with 'psychotic excitement' (Cade, 1949). Lithium had been used in the nineteenth century to treat gout and mood disorders but Cade's paper triggered renewed interest in lithium. In Denmark Mogens Schou and colleagues conducted the first randomized placebo-controlled trial of lithium demonstrating its efficacy in acute mania (Schou et al., 1954). In the late 1960s and early 1970s a series of trials showed the efficacy of lithium in the maintenance phase of bipolar illness (Angst et al., 1970; Baastrup & Schou, 1967; Baastrup et al., 1970). Current clinical guidelines for the management of bipolar disorder, from the National Institute for Health and Care Excellence (NICE, 2014) and the British Association for Psychopharmacology (Goodwin et al., 2016), regard lithium as the first-line option for maintenance treatment (see Chapter 11).

The world's first antipsychotic drug was chlorpromazine, a phenothiazine. It was synthesized in 1950 by Paul Charpentier, a chemist working for the French pharmaceutical company Rhône-Poulenc. It was developed as part of the company's antihistamine development programme. In keeping with contemporary practice, the company gave samples to interested clinicians so that they could report on its clinical effects. The French naval surgeon Henri Laborit noted that when it was used as a pre-anaesthetic agent it produced calming without excessive sedation and suggested its possible use in psychiatry. In 1952 Jean Delay and Pierre Deniker (Figure 1.1), working at St Anne's Hospital in Paris, reported on chlorpromazine's beneficial effects in treating psychotic patients with disturbed behaviour (Delay et al., 1952). Originally it was thought that chlorpromazine worked by inducing 'artificial hibernation' and so ice packs were used at St Anne's Hospital to enhance its effects, but it quickly became apparent that therapeutic effects were due to the drug alone (Thuillier, 1999). At the same time as Delay and Deniker's work, several other psychiatrists published case reports that supported the efficacy of chlorpromazine (e.g. Hamon et al., 1952).

Delay and Deniker organized an international colloquium on the psychiatric uses of chlorpromazine in Paris in 1955 that was attended by 257 participants from 19 countries. Clinicians were impressed by the drug's benefits and felt that a new era of treatment was starting (Swazey, 1974). Chlorpromazine was quickly adopted as a treatment by psychiatrists working throughout Europe and North America. At the same time chlorpromazine

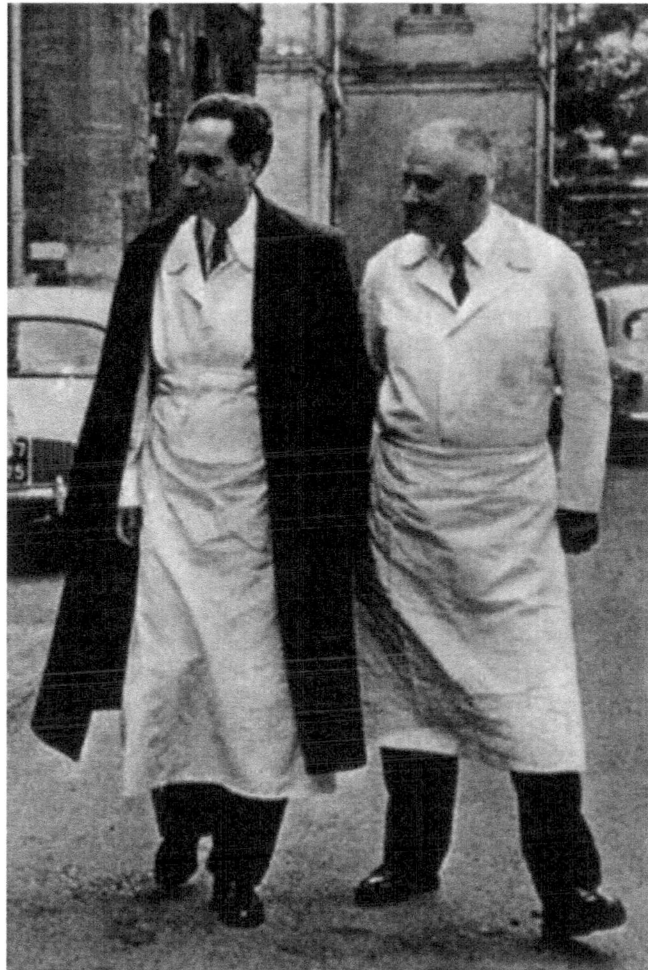

Figure 1.1 Jean Delay (left) and Pierre Deniker (right).

was also being promoted for various non-psychiatric indications including as an antiemetic. The success of chlorpromazine in the large state psychiatric hospitals in the United States (US) partly reflected an extensive marketing campaign by Smith Kline & French who owned the US licence (Swazey, 1974) (Figure 1.2). In the UK, chlorpromazine was marketed as Largactil and in North America as Thorazine. In 1957 the American Public Health Association presented a Lasker Award jointly to Henri Laborit, Pierre Deniker and Heinz Lehmann to recognize their work in introducing chlorpromazine as a treatment for schizophrenia. The term antipsychotic was not used in the 1950s; instead chlorpromazine and related drugs were referred to as 'neuroleptics', 'ataraxic drugs' or 'tranquillisers'. Following the introduction of the benzodiazepines in the 1960s, antipsychotics started being referred to as 'major tranquillisers' to differentiate them from the benzodiazepines which were termed 'minor tranquillisers'. The term antipsychotic appears to have first been used in print by Himwich (1958).

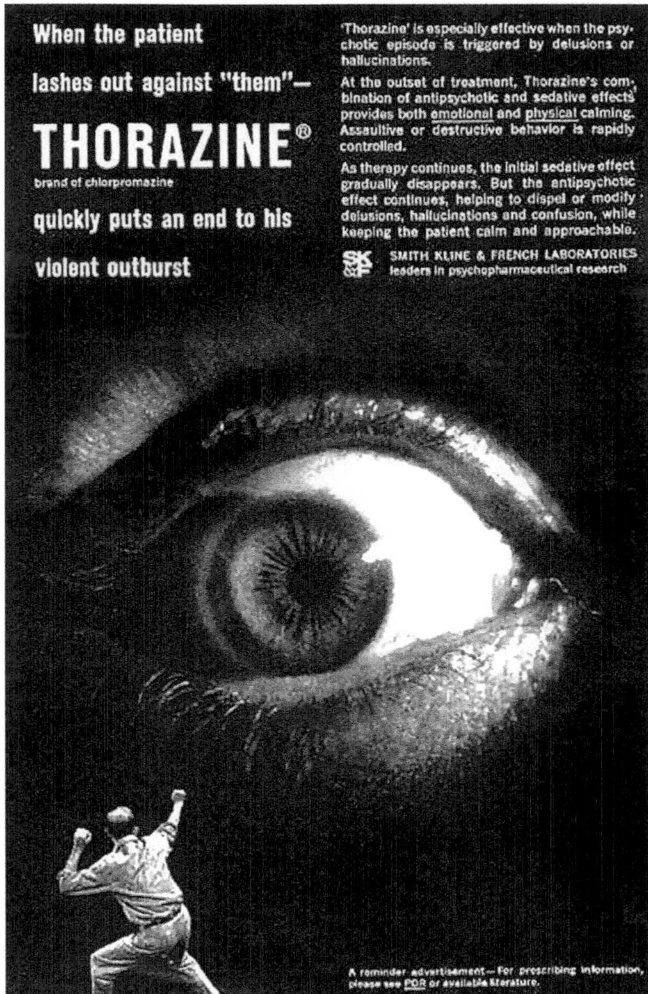

Figure 1.2 Advert for Thorazine (chlorpromazine) from the early 1960s.

The commercial success of chlorpromazine led other companies to develop other phenothiazine antipsychotics, and also, most notably, the butyrophenone compound haloperidol, synthesized in 1958 by Janssen Pharmaceutica.

The development of phenothiazine-related compounds by Geigy resulted in a further unexpected development. The clinical evaluation of imipramine, a drug structurally similar to chlorpromazine (Figure 1.3), failed to detect any noticeable antipsychotic effect, but the psychiatrist Roland Kuhn, working in Munsterlingen, Switzerland, reported that it had antidepressant effects (Brown & Rosdolsky, 2015; Kuhn, 1958). This observation was pivotal in Geigy introducing imipramine as a treatment for depression in Europe in 1958 and in the USA the following year. It was the first TCA and led to other companies developing and marketing TCAs and closely related compounds. By the early 1970s randomized placebo-

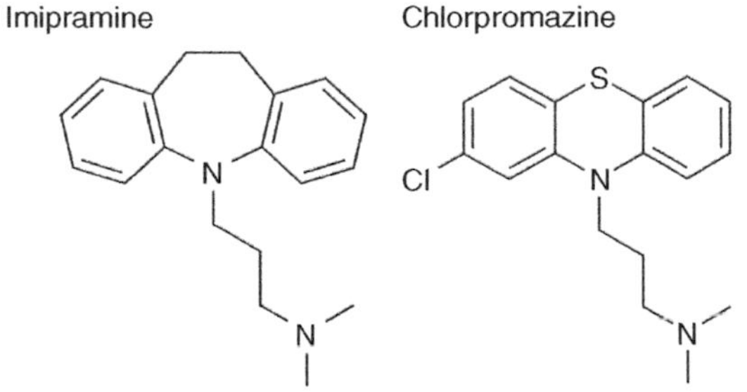

Figure 1.3 Chemical structures of imipramine and chlorpromazine.

controlled trials had demonstrated the benefit of maintenance treatment with TCAs in reducing the risk of relapse of depression (Mindham et al., 1972).

In 1957 Nathan Kline, working in New York, reported that iproniazid, an anti-tuberculous drug, had antidepressant effects (Loomer et al., 1957). Iproniazid was the first MAOI and was followed by others including phenelzine (Figure 1.4), isocarboxazid and tranylcypromine. In the 1960s, the MAOIs fell out of favour partly due to concerns about both hepatotoxicity and their interactions with foodstuffs and other medications (Blackwell, 1963). A Medical Research Council-sponsored trial also cast doubts on their efficacy, though this may have partly reflected under-dosing of phenelzine, the MAOI used in the study (Medical Research Council, 1965). Today, the use of MAOIs is restricted to treatment-resistant depression, with prescribing tending to be limited to clinicians experienced in their use and who often work in tertiary affective disorder centres. Anecdotally it seems that some patients with depression respond to MAOIs when they have failed to respond to other antidepressants and it has been argued that MAOIs are currently under-used by psychiatrists.

Although the first trials of antidepressants, antipsychotics and lithium focused in demonstrating their acute efficacy, subsequent randomized controlled trials (RCTs) showed that continued treatment with each of these drugs reduced the risk of relapse in people who had initially responded to acute treatment with that medication. This meant that for the first time it was possible to prevent the recurrence of major psychiatric illness. Furthermore, this benefit applied to people with depression, schizophrenia and bipolar disorder.

The year 1955 saw the launch of meprobamate for the management of anxiety though it was also promoted to treat other psychiatric disorders including psychosis (Green et al., 2018a). Its trade name was Miltown, named after Milltown, a village near the Wallace laboratories in New Brunswick, USA, where it was synthesized. It was the first 'blockbuster' drug in psychiatry and initially promoted as a safer anxiolytic than the barbiturates which were dangerous in overdose. However, by the 1960s the addictive potential of meprobamate was recognized and by 1970 it was listed as a controlled drug in the USA. In 2012 the European Medicines Agency withdrew the marketing authorization in the European Union for all medicines containing meprobamate due to concerns about adverse effects including addiction (European Medicines Agency, 2012). A recurrent theme in the history of anxiolytic drugs is delayed recognition of the potential of a new drug to be associated with dependence and also recreational misuse; this was first seen with the barbiturates and later repeated with meprobamate, the benzodiazepines and most recently pregabalin (Schjerning et al., 2016).

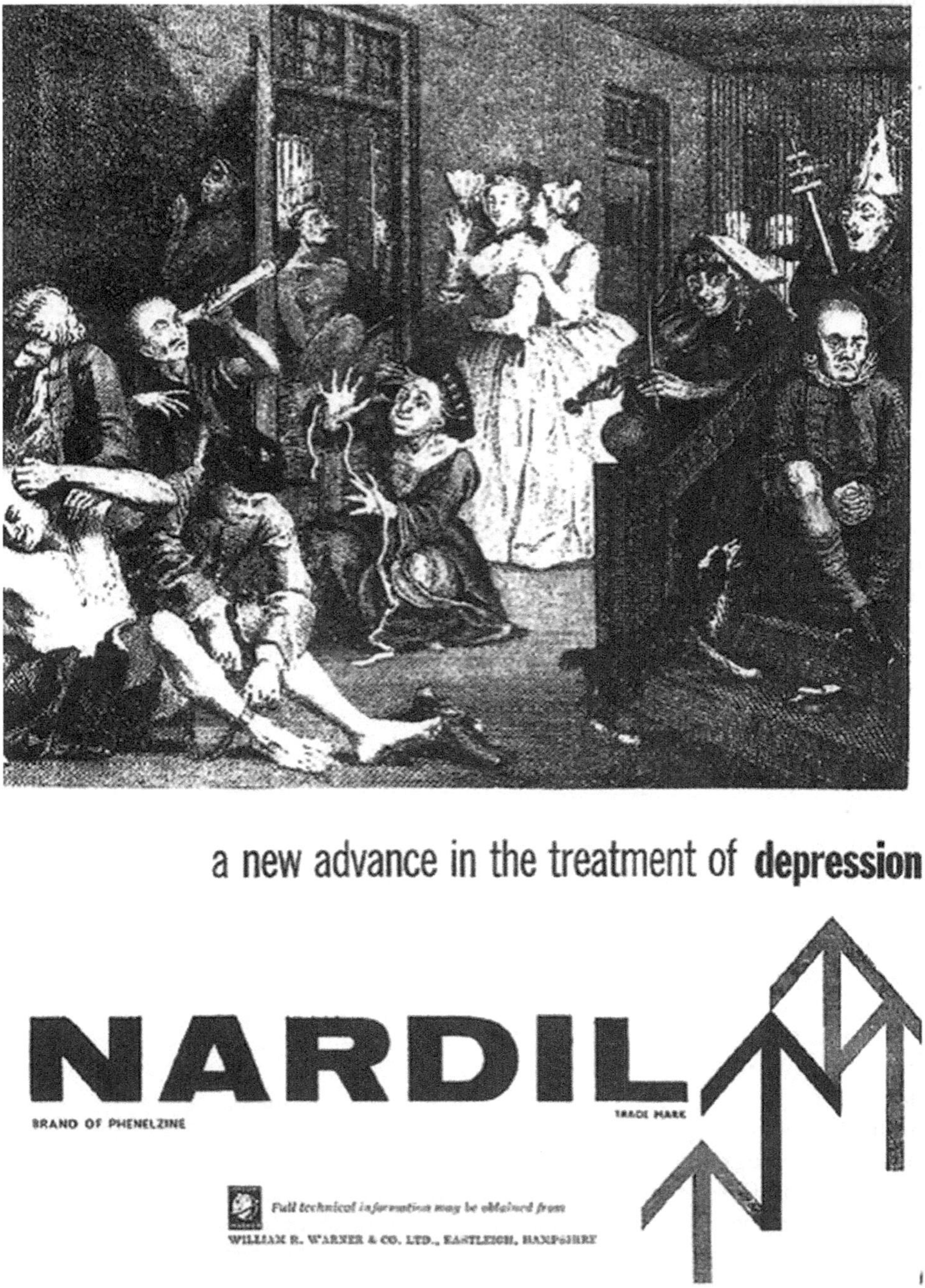

a new advance in the treatment of depression
NARDIL
BRAND OF PHENELZINE
TRADE MARK

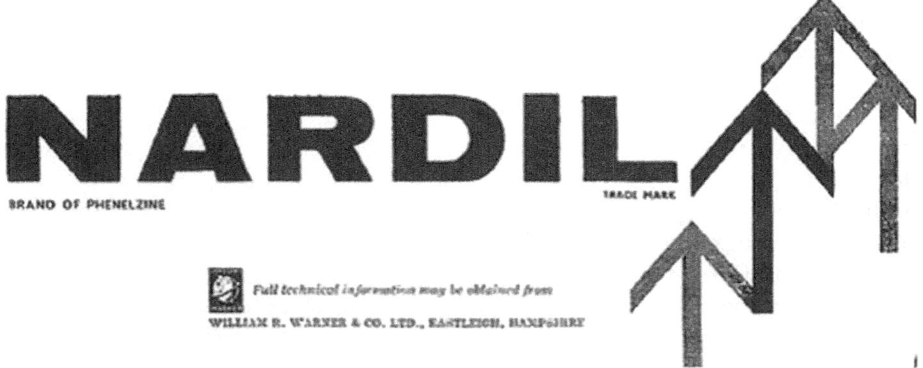

Figure 1.4 Advert for Nardil (phenelzine) from *British Medical Journal* (1960).

The introduction of chlorpromazine, imipramine and iproniazid into psychiatric practice each resulted from clinicians observing a benefit of the drug in patients with conditions different to those the manufacturer had originally proposed. All three drugs entered clinical practice without any supporting placebo-controlled RCTs, reflecting the much less rigorous process for drug development and approval in the 1950s compared with today. One often reads that these drug discoveries were 'serendipitous' but this is oversimplistic. Each reflected far more than chance or accident; there was a rationale as to why the company developed the drug and why it was first used in psychiatric patients. Astute clinical observations, not chance, led to a benefit being observed. In addition, the very basic understanding of pharmacology in the 1950s and 1960s meant that the 'discovery' of many drugs at that time, in all branches of medicine, followed a similar path. It was only decades later that technology and pharmacological knowledge were sufficient to design drugs in the laboratory to act on specific receptors and other pharmacological targets (see Chapter 2). With regard to the discovery of the psychiatric benefits of chlorpromazine, Rhône-Poulenc had been developing sedative antihistamines for many years. They had reason to suspect that a more centrally acting compound could have clinical applications as a pre-anaesthetic agent, partly based on clinical reports from Laborit regarding their earlier drug promethazine. As a result, the more lipophilic analogue chlorpromazine was synthesized. As already described, Laborit observed that it caused calming without sedation and this led to several psychiatrists using it in patients with marked behavioural disturbance. The detailed reports of Delay and Deniker and their contemporaries confirmed the drug's benefits in the treatment of patients with mania and schizophrenia. As Sir John Gaddum, the father of monoamine neurotransmitter research in the UK, commented '*It is true that many discoveries* [in pharmacology] *have been accidents, but these accidents would not have occurred to anyone who was not engaged in a systematic research for new knowledge, and without the techniques and apparatus of modern science they would usually have passed unheeded in the modern world*' (Gaddum, 1954).

Finally, it is notable that recent investigations, using advertising in the *British Medical Journal* during the 1950–80 period as an index of the rise of modern pharmaceuticals in several major therapeutic areas (cardiovascular, respiratory, gastrointestinal and central nervous system (CNS) diseases), observed that one of the first areas to benefit from the launch of novel effective medications was psychiatry (Green et al., 2018a, 2018b). A significant number of these drugs, or their related descendants, are still widely used today.

1.5 Clinical Psychopharmacology 1960 to 1979

The 1960s saw the results of the first large, double-blind, placebo-controlled RCTs in psychiatry. Of particular note was a series of RCTs that supported the efficacy of antipsychotic drugs in schizophrenia. These included two RCTs conducted in Veterans Administration (VA) centres that demonstrated that phenothiazines were superior to placebo in treating overall symptoms in chronic inpatients (Adelson & Epstein, 1962; Casey et al., 1960). More impressive still were the data in one of those studies relating to the proportion of patients deemed well enough for discharge when the study ended and blinding was broken; 36% in the antipsychotic-treated group versus 5% in the placebo-treated group (Adelson & Epstein, 1962). A weakness of both VA studies was that the participants were all long-term inpatients. This was overcome when a third trial, conducted by the National Institute of Mental Health (NIMH), was published in 1964 showing the superiority of antipsychotics compared with placebo in acute inpatients with schizophrenia (National Institute of Mental Health Psychopharmacology Service Center Collaborative Study Group, 1964). This study also showed that the benefit of antipsychotics extended beyond treating overactivity and behavioural disturbances, i.e. antipsychotics were shown to be effective in treating a wide range of symptoms of schizophrenia including auditory hallucinations, ideas of persecution, hebephrenic symptoms and incoherent speech, as well as irritability and hostility.

Soon after the antipsychotics were introduced it became apparent that many patients with schizophrenia who were discharged from the asylums stopped their oral antipsychotics and subsequently relapsed. To try and improve adherence, and reduce the risk of relapse, long-acting intramuscular injections of antipsychotics were developed. These were originally referred to as depots though the term long-acting injectable (LAI) antipsychotic is often used today. Fluphenazine enanthate, the first LAI antipsychotic, was introduced in 1966 (Johnson, 2009), and other LAIs followed. Whether LAIs reduce relapse rates compared to oral antipsychotics remains a subject of contention, with the most recent meta-analysis of RCTs (Kishimoto et al., 2014) showing no difference in relapse between those randomized to oral antipsychotic versus those randomized to LAIs, but with observational studies, including mirror-image studies (Kishimoto et al., 2013b) and cohort studies (Kishimoto et al., 2018), usually showing superiority for LAIs. These conflicting results seem to partly reflect trial methodology. Irrespective of their comparative effectiveness, the main advantage of LAI antipsychotics over oral antipsychotics is that LAIs make adherence transparent. Although some patients find a LAI more convenient than taking an oral antipsychotic, others do not like to receive their medication this way for various reasons, including a loss of autonomy.

The first benzodiazepine, chlordiazepoxide, was introduced in 1960 by Hoffmann–La Roche (now Roche) to treat anxiety. Diazepam was launched in 1963 and was followed by many other benzodiazepines. Some benzodiazepines with a shorter half-life, such as temazepam, were promoted as hypnotics. The benzodiazepines have a wide range of actions, including sedative, hypnotic, anxiolytic, anticonvulsant and muscle relaxant. They also have amnesic properties. Their main advantage in comparison with the earlier barbiturates was that they were much less dangerous in overdose. However, the benzodiazepines, like the barbiturates, can cause tolerance and dependence and are associated with misuse, although the extent of these problems was not initially recognized by the medical profession, leading to a serious problem with iatrogenic benzodiazepine dependence. This problem was compounded by over-marketing and overprescribing. For example, a 1963 advert for Valium stated that it was for '*prisoners of the society of stress*' with the illustration showing a woman shopping. Diazepam sales peaked in the United States in the mid-1970s and since then levels of benzodiazepine prescribing have fallen. Nevertheless, a large proportion of benzodiazepine prescribing continues to be off-label. That is, it is either for disorders not specified in the drug's marketing authorization or at doses and for durations that exceed those that are approved (Lader, 2014). The overprescribing of benzodiazepines and the delayed recognition of benzodiazepine dependence remain salutary lessons for psychiatry and psychopharmacology today.

1.6 Clinical Psychopharmacology 1980 to 1999

The 1980s saw the introduction of a new antidepressant class, the selective serotonin reuptake inhibitors (SSRIs). The SSRIs were the first class of psychiatric drugs that were designed to act on a selective pharmacological target, in this case the serotonin reuptake transporter. As the SSRIs had little action at other pharmacological sites, they were associated with fewer side effects than the earlier TCAs which had anticholinergic, antihistaminergic and α_1-adrenoceptor-blocking actions. The first SSRI to be introduced was zimeldine in 1982. It was manufactured by Astra and withdrawn soon after its launch due to an association with Guillain–Barré syndrome (Fagius et al., 1985). The next two SSRIs to be approved were fluvoxamine, licensed in Europe in 1983, and fluoxetine, licensed in the USA in 1987. Other SSRIs followed including paroxetine, sertraline, citalopram and escitalopram.

The improved tolerability of the SSRIs meant that they could be started at a therapeutic dose, a major advantage compared with the TCAs, which had to be started at a subtherapeutic dose with the dose subsequently being gradually stepped up to allow the patient to develop tolerance to side effects such as sedation and dry mouth. The SSRIs were also much less toxic than the TCAs in overdose. Although the efficacy of the SSRIs in depression is similar to that of the TCAs, their advantages in terms of fewer side-effects, safety in overdose and ease of use meant that they were a major advance in the treatment of depression. The quality and number of RCTs that accompanied the SSRIs was superior to that for the TCAs. RCTs subsequently demonstrated the efficacy of specific SSRIs in treating a range of anxiety disorders, including obsessive-compulsive disorder, panic disorder, social anxiety disorder, generalized anxiety disorder and post-traumatic stress disorder. The SSRIs remain first-line options today for the treatment of, and prevention of recurrence in, moderate and severe major depressive disorder. They also have an important role in the treatment of more severe anxiety disorders. Psychological interventions are generally the treatment of choice for mild depressive disorders and less severe anxiety disorders.

In 1988 a trial by John Kane and colleagues showed that clozapine was more effective than chlorpromazine in treatment-resistant schizophrenia (Kane et al., 1988). Clozapine was originally synthesized by the Swiss pharmaceutical company Wander in the 1950s but was not introduced as an antipsychotic until 1972 when it was launched in several European countries. This delay has been attributed to its lack of extrapyramidal side-effects (EPSE) leading some to doubt it was an effective antipsychotic. During the 1950s there was a commonly held view that EPSE and antipsychotic efficacy were closely linked, a view that was only disproved when the NIMH antipsychotic study was published in 1964 (National Institute of Mental Health Psychopharmacology Service Center Collaborative Study Group, 1964). The delay in the initial launch of clozapine is also likely to have reflected concerns about its propensity to cause postural hypotension and grand mal seizures. Clozapine was voluntarily withdrawn by Sandoz in 1975 after a series of cases of agranulocytosis were reported in Finland (Idanpaan-Heikkila et al., 1975). The 1988 trial of Kane and colleagues, and subsequent confirmatory studies, resulted in clozapine being licensed in 1989 by the Food and Drug Administration (FDA) for the treatment of treatment-resistant schizophrenia, with close haematological monitoring being a mandatory condition for its use. Clozapine remains the only drug licensed for treatment-resistant schizophrenia. Its superiority in this condition has been demonstrated by meta-analysis (Siskind et al., 2016) and in two large trials that recruited patients from a range of clinical settings, Phase II of the Clinical Antipsychotic Trials of Intervention Effectiveness (CATIE) (Lieberman et al., 2005) and Cost Utility of the Latest Antipsychotic Drugs in Schizophrenia Study (CUtLASS) (Jones et al., 2006; Lewis et al., 2006). In the UK, NICE (2014) recommends that clozapine is offered to patients with schizophrenia who have not responded sufficiently to the sequential use of at least two different antipsychotic drugs prescribed at adequate doses, at least one of which should be a non-clozapine second-generation antipsychotic.

In 2002 the FDA approved clozapine for the treatment of recurrent suicidal behaviour in schizophrenia and schizoaffective disorder; it is not approved for this indication in Europe. The US approval for suicidal behaviour reflected the results of the International Suicide Prevention Trial (Inter SePT), a multi-centre trial that randomized nearly 1000 people with schizophrenia or schizoaffective disorder, who were judged at high risk of suicide, to treatment with either clozapine or olanzapine (Meltzer et al., 2003). During the two-year follow-up period, the proportion of people who attempted suicide was significantly lower among those treated with clozapine. Chapter 10 provides a detailed review of the pharmacology and clinical uses of clozapine.

In 1994 risperidone was approved by the FDA and became the first of the so-called second-generation antipsychotics (SGAs). Other SGAs followed, including olanzapine (FDA approval for schizophrenia, 1996) and quetiapine (FDA approval for schizophrenia, 1997), and most recently lurasidone (FDA approval for schizophrenia, 2014). The SGAs were originally thought to offer superior efficacy to the first-generation antipsychotics (FGAs), especially in the treatment of negative symptoms, and to have a reduced risk of causing EPSE. Research in the 2000s, most notably the CATIE (Lieberman et al., 2005) and CUtLASS (Jones et al., 2006; Lewis et al., 2006) studies, showed no efficacy advantage for the SGAs over the FGAs in acute schizophrenia and that the situation regarding side effects was more complex, with comparisons needing to be made at the level of individual drugs rather than comparing broad pseudo-classes such as FGAs and SGAs. Some of the second-generation drugs, especially olanzapine, carry a high relative risk of weight gain and metabolic abnormalities (i.e. elevation of plasma glucose and lipids) that was not recognized when they were initially approved. These events highlight the importance of clinicians being sceptical of marketing claims made for new products, especially before there is sufficient post-marketing surveillance, including Phase IV studies, and independent clinical trials. Now rather than calling them SGAs the preferred pharmacology term in Neuroscience-based Nomenclature (NbN) is dopamine/serotonin blockers (see Editor's Note on Nomenclature).

In 1993 tacrine, a centrally acting acetylcholinesterase inhibitor, became the first drug to be licensed for the symptomatic treatment of Alzheimer's disease (Crismon, 1994). It was withdrawn from the US market in 2012 due to concern about hepatic adverse effects. Subsequently, several other acetylcholinesterase inhibitors were approved for the symptomatic treatment of mild to moderate Alzheimer's disease including donepezil (approved 1996), rivastigmine (approved 2000) and galantamine (approved 2000). Rivastigmine was subsequently approved for the symptomatic treatment of mild to moderately severe dementia in patients with idiopathic Parkinson's disease.

1.7 Psychopharmacology in the New Millennium

Two landmark studies in schizophrenia that were published in the first decade of the new millennium were the CATIE study (Lieberman et al., 2005), conducted in the United States, and the CUtLASS study (Jones et al., 2006; Lewis et al., 2006), conducted in the UK. Both studies found that there was little difference in efficacy between FGAs and SGAs in the treatment of acute schizophrenia, the exception being clozapine, which was superior in treatment-resistant schizophrenia. Both studies also found that there was little difference in the risk of EPSE between the specific first- and second-generation drugs that were studied. The results of CATIE and CUtLASS surprised many clinicians who had assumed that the SGAs were superior in efficacy, and had a lower EPSE risk, compared to the FGAs. The assumption that SGAs had a lower propensity than FGAs to cause EPSE probably stems from most SGA registration studies adopting haloperidol as the FGA comparator. Haloperidol has a high relative risk of EPSE while many other FGAs, such as chlorpromazine and perphenazine, have a lower risk (Leucht et al., 2013). In summary, the high risk of EPSE seen with haloperidol in many RCTs seems to have been incorrectly extrapolated to FGAs in general. Although antipsychotics differ little in terms of acute efficacy (the exception being clozapine, which is more effective in treatment-resistant schizophrenia), they differ significantly in their propensity to cause EPSE and a wide range of other side effects including weight gain, sedation, prolactin elevation, metabolic dysregulation and QTc prolongation. The differential risks of a range of antipsychotic adverse effects in people with schizophrenia have been quantified by meta-analysis (Leucht et al., 2013).

The introduction of the SGAs did have some advantages. In particular, the quality of the supporting RCTs was far superior to that of the FGA studies, some of which had been conducted more than three decades earlier. Meta-analysis showed a small advantage for SGAs versus the FGAs in the maintenance treatment of schizophrenia, the risk of relapse being slightly lower for SGAs (Kishimoto et al., 2013a). In addition, several SGAs were shown to be effective in disorders other than schizophrenia. For example, RCTs showed that several SGAs were effective in augmenting antidepressants in the treatment of major depressive disorder (Nelson & Papakostas, 2009). One SGA, quetiapine, was shown in placebo-controlled RCTs to be effective in the acute treatment of bipolar depression (Suttajit et al., 2014) and in a further RCT to reduce the risk of relapse of bipolar depression (Weisler et al., 2011). Although all antipsychotics are effective in treating acute mania and reducing the risk of manic relapse, the efficacy of quetiapine in the acute and maintenance treatment of bipolar depression is not a class effect shared by other antipsychotics. An added advantage of the quetiapine bipolar maintenance study was the inclusion of a lithium comparator arm, in addition to the quetiapine and placebo arms (Weisler et al., 2011). As such, this study, designed primarily to investigate the long-term efficacy of quetiapine, was also the largest placebo-controlled trial of lithium maintenance treatment in bipolar disorder ever conducted. It showed that lithium was superior to placebo in reducing the risk of relapse of bipolar depression as well as of mania. Previously it had been thought that lithium's benefits in the long-term treatment of bipolar disorder were largely restricted to reducing the risk of recurrence of mania rather than depression.

In 2002 the NMDA (*N*-methyl-D-aspartate) receptor antagonist memantine received European marketing approval for use in moderate to severe Alzheimer's disease, thereby becoming the first drug other than an acetylcholinesterase inhibitor to reach the market for this indication.

In 2002 the FDA approved aripiprazole for the treatment of schizophrenia. Subsequently, it received FDA approval in the USA for the treatment of bipolar I disorder (mania and mixed episodes and as a maintenance treatment) (2004), the treatment of irritability associated with autistic disorder (2009), the treatment of Tourette's disorder (2014) and as an adjunctive treatment for major depressive disorder (2006). In the UK aripiprazole is only licensed for the treatment of schizophrenia and the treatment of manic episodes and the prevention of a new manic episode in bipolar I disorder. Aripiprazole was the first antipsychotic drug to be marketed that was a D_2 partial agonist; all previous antipsychotics are full D_2 antagonists. Subsequently, two other D_2 partial agonists, brexpiprazole and cariprazine, received FDA approval. Brexpiprazole was approved for the treatment of schizophrenia and adjunctive treatment of major depressive disorder and cariprazine for the treatment of schizophrenia and the acute treatment of manic or mixed episodes in bipolar I disorder. The three currently available dopamine partial agonists differ not only in their indications but also in the formulations, pharmacodynamics, pharmacokinetics and side-effect profiles (Frankel & Schwartz, 2017). Overall, the dopamine partial agonists have a relatively low risk of causing prolactin elevation, metabolic side effects and EPSE other than akathisia.

In 2019 eskatamine, an intranasal formulation of ketamine, an NMDA receptor antagonist, received FDA approval for use in combination with a newly commenced antidepressant in adults with treatment-resistant depression. This represents a treatment for depression that is not reliant on modulating the monoamine system and benefit can occur within hours of administering the first dose, representing a far quicker onset of action than with traditional antidepressant drugs. The FDA approval reflected positive results from short- and long-term clinical trials (Janssen, 2019). Ketamine has a number of potential drawbacks including that its effects seem transient. Its place in clinical practice is yet to be determined.

At the time of writing, a large range of psychiatric drugs are under development. For example, a recent review identified 112 agents in the current pipeline for the treatment of Alzheimer's disease (Cummings et al., 2018). Much research is also focused on the treatment of depression (Garay et al., 2017) and schizophrenia (Garay et al., 2016). One area of development in treatment-resistant depression relates to drugs that modulate the opiate system. Recent RCTs of opiate-modulating drugs in depression have produced somewhat inconsistent results (Fava et al., 2016; Zajecka et al., 2019) but overall the field remains promising and further work is warranted. Another area of interest relates to the use of psilocybin and lysergic acid diethylamide (LSD) to treat addiction, anxiety disorders and treatment-resistant depression (Dos Santos, 2018). The work on psychedelics is largely based on small open studies of a short duration (e.g. Carhart-Harris et al., 2016) but a large Phase IIb dose-ranging study of psilocybin in treatment-resistant depression is currently underway in Europe and North America (ClinicalTrials.gov Identifier: NCT03775200). Psychedelics appear only to need one or two doses to be effective and there is the suggestion that they allow brain networks to be reset (Carhart-Harris & Nutt, 2017). Caution is needed when considering any drugs in the pipeline as the failure rate in drug development in all branches of medicine is high (see Chapter 2).

1.8 Preclinical Psychiatric Drug Development 1950 Onwards

1.8.1 Introduction

It is apparent to anyone reading the earlier sections on clinical psychopharmacology and drug development in the 1950–60 era that the first drugs that became available for the treatment of both depressive illness and schizophrenia during that period (and indeed well beyond) did not emanate from a rational drug discovery process. Indeed, neither chlorpromazine nor imipramine were developed for these respective indications. However, their appearance on the market and evidence for their efficacy came concomitantly with the realization that certain neurotransmitters in the brain might play a role in mood disorders. Consequently, during the 1960s there was a flood of investigations on the ways that psychiatric drugs altered neurotransmitter concentrations and function in the brain of experimental animals. This discovery process was assisted by the increasingly accurate and rapid methods, primarily spectrofluorimetry, for measuring monoamines in cerebral tissue. Such studies both enhanced our understanding of the possible mechanisms by which the drugs might be producing their therapeutic effect but also, to some extent, resulted in the proliferation of drugs with the same probable mechanism of action, the so-called 'me too' drugs, as will be discussed later.

The suggestion that psychoactive drugs might be achieving their therapeutic effect through an action on brain neurotransmitters was enunciated in the early years of the 1950s. The structural characterization of the vasoconstrictive substance 5-hydroxytryptamine (5-HT; serotonin) was published in 1948 by Maurice Rapport in the USA (Rapport et al., 1948), and only four years later it was reported that this compound was present in mammalian brain by both John Gaddum in Edinburgh and Irvine Page in Cleveland, Ohio. Gaddum noted that the action of 5-HT on peripheral tissue preparations was antagonized by LSD, and in a seminal publication he suggested that since LSD produced mood change it was reasonable to speculate that cerebral 5-HT was involved in controlling mood (Amin et al., 1954). The same conclusion was reached independently in the USA by Woolley and Shaw (1954) who had observed the structural similarity between the 5-HT and LSD molecule (Figure 1.5).

The other two major monoamine neurotransmitters now known to be closely associated with the actions of psychoactive drugs were also identified in the brain in the 1950s. Marthe Vogt in Edinburgh, both identified and mapped noradrenaline (norepinephrine) in the mammalian brain (Vogt, 1954), while dopamine, a known precursor of noradrenaline, was reported in 1957 to be acting as a neurotransmitter in the brain in its own right by groups working independently in Sweden and the UK (Björklund & Dunnett, 2007).

Although the idea that alteration of brain chemistry could have an effect on mood is now generally accepted by psychiatrists, this was not the case in the 1960s. So much so that in the introduction to his review 'The biochemistry of affective disorders' Alec

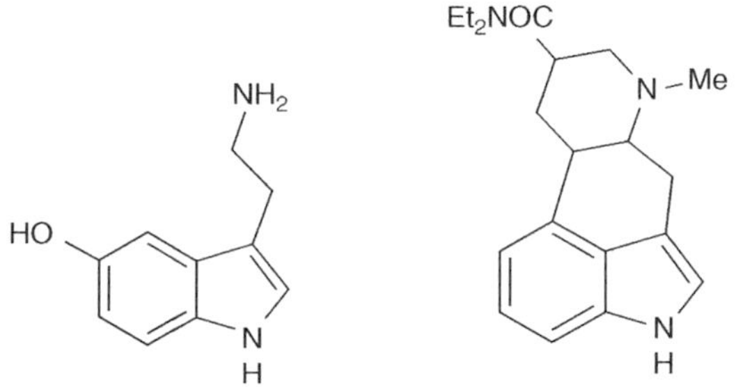

Figure 1.5 Chemical structures of 5-HT and LSD.

Coppen stated: '*The title of this review would be regarded by some psychiatrists as provocative; they would relegate the biochemical concomitants of depression and mania to a secondary position and deny the biochemical changes have any place in the aetiology of these conditions*' (Coppen, 1967).

The preclinical development of new drugs in these early days was reliant on two fundamental approaches. One was to use medicinal chemistry to synthesize structurally similar compounds to an existing therapeutically active drug to mimic the known biochemical and behavioural actions of that compound with the hope that the new compound would have greater efficacy and possibly fewer adverse effects. The other was to examine the preclinical pharmacology of the known compound and integrate this information with the expanding clinical knowledge of this drug to try and understand its mechanism of action and again produce compounds acting similarly. This latter approach is termed translational and reverse translational pharmacology. This tended to work successfully until the 1970s as there were fewer regulatory controls on clinical investigations compared to today, and small experimental studies on patients could be conducted and information fed back to initiate further preclinical studies (Sjoerdma, 2008). Such studies are now impossible as small-scale 'look see' studies on patients are not permitted for ethical reasons. Nevertheless, greater day-to-day collaboration between preclinical and clinical psychopharmacologists can still be valuable and its loss in many academic centres is unfortunate. It has been suggested that its re-emergence would enhance the discovery process in both psychiatry and other therapeutic areas (Green & Aronson, 2012).

1.8.2 Depression and the Monoamine Hypothesis of Affective Disorders

The preclinical development of antidepressant drugs in the 1950s to 1980s followed the path of good clinical observation of unexpected therapeutic activity, followed by development of related drugs and greater understanding of their possible mechanism of action. Iproniazid was first discovered to be a MAOI by Zeller et al. (1952) and later reported to have an antidepressant action by Nathan Kline (Loomer et al., 1957), among others. This led to several companies synthesizing other hydrazine derivatives and the hypothesis that raising the concentration of brain monoamines (5-HT and noradrenaline) by inhibiting their breakdown by MAO would lead to an antidepressant action. The toxicity of hydrazines meant that most of these drugs were removed from the marketplace fairly soon after launch. As it happened, another class of drug, the TCA, started to appear at much the same time and these drugs rapidly replaced the MAOIs, although it took preclinical psychopharmacologists several years to clarify how they might be acting.

The first TCA (imipramine) was structurally related to the phenothiazines antipschotics (Figure 1.3) and was found empirically to act as an antidepressant. Structurally related compounds from other companies followed, but with little idea as to any possible mechanism of action. However, during the mid-1960s onwards there was the discovery that monoamines were inactivated by their reuptake into the nerve ending (Iversen, 1971) and that several drugs, but notably the TCAs, inhibited the noradrenaline and 5-HT reuptake pumps. Their potency at these uptake sites varied, with desipramine being relatively selective at the noradrenaline site, and clomipramine at the 5-HT site, while amitriptyline was equipotent at both sites (see Grahame-Smith & Aronson, 1992).

These major observations, together with the suggestion that the amine-depleting drug reserpine (used to treat hypertension) could produce a depressive episode, resulted in the development of the 'monoamine hypothesis of affective disorders'. Basically, this stated that increasing monoamine function, either by inhibiting the enzyme inactivating monoamines and thereby increasing the monoamine concentration (MAOIs), or by blocking the uptake pump to increase synaptic concentration (TCAs), resulted in an antidepressant effect, while lowering monoamine concentrations (reserpine) could induce depression. Most TCAs inhibit the uptake of both 5-HT and noradrenaline, although the ratio of activity varies (dopamine uptake is generally little affected). The involvement of 5-HT in the antidepressant action of TCAs was championed in the UK (Coppen, 1967), while the importance of noradrenaline held sway in the USA (Schildkraut, 1965).

The finding by Coppen et al. (1963) that the antidepressant activity of a MAOI could be enhanced by administration of the 5-HT precursor L-tryptophan further strengthened the hypothesis, so much so that today the simplistic statement that antidepressants increase the *amount* of 5-HT in the brain can often be read in the popular press, even though it is nonsense as TCAs do no such thing.

The idea that making antidepressant drugs more selective at the 5-HT or noradrenaline uptake site might maintain the therapeutic action but decrease adverse effects (most TCAs had both antihistaminic and anticholinergic activity) resulted in the development of drugs that were more selective at either inhibiting noradrenaline or serotonin uptake. In the 1970s two drugs that were selective noradrenaline reuptake inhibitors entered the market. One, nomifensine, also inhibited dopamine reuptake, and while it had antidepressant activity it was withdrawn by the manufacturers in 1986 following reports of an association with haemolytic anaemia (Committee on Safety of Medicines, 1986). This association was largely identified through the 'Yellow Card', a UK system for recording adverse incidents with medicines. The second was maprotiline, which was discontinued in the UK in 2006. Interestingly, neither compound has the tricyclic structure. Drugs that are selective as serotonin reuptake inhibitors (SSRIs) entered the market during the 1980s and early 1990s and included fluoxetine, fluvoxamine, paroxetine and citalopram. These became extensively prescribed and remain widely used today. The SSRI drugs are clinically effective and safer in overdose than the TCAs. However, individual SSRIs show similar efficacy to each other and also to both the earlier non-selective drugs and also later drugs such as venlafaxine that have activity at both 5-HT and noradrenaline uptake sites (there is some evidence that certain antidepressants may be slightly more efficacious than others but the differences are marginal – for a further discussion see Cleare et al., 2015). Targeting a selective neurochemical site therefore predominantly produced more 'me-too' drugs in terms of postulated mechanism of action.

Although the monoamine hypothesis (increasing the synaptic concentration of monoamines) proved to be an effective marketing story, its weaknesses were apparent by the later 1980s. Firstly, later antidepressant drugs such as mianserin and iprindole had little effect on monoamine uptake, although they do have actions at monoamine receptors. Secondly, the TCAs and MAOIs could be shown to have a rapid biochemical effect in both rats and humans, but significant clinical improvement is often delayed for two to three weeks. Recent meta-analysis has challenged the idea of 'delayed' antidepressant action by showing that symptom improvement with SSRIs starts within one week of initiating treatment with the improvement building up over subsequent weeks (Taylor et al., 2006). The difference between this and the earlier view of delayed clinical effect probably reflects the sensitivity of methods used to measure change and how one defines a significant improvement. Nevertheless, the point remains that clinical improvement is slower than the changes seen in monoamine chemistry in animal models. Thirdly, administration of TCAs actually inhibits monoamine synthesis through a regulatory feedback inhibition process, and this is probably what was seen in the Sulser (1984) studies on β-adrenoceptor down-regulation that were some of the earliest to focus on the consequences of longer-term dosing in animals. It has been suggested that the initial changes in monoamine biochemistry may initiate longer-term mechanisms that result in the antidepressant effect, particularly as such adaptive mechanisms can be seen in other therapeutic areas (Grahame-Smith, 1997).

Despite the fact that the simple monoamine hypothesis of antidepressant action has now been abandoned (by psychopharmacologists at least) it is hard to deny that 5-HT is playing a role somewhere in the mechanism of many psychiatric drugs (Cowen, 2008). The top five selling drugs active on the CNS in the new millennium all modulated 5-HT function (Jones & Blackburn, 2002). The real problem for experimental psychopharmacology research is not merely that we still have relatively little understanding of how the drugs actually achieve their therapeutic effect, but rather that although the newer drugs such as the SSRIs produce fewer adverse effects, and have greater safety in overdose, the holy grail of producing a drug that has efficacy significantly greater than the older antidepressants such as amitriptyline has proved elusive. It is generally accepted that in the treatment of severe depression, ECT has the highest efficacy of all available treatments and experimental studies have been conducted to examine changes in brain neurochemistry produced when repeated electroconvulsive shocks (ECS) are given to rats (five to eight treatments spread out over a couple of weeks). Results demonstrated that ECS treatment actually produced many of the changes seen when antidepressant drugs were given, particularly altered 5-HT function. One notable change was in 5-HT$_{1A}$ receptor function in rats, as this effect lasted for almost a month after the last ECS (Goodwin et al., 1985). However, despite this and related work, there remains no consensus as to the mode of action of ECT.

Some preclinical studies attempted to move away from the simple monoamine hypothesis. Such investigations included studies on peptides such as thyrotrophin-releasing hormone (TRH) and cholecystokinin (CCK), the β-adrenoceptor agonist salbutamol and β-adrenoceptor antagonist propranolol and drugs acting at 5-HT receptor subtypes, but none has resulted in clinically useful drugs, which does make one wonder whether the non-specific effect of uptake inhibitors releasing 5-HT onto all receptor subtypes is essential. One important recent area of investigation has been the role of glutamatergic drugs but whether this will lead to effective new drugs remains unclear (Naughton et al., 2014).

1.8.3 Antipsychotics and the Dopamine Theory

The situation with regard to the preclinical studies on the mechanism of antipsychotic drugs is, in some ways, less complex. The first clear indication that they might be acting through a defined neurochemical mechanism came in the report of Carlsson and Lindqvist (1963) that chlorpromazine and haloperidol, two effective antipsychotics but with markedly different chemical structures, both increased dopamine turnover, an effect that suggested dopamine receptor blockade. In addition, behavioural studies in rats observed that amphetamine-induced locomotor activity was antagonized by antipsychotic drugs. Since amphetamine was found to release dopamine in the brain, this strengthened the idea that antipsychotic action probably involved decreasing dopaminergic function.

The next major finding supporting this hypothesis was that there was a strong correlation between the potency of a wide range of antipsychotic drugs to act as antagonists at the dopamine D_2 receptor subtype and the average effective clinical dose (Enna et al., 1976). The idea that dopamine D_2 receptor antagonism resulted in anti-schizophrenic action in turn led some companies to focus on developing selective D_2 receptor antagonists (notably Astra with remoxipride and Janssen with risperidone). Although clinically effective, the failure of such drugs to treat schizophrenia more successfully than earlier drugs, at least in terms of treating both positive and negative symptoms, has helped to destroy any concept of dopamine selective activity being the only requirement. Indeed, the most successful drug for treatment-resistant schizophrenia is clozapine, a drug that has affinity for a wide range of dopamine and 5-HT receptor subtypes. More recent antipsychotics such as quetiapine also lack receptor specificity (Green & Aronson, 2012).

1.8.4 Drugs for Anxiety

The problem of producing a novel anxiolytic drug that was an improvement on those already on the market became evident after the late 1960s. Barbiturates were first discovered in the early years of the last century and available thereafter, with their use in the UK peaking in the 1950s. Their addictive properties and toxicity in overdose were known and seen as a major limitation to their use. The launch of chlordiazepoxide, the first benzodiazepine, was therefore a major step forward as the drug was effective, relatively safe and not thought to produce dependence problems. Its discovery resulted from re-testing in animal models a drug that had sat on the shelf of Hoffmann–La Roche for some time; another example of a highly successful drug that did not result from a structured drug discovery programme. Chlordiazepoxide was followed by the much more potent diazepam, and the shorter-acting nitrazepam; the latter was therefore marketed as a hypnotic. Preclinical studies indicated that the benzodiazepines acted via an action on the inhibitory neurotransmitter gamma-aminobutyric acid (GABA). Interestingly, both barbiturates and meprobamate also act through a GABAergic mechanism. What was fascinating was the identification of a specific benzodiazepine binding site on the GABA receptor (Braestrup & Squires, 1977), raising the possibility that the brain has an endogenous benzodiazepine. A variety of peptides and other compounds have been suggested to act at the site, the so-called endozepines (Farzampour et al., 2015). Moreover, the molecular biology of the $GABA_A$ receptor has revealed several functional subtypes with different distributions in the brain. The α_1 subtype is especially expressed in cortex and is the target of the first subtype-selective hypnotic zolpidem.

1.8.5 Drugs for Alzheimer's Disease

One neuropsychiatric disease where drug development was initiated as the result of preclinical observations is Alzheimer's disease. The first discovery that some of the clinical problems were neurochemical was the seminal report by David Bowen and colleagues of a loss of cholinergic neurons in the senile dementia brain (Bowen et al., 1976). This finding led to the use of cholinesterase inhibitors such as tacrine and rivastigmine. Post-mortem studies subsequently identified other neurotransmitter abnormalities including 5-HT and glutamate (Francis, 2009). These studies resulted in the clinical use of memantine, a glutamate NMDA receptor subtype antagonist. However, the fact that these approaches were merely symptomatic has resulted in most research now focusing on pharmacological ways to prevent the neurodegenerative changes, primarily the formation of plaques and tangles in the brain.

1.8.6 Animal Models in Psychopharmacology

A fundamental problem that runs through all preclinical psychopharmacology studies is the weakness of animal models. The validity of animal studies can be a problem in other therapeutic areas but is particularly troublesome in psychiatric disorders where there remains substantial ignorance of their causes and pathology.

Animal models can simplistically be divided into two basic types; those that can be used as screens to detect possible therapeutic value for a specific indication and those that try to mimic the clinical condition. Most early models were those for drug screening and to show responses to acute drug administration even though the drugs themselves are only clinically effective after longer-term administration. Acute tests include the Porsolt test for antidepressants (Porsolt et al., 1978) and its related tests, the elevated plus maze for anxiolytics (Cryan & Sweeney, 2011) and prepulse inhibition of the acoustic startle for antipsychotic drugs (Jones et al., 2011). The behaviour evoked in response to a provoking stimulus in these tests, given as it is to a 'normal' animal, probably involves different neuronal circuits and neuropharmacology from that required to treat a psychiatric disorder in the human brain. Furthermore, many screening animal models will only detect drugs that act through a specific neurochemical mechanism, whereas the symptoms of psychiatric disorders are many and this probably reflects multiple mechanisms. Consequently, novel compounds may not be detected. For example, SSRI drugs show up poorly in most animal models of anxiety (Cryan & Sweeney, 2011).

To try and deal with this problem there have been substantial efforts made to model psychiatric disorders. Psychopharmacology presents particular problems because, as Horrobin (2003) pointed out: '*An animal model of disease can be said to be congruent with the human disease only when three conditions have been met: we fully understand the animal model, we fully understand the human disease and we have examined the two cases and found them to be substantially congruent in all important respects.*' Ignorance of the causes and pathology of the major psychiatric diseases emphasizes that these conditions cannot be met. Models only partly replicate the full clinical condition or pathology of the disorder. In an attempt to deal with this problem, the MATRICS (Measurement and Treatment Research to Improve Cognition in Schizophrenia) initiative recommended a battery of rodent behavioural tasks with translational relevance to most of the seven cognitive domains affected in schizophrenia. MATRICS also recommended a specific neuropsychological test battery to characterize these domains (Kern et al., 2008; Nuechterlein et al., 2008).

There is a need for new animal models that accurately reflect the pathophysiology of the disease, as emphasized by Spedding et al. (2005), and newer models of schizophrenia (Jones et al., 2011), anxiety (Cryan & Sweeney, 2011) and depression (Robinson, 2018) are available, albeit only reflecting some of the pathology, as might be expected.

1.8.7 Conclusions Regarding Preclinical Research Studies

Since the late 1980s research approaches in psychopharmacology have changed from often undertaking 'look see' experiments to examine whether a compound might have an effect in an animal model (sometimes with no seriously developed hypothesis) or even sometimes clinically, to that of proposing a possible mechanism of action (for example, an interaction with a neurotransmitter receptor) and synthesizing further compounds that interact with that target site. This emphasis on target identification ('targetophilia') has produced novel drugs, and high throughput screening (HTS) has speeded up the process of identifying potentially useful new compounds. However, it has not enhanced the drug discovery process, and it may even have slowed the discovery process down as it '*requires a good understanding of target physiology and its integration with the target organ, with a hierarchical integration from in vitro cellular and functional tissue studies to animal models that reasonably predict human responses*' (Enna & Williams, 2009). In the case of CNS disorders, researchers were unable to meet this requirement 25 years ago, when targetophilia first became extensively used in the pharmaceutical industry, and are only modestly closer now. A single target approach will only work if the mechanism being targeted is the final step in the pathway that leads to the pathology. Given the complexity of psychiatric illness and evidence suggestive of multiple causative factors (both genetic and environmental), a final common pathway seems unlikely in most cases. Preclinical psychopharmacology has made enormous advances over the years, giving us greater understanding of the neurochemical changes produced by psychoactive drugs and suggesting possible mechanisms by which they produce their therapeutic effects. Nevertheless, a lack of understanding of the mechanisms involved in psychiatric disorders has meant that existing drugs are treating symptoms, not the underlying initiating factors. In terms of failure of new drugs, neuropsychiatry does not have a worse attrition rate than several other therapeutic areas companies still support and various new scientific approaches have been proposed to get the industry re-engaged with this vital area of public health (Green & Marsden, 2013).

To date, all drugs approved to treat depression and psychosis manipulate monoamine transmission, though some have additional actions. Developing drugs to treat depression and schizophrenia that have alternative mechanisms of action has proved disappointing with several notable failures including Group II metabotropic glutamate receptor ($mGlu_{2/3}$) agonists to treat schizophrenia (Li et al., 2015). One reason may be that trials recruit too broad a range of patients. People with both depression and schizophrenia almost certainly encompass subgroups with different neurotransmitter abnormalities. This argues that in clinical trials, and later in clinical practice, medications should be matched to different underlying disease mechanisms. For example, it may be that some people with schizophrenia have a primary dopaminergic abnormality and others a primary glutaminergic abnormality. The process of matching drugs to the presumed underlying pathophysiology is termed stratification. It requires the identification of reliable biomarkers (e.g. genetic, neuroimaging, electrophysiological, neurochemical) to identify underlying disease mechanisms and thereby predict response to specific medications. At present work adopting this approach is in very early stages but it appears an important avenue for future preclinical research and clinical practice. Drug development is discussed in detail in Chapter 2 of this book.

1.9 The Legacy of the Psychopharmacology Revolution

In the first half of the twentieth century care for those with severe mental illness in North America, Australia, New Zealand and most European countries was largely provided by asylums. Underfunding, understaffing and overcrowding meant that standards of care were low despite the good intentions of many staff. Up to 1949 there were no effective treatments for major mental illness. Many patients in asylums displayed severe psychotic symptoms and behavioural disturbance (Norton, 1979). Medications that were available could only treat anxiety, provide sedation and help control disturbed behaviour. The introduction of antipsychotic drugs in the 1950s allowed mania and schizophrenia to be treated effectively for the first time and contributed to the demise of ineffective treatments including psychosurgery, insulin-coma treatment and ECT to treat schizophrenia.

The introduction of effective psychiatric drugs in the 1950s had widespread ramifications. It became apparent that scientific methodology was required to assess their clinical impact and this led to the development of RCTs in psychiatry. One of the earliest randomized trials in psychiatry compared lithium to placebo in the treatment of mania (Schou et al., 1954). This was a small study with less than 40 participants. Some were treated double blind but others received open treatment. The study utilized a cross-over design in which subjects received treatment with lithium and then treatment with placebo or vice versa. By the early 1960s several large double-blind randomized studies, with parallel treatment arms, had been published comparing phenothiazines to placebo in the treatment of schizophrenia (Adelson & Epstein, 1962; Casey et al., 1960; National Institute of Mental Health Psychopharmacology Service Center Collaborative Study Group, 1964). To allow the systematic assessment of treatment outcome in trials, symptom rating scales were developed as were rating scales to assess medication side effects. Today, RCTs are not only the benchmark for establishing the efficacy of pharmacological treatments, but also of psychological treatments and competing methods of service delivery. RCTs alone cannot answer all the questions regarding drug safety and furthermore they assess efficacy, i.e. the ability of a drug to treat a condition in ideal circumstances. Observational studies are necessary to assess effectiveness, i.e. how well a drug works in real-world clinical practice. Post-marketing surveillance plays a vital role in monitoring drug safety.

The introduction of new psychiatric drugs in the 1950s helped to reduce the stigma of mental illness. The fact that mental illnesses could be treated with medicines put them, to a degree, on a par with medical conditions such as diabetes and hypertension. The new treatments also served to generate hope among patients, families and mental health staff. Prior to the introduction of the antidepressants and antipsychotics in the 1950s, care in the asylums for those with severe mental illness often came down to containment. It is important to acknowledge that some people find the idea of having to take a medication to treat a mental health condition stigmatizing in its own right. Similarly, although many people find it helpful to know that there are biological factors at play in the genesis of a mental illness, if the concept is misunderstood it may incorrectly help foster a view that self-help is not possible.

The second half of the twentieth century saw a massive reduction in the number of psychiatric inpatient beds in many countries and the parallel development of community psychiatric services, a process termed deinstitutionalization. In England the number of psychiatric beds peaked at approximately 150 000 in 1955 and had fallen to around 22 000 in 2012 (The Kings Fund, 2015). In the United States the number of inpatients in state mental hospitals peaked at 559 000 in 1955 and had fallen to 57 000 by 1998 (Lamb & Bachrach, 2001). The causes of deinstitutionalization, and whether the introduction of the antipsychotics contributed, have been the subject of much debate. The two extremes are represented by the argument that the antipsychotics were 'wonder drugs' that almost single-handedly emptied the asylums versus the view that deinstitutionalization was solely a social phenomenon. Most authorities, including the authors, take an intermediate view regarding deinstitutionalization as the result of multiple factors of which the antipsychotics were one (Grob, 1991; Shorter, 1997). It is reasonable to suggest that the antipsychotics contributed in several ways. Their effectiveness in treating severe psychiatric symptoms (hallucinations, delusions, manic excitement, thought disorder and agitation) facilitated the discharge of some patients. They also allowed a greater proportion of hospital patients to engage and benefit from rehabilitation. Some patients in the community could be treated with antipsychotics without the need for admission. Finally, the antipsychotics probably played an indirect role by giving policymakers a rationale to move care from the asylums to the community, making this process more publicly acceptable and giving clinicians a greater confidence in providing community services.

Social factors were without doubt also an important contributor to deinstitutionalization. In both the USA and UK, a change in government policy aimed to drastically cut the asylum population and shift mental health care to the community. In addition, changes to mental health law meant that informal admission to psychiatric inpatient units became the norm. The introduction of Medicaid in the USA in 1965 provided a financial incentive to move care from the state-funded asylums to federally funded institutions including nursing homes and psychiatric wards attached to general hospitals (Gronfein, 1985). Additional factors that contributed to the closure of the asylums included increasing public awareness of scandals and poor care in asylums, recognition of the problems caused by long-term hospital admission, including institutionalization, and a greater appreciation among professionals of social and psychological treatments. Views on the success of community-care for the mentally ill vary and critics argue that deinstitutionalization was followed by an increasing population of people with mental illness in prisons, supported housing and forensic psychiatric units (Priebe et al., 2005).

The psychopharmacology revolution stimulated research into the biological nature of psychiatric illness and led to the creation of psychopharmacology as a discipline. For example, the introduction of the MAOIs and TCAs led to the monoamine theories of depression (Coppen, 1967; Schildkraut, 1965) and schizophrenia (Carlsson & Lindqvist, 1963) being proposed. Both theories of depression have been modified over time (e.g. Cowen, 2008; Howes & Kapur, 2009) and have faced criticism. The issue here is not to what extent they are right or wrong, but to emphasize that drug development led to theories being proposed that could then be tested in a scientific manner.

In summary, the psychopharmacology revolution changed the practice of psychiatry and led to the creation of psychopharmacology as a new scientific discipline. However, psychopharmacology is not without its critics or its problems as will be discussed in the following two sections.

1.10 Controversies in Psychopharmacology

Some of the most strident criticism of psychopharmacology, as well as drug treatment in other disease areas, has related to the actions of pharmaceutical companies. The role of pharmaceutical companies in developing new medications to treat psychiatric and medical disorders has helped revolutionize medicine over the last 50 years, improving quality of life for countless people. In many disease areas the advantages of pharmacological treatment are apparent in terms of increased life expectancy. The expertise and finance necessary to bring one new drug to market is huge, recently estimated at $1.2 billion (Adams & Brantner, 2010). As such, it is difficult to conceive further advances in drug development occurring without the involvement of the pharmaceutical industry.

A major problem affecting pharmacological treatment was that until fairly recently there was no requirement to register or publish the results of RCTs. Consequently, licensing decisions and systematic reviews could be based on a skewed evidence base because negative trials are less likely to be published. At its worst this could represent a drug company deliberately suppressing a negative study, but the problem also encompasses independent research groups whose priorities may lie in publishing positive studies rather than negative ones. In addition, journals are more likely to publish positive studies with the result that negative studies are often reported briefly or only as conference abstracts. To prevent this problem, clinical trials registries, such as Clinical .Trials.gov run by the United States National Library of Medicine, allow RCTs, industry sponsored or otherwise, to be registered, and the results made available within a short period of completion. In the United States and many other countries registration of Phase II to IV clinical trials is now mandatory. This has partly addressed the concern of unpublished trial data, although recent research shows that adherence to registry guidelines is far from perfect (Jones et al., 2013).

Other problems related to industry-sponsored research have included companies failing to make data available to independent researchers, controversy about the methodology and statistical analysis used in trials, industry promotion of drugs beyond their licence and failure to declare conflicts of interests by authors and researchers. These are all serious issues that are now being addressed. They apply to all branches of pharmacological research and not just psychopharmacology. Parallel issues apply to research on psychological treatments, but this has attracted less attention.

Some critics have argued that psychiatric drugs are overprescribed and do more harm than good (Gøtzsche et al., 2015). There is no doubt that some psychiatric medications have been used inappropriately. Examples include the overprescription of benzodiazepines leading to iatrogenic dependence (Lader, 2014) and the excessive use of antipsychotic drugs in nursing homes to manage behavioural disturbance (Tjia et al., 2012). However, one cannot generalize from these examples to all psychotropic prescribing and all psychiatric disorders. Many factors can drive the inappropriate use of psychiatric drugs. These include overpromotion by drug companies, an unquestioning approach by doctors to the information they receive from companies, a desire from some patients and relatives for a 'simple fix' for emotional distress and psychiatric problems, a widening of diagnostic criteria and clinicians applying diagnostic criteria too loosely so that an increasing proportion of individuals are deemed 'ill' and prescribed for. Lack of availability of psychosocial interventions may also mean that a pharmacological approach is the only intervention available to a clinician and patient. Public information, training for doctors, guidelines for company advertising of drugs and clinical guidelines all have a role to play in ensuring that prescribing is appropriate and evidence-based.

The introduction of evidence-based clinical guidelines has been a major development in recent decades leading to greater uniformity in the quality of treatment. Psychological treatments are first-line treatments for many psychiatric disorders including anxiety disorders and major depressive disorder that are of mild to moderate severity. However, critics of psychopharmacology often seem to lack awareness of the severity, persistence and disability associated with psychiatric illnesses such as schizophrenia, bipolar disorder and severe major depressive disorder that psychiatrists deal with every day, and of the benefits that can come from appropriate prescribing that is part of a comprehensive package of care that incorporates psychosocial treatments.

Another criticism levelled at psychopharmacology is that the evidence base supporting long-term treatment is flawed. Trials that support the long-term efficacy of psychiatric drugs usually have a continuation design in which those with an acute illness who respond to a drug are randomized to stay on that drug, or switch to placebo. It has been suggested that in some cases the switch from active drug to placebo may trigger a drug 'withdrawal' reaction which is misdiagnosed as a relapse; that is, in some patients the recurrent nature of mental illness may be partly an iatrogenic effect (Montcrieff, 2006). In the case of schizophrenia this has been linked to antipsychotics causing dopamine receptor supersensitivity. This hypothesis warrants further research; there is evidence of withdrawal effects with many psychiatric drugs and rebound psychosis has been recognized to occur with clozapine. However, a meta-analysis of randomized antipsychotic maintenance trials (trials in which stable patients with schizophrenia are randomized to continue or withdraw from their current antipsychotic) showed that the benefit of antipsychotics in reducing relapse was not affected by how quickly the antipsychotic was withdrawn in those randomized to placebo (Leucht et al., 2012). This contrasts to the findings of an earlier and less comprehensive analysis by Viguera et al. (1997) in which the risk of relapse was higher after abrupt discontinuation of oral antipsychotics compared to gradual discontinuation of oral antipsychotics or stopping depot injections. The Leucht et al. (2012) finding is not consistent with an iatrogenic explanation of relapse. Nevertheless, it does not rule out the possibility that a drug withdrawal effect may contribute to relapse in a minority of patients. It has also been argued that tolerance to the maintenance effect of antipsychotics develops over time. In support, Leucht et al. (2012) noted that the effect of antipsychotics in reducing relapse, compared to placebo, reduced with increasing study duration. However, as the authors point out, there are other explanations of this finding; it could reflect antipsychotic non-adherence which tends to increase with increasing duration of treatment, or that the severity of illness and potential for relapse varies between those enrolled in short-term and long-term trials. Ultimately, a scientific approach and further research is the only way to answer these and related questions.

In summary, psychopharmacology has attracted both criticism and controversy. Similar issues have been seen in many parts of medicine and other aspects of psychiatry, though this is not in any way to downplay these issues. Positive criticism is helpful and can lead to clinical and research issues being seen from a different perspective. Open discussion and continuing research, education and collaboration with other organizations and the public are among the important ways to deal with these areas.

1.11 Current Problems Facing Psychopharmacology Research

Since the 1950s knowledge of CNS transmitter systems and their interplay with other bodily systems and genetics has increased at an incredible rate. It has been accompanied by the introduction of in vitro and in vivo techniques including the ability to image receptors and brain activity in living subjects. Unfortunately, this explosion of scientific knowledge has not been matched by the introduction of more effective psychiatric drugs. In particular, the efficacy of drugs to treat depression and schizophrenia (with the exception of clozapine) has not changed significantly since imipramine and chlorpromazine were introduced in the 1950s. The reasons for this are many but include the complexity of the CNS, deficiencies in current animal models used for preclinical research and weaknesses in the design of clinical trials including recruiting too broad a range of patients. Ideally in a clinical trial, one would aim to recruit a subset of patients on the basis of reliable genetic, neuroimaging or other biomarkers that were postulated to predict response to the drug being investigated. If the trial was successful, then similar stratification could also be adopted in clinical practice. Currently, the ability to target treatments in this way is in its infancy. A related approach is to develop drugs that target specific symptom domains of a clinical syndrome, for example cognitive dysfunction or primary negative symptoms in schizophrenia, and investigate putative treatments in samples enriched for the symptom domain in question. Another contributing factor to the paucity of new compounds is the relative underfunding of CNS research relative to other disease areas. When disability and economic burden are considered, neuroscience research is underfunded in comparison with research for cancer and coronary heart disease (Green & Marsden, 2013; Luengo-Fernandez et al., 2012).

The prospect for developing improved drugs for CNS disorders has taken a further setback in recent years as most major drug companies with an interest in this field have scaled back their research and development programmes or moved away from the area totally. This reflects the complexity and difficulty of developing new and more effective CNS treatments. The recent failure of a number of drugs in development, including glutamatergic drugs for schizophrenia, and the fact that most health services require increasingly strong evidence that new drugs offer advantages in efficacy or safety before approving use, has further weakened confidence in companies wishing to invest in research on psychiatric disorders. However, failures in drug development in the CNS are not clearly worse than in some other therapeutic areas (Green & Marsden, 2013).

Reduced investment in psychopharmacology research and development is particularly worrying given the high disability associated with CNS disease. Fineberg et al. (2013) estimated that in 2010 there were approximately 45 million cases of brain disorders in the UK, with an annual cost of €134 billion. This comprised 27% direct healthcare costs (i.e. cost of healthcare professionals, hospitalization, investigations, medication and other treatments), 27% non-medical direct costs (e.g. cost of social services and special accommodation) and 46% indirect costs (i.e. lost productivity due to work absence and early retirement). The five costliest disorders were dementia, psychotic disorders, mood disorders, addiction and anxiety disorders. The coming decades are likely to see an increase in the incidence and cost of brain disorders in the UK due to an increasing elderly population. For this reason, and to reduce individual suffering and to improve quality of life, there is a pressing need to develop new and more effective treatments, including new medications. This will require investment in translational neurosciences research and close collaboration between the healthcare sector and preclinical and clinical scientists (Green & Aronson, 2012).

References

Ackner B, Harris A, Oldham, AJ (1957). Insulin treatment of schizophrenia; a controlled study. *Lancet*, ii, 607–611.

Adams CP, Brantner, VV (2010). Spending on new drug development. *Health Econ*, 19, 130–141.

Adelson D, Epstein LJ (1962). A study of phenothiazines with male and female chronically ill schizophrenic patients. *J Nerv Ment Dis*, 134, 543–554.

Akers BP, Ruiz JF, Piper A, Ruck CAP (2011). A prehistoric mural in Spain depicting neurotropic psilocybe mushrooms? *Econ Bot*, 65, 121–128.

Amin AH, Crawford TBB, Gaddum JH (1954). The distribution of substance P and 5-hydroxytryptamine in the central nervous system of the dog. *J Physiol*, 125, 596–618.

Angst J, Weis P, Grof P, et al. (1970). Lithium prophylaxis in recurrent affective disorders. *Br J Psychiatry*, 116, 604–614.

Baastrup PC, Schou M (1967). Lithium as a prophylactic agent. Its effect against recurrent depressions and manic-depressive psychosis. *Arch Gen Psychiatry*, 16, 162–172.

Baastrup PC, Poulsen JC, Schou M, et al. (1970). Prophylactic lithium: double blind discontinuation in manic-depressive and recurrent-depressive disorders. *Lancet*, 2, 326–330.

Ban TA, Ray OS (1996). *A History of the CINP*. Brentwood TN: JM Productions, pp. 457.

Björklund A, Dunnett SB (2007). Fifty years of dopamine research. *Trends Neurosci*, 30, 185–187.

Blackwell B (1963). Hypertensive crises due to monoamine inhibitors. *Lancet*, ii, 849–851.

Board of Control for England and Wales (1947). *Prefrontal Leucotomy in 1,000 Cases*. London: HMSO.

Bowen DM, Smith CB, White P, Davison AN (1976). Neurotransmitter-related enzymes and indices of hypoxia in senile dememeentia and other abiotrophies. *Biochem J*, 99, 459–496.

Bradley C (1937). The behavior of children receiving benzedrine. *Am J Psychiatry*, 94, 577–581.

Bradley C, Bowen M (1940). Amphetamine (Benzedrine) therapy of children's behavior disorders. *Am J Orthopsychiatry*, 11, 92–103.

Braestrup C, Squires RF (1977). Stereospecific benzodiazepine receptors in rat brain characterized by high affinity (3H)-diazepam binding. *Proc Natl Acad Sci USA*, 74, 3805–3809.

Brown WA, Rosdolsky M (2015). The clinical discovery of imipramine. *Am J Psychiatry*, 172, 426–429.

Cade JFJ (1949). Lithium salts in the treatment of psychotic excitement. *Med J Aust*, 2, 349–352.

Carhart-Harris RL, Nutt DJ (2017). Serotonin and brain function: a tale of two receptors. *J Psychopharmacol*, 31, 1091–1120.

Carhart-Harris RL, Bolstridge M, Rucker J, et al. (2016). Psilocybin with psychological support for treatment-resistant depression: an open-label feasibility study. *Lancet Psychiatry*, 3(7), 619–627.

Carlsson A, Lindqvist M (1963). Effect of chlorpromazine and haloperidol on formation of 3-methoxytyramine and normetanephrine on mouse brain. *Acta Pharmacol Toxicol*, 20, 140–144.

Casey JF, Bennett IF, Lindley, CJ, et al. (1960). Drug therapy in schizophrenia. A controlled study of the relative effectiveness of chlorpromazine, promazine, phenobarbital, and placebo. *AMA Arch Gen Psychiatry*, 2, 210–220.

Cleare A, Pariante CM, Young AH, et al. (2015). Evidence-based guidelines for treating depressive disorders with antidepressants: a revision of the 2008 British Association for Psychopharmacology guidelines. *J Psychopharmacol*, 29, 459–525.

Committee on Safety of Medicines (1986). CSM Update: withdrawal of nomifensine. *Br Med J (Clin Res Ed)*, 293, 41.

Coppen A (1967). The biochemistry of affective disorders. *Br J Psychiatry*, 113, 1237–1264.

Coppen A, Shaw DM, Farrell JP (1963). Potentiation of the antidepressive effect of a monoamine-oxidase inhibitor by tryptophan. *Lancet*, 281, 79–81.

Cowen PJ (2008). Serotonin and depression: pathophysiological mechanism or marketing myth? *Trends Pharmacol Sci*, 29, 433–436.

Crismon ML (1994). Tacrine: first drug approved for Alzheimer's disease. *Ann Pharmacother*, 28, 744–751.

Cryan JF, Sweeney FF (2011). The age of anxiety: role of animal models of anxiolytic action in drug discovery. *Br J Pharmacol*, 164, 1129–1161.

Cummings J, Lee G, Ritter A, Zhong K (2018). Alzheimer's disease drug development pipeline: 2018. *Alzheimers Dement (N Y)*, 4, 195–214.

Delay J, Deniker P, Harl JM (1952). Utilisation en thérapeutique d'une phénothiazine d'action centrale selective. *Ann Med Psychol (Paris)*, 110, 112–117.

Dos Santos RG, Bouso JC, Alcázar-Córcoles MÁ, Hallak JEC (2018). Efficacy, tolerability, and safety of serotonergic psychedelics for the management of mood, anxiety, and substance-use disorders: a systematic review of systematic reviews. *Expert Rev Clin Pharmacol*, 11(9), 889–902.

El-Seedi HR, De Smet PA, Beck O, Possnert G, Bruhn JG (2005). Prehistoric peyote use: alkaloid analysis and radiocarbon dating of archaeological specimens of *Lophophora* from Texas. *J Ethnopharmacol*, 101, 238–242.

Enna SJ, Williams M (2009). Challenges in the search for drugs to treat central nervous system disorders. *J Pharmacol Exp Ther*, 329, 404–411.

Enna SJ, Bennett JP Jr, Burt DR, Creese I, Snyder SH (1976). Stereospecificity of interaction of neuroleptic drugs with neurotransmitters and correlation with clinical potency. *Nature*, 263, 338–341.

European Medicines Agency (2012). Questions and answers on the suspension of the marketing authorisations for oral meprobamate containing medicines. Available at: www.ema.europa.eu/docs/en_GB/document_library/Referrals_document/meprobamate_107/WC500120737.pdf (last accessed 29.4.18).

Fagius J, Osterman PO, Sidén A, Wiholm BE (1985). Guillain-Barré syndrome following zimeldine treatment. *J Neurol Neurosurg Psychiatry*, 48(1), 65–69.

Farzampour Z, Reimer RJ, Huguenard J (2015). Endozepines. *Adv Pharmacol*, 72, 147–164.

Fava M, Memisoglu A, Thase ME, et al. (2016). Opioid modulation with buprenorphine/samidorphan as adjunctive treatment for inadequate response to antidepressants: a randomized double-blind placebo-controlled trial. *Am J Psychiatry*, 173, 499–508.

Fineberg NA, Haddad PM, Carpernter L, et al. (2013). The size, burden and cost of disorders of the brain in the UK. *J Psychopharmacol*, 27, 761–770.

Francis PT (2009). Altered glutamate neurotransmission and behaviour in dementia: evidence from studies of memantine. *Curr Mol Pharmacol*, 2, 77–82.

Frankel JS, Schwartz TL (2017). Brexpiprazole and cariprazine: distinguishing two new atypical antipsychotics from the original dopamine stabilizer aripiprazole. *Ther Adv Psychopharmacol*, 7(1), 29–41.

Gaddum JH (1954). Discoveries in therapeutics. *J Pharm Pharmacol*, 6, 497–512.

Garay RP, Citrome L, Samalin L, et al. (2016). Therapeutic improvements expected in the near future for schizophrenia and schizoaffective disorder: an appraisal of phase III clinical trials of schizophrenia-targeted therapies as found in US and EU clinical trial registries. *Expert Opin Pharmacother*, 17(7), 921–936.

Garay RP, Zarate CA Jr, Charpeaud T, et al. (2017). Investigational drugs in recent clinical trials for treatment-resistant depression. *Expert Rev Neurother*, 17(6), 593–609.

Goodwin GM, DeSouza RJ, Green AR (1985). Presynaptic serotonin-mediated response in mice attenuated by antidepressants and electroconvulsive shock. *Nature*, 317, 531–533.

Goodwin GM, Haddad PM, Ferrier IN, et al. (2016). Evidence-based guidelines for treating bipolar disorder: revised third edition recommendations from the British Association for Psychopharmacology. *J Psychopharmacol*, 30, 495–553.

Gøtzsche PC, Young AH, Crace J (2015). Maudsley Debate. Does long term use of psychiatric drugs cause more harm than good? *BMJ*, 350, h2435.

Grahame-Smith DG (1997). 'Keep on taking the tablets': pharmacological adaptation during long-term drug therapy. *Br J Clin Pharmacol*, 44, 227–238.

Grahame-Smith DG, Aronson JK (1992). *Oxford Textbook of Clinical Pharmacology and Drug Therapy*. Oxford: Oxford University Press.

Green AR, Aronson JK (2012). From basic to clinical neuropharmacology: targetophilia or pharmacodynamics. *Br J Clin Pharmacol*, 73, 959–967.

Green AR, Haddad PM (2016). *The British Association for Psychopharmacology: The First 40 Years*. Cambridge: British Association for Psychopharmacology.

Green AR, Marsden CA (2013). How do we re-engage the pharmaceutical industry in research on serotonin and psychiatric disorders? *ACS Chem Neurol*, 4, 9–12.

Green AR, Aronson JK, Haddad PM (2018a). Examining the 'psychopharmacology revolution' (1950–1980) through the advertising of psychoactive drugs in the *British Medical Journal*. *J Psychopharmacol*, 32, 1056–1066.

Green AR, Haddad PM, Aronson JK (2018b). Marketing medicines: charting the rise of modern therapeutics through a systematic review of adverts in UK medical journals (1950–1980). *Br J Clin Pharmacol*, 84, 1668–1685.

Griesinger W (1861). *Pathologie und Therapie der psychischen Krankheiten* (*Mental Pathology and Therapeutics*), Stuttgart: Krabbe, 1845; second edition, Braunschweig, 1861.Translated by C Lockhart Robertson and James Rutherford, New York: William Wood and Company, 1882. Available at: https://archive.org/stream/mentalpathology00ruthgoog#page/n6/mode/2up (last accessed 2.8.19).

Grob GG (1991). *From Asylum to Community Mental Health Policy in Modern America*. Princeton, NJ: Princeton University Press.

Gronfein W (1985). Incentives and intentions in mental health policy: a comparison of the Medicaid and community mental health programs. *J Health Soc Behav*, 26, 192–206.

Hamon J, Paraire J, Velluz J (1952). Remarques sur l'action du 4560 RP sur l'agitation maniaque. *Ann Med Psychol (Paris)*, 110, 331–335.

Himwich HE (1958). Psychopharmacologic drugs. *Science*, 127, 59–72.

Hippius H (1999). A historical perspective of clozapine. *J Clin Psychiatry*, 60(Suppl 12), 22–23.

Holden TJ, Cavanagh WG (1987). Use of paraldehyde. *Br J Psychiatry*, 150, 564–565.

Horrobin DF (2003). Modern biomedical research: an internally self-consistent universe with little contact with medical reality? *Nat Rev Drug Discov*, 2, 151–154.

Howes OD, Kapur S (2009). The dopamine hypothesis of schizophrenia: version III – the final common pathway. *Schizophr Bull*, 35, 549–562.

Hutton EL, Fleming, GWTH, Fox EE (1941). Early results of prefrontal leucotomy. *Lancet*, ii, 3–7.

Idanpaan-Heikkila J, Alhava E, Olkimora M, Palva J (1975). Clozapine and agranulocytosis. *Lancet*, 2, 611.

Iversen LL (1971). Role of transmitter uptake systems in synaptic neurotransmission. *Br J Pharmacol*, 41, 571–591.

Janssen (2019). SPRAVATO (esketamine) nasal spray, CII Prescribing information. Available at: www.janssenlabels.com/package-insert/product-monograph/prescribing-information/SPRAVATO-pi.pdf (last accessed 25.5.19).

Johnson DAW (2009). Historical perspective on antipsychotic long-acting injections. *Br J Psychiatry*, 195, S7–S12.

Jones BJ, Blackburn TP (2002). The medical benefit of 5-HT research. *Pharmacol Biochem Behav*, 71, 555–568.

Jones CA, Watson DJG, Fone KCF (2011). Animal models of schizophrenia. *Br J Pharmacol*, 164, 1162–1194.

Jones CW, Handler L, Crowell KE, et al. (2013). Non-publication of large randomized clinical trials: cross sectional analysis. *BMJ*, 347, f6104.

Jones K (2000). Insulin coma therapy in schizophrenia. *J R Soc Med*, 93, 147–149.

Jones PB, Barnes TR, Davies L, et al. (2006). Randomized controlled trial of effect on quality of life of second- vs first-generation antipsychotic drugs in schizophrenia. Cost Utility of the Latest Antipsychotic Drugs in Schizophrenia Study (CUtLASS 1). *Arch Gen Psychiatry*, 63, 1079–1087.

Kane J, Honigfield G, Singer J, et al. (1988). Clozapine for the treatment-resistant schizophrenic; a double-blind comparison with chlorpromazine (Clozaril Collaborative Study). *Arch Gen Psychiatry*, 45, 789–796.

Kern RS, Nuechterlein KH, Green MF, et al. (2008). The MATRICS Consensus Cognitive Battery, part 2: co-norming and standardization. *Am J Psychiatry*, 165, 214–220.

Kishimoto T, Agarwal V, Kishi T, et al. (2013a). Relapse prevention in schizophrenia: a systematic review and meta-analysis of second-generation antipsychotics versus first-generation antipsychotics. *Mol Psychiatry*, 18, 53–66.

Kishimoto T, Nitta M, Borenstein M, Kane JM, Correll CU (2013b). Long-acting injectable versus oral antipsychotics in schizophrenia: a systematic review and meta-analysis of mirror-image studies. *J Clin Psychiatry*, 74, 957–965.

Kishimoto T, Robenzadeh A, Leucht C, et al. (2014). Long-acting injectable vs oral antipsychotics for relapse prevention in schizophrenia: a meta-analysis of randomized trials. *Schizophr Bull*, 40, 192–213.

Kishimoto T, Hagi K, Nitta M, et al. (2018). Effectiveness of long-acting injectable vs oral antipsychotics in patients with schizophrenia: a meta-analysis of prospective and retrospective cohort studies. *Schizophr Bull*, 44, 603–619.

Kuhn, R. (1958). The treatment of depressive states with G22355 (imipramine hydrochloride). *Am J Psychiatry*, 115, 459–464.

Lader M (2014). Benzodiazepine harm: how can it be reduced? *Br J Clin Pharmacol*, 77, 295–301.

Lamb HR, Bachrach LL (2001). Some perspectives on deinstitutionalization. *Psychiatr Serv*, 52, 1039–1045.

Lange KW, Reichl S, Lange KM, et al. (2010). The history of attention deficit hyperactivity disorder. *Atten Defic Hyperact Disord*, 2, 241–255.

Lehmann HE (1993). Before they called it psychopharmacology. *Neuropsychopharmacology*, 8, 291–303.

Leucht S, Tardy M, Komossa K, et al. (2012). Maintenance treatment with antipsychotic drugs for schizophrenia. *Cochrane Database Syst Rev*,(5), CD008016.

Leucht S, Cipriani A, Spineli L, et al. (2013). Comparative efficacy and tolerability of 15 antipsychotic drugs in schizophrenia: a multiple-treatments meta-analysis. *Lancet*, 382, 951–962.

Lewis SW, Barnes TR, Davies L, et al. (2006). Randomized controlled trial of effect of prescription of clozapine versus other second-generation antipsychotic drugs in resistant schizophrenia. *Schizophr Bull*, 32(4), 715–723.

Li ML, Hu XQ, Li F, Gao WJ (2015). Perspectives on the mGluR2/3 agonists as a therapeutic target for schizophrenia: still promising or a dead end? *Prog Neuropsychopharmacol Biol Psychiatry*, 60, 66–76.

Lieberman JA, Stroup S, McEvoy JP, et al.; Clinical Antipsychotic Trials of Intervention Effectiveness (CATIE) Investigators (2005). Effectiveness of antipsychotic drugs in patients with chronic schizophrenia. *N Engl J Med*, 353, 1209–1223.

Loomer HP, Saunders IC, Kline NS (1957). A clinical and pharmacodynamics evaluation of iproniazid as a psychic energizer. *Psychiatr Res Rep Am Psychiatr Assoc*, 8, 129–141.

Luengo-Fernandez R, Leal J, Gray AM (2012). UK research expenditure on dementia, heart disease, stroke and cancer: are levels of spending related to disease burden? *Eur J Neurol*, 19, 149–154.

Macht DJ (1920). Contributions to psychopharmacology. *Johns Hopkins Hosp Bull*, 31, 167.

McCrae N (2006). A violent thunderstorm: cardiazol treatment in British mental hospitals. *Hist Psychiatry*, 17(65 Pt 1), 67–90.

McGovern PE, Zhang J, Tang J, et al. (2004). Fermented beverages of pre- and proto-historic China. *Proc Natl Acad Sci U S A*, 101, 17593–17598.

Medical Research Council (1965). Report by the Clinical Psychiatry Committee. Clinical trial of the treatment of depressive illness. *Br Med J*, 1, 881–886.

Meltzer HY, Alphs L, Green AI, et al. (2003). International Suicide Prevention Trial (InterSePT). *Arch Gen Psychiatry*, 60, 82–91.

Mindham RHS, Howland C, Shepherd M (1972). Continuation therapy with tricyclic antidepressants in depressive illness. *Lancet*, 2, 854–855.

Moncrieff J (2006). Why is it so difficult to stop psychiatric drug treatment? It may be nothing to do with the original problem. *Med Hypotheses*, 67, 517–523.

Moreau JJ (1845). *Du hachisch et de l'aliénation mentale: études psychologiques*. Paris: Fortin Masson. English translation: Moreau JJ (1973). *Hashish and Mental Illness*. New York: Raven Press.

National Institute for Health and Care Excellence (NICE) (2014). *Bipolar disorder: assessment and management*. Clinical guideline [CG185]. London: National Institute for Health and Care Excellence.

National Institute of Mental Health Psychopharmacology Service Center Collaborative Study Group (1964). Phenothiazine treatment in acute schizophrenia effectiveness. *Arch Gen Psychiatry*, 10, 246–261.

Naughton M, Clarke G, O'Leary OF, Cryan JF, Dinan TG (2014). A review of ketamine in affective disorders: current evidence of clinical efficacy, limitations of use and pre-clinical evidence on proposed mechanisms of action. *J Affect Disord*, 156, 24–35.

Nelson JC, Papakostas GI (2009). Atypical antipsychotic augmentation in major depressive disorder: a meta-analysis of placebo-controlled randomized trials. *Am J Psychiatry*, 166, 980–991.

Norton A (1979). Depression. *Br Med J*, 2, 429–430.

Nuechterlein KH, Green MF, Kern RS, et al. (2008). The MATRICS Consensus Cognitive Battery, part 1: test selection, reliability, and validity. *Am J Psychiatry*, 165, 203–213.

Nutt DJ (1990). The pharmacology of human anxiety. *Pharmacol Ther*, 47, 233–266.

Ohlow MJ, Moosmann B (2011). Phenothiazine: the seven lives of pharmacology's first lead structure. *Drug Discov Today*, 16, 119–131.

Oxford English Dictionary Online (2018). Oxford University Press. Available at: https://en.oxforddictionaries.com/definition/psychopharmacology (last accessed 13.10.18).

Pearce JMS (2002). Bromide, the first effective antiepileptic agent. *J Neurol Neurosurg Psychiatry*, 72, 412.

Physicians' Desk Reference (1956). *Methylphenidate*, 11th ed. Oradell, NJ: Medical Economics, pp. 441–442.

Porsolt RD, Anton G, Blavet N, Jalfre M (1978). 'Behavioural despair' in rats: a new model sensitive to antidepressant treatments. *Eur J Pharmacol*, 47, 379–391.

Priebe S, Badesconyi A, Fioritti A, et al. (2005). Reinstitutionalisation in mental health care: comparison of data on service provision from six European countries. *BMJ (Clin Res Ed)*, 330(7483), 123–126.

Rapport MM, Green AA, Page IH (1948). Serum vasoconstrictor, serotonin; isolation and characterization. *J Biol Chem*, 176, 1243–1251.

Ray OS (2007). About the American College of Neuropsychopharmacology. *Acad Psychiatry*, 31, 122–124.

Robinson ES (2018). Translational new approaches to investigating mood disorders in rodents and what they may reveal about the underlying neurobiology of major depressive disorder. *Philos Trans R Soc Lond B Biol Sci*, 373, 20170036.

Schildkraut JJ (1965). The catecholamine hypothesis of affective disorders: a review of supporting evidence. *Am J Psychiatry*, 122, 509–522.

Schjerning O, Rosenzweig M, Pottegård A, et al. (2016). Abuse potential of pregabalin: a systematic review. *CNS Drugs*, 30, 9–25.

Schou M, Juel-Nielsen N, Strömgren E, Voldby H (1954). The treatment of manic psychoses by the administration of lithium salts. *J Neurol Neurosurg Psychiatry*, 17, 250–260.

Shorter S (1997). *A History of Psychiatry: From the Era of the Asylum to the Age of Prozac*. New York: John Wiley & Sons.

Siskind D, McCartney L, Goldschlager R, Kisely S (2016). Clozapine v. first- and second-generation antipsychotics in treatment-refractory schizophrenia: systematic review and meta-analysis. *Br J Psychiatry*, 209, 385–392.

Sjoerdsma AG (2008). *Starting with Serotonin*. Silver Spring, MD: Improbable Books, pp. 617.

Spedding M, Jay T, Costa e Silva J, Perret L (2005). A pathophysiological paradigm for the therapy of psychiatric disease. *Nat Rev Drug Discov*, 4, 467–474.

Stokes JH, Sternberg T, Schwartz W, et al. (1944). The action of penicillin in late syphilis. *JAMA*, 126, 73–80.

Sulser F (1984). Regulation and function of noradrenaline receptor systems in brain. Psychopharmacological aspects. *Neuropharmacology*, 23(2B), 255–261.

Suttajit S, Srisurapanont M, Maneeton N, Maneeton B (2014). Quetiapine for acute bipolar depression: a systematic review and meta-analysis. *Drug Des Devel Ther*, 8, 827–838.

Swazey JP (1974). *Chlorpromazine in Psychiatry: A Study of Therapeutic Innovation*. Cambridge, MA: MIT Press.

Taylor MJ, Freemantle N, Geddes JR, Bhagwagar Z (2006). Early onset of selective serotonin reuptake inhibitor antidepressant action, systematic review and meta-analysis. *Arch Gen Psychiatry*, 63, 1217–1223.

The Kings Fund (2015). Briefing: Mental health under pressure. Available at: www.kingsfund.org.uk/sites/default/files/field/field_publication_file/mental-health-under-pressure-nov15_0.pdf (last accessed 3.11.18).

Thuillier J (1999). *Ten Years That Changed the Face of Mental Illness*. London: Dunitz.

Tillim SJ (1952). Bromide intoxication. *Am J Psychiatry*, 109(3), 196–202.

Tjia J, Gurwitz JH, Briesacher BA (2012). Challenge of changing nursing home prescribing culture. *Am J Geriatr Pharmacother*, 10, 37–46.

Tooth GC & Newton MP (1961). *Leucotomy in England and Wales 1942–1954. Reports on Public Health and Medical Subjects No. 104*. London: HMSO.

Tsay CJ (2013). Julius Wagner-Jauregg and the legacy of malarial therapy for the treatment of general paresis of the insane. *Yale J Biol Med*, 86, 245–254.

Viguera AC, Baldessarini RJ, Hegarty JD, van Kammen DP, Tohen M (1997). Clinical risk following abrupt and gradual withdrawal of maintenance neuroleptic treatment. *Arch Gen Psychiatry*, 54, 49–55.

Vogt M (1954). The concentration of sympathin in different parts of the central nervous system under normal conditions and after the administration of drugs. *J Physiol*, 123, 451–481.

Weisler RH, Nolen WA, Neijber A, et al.; Trial 144 Study Investigators (2011). Continuation of quetiapine versus switching to placebo or lithium for maintenance treatment of bipolar I disorder (Trial 144: a randomized controlled study). *J Clin Psychiatry*, 72, 1452–1464.

Windholz G, Witherspoon LH (1993). Sleep as a cure for schizophrenia: a historical episode. *Hist Psychiatry*, 4(13, Pt 1), 83–93.

Wolman BB (1977). *International Encyclopedia of Psychiatry, Psychology, Psychoanalysis and Neurology*. New York: Aesculapius Publishers, p. 267.

Woolley DW, Shaw E (1954). A biochemical and pharmacological suggestion about certain mental disorders. *Proc Natl Acad Sci U S A*, 40, 228–231.

Zajecka JM, Stanford AD, Memisoglu A, Martin WF, Pathak S (2019). Buprenorphine/samidorphan combination for the adjunctive treatment of major depressive disorder: results of a phase III clinical trial (FORWARD-3). *Neuropsychiatr Dis Treat*, 15, 795–808.

Zeller EA, Barsky J, Berman JR, Fouls JR (1952). Action of isonicotinic acid hydrazide and related compounds on enzymes involved in the autonomic nervous system. *J Pharmacol Exp Ther*, 106, 427–432.

Psychiatric Drug Discovery and Development

Mohammed Shahid, Joanna C. Neill and John Hutchison

2.1 Introduction

This chapter reviews the process of psychiatric drug discovery and development. People suffering from mental illness need better drugs with improved efficacy and reduced side-effect burden than those currently available. The aim of drug discovery and development in this area is to manage illness, improve quality of life, and to reduce burden on carers and on the economy. Long-term disability associated with incomplete treatment response profoundly compromises the ability of affected individuals to function properly and significantly reduces their quality of life. This in turn has societal consequences in terms of the cost burden associated with the high prevalence of psychiatric disorders. Brain disorders cost €141 billion per annum in the UK 2010, with a total 2010 cost (in million € purchasing power parity) of psychotic disorders of €16 717 (Fineberg et al., 2013). Of this cost, direct health care accounted for only 25%; the major spend was due to indirect costs (50%, mostly due to loss of productivity) and direct, non-medical costs (25%). Consequently, the pharmaceutical industry continues to be attracted to investing in further research and development (R&D) with the aim of producing better, more efficacious psychopharmacological therapies. However, it is important to note that the level of commitment towards developing new medicines for psychiatric disorders has come under intense pressure over the past decade with the result that many pharmaceutical companies have ceased R&D activity in psychiatry. High attrition associated with central nervous system (CNS) drug discovery and numerous late stage, and hence costly, failures have provoked the current situation (see Kola, 2008; Talpos, 2017). Multiple factors are likely to be involved in the failure of clinical trials, some of which we describe later in this chapter, but lack of reproducible efficacy, responsible for 50–60% of failure, is a key driver (Waring et al., 2015) as is lack of biomarker identification (Bespalov et al., 2016). This has primarily been due to a rather limited insight into the molecular pathology associated with these diseases and hence the high failure rate in clinical development efforts. Consequently, there is a need for an improved translational approach, providing an enhanced relationship between what is done in early drug discovery, i.e. preclinically, and then subsequently, in clinical development. This requires both forward (laboratory to patient) and reverse (patient to laboratory) translational approaches particularly towards identification and development of reliable biomarkers enabling patient stratification and test of proof of concept (PoC). However, in spite of these caveats, significant progress has been made in R&D in psychiatry, which we describe in some detail in this chapter.

Advancement has been made in identification of promising new categories of therapeutic modalities different from the traditional small molecule-based approaches. Some examples of these include proteins (e.g. monoclonal antibodies), peptides, ribonucleic acid (e.g. aptamers, antisense), gene and cell-based therapies which represent promising avenues recently being explored (Bishop, 2017; Choudhury et al., 2017; Fosgerau & Hoffman, 2015; Freskgård & Urich, 2017). Biological drugs such as monoclonal antibodies in particular have established a profound successful track record in a number of challenging disease areas including chronic inflammatory disease and cancer. While such modalities are also potential approaches for psychiatric indications, particularly for impact beyond symptomatic relief (e.g. alteration of disease progression or development), significant technological barriers remain. Brain penetration, formulation and safety concerns pose a significant hurdle for the non-small molecule-based therapeutics for psychiatric diseases. Thus, pragmatically, the scope and focus of the current chapter is restricted to small molecule-related drug discovery and development. However, it is important for the reader to be aware that a humanized monoclonal antibody against the interleukin 6 receptor, tocilizumab, licensed for treating rheumatoid arthritis, failed to improve symptoms in a small trial in schizophrenia patients (Girgis et al., 2018). Furthermore, natalizumab, licensed for the treatment of multiple sclerosis, is currently being tested for efficacy in schizophrenia (https://clinicaltrials.gov/ct2/show/NCT03093064).

The pharmceutical R&D process (schematically illustrated in Figure 2.1), in general, is aimed at testing scientific hypotheses, both at the preclinical and clinical level, and building confidence towards product-related technical feasibility as well as addressing therapeutic value to the target patient population. The overall process for an individual drug can take 10–15 years to complete and cost in excess of $2 billion. In terms of the R&D process used by most pharmaceutical companies, this is similar, albeit, with elements of organization and perhaps therapeutic area-related differences. Drug discovery (also referred to as preclinical research) followed by

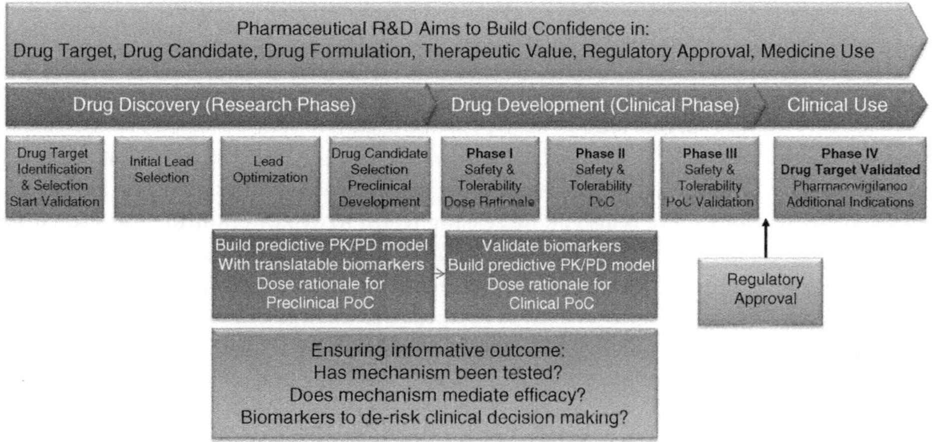

Figure 2.1 Typical drug discovery and drug development process.

drug development (encompassing clinical trials, registration and product introduction) are the two large steps involved and rely on effective engagement of cross-functional multidisciplinary teams. Technological advances over the past three decades, in molecular biology, as well as in automation and information technology have helped to reshape the early process of drug discovery in particular. In this chapter we describe each of these processes in some detail, starting with drug discovery, and provide relevant examples where appropriate.

2.2 Drug Discovery

The focus during the drug discovery (or preclinical research) phase is directed towards addressing two needs: confidence in the biological drug target (mode of action; therapeutic rationale) and confidence in the candidate drug molecule (suitability for clinical development; technical feasibility). A third, interlinked, domain is translational drug target biomarkers (disease related) enabling PoC evaluation in animals and then subsequently in humans. These aspects are central considerations during evaluation and inform a go/no go outcome at key decision points during the drug discovery phase.

Many variations of the drug discovery process have been described but essentially these consist of similar steps in terms of selection and decision point, involving: drug target selection, initial chemical lead generation, lead optimization and drug candidate selection for clinical development (Figure 2.1). For a historical perspective as well as detailed presentation of modern trends and challenges in drug discovery the recent book edited by Nielsch et al. (2016) may be a useful resource.

2.2.1 Drug Target Selection

Drug target selection is, arguably, the most important step in the whole drug discovery and development process, and is summarized in Figure 2.2. It is the basis for the mode of action, scientific concept, therapeutic hypothesis, differentiation and putative therapeutic value. Indeed, 50–60% of failures during Phase II clinical development are due to efficacy-related issues (Harrison, 2016), emphasizing the need for greater rigour in scrutiny and quality testing during drug target selection and subsequent validation. The majority of drug targets tend to be proteins, the function of which can be modulated by small chemical ligands which, relatively specifically, alter the activity in a biological pathway of some relevance to disease pathology. However, as indicated earlier, due to enhanced technology there is also an increasing trend to explore non-protein modalities as well as large molecule ligands. Drug target identification, combined with initial evaluation, drive the decision whether to select that particular candidate for further drug discovery work. Gashaw et al. (2012) provide an interesting overview detailing approaches towards target identification as well as key characteristics of an 'ideal' drug target and Hutson et al. (2017) provide a useful summary of the challenges specifically associated with psychiatric drug target identification and validation. Generally, initial target evaluation can take one to two years but given the critical importance of this process towards the rationale for efficacy, more time may be required for attaining higher confidence and making an evidence-based decision. The initial decision to select is the first step in the long drug target validation process, through a series of confidence building steps, as illustrated in Figure 2.2. This can only be achieved with the approval and use of medicinal product.

Drug targets can be identified from a variety of sources including proprietary and/or public sources. Powerful new technologies to probe the genetic underpinning of disease have had a major impact on the search for disease relevant pathways and new treatments. This has perhaps been most apparent in disease states with a single or dominant gene dysfunction (e.g. cystic fibrosis, see Marson et al., 2017). Nevertheless, genetic-based approaches have also provided new insight into genetic elements that may be predisposing factors in psychiatric disorders, which tend to be multigenic in nature. For example, a recent large-scale genome-wide association

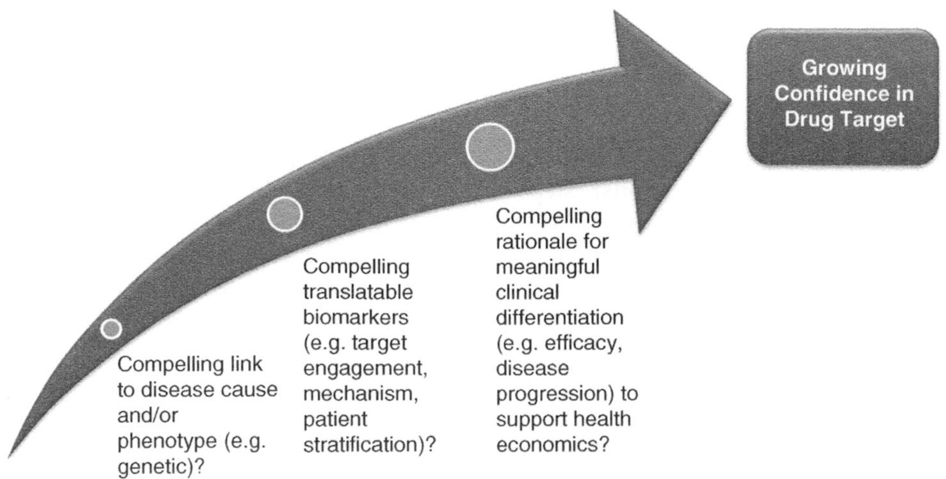

Figure 2.2 Compelling questions driving confidence in drug target.

study (GWAS), conducted by Psychiatrics Genomics Consortium (PGC), analyzed and compared single nucleotide polymorphism (SNP) frequency for schizophrenia and control subjects to identify potential risk or safety alleles. The data were presented in a landmark publication by the PGC in 2014 (see Schizophrenia Working Group of the Pyschiatric Genomics C, 2014; as well as Foley et al., 2017 for updated review). This identified 108 candiate risk factor genes for schizophrenia, including known targets (e.g. dopamine D_2 receptor and glutamate system-related genes) but also surprising new genes such as those involved in immune system regulation (e.g. the major histocompatibility complex).

The introduction of a range of so-called 'omics' platforms such as genomics, transcriptomics, proteomics and metabolomics has also been used to identify potential disease predisposing targets and pathways as well as biomarkers (Matthews et al., 2016). Data from these approaches have been assembled into a variety of both public and proprietary databases which can be mined for target identification and interrogation to determine their influence on disease-related biological pathways. The degree of curation and accuracy can be an issue with some sources and must be considered accordingly. Literature databases with recent research publications (e.g. PubMed and Web of Science) are still important sources of ideas for new drug targets. However, the rather limited value of research publications for this purpose is being recognized as a growing issue for concern, with estimates of up to 50–80% of published academic data not being reproduced by industry (Prinz et al., 2011). Indeed, industry is now taking steps to deal with this uncertainity (Frye et al., 2015). This, combined with publication bias towards positive results is an increasingly acknowledged limitation of peer-reviewed research work (Munafò & Neill, 2016). In the academic setting, pressure to produce impactful, highly cited publications, lack of funding for replication studies and the intense competition for research grants is a likely contributor to this unfortunate situation.

A high degree of novelty and a differentiating mode of action has become standard practice, and is an important element for a putative new drug target. A shift away from the historical 'me too' type of approach is anticipated to facilitate the discovery of first-in-class therapeutic agents with better efficacy, at least in the relevant stratified patient subpopulation. Most of the attempts in this direction for psychiatric diseases have, however, so far met with a high rate of failure. Indeed, lack of a precision medicine approach for psychiatry drug discovery is increasingly recognized as a weakness that needs to be addressed (see Clementz et al., 2016 for recent work in psychosis). Consequently, recent approvals have tended to be incremental improvements over existing therapeutic agents, such as reduced side-effect burden and long-acting injectable formulations of existing oral antipsychotics for the management of schizophrenia. However, these do provide additional options to patients whose treatment needs may not be adequately addressed by available drugs. Healthcare budget holder or payer support for access to new treatment options with improvements in tolerability but modest gain in efficacy is a growing challenge for drug developers.

Having identified a potential drug target, the process of further, usually limited, evaluation is necessary to enable selection. This may also be considered as an initial stage in the long process of target validation. This stage of target evaluation aims to test whether initial proof of idea or concept can be established and to build confidence in continuing with the drug target. Ideally, a combination of different approaches (e.g. bioinformatics, molecular biology, 'omics', pharmacology) using pathophysiologically relevant animal and, where possible and most importantly, human tissue systems should be used. The latter is a particular challenge for brain diseases for obvious reasons. However, considerable advances have been made, using modern cell biology approaches in recent times to enable access to close surrogates of human brain. A good illustration is the application of stem cell technology; human-induced pluripotent stem cells (iPSCs) provide a promising avenue generating patient-derived (thus genetically loaded) cells for evaluating new drug targets but also for more valid in vitro disease relevant assays (see Seshadri et al., 2017; Soliman et al., 2017; Wen et al., 2016 for recent reviews). The study of Pak et al. (2015) provides an interesting illustration on the application of stem cell technology towards investigating the role of heterozygous mutations in the cell adhesion molecule neurexin-1 gene (*NRXN1*) which has been linked to schizophrenia and autism. In contrast to the data from genetically modified mouse cortical neurons, showing a lack of impact on excitatory neurotransmission, stem cell-derived human neurons displayed a *decrease* in spontaneous miniature excitatory postsynaptic currents and the possibility of interefering with neurotransmitter release. Multivariate approaches, pointing towards a similar outcome, will enhance the level of confidence in the quality of evaluation, subsequent conclusion and likelihood of drug target selection. Key issues for investigation at this stage include:

- Link to disease biology of the intended patient population (e.g. based on genetics, tissue expression and function, mode of action of existing therapeutics, role and activity in disease models).
- Potential side effects and any safety risks (e.g. based on pharmacological profile, transgenic animal-based analysis).
- Technical feasibility (e.g. suitable screening assay, druggability (how easy it is to design a molecule to interact with the target), regulatory issues).
- Potential for clinically meaningful differentiation and therapeutic value (e.g. degree of novelty of mode of action, impact on unmet medical need, health economic justification).

For a compelling data package, evidence from both traditional (e.g. pharmacological tool compound) and more modern molecular and cell biology (e.g. genetic manipulation of drug target expression and/or function preferably using both in vitro and in vivo techniques) needs to be assembled. Optogenetic approaches are a particularly interesting innovation in this respect for CNS drug discovery (see Zhang & Cohen, 2017). This technology provides a powerful method for evalutating drug target evaluation in a specific manner and more importantly in a physiologically relevant background. Furthermore, if applied in combination with patient-derived cells (e.g. iPSC neurons) it can enable insight on the relationship between particular genotype and individual patient phenotype as well as disease mechanisms. Consequently, iPSC-based optogenetics could also aid patient selection and stratification for clinical trials.

Given the nature of the issues to be addressed, it is clear that a multidisciplinary and cross-functional input should be sought to assist a good quality decision on target selection. This also ensures buy-in from key stakeholders likely to be involved, as the drug target-related project progresses through the R&D process. In view of the fact that efficacy failure is a key driver for the high level of attrition in CNS drug discovery, it is essential that thorough evaluation coupled with the compelling nature of available data is engaged to guide an evidence-based target selection decision. Part of the argument should take into account and address any failed attempts with the same or similar drug targets or pathway, e.g. there have been some recent costly, high profile failures in large-scale Phase III clinical trials with novel drug targets. For example (i) for cognitive impairment in schizophrenia, encenicline, a partial agonist at nicotinic α7 receptors (www.alzforum.org/therapeutics/encenicline); (ii) for negative symptoms in schizophrenia, bitopertin, a glycine transporter-1 (GlyT-1) inhibitor (Bugarski-Kirola et al., 2017); and (iii) for psychosis, LY2140023, an agonist at glutamatergic $mGlu_{2/3}$ receptors (Downing et al., 2014).

Reviewing recent psychiatric drug approvals, it is clear that very limited progress has been made in the introduction of highly novel first-in-class treatments. Agents that have been introduced may provide new treatment options but are basically still variations on a standard mode of action and target pathways. Thus for schizophrenia and bipolar disorder (e.g. asenapine, lurasidone, cariprazine, brexpiprazole) as well as depression (e.g. vortoxetine) several new treatments have been introduced but their mechanism of action is still through modulation of monoaminergic (dopamine, noradrenaline, serotonin) neurotransmission and thus represents an evolution, or new generation, that is firmly based on older agents (Millan et al., 2015; Zohar et al., 2015). While these agents show some gains in benefit-risk profile compared with their predecessors, this seems to be primarily driven by improvement in adverse effect liability. Ambitious attempts to establish differentiated efficacy were made with several compounds including asenapine, bitopertin and cariprazine for negative symptom of schizophrenia (see detailed illustration in Box 2.1) and with vortioxetine for cognitive impairment in major depression.

It is important to recognize that novelty does not necessitate a wholly novel drug target, it could also be a new mode of modulation of a well-known drug target. An illustration in this respect is the atypical antipsychotic pimavanserin which gained first-in-class approval from the Food and Drug Administration (FDA) for treatment of psychotic symptoms associated with Parkinson's disease (Sahli & Tarazi, 2018). Its mode of action is thought to rely on inverse agonism (though see Nutt et al., 2017) at the $5\text{-}HT_{2A}$ receptor which is a known target for both atypical antipsychotics and antidepressants. Given the rather rich armamentarium of first-, second- and third-generation monoamine-based agents for psychiatric disease, the focus for future R&D is very much on novel signalling pathways (Keshavan et al., 2017). Thus, there has been a concerted industry-wide effort with regards to the glutamate system, with notable disappointments (e.g. $mGlu_{2/3}$ agonists, GlyT-1 inhibitors for schizophrenia, see above) as well as some positive signs of progress towards signals for efficacy (e.g. α-amino-3-hydroxy-5-methyl-4-isoxazolepropionic acid (AMPA) receptor potentiators, NMDA receptor antagonists for depression).

Ketamine, an old drug and an NMDA receptor blocker, seems to be particularly promising in this context, with reproducible evidence of efficacy in treatment-resistant depression characterized by rapid onset of action (see Sanacora et al., 2017; Singh et al., 2017). These data have re-invigorated interest in the NMDA receptor as a drug target for more effective antidepressants (Wilkinson & Sanacora, 2019). Another new particularly promising approach is targeting potassium ion channels (KV3.1/3.2) located on fast-spiking gamma-aminobutyric acid (GABA)

Box 2.1 Aiming for meaningful clinical differentiation: targeting persistent negative symptoms of schizophrenia

While the positive symptoms of schizophrenia and secondary negative symptoms, due to psychosis, are on the whole adequately managed by current antipsychotics, these agents in general, when given alone, do not resolve the more enduring cognitive impairment or the persistent negative symptoms. Both of these symptom domains are thought to be important drivers for long-term disability, functional impairment and diminished quality of life. Consequently, the treatment of these deficit symptoms represents an important unmet medical need and a point of focus for the discovery of new treatment options. Several interesting attempts have been made recently notably with a first-in-class drug candidate bitopertin (Bugarski-Kirola et al., 2017), a GlyT-1 inhibitor and a third-generation atypical antipsychotic, asenapine, with a promising multi-fuctional pharmacology (see Tarazi & Neill, 2013; Tarazi & Shahid, 2009). Bitopertin despite initial promising signal in a PoC study failed to show replication in two Phase III studies. Asenapine in contrast showed an interesting signal indicative of potential use in the treatment of persistent negative symptoms. The profile of asenapine is summarized in this section to provide an illustration of an attempt to establish clinically meaningful differentiation as well as the magnitude of the drug discovery challenge and learnings for the future.

Asenapine: A novel atypical antipsychotic with a promising multifunctional pharmacology (Shahid et al., 2009; Tarazi & Neill, 2013; Tarazi & Shahid, 2009). Novel features:

- Promising tetracyclic chemistry related to and encompassing key pharmacological features of the antidepressant mirtazapine.
- Core pharmacology: exceptional subnanomolar affinity for and antagonism at a broad panel of serotonin, noradrenaline and dopamine receptors (see Figure 2.3).
- Formulation: first-in-class sublingual mode of administration.

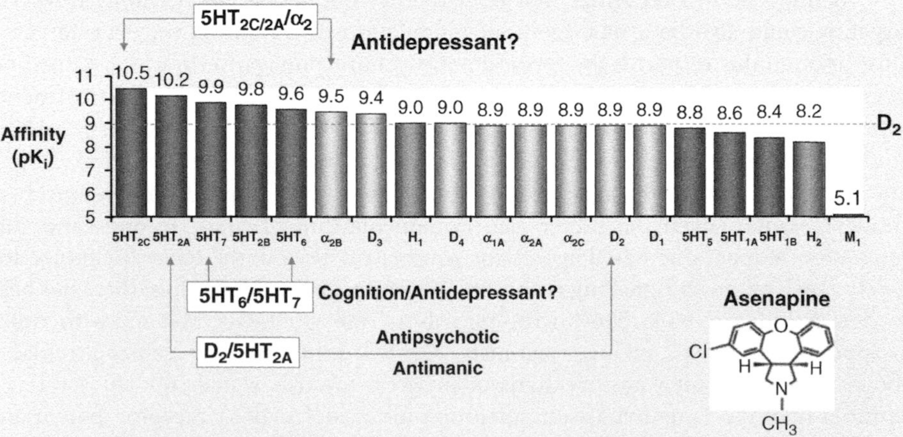

Figure 2.3 Multifunctional pharmacology of asenapine: cloned human receptor binding profile of asenapine. Adapted from Shahid et al. (2009).

Working hypothesis for potential clinical efficacy:

- D_2/5-HT_{2A} antagonism: may confer atypical antipsychotic and antimanic properties
- 5-HT_{2A}/α_2 antagonism: analogous to mirtazapine may confer antidepressant. properties and treatment of negative symptoms based on clinical studies showing improvement of these symptoms with mirtazapine plus antipsychotic combination

(Möller & Czobor, 2015). Supported by initial proof of concept study with asenapine showing differential efficacy compared to risperidone (Potkin et al., 2007).

Phase III Clinical Development: key efficacy studies

- Dose (5–10 mg bid, sublingual) selection based on 70–80% D_2 receptor occupancy and PK/PD modelling. The dose range predicts similar or higher occupancy of serotonin and α_2-adrenoceptors.
- Demonstration of efficacy in the treatment of acute exacerbation of schizophrenia.
- Demonstration of efficacy in the treatment of acute exacerbation of bipolar I disorder associated mania.
- Demonstration of efficacy in the treatment of persistent (primary) negative symptoms of schizophrenia.

Design and outcome of dedicated study to examine effects on persistent negative symptoms (see Buchanan et al., 2012; Potkin et al., 2013):

- Two global multi-centre 26-week double-blind randomized controlled trials comparing flexible-dose asenapine (5 or 10 mg bid) with olanzapine (5–20 mg, qd) in patients clinically stable in terms of positive or depressive symptoms for at least five months.
- Completers were enrolled in a 26-week extension for each trial on the same treatment.
- Change in negative symptom assessment (NSA)-16 scale at week 26 was the prespecified efficacy measure using mixed model analysis.
- Both treatments reduced negative symptoms with no significant difference at week 26 but asenapine was significantly superior at week 52.
- In the extension population a significant difference in favour of asenapine was observed at week 30 and continued through to week 52.
- Asenapine differentially improved expressive gestures, social drive and interest NSA-16 items.
- Interpretation complicated by higher dropout rate with asenapine compared to olanzapine.
- Authors concluded asenapine may be a useful option for patients with prevalence of persistent negative symptoms.

Learnings and issues:

- Possible to study persistent negative symptoms in a specific manner but can take up to 12 months of treatment to see an effect when comparing to standard treatment.
- Could the differential effect on α_2 pharmacology be one of the drivers for difference from olanzapine? However, need more direct evidence supporting differential target engagement. Is there still mileage in monoamine-based targets, e.g. α_2 subtypes?
- How to limit strong placebo effect of increased patient attention and care.
- Clinical significance of effect on NSA-16 in terms of functional outcome needs further evaluation.
- Further need for biomarker-driven patient stratification with predictors of response.
- Promising data with another third-generation atypical antipsychotic, cariprazine (Németh et al., 2017), showing differentiation from risperidone, were reported recently. Lack of success with new drug targets, such as Gly-T1, raises questions about the effectiveness of preclinical to clinical translation as well as reproducibility during clinical development.

interneurons to restore the balance in brain circuitry disrupted in schizophrenia. The lead molecule, AUT00206, is currently being developed by Autifony Therapeutics. At the time of writing it is undergoing Phase IB clinical trial evaluation in patients with schizophrenia, having successfully completed preclinical and Phase IA evaluations (see Section 2.2.3).

The cholinergic system has also been a strong point of interest and many ligands targeting muscarinic and nicotinic receptors have been evaluated, unfortunately however, with no clinical breakthrough so far. Intracellular targets such as cyclic nucleotide phophosdiesterase isoenzyme (e.g. PDE10) selective inhibitors have also been investigated by several companies but again, without success (see Geerts et al., 2017). Genetic analysis of patient samples has also provided clues towards new pathways for depression (e.g. neurotrophic factors, inflammatory mediators) and schizophrenia (e.g. disrupted in schizophrenia 1 gene, inflammatory processes, e.g. see Chaudhry et al., 2015 and most recently, neurodevelopmental processes, Birnbaum & Weinberger, 2017). The latter trend is anticipated to grow in the future and perhaps represents the most promising and productive path forward for identifying drug targets with compelling disease validity. A better understanding of disease-related molecular pathology should help open a new era of target-focused drug discovery, delivering more effective treatments for not only managing symptoms but hopefully impacting disease progression.

2.2.2 Drug Candidate Selection

The initial search for small molecule ligands can involve multiple approaches although the default option involves some level of high throughput screening (HTS). To enable this, the drug target must be amenable to an assay format suitable for HTS. Huge proprietary compound libraries ranging from thousands to millions of individual samples have been developed by many pharmaceutical companies and are also provided by commercial vendors. Hit compounds are validated for activity, for example to rule out false positives, and are examined for drug-like features (e.g. molecular weight, physicochemical properties, toxicophores) to qualify as promising hits.

In addition to the drug target-led HTS approach, more traditional phenotypic screening has seen a resurgence in recent times, partly to address the productivity challenge faced by the pharma industry (see Zheng et al., 2013). This type of methodology usually requires a cellular assay with a strong disease relevance (e.g. based on patient genetics and/or patient-derived cells). Advantages of phenotypic screening include facilitating seredipitious discovery of new drug targets and novel chemical hits. However, it suffers from the significant issue of extra effort to deconvolute mode of action without which it can be highly challenging to generate a structure–activity relationship.

These hits are then usually subjected to a limited programme of medicinal chemistry to gain insight into the scope for optimization and feasibility for structure–activity relationship generation, preferably across multiple chemical series. This initial phase of lead development can typically take one to two years. If this looks promising, the effort is substantially expanded into a major lead optimization programme aimed at identifying potential candidates for clinical development. Depending on the quality of the chemical starting points, the lead optimization phase can take two to three years to complete. The focus is not just on optimizing chemistry (e.g. physicochemical properties such as solubility) and pharmacology (e.g. affinity, potency, selectivity, efficacy) but also strongly on metabolism and pharmacokinetic properties (e.g. plasma exposure and half-life, brain penetration bioavailability, metabolites) and ease of formulation. Recent drug candidate attrition analysis from four major pharmaceutical companies has highlighted the importance of physicochemical quality as being a key driver of termination (Waring et al., 2015). In addition, the safety profile (e.g. cardiotoxicity, genotoxicity, hepatotoxicity) may also need design effort.

Promising optimized molecules, preferably from different chemical series, are then evaluated for synthetic scale-up and more extensive pharmacokinetic and initial safety testing in at least two different species in accordance with regulatory agency requirements. In parallel, pharmaceutical development feasibility is conducted to prepare an active pharmaceutical ingredient (API) for human clinical trials. High-quality molecules surviving these initial evaluations form the basis for drug candidate selection (see Figure 2.1). Once a candidate is selected in this manner, it will be assessed in a range of animal models in order to predict efficacy in the clinical population as described below.

2.2.3 Evaluation in Animal Models

The traditional means to evaluate efficacy of a new chemical entity prior to clinical evaluation is by thorough testing in one or more validated animal models. This process is conducted to assess whether the new compound will produce the desired therapeutic benefit in patients. Of course, the animal model must have relevance for the disorder, i.e. it must be translational as described in the previous section. Constructing a valid animal model for a psychiatric disorder is particularly challenging in view of the complexity of these disorders, lack of complete understanding of their pathophysiology, varied neurobiology, heterogeneity within a given population, mixed aetiologies including of course a complex interplay between genetic and environmental factors. It is important to be clear that the animal model is only a representation of one or more features of the human condition and cannot replicate the human disease state in its entirety.

2.2.3.1 Ethical and Legal Considerations

Typically, rodents are used initially. There are several advantages to using rodents, they breed well and thrive in captivity, they are robust and relatively small and do not require special maintenance beyond that provided by a well-run biological services facility. Most universities that teach biological subjects will have a facility, the size and capability of these varies enormously. Usually, but not always, the size of the facility reflects the size of the institution. Likewise, most pharmaceutical companies will have a facility where the animals may be bred, are maintained and experimental procedures carried out, including humane euthanasia at the end of the study. If animals are not bred in-house, they must be purchased from a registered breeding facility; in the UK the main suppliers are Charles River and Envigo. In the UK, anyone using animals for experimental procedures must be compliant with the Animals Scientific Procedures Act 1986; full training and proficiency is a legal requirement and this is often provided in-house. In the UK, few facilities now house non-human primates, again their use is regulated by the UK Home Office, under the 1986 Act. Primates are much more expensive to keep and maintain as they require more space and specialized environments.

All facilities in the UK are regularly inspected by the UK Home Office. Home Office Inspectors also assist with design of studies and maximizing welfare for the animals within the constraints of the purpose of the experiments. When designing experiments, particular attention is taken to the principles of the 3Rs (www.nc3rs.org.uk/the-3rs), Replacement, Reduction and Refinement; *reduction* in numbers used, *refinement* of techniques to minimize pain, distress and suffering and ultimately to *replace* animals completely. This final goal of replacement is hard to envisage for a CNS disorder affecting brain and behaviour, but may be feasible for other human disorders. However, there are of course alternative approaches, including the use of human-derived iPSCs, as described in Section 2.2.1, and certain studies in human patients that reduce the requirement for efficacy testing in animals (e.g. see Pringle & Harmer, 2015). Researchers are strongly encouraged to follow the ARRIVE guidelines (Animal Research: Reporting of *In Vivo* Experiments; www.nc3rs.org.uk/arrive-guidelines) which aim to improve the reporting of research involving animals, usually in peer-reviewed publications in scientific journals. The overall aim is to enhance the quality of the information presented and so avoid unnecessary studies being performed. Another issue in this respect is reporting of negative results as previously mentioned (Munafò & Neill, 2016). A recent investigation into publications on animal models for Alzheimer's disease and schizophrenia revealed that 95% of papers published in a five-year period, between 2012 and 2017, reported positive results (Wishart & Neill, unpublished report, 2017). This type of publication bias is particularly problematic for transparency in research and leads to unnecessary experimental procedures being carried out.

2.2.3.2 Welfare, Sex Differences and Ethology

For drug discovery in psychiatry, the principal features of the illness that can be mimicked are changes in brain function leading to alterations in behaviour. For successful evaluation of behavioural changes due to perturbation of brain function, several principles must be adhered to in order to ensure successful outcome as for any animal research. Welfare is critical, if the animal is stressed or unwell, the results from experiments will be meaningless. In most animal facilities, this is a key component of management of the facility and environmental enrichment is a mandatory requirement. Applications must be made to the UK Home Office for any alterations in welfare such as food restriction (to motivate animals to make responses for food reinforcement). Another key principle is ethological analysis of behaviour. The experimenter must have a good understanding of the natural behaviour patterns of the species under study, i.e. instincts. In the UK, our best-known ethologist is Sir David Attenborough who has made several documentaries for the BBC. Instincts are not lost by the breeding of successive generations. In a key experiment to test this hypothesis, Manuel Berdoy, a vet and researcher from Oxford University, let two strains of rat commonly used in CNS research, Lister Hooded and Wistar, into a simulated wild environment and monitored their behaviour patterns for six months (www.ratlife.org). He demonstrated that they formed a successful colony through mating, constructing housing, foraging for food and avoiding predators. In short, they used instincts to survive and adapted to a wild environment. This shows that researchers can use these instincts to devise appropriate test paradigms for drug discovery for all human disorders, and enable a deeper understanding of the species we are studying.

Another important factor is the sex of animal under investigation. There has been an unfortunate reliance on males of the species in drug discovery for all human disorders, in clinical trials and at all stages of drug discovery and development. This situation is currently being addressed by the US National Institutes of Health (Clayton, 2017; Clayton & Collins, 2014). At least half of the human population are female, women and men have different risks for developing neurological and psychiatric disorders, respond differently to drug treatments and express differential symptomatology (see Bale & Epperson, 2017; Cahill, 2014 and Neill & Kulkarni, 2011 for reviews). For a review of sex differences in cognition in schizophrenia, and the similarities between animals and humans, see Leger and Neill (2016). In short, both sexes should be used wherever possible, in some cases one sex is preferred, but this should be clearly justified. Several other factors are important and can alter the outcome of drug discovery animal work, i.e. housing, lighting schedule (rodents, unlike primates, are nocturnal), strain of animal, circadian variation of neurotransmitters and hormones. Detailed discussion is beyond the scope of this chapter but it is important that the reader is aware of these. Overall, the experimenter is required to have a clear understanding of the capability of the species being used (not all rodents are the same, especially rats and mice, which are most widely used) and of the pathophysiology and behaviour of the human disorder being investigated.

2.2.3.3 A Model Versus a Test

It is important to be clear of the difference between an animal model and a test. A model attempts to recreate certain aspects of the pathophysiology and behaviour of a human disease state, e.g. a genetically modified animal (Moran et al., 2016), a pharmacologically altered animal (see the sub-chronic phencyclidine (scPCP) model example provided in Box 2.2), a developmental model (e.g. offspring of a dam treated with a viral mimetic, see Knuesel et al., 2014) or a combination thereof. In contrast, a test assesses the capability of the animal to perform a specific task, or evaluation of its behaviour under specific test conditions, e.g. maze learning for memory, avoidance of predator odour or open spaces for anxiety, self-administration of psychoactive substances for drug taking. These tests have been refined in recent years, with improved technology and enhanced translation to the clinic. A good example of this is the implementation of touchscreens for cognitive behaviour and the Birrel and Brown attentional set shifting task for executive function, back tanslated from the human version (see Section 2.2.3.5). See Cadinu et al. (2018) for a recent comparison of the various tests for assessing cognition in animals.

2.2.3.4 Validation of Animal Models

Historically, validity of an animal model is considered at three levels: face, construct and predictive validity (Willner, 1984). Willner's definition was based on the features desired for an animal model for depression. Briefly, face validity concerns the phenomenological or apparent similarities between the model and the disorder; construct validity refers to the similarities between the methods used to construct the model and the disorder, specifically how well the model incorporates the aetiology of the illness; and predictive validity refers to how well the model predicts therapeutic strategies, current and novel. These validity criteria have since evolved to place less emphasis on therapeutic predictive validity, and expanded this aspect to incorporate induction validity as explained by Belzung and Lemoine (2011). Thus, the model should not be limited to prediction of

Box 2.2 Building a disease model to support novel drug discovery for schizophrenia: scPCP rat model for cognition and negative symptoms

The Neill laboratory at the University of Manchester (Manchester, UK) have thoroughly validated a pharmacological model for cognitive impairment associated with schizophrenia (CIAS) and aspects of negative symptomatology such as social withdrawal and negative affect. These are two clinical unmet needs, not adequately treated with current antipsychotics, highly disabling for patients and greatly reducing quality of life for them and their carers.

Clinical basis:

- The non-competitive NMDA receptor antagonist phencyclidine (PCP), when given to healthy volunteers, can produce behavioural disturbances closely resembling positive and negative symptoms as well as cognitive impairment seen in schizophrenia patients.
- PCP can exacerbate pathology in schizophrenia patients.

Key features and use of sub-chronic PCP (scPCP) model:

- See Cadinu et al. (2018) and Neill et al. (2010, 2014) for reviews and Reynolds and Neill (2016) for commentary on the scPCP model.
- Involves treating adult female Lister Hooded rats with a seven-day PCP (2 mg/kg, bid) treatment regimen, adapted from that originally described by Jentsch and Roth (1999), followed by at least seven days washout.
- Animals develop robust and subtle cognitive deficits of relevance to schizophrenia in a range of tests including: attentional set shifting for executive function, operant reversal learning for problem solving and reasoning, 5 Choice Continuous Performance test (5C-CPT) for attention and vigilance, novel object recognition (NOR) for visual learning and memory.
- Animals also show reduced affect, impaired social behaviour as well as several neuropathological features associated with schizophrenia patients including:
    - reduced parvalbumin, a calcium binding protein found in GABA interneurons in hippocampus and prefrontal cortex (PFC), brain areas essential for cognitive function and affected in the illness
    - reduced N-acetyl aspartate (NAA; a marker of neuronal integrity) and reduced release of dopamine in PFC
    - reduced cortical thickness and grey matter density in the hippocampus and amygdala (Barnes et al., 2014).
- Robustness and reliability, run by several Pharma and academic laboratories, and used to evaluate up to 100 new molecules for CIAS and negative symptoms and has enabled the licensing of new antipsychotics; lurasidone, cariprazine and asenapine.
- Currently being used to evaluate efficacy of the new drug molecule, AUT00206, a KV3.1/3.2 channel modulator, for schizophrenia.
- A well-validated animal model with good face and construct validity for schizophrenia.
- With regards to predictive validity efficacy is observed with low doses of atypical antipsychotics (at non-dopamine D_2 receptor-blocking doses), which target non-dopamine mechanisms, but not by typical antipsychotics, antidepressants or anxiolytic agents (see Cadinu et al., 2018 and Neill et al., 2014 for discussion of this issue). It also detects efficacy of several novel drug targets and we believe it provides a very good example of a useful animal model for CIAS (see Figure 2.4 for an overview).

Limitations:

- Pharmacological challenge model, and does not incorporate genetic or developmental features known to be involved in the aetiology of schizophrenia; a neurodevelopmental animal model for schizophrenia is provided by maternal immune activation (see Knuesel et al., 2014 for review) and genetic models through the use of transgenic mice, e.g. DISC1, COMT, reelin, neuregulin (see Ayhan & Pletnikov, 2016 and Moran, 2016 for recent reviews).
- Not routinely used for assessing efficacy for psychosis.

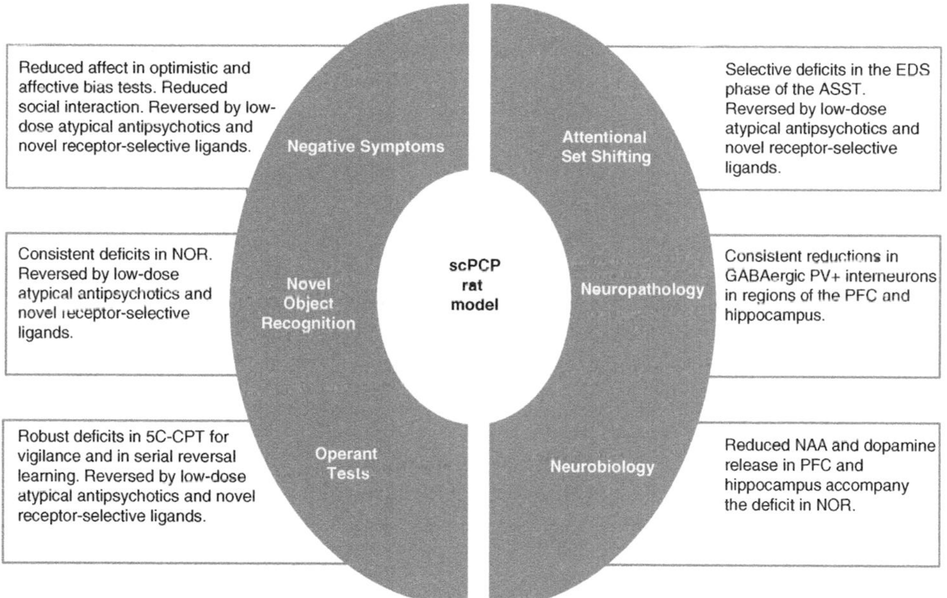

Figure 2.4 The sub-chronic PCP (scPCP) rat model is widely used for studying negative symptoms, cognitive and neurobiological deficits of relevance to schizophrenia. Abbreviations: NOR, novel object recognition; EDS, extra-dimensional shift; ASST, attentional set shifting task; PV+, parvalbumin positive; PFC, prefrontal cortex; NAA N-acetyl aspartate; 5C-CPT 5 Choice Continuous Performance Test.

efficacious treatments through response only but also by biomarkers and aetiological factors. The model should resemble the illness in terms of its induction and the way it can predict certain markers of the disease which are then influenced by treatment. Indeed, models designed to detect current pharmacotherapies through response only are unlikely to detect treatments with a novel mechanism of action (see Hendrie & Pickles, 2013 for further discussion of this issue and Neill et al., 2014 for discussion of predictive validity of the scPCP model described in Box 2.2).

Belzung and Lemoine (2011) propose five levels of validity: homological, pathogenic, mechanistic, face and predictive validity. Homological validity refers to the choice of species and strain, as discussed above, pathogenic validity refers to the similarity between the pathogenesis of the disorder and the animal model, incorporating relevant and appropriate interventions both at developmental stages and in adulthood, often called two hit models. Mechanistic validity refers to the similarities between the neurobiology of the illness and that produced in the animal model by these interventions. The authors extend face validity to incorporate ethological (as described above) and biomarker or biological features (discussed below). These authors also frame their suggested criteria around animal modelling for depression, as Willner did in his original classification.

2.2.3.5 Translation to Humans

Of course one issue with face validity is the imprecise nature of the diagnosis of psychiatric disorders and definitions in the DSM (*Diagnostic and Statistical Manual of Mental Disorders*, now in its fifth edition) or ICD-10 (the 10th revision of the International Statistical Classification of Diseases and Related Health Problems) do not always help the animal researcher. For example, for schizophrenia, symptoms such as delusions, hallucinations and disorganized speech cannot be recreated in animals or easily measured. This led to establishment of behavioural endophenotyping, as described elegantly by Paula Moran in a recent review (Moran, 2016). As she explains, for delusions and hallucinations, likely caused by disturbed sensorimotor gating, we can measure equivalent behavioural processes in animals and humans through prepulse inhibition of the startle reflex (PPI). Cognitive disruption in psychiatric illness is more straightforward to model in animals and tests to measure, for example, executive function and vigilance have been back translated from humans to animals and versions of the tests appropriate for animals have been developed (e.g. attentional set shifting for executive function, see Goetghebeur & Dias, 2014 for its role in drug discovery for schizophrenia, and the Continuous Performance Task for vigilance, see Bhakta & Young, 2017).

A good example of a more recent approach is the RDoC (Research Domain Criteria, supported by the National Institute of Mental Health, NIMH; Cuthbert, 2015). The aim of the RDoC is to remove ambiguity in diagnosis and improve the classification of psychiatric symptoms focusing on a dimensional approach. Human behaviour is divided into five categories termed domains, such as positive and negative valence and cognitive systems. This suggests investigating specific aspects of behaviour impaired across a range of disorders, e.g. attention which is compromised in several psychiatric conditions such as attention deficit hyperactivity disorder (ADHD), schizophrenia and depression. Drug discovery would then aim to treat these domains from a knowledge of their underpinning neurobiology rather than an entire illness (Insel et al., 2010; Kas et al., 2019). It is likely that a combination of approaches will lead to the most robust and thorough evaluation of putative efficacy in validated animal models, which will lead to successful clinical evaluation, as described in subsequent sections of this chapter.

At the time of writing, as described earlier, there has been a lack of success in developing molecules with a novel mechanism of action for schizophrenia (see Talpos, 2017 for review). The most recent drugs to receive a licence for schizophrenia, asenapine (Saphris™, Plosker & Deeks, 2016), cariprazine (Vrylar™, Scarff, 2017) and lurasidone (Latuda™, Pompili et al., 2017) (see Box 2.2), have a dopamine D_2 receptor mechanism of action, albeit alongside other pharmacology that may improve certain symptoms, e.g. negative symptoms, and reduce the side-effect burden. The reasons for lack of success in schizophrenia drug discovery for molecules with a novel mechanism of action or for the unmet clinical needs of cognition and negative symptoms have been discussed previously by us (Cadinu et al., 2018) and others

(Bespalov et al., 2016). It is a similar case for depression; however, the multimodal drug, vortioxtine does appear to show some enhanced clinical efficacy for certain aspects of the illness, particularly cognition (see Sanchez et al., 2015 for review). Briefly, Bespalov and colleagues (2016) explain that one key issue is lack of target engagement to identify the correct dose and drug candidate to be taken forward into clinical trials. They conducted an in-depth analysis of 72 novel drugs and revealed that in 80% of the studies they could not find any evidence for dose selection based on target engagement or through biomarker evaluation (using e.g. PET (positron emission tomography), MRI (magnetic resonance imaging) or EEG (electroencephalography)). Incorporating careful dose selection work prior to clinical trials, biomarker evaluation, along with patient stratification strategies as described by Carol Tamminga and colleagues (Clementz et al., 2016) could radically improve clinical trial outcome in this area.

In summary, an animal programme for psychiatric drug discovery should incorporate mechanistic studies, target engagement and biomarker work, and the use of more than one animal model representing different biotypes and aetiologies. If these principles are adhered to in preclinical studies and appropriate target engagement and biomarker studies, as described below, are conducted prior to Phase II clinical trials, enhanced success in this area is likely. An example of good practice at the time of writing is development of AUT00206, briefly described above. This molecule has been thoroughly evaluated in preclinical studies (see Leger et al., 2015; Reynolds & Neill, 2016) in more than one animal model, and is currently undergoing the target engagement and biomarker studies recommended by Bespalov and colleagues (2016) in humans. It remains to be determined whether this will lead to success in the clinic. However, if not, this will not be due to insufficient evaluation in preclinical or early clinical studies and could provide a gold standard for hypothesis-driven drug discovery in psychiatry in the future.

2.2.4 The Need for Translational Thinking and Science

As mentined above, a clear focus on translational science is an essential requirement of modern-day drug discovery and drug development. The goal is to enable a more effective connection between drug discovery and drug development phases in the search for a new medicine. Ideally this should operate both in a forward and backward direction as described above. As much as possible, drug discovery research should be engineered closely towards addressing the needs of clinical development and in particular, towards testing PoC. It is important to engender a translational mindset from the first step in the process of target identification and selection. This will then grow into plans and action during subsequent steps in drug discovery, particularly during lead optimization for identification of putative drug candidates. Indeed, in recent times, the early drug discovery process has been realigned, to a significant extent, to more effectively address the aims and requirements of exploratory clinical development and PoC studies. This has also been driven by attempts to understand the factors contributing to attrition in clinical development (Kola, 2008). A number of interesting analyses have been reported (Cook et al., 2014; Dolgos et al., 2016; Morgan et al., 2012) of which perhaps the 'three pillars' approach (Morgan et al., 2012; Figure 2.5) is particularly interesting. This was an analysis of 45 clinical projects examining factors facilitating survival during PoC and progression into Phase III clinical development. The authors proposed an evidence-driven three question-based approach ('three pillars') which should be addressed during exploratory clinical development (see Section 2.3.1.3 for further details).

- Arose from Pfizer 44 project evaluation of factors influencing attrition from Phase II to Phase III clinical development (Morgan et al., 2012)
- Pillar 1: exposure at the target site of action (for a desired period of time)
- Pillar 2: binding to the pharmacological target (as expected for its mode of action)
- Pillar 3: expression of pharmacology (effect – commensurate with the demonstrated target exposure and target binding)
- Used to manage risk in Phase II clinical development

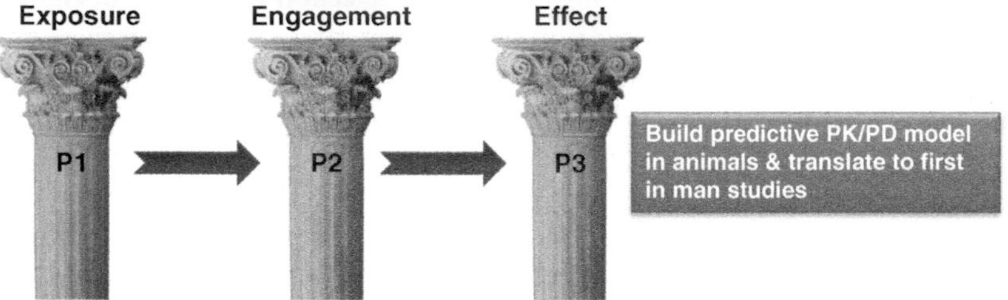

Figure 2.5 Three pillars concept: addressing confidence in drug candidate.

With a strong data package addressing these questions, reasonable confidence that the scientific concept has been adequately examined in the test patient population is achieved. Thus, even if the PoC trial is negative, it can still serve a useful purpose in providing an informative failure. The Pfizer attrition-based analysis (Morgan et al., 2012), and similar analyses from other large pharma, have encouraged reverse translation so that the three pillars type of approach is developed and applied during drug discovery and drug candidate evaluation: firstly, to address whether adequate testing of preclinical PoC has been achieved, and secondly, to support this approach in exploratory clinical development. For the latter aspect, key elements that should be included in a preclinical package for a putative drug candidate include:

- Translational biomarkers for
  - target engagement
  - expression of target-related pharmacology
  - patient stratification
  - response and side-effect prediction.
- Translational PK/PD model to provide
  - rationale for human dose selection
  - insight into safety margin.

Identification of biomarkers, particularly amenable to translation, can be challenging and time-consuming so it is important to start this work as early as possible in the drug discovery process and certainly during lead optimization. Lastly, ongoing drug target validation-related work may also have additional and specific translational requirements.

In the next sections we describe the clinical evaluation process. We attempt to explain how this works and how it leads to the development and licensing of new drugs for psychiatric disorders which then become available for clinicians and patients.

2.3 Drug Development

2.3.1 Phase I Clinical Studies

Phase I comprises the first stage of clinical drug development, usually, but not always, conducted in healthy volunteer subjects. The primary aim is to establish the safety and tolerability of the new chemical entity, including its pharmacokinetic, pharmacodynamic and metabolic behaviour in man. Some of these parameters will have been predicted from modelling of preclinical studies but nonetheless need to be confirmed in humans. Biomarkers of pharmacodynamic activity are increasingly used to guide decision making and further development of CNS drugs and include imaging (Borsook et al., 2013), cognitive function (Newhouse et al., 2017), saccadic eye movements (Chen et al., 2017), electroencephalogram (EEG) and pharmaco-EEG with evoked potentials (Grünberger et al., 1985; Heekeren et al., 2008; Picton, 1992) and many more currently under evaluation.

2.3.1.1 Selection of First-in-Human Starting Dose

There are several methods for estimating a safe human starting dose and most companies will apply more than one method and adopt the most conservative one. A traditional approach is described in guidance from the FDA (2005a), which provides an algorithm for estimating the maximum recommended starting dose (MRSD) based on conversion of the no observed adverse effect level (NOAEL) in the most sensitive toxicological species to a human equivalent dose (HED), using alimetric scaling. Normally a 10-fold safety margin is then applied, guided by the severity and reversibility of the toxicology findings. Using this method, the starting dose is selected solely on the basis of a toxicological outcome. In 2007 the European Medicines Agency (EMA) issued guidance (EMEA/CHMP/SWP/28367/07) on strategies to reduce risk in first-in-human trials (European Medicines Agency, 2018), arising from an investigation prompted by a major incident in the UK in which volunteers were severely injured as result of a cytokine storm provoked by a novel monoclonal antibody (Suntharalingam, 2006). This methodology encompasses the traditional toxicological approach but extends the scope to include an assessment of pharmacological activity of the compound. The minimum anticipated biological effect level (MABEL) is compared to the NOAEL and usually the most sensitive of the two is chosen for human starting dose estimation. The development of techniques such as physiologically based pharmacokinetic (PBPK) modelling, utilizing data from a variety of preclinical experiments, provides additional data to estimate an appropriate starting dose (Jones et al., 2013). The 2007 EU guidance has now been updated to accommodate adaptive first-in-human clinical trial designs with multiple components, as described below.

2.3.1.2 Phase I Study Designs

Traditionally, first-in-human studies are conducted in young healthy adults, starting with single administrations and moving to multiple dosing (if appropriate). Cohorts of six to eight subjects receive progressively higher doses of the investigational product (or placebo), with safety and pharmacokinetic monitoring, until predefined safety or exposure endpoints are achieved. Very often the multiple dose part of the study will run contemporaneously with the single-dose cohorts (so called inter-leaving), but only at dose levels previously shown to be safe after a single administration. At the beginning, sentinel subjects (usually two individuals) will be dosed alone on separate days to limit first dose risk. Dose escalation in the single and multiple parts of the study is only continued following full review of the safety and exposure data from the previous dose, and may follow a preordained pattern based on modelling. Protocols are written flexibly to allow repeated dosing at the same level, or dose de-escalation if necessary, and hence a real-time adaptive trial design approach is adopted. Stopping criteria usually involve changes in safety measures (adverse events, laboratory variables or other safety parameters), predetermined levels of exposure being achieved, or achievement of a biomarker endpoint believed to predict for clinical effects. Normally one tries to achieve supra-therapeutic exposure levels in Phase I to provide a margin of safety for later studies, assuming this can be done within the confines of the preclinical safety window. Modern Phase I trial protocols often include multiple elements in addition to single and multiple dosing components, including food effect, males and females, different age ranges and sometimes more than one formulation of the product, for which EMA guidance (EMA/CHMP/SWP/28367/07 Rev 1) has been issued (European Medicines Agency, 2018).

2.3.1.3 Three Pillars of Survival

This term has been coined (Morgan et al., 2012) to describe three tenants of early development aimed at ensuring that a new chemical or biological entity has a chance of demonstrating efficacy later on, and is described in the Drug Discovery section (Section 2.2) of this chapter. In short, the questions, as described above are: (i) can the drug access the intended target; (ii) can it engage with it; and (iii) does that engagement lead to a functional outcome? In practice, Phase II results may be required to answer all three questions, but it is prudent to go as far as possible in healthy human volunteers. The challenge is particularly tough for drugs intended for CNS disease as the target is usually sitting on the wrong side of the blood–brain barrier. Some companies favour measuring cerebrospinal fluid (CSF) drug levels as an indicator of central penetration, but this can be misleading as CSF may not be in equilibrium with extracellular fluid, which is the physical compartment the astrocytes and neurons are exposed to and can only be accessed via central microdialysis (Shannon et al., 2013). PET is a technique that has been used successfully for confirming target access for dopaminergic drugs (Catafau & Bullich, 2013), as radioligands are readily available and brain occupancy levels associated with efficacy in schizophrenia have been established for dopamine antagonists (Takano, 2010). The recent emergence of [11C UCB-J] as a PET ligand for synpatic vesicular protein 2a (SV2a) is a valuable addition in the neurodegenerative disease research field, as it permits direct visualization of synaptic density (Finnema et al., 2016) as a marker of disease progression. Biomarkers of activity are also popular and provide considerable mechanistic value, particularly for established mechanisms. For example, changes in saccadic eye movement provides a reliable biomarker for GABAergic activity (Chen et al., 2017), and many psychoactive drugs have a characteristic signature on the power spectral analysis of pharmaco-EEG (Herrmann et al., 1979). These may all help with dose selection and estimation of duration of effect. Psychostimulants often give rise to changes in tests of cognitive function (Baroni & Castellanos, 2015), which are more or less used routinely in CNS drug development as safety and/or efficacy measures.

2.3.1.4 Phase I Challenge Studies

In the absence of a measurable abnormality in healthy volunteers upon which to test a drug, it may be possible to generate one by way of a challenge test. For example, both ketamine (schizophrenia), and scopolamine (cognition) have been used in animals and humans to create specific deficits (Doyle et al., 2013; Snyder et al., 2005) upon which the novel treatment can be overlaid to produce a reversal of the induced effect. In the field of epilepsy, it has been possible to show in volunteers with photosensitive epilepsy that flicker-induced EEG abnormalities can be reversed with novel agents destined to become anticonvulsants (French et al., 2014; Yuen & Sims, 2014). Pain is an area where challenge studies in human volunteers are used commonly, although their relevance to non-inflammatory chronic pain conditions may be limited (Olesen et al., 2012; Staahl & Drewes, 2004). Activation of superficial and deep nociceptors in human volunteers can be achieved by induction of local ischaemia, by application of mechanical or chemical stimuli, by ultraviolet (UV) burn and by electrical stimulation. However, all these tests, with the exception of delayed hypersensitivity to UV burn, are models of acute pain and do not necessarily recreate the neuronal hypersensitivity associated with spinal cord wind-up, which is believed to be a significant factor implicated in the hyperalgesia of neuropathic pain, for example (Herrero et al., 2000).

2.3.1.5 Ancilliary Phase I Investigations

Phase I studies continue during the course of drug development to provide information to support marketing authorization registration packages. These studies further evaluate drug metabolism (identifying human metabolites for qualification), and investigate special groups such as elderly subjects, children and the effects of organ impairment. Other studies specific to the new chemical entity under evaluation may include drug–drug interaction studies, abuse liability and impairment of driving performance. While these investigations have become more sophisticated with improvements in methodologies, none is particularly new in concept. However, one technique that has emerged in the recent past, and is fast becoming mainstream in drug development, is PBPK, to the extent that there is now guidance from the FDA (FDA, 2018) and EU (European Medicines Agency, 2016) as to its use, including handling and the presentation of data. This technique models and simulates human physiology, population kinetics and other characteristics of a drug's perfomance (small molecule or biological) to mechanistically predict likely pharmacokinetic and pharmacodynamic behaviours of the drug in different populations. It is a valuable supplement to conventional modelling at both ends of the development spectrum; calculating a safe starting dose in man by reaching back into preclinical data, and predicting drug behaviour in small or rare human populations that might not be well represented in the final registration package (Jones & Rowland-Yo, 2013; Jones et al., 2013). Currently, the FDA considers PBPK data on a case-by-case basis when used to support dosing recommendations in product labelling, for example when drug–drug interactions might be predicted.

2.3.2 Phase II Clinical Studies

Many companies view Phase II in two parts, with quite distinct and separate objectives. A key determinant for future investment in a drug relies on the establishment of efficacy, or a reasonable surrogate for it, in patients. Some confidence of target engagement or activity may have been established in Phase I, but clearly establishing the pharmacodynamic effects of the drug in the intended patient population is a critical defining point. Some mechanisms of action may lend themselves to more than one putative clinical indication, and more than one PoC study may be conducted in early Phase II (so-called Phase IIa) in an attempt to establish the most promising route for further evaluation. Where therapies already exist for the target disease indication, these early studies may also include a comparator drug to confirm that there is a chance of meaningful improvement over the existing standard of care, particularly as a major investment decision often depends on the PoC outcome. As PoC studies are often used for decision making, it is as important in these as it is in subsequent studies to ensure that the endpoints chosen are valid for the disease under investigation, and that there is sufficient statistical power to detect a treatment difference if it exists.

In these (generally small) patient trials it is usual to include a number of biomarkers. Typically in the CNS one might consider some of the following for inclusion: pharmaco-EEG with or without evoked potentials (Erickson et al., 2016; Yener & Basar, 2013), cytokine measurement (Kothur et al., 2016), histamine and other immune mediators (Cacabelos et al., 2016), glial biomarkers (Garden & Campbell, 2016), microRNA (Rao et al., 2013), and one might predict that neurotransmitter measurement is set to enjoy a resurgence with the emergence of ever more miniaturized and sensitive analytical probes (Chandra et al., 2017). For many years, brain imaging has also played a major part in early stage drug evaluation with conventional and functional MRI, PET and single photon emission computed tomography (SPECT) all considered useful in certain circumstances, set alongside the more conventional clinical endpoint measurement (for a comprehensive review of central imaging techniques used in drug development see Matthews et al., 2012; Wong et al., 2008).

The second part of Phase II, generally referred to as IIb, is designed to provide registration data on dose (or concentration) response, to establish the active dose range taking tolerability into account (Schmidt, 1988). Essentially, these studies are larger than those that have gone before and patients may be randomized to one of a range of doses or placebo. As before, some may also include a positive control. A variety of statistical regression analysis methods (Rekowski et al., 2017) are used to maximize the information obtained and help select the doses to be taken forward in Phase III. The endpoints used for dose selection are usually clinical endpoints intended to be used for drug registration, although others, including exploratory outcomes, may also be included at this stage. Adaptive designs may allow patients to switch dose based on predetermined dosing algorithms, often involving one or more interim analyses.

In order to establish the best dose(s) going forward, the trials in Phase II are usually tightly controlled in terms of patient inclusion/exclusion criteria, in an attempt to reduce variability (noise) by restricting the patient population and limiting potential confounders. Phase IIb may explore subpopulations of the intended patient population, either by stratification of the trial participants, or by conducting entirely separate clinical studies, for example enrolling different stages of a disease. A good example may be found in the draft EMA guidance (European Medicines Agency, 2014) on conducting drug trials in Alzheimer's disease, where the early stages of the disease are mostly characterized by cognitive symptoms, but in the later stages, behavioural and psychiatric symptoms may become more problematic. The outcome from studying subpopulations may also inform decisions about Phase III, particularly if some characteristic that leads to enhanced response can be identified.

Schizophrenia is another example where the approach to Phase II could be quite varied depending on which aspect of the disease is the primary focus for treatment. Most current antipsychotic drugs for schizophrenia have traditionally targeted 'positive' symptoms in relatively short-term trials (four to six weeks), with longer trials to demonstrate lack of symptom recurrence coming later on. More recently, some novel approaches to treating schizophrenia are now targeting 'negative' and/or 'cognitive' symptoms, which remain problematic with current therapy (Keefe et al., 2007). Clinical trials designed to show improvements in these features of the disease tend to be longer (three to six months), and would include different subsets of patients compared to trials aimed at acute treatment of psychosis. Such trials typically add the new molecule on to existing treatment and use cognitive function tests and negative symptom rating scales as primary endpoints. At the end of Phase II, the novel drug will typically be measured against a 'product profile', a detailed description of what the drug needs to achieve across a wide range of performance measures in order to be successful in the marketplace. Many fail at this stage. Indeed, as we describe above, to date no drug has received a licence for cognition in schizophrenia, in spite of several reaching late stage clinical trials (Talpos, 2017).

2.3.3 Phase III Clinical Studies

Phase III is the most expensive part of the process of developing a new drug, not only because of the scale of the clinical trials but also because of the concurrent investment in drug safety, and development of drug substance and drug product manufacturing to a commercial scale. Niche or orphan indications may be something of an exception, and have become popular of late, but even so, the Phase III is still something of a major undertaking. For example, in 2014 the overall costs of gaining market approval for a new drug was estimated at $2.56 billion, including $1.34 billion of direct costs (Grabowski & Hansen, 2014), with the process from Phase I to registration taking 7–10 years. A large proportion of the cost would have to be committed by the time Phase III commences, explaining why late stage failures have such a major economic impact on even the largest pharmaceutical companies.

The efficacy trials in Phase III generally involve observing patients for longer than in Phase II (three or six months for chronic indications) and may include up to one year of treatment where an indication for disease modification is being sought. The safety studies may run for a number of years, dependent on the indication, and accumulate hundreds of 'patient years' of safety information.

The general aim in Phase III is to provide two positive controlled trials confirming efficacy, with sufficient safety information to confirm a suitable benefit–risk assessment and to support the anticipated duration of use. For mainstream indications, Phase III generally involves 3000–5000 patients, compared to around 100 in Phase I and up to 500 in Phase II. In addition to at least two confirmatory trials, there are usually a host of other studies providing information for the product label, for commercial claims and advertising, and also for pricing and reimbursement (e.g. comparator trials with established drugs). For conditions which are also relevant to younger age groups, a full paediatric programme of clinical studies will also be ongoing at this time. These large-scale trials are designed to encompass real-world patients (i.e. not so tightly selected as in Phase II) and generally include additional clinical measures, such as patient reported outcomes (PROs), which endeavour to assess some impact of the drug on the patients' lives by asking them to report on aspects of their disease directly.

Success in Phase III paves the way for regulatory submissions (a New Drug Application in the USA, a Marketing Authorisation Application in the EU), whereas failure leads to huge disappointment, not only for the company developing the drug, but also for the physicians and patients who have invested time and effort in supporting the trials. This is particularly true for serious diseases and for those where there may not be an alternative therapy.

2.3.4 Phase IV Clinical Trials

The definition of a Phase IV trial is that it commences once the drug has been approved for marketing. The reasons to conduct these trials are diverse, and the number of patients studied over the lifetime of the drug can ultimately exceed the original development programme, as theoretically there is no point at which Phase IV stops. Nonetheless, the majority of Phase IV trials are normally performed within a few years of marketing approval, while there is significant patent life left.

A common reason for conducting a Phase IV trial is that it is a post-approval commitment agreed between the Sponsor company and the regulator at the time of approval. Typically, this might be to monitor identified risks and to quantify infrequent adverse events, which may or may not have been seen during the development programme. EU and US approval dossiers contain a plan for risk management which describes the procedures in place to identify and manage potential risks once the drug is on the market. An observational trial for a specific safety risk would not be unusual; however, the ethics and privacy concerns with respect to the use of patients' data in this way do need to be considered, respected and preserved (Evans, 2012).

Commercialization of a new drug is a sophisticated process and Phase IV studies are often conducted to ensure that a new drug has access to its markets. A key objective of this research, which often begins preregistration, is to establish cost-effectiveness of the new, in comparison to other, treatment modalities. The requirements may differ between countries such that local domestic clinical trials are required. Obtaining a position on formularies and gaining reimbursement for patients from healthcare providers often require specific instruments to assess a new drug's value, set against other healthcare costs (Khoury et al., 2015).

Another reason to conduct Phase IV trials is to extend the indications to a wider group of patients than the drug was originally approved for, which requires a supplementary application to the marketing authorities. A good example would be Pfizer's gabapentin, originally approved in 1994 as adjunctive treatment for control of partial onset epileptic seizures in adults, but later found to be of benefit in neuropathic pain, obtaining a licence for post-herpetic neuralgia in the United States in 2002 (Sirven, 2010).

Finally, as part of the management of the 'life cycle' of the drug, new formulations may be developed with the aim of making the drug more effective or user-friendly. Examples might include slow-release versions to reduce the amount of administrations required per day, fast-melt formulations if rapid absorption is a benefit, depot formulations to improve compliance and combination therapy where there is a rationale to combine two or more drugs (e.g. Parkinson's disease). If sufficiently novel, a new formulation may extend a product's patent life.

2.4 Drug Registration

The pharmaceutical industry is one of the most highly regulated international businesses, such that each step of the process from discovery to approval and commercialization is subject to external scrutiny. In this section we will consider the process of obtaining marketing approval. Until 1990, the process for developing and registering drugs for approval was highly devolved, with different rules and requirements from country to country. Coupled with the fact that many registration dossiers were submitted in hard copy (as most registration authorities had no way of handling electronic submissions), the process of registering a new drug internationally was cumbersome and time-consuming, with much repetition and redundancy. As most territories assessed the dossiers independently, the diversity of the resultant product labels (Product Information Sheets) could lead one to wonder whether the same product dossier had been assessed by the different authorities.

In 1990, the USA, EU and Japan came together as the International Commission for Harmonisation of Technical Requirement for Registration of Pharmaceuticals for Human Use (ICH) to provide Sponsors with guidance on the contents and presentation of a Common Technical Dossier (CTD). Since then, ICH has addressed many facets of the drug development process and provided guidance on process improvements, such as the introduction of electronic submissions. This has dramatically improved the operational efficiency for both the compilation and submission of approval dossiers and their regulatory review. In its most recent incarnation (2015), ICH represents the International Council for Harmonisation, a non-profit organization based in Switzerland, and comprising Canada, Brazil and Switzerland, in addition to the three founder members. Many other countries are represented by observers. While many other challenges remain, the ongoing ICH initiative must be regarded as one of the success stories of modern drug development and regulation (www.ich.org).

Amongst the guidance to Sponsors provided by ICH (and which has been adopted into law in the EU), one of the first guidance proposals to be unveiled was the minimum requirements for submission of a preclinical package (safety and manufacturing) prior to first human exposure (ICH-M3), which was inaugurated in 1995. Around this time, guidance was provided both on the standard required for the conduct of clinical trials (Good Clinical Practice ICH-E6, 1996) and a standardized trial reporting format (ICH-E3, 1996).

While individual authorities still differ on some aspects of the process, the basic principle of seeking expert advice at key points in the development cycle is common and is expected. Typically, these advisory meetings might occur prior to first human exposure, at the end of Phase II and sometimes prior to the submission of a marketing authorization (often to discuss the detailed format of the dossier). In addition, for disease indications relevant to children, advice will be sought of the design and content of the paediatric development programme (Turner et al., 2014). Further assistance can be sought in guidance documents provided by individual authorities on aspects of drug development, perhaps regarding the design of clinical trials for a particular disease, or the use of biomarkers for example. The NIMH in the USA is particularly active in assisting industry to develop and validate new clinical endpoint instruments; the MATRICS cognitive assessment scale for schizophrenia being one example (Marder, 2006). This is a highly evolving field and companies, referred to in regulatory parlance as Sponsors, are well advised to remain up-to-date.

In the 1980s the FDA recognized the need to encourage Sponsors to develop medicines for rare diseases, where the market is, by definition, much smaller than for common conditions. The Orphan Drug Act was passed in 1983 (Kesselheim, 2010) which incentivized companies to consider rare disease indications (rare being defined as less than 200 000 patients in the USA), and similar legislation was adopted in the EU sometime later. While it arguably took over a decade or so to catch on, the number of companies, both large and small, with orphan drugs in development has multiplied to the extent that many mid to large pharmaceutical companies have at least one orphan programme. Notable success has been achieved for patients with inborn errors of metabolism using enzyme replacement therapy, and the emergence of gene editing technology holds great promise for patients with identified single gene mutations.

The USA has led the way in creating initiatives for the accelerated development of drugs for serious diseases where no alternatives exist, prompted by the AIDS crisis. There are various regulatory and legal instruments to achieve this, including the most commonly quoted 'Fast Track' initiative. The key to success with these initiatives is early dialogue, as the Sponsor may not have chosen the most expeditious route for the product, and what can and cannot be done is often a matter for dialogue and negotiation. The concept of Conditional Approval, adopted in the EU in 2006, permits sales of drug, where the benefit side of the benefit–risk assessment is not fully established, but garners sufficient confidence for a product to be released onto the market while its efficacy and safety evaluation continues. Of the 26 products authorized up to 2015 by this route, 14 remain conditional. This has led to questions regarding how much the post-marketing studies contribute to the overall body of knowledge of a product approved conditionally (Banzi et al., 2017). With regard to the CNS, fampridine was conditionally approved for multiple sclerosis in 2011 (and remains conditional), and stirpentol was conditionally approved for juvenile myoclonic epilepsy in 2007, and now has full approval. As with all new products, a robust risk monitoring plan must be in place prior to drug approval, regardless of territory, as the true profile of a drug cannot be established until it has been marketed for a number of years. This is called post-marketing surveillance.

2.5 Post-Marketing Surveillance and Risk Management

Pharmacovigilance is an established tenant of drug safety monitoring, starting in Phase I and continuing throughout the lifetime of a drug. Over the last decade or so an increasing emphasis has been placed on monitoring the risks of a drug once it is released to the market, such that presentation of a risk management and monitoring plan is a major component of an approval dossier.

The concept of pharmacovigilance originated as a discipline in the early 1960s following the thalidomide disaster in 1956, in which hundreds of newborns were found to have limb deformities after their mothers had taken the drug during pregnancy to control nausea (Caron et al., 2016). Systems were set up to track the safety of new drugs by asking practitioners to report adverse findings to a central authority. In Great Britain this was known as the Yellow Card system, reflecting the colour of the form on which reports were to be made. This system, established in 1964, has undergone many improvements over time and is maintained today (www.dmrc@mhra.gov.uk). Reports are sent to the healthcare regulator and the manufacturer whose joint responsibility is to look for trends and take any appropriate action, ranging from changes to the product labelling to placing restrictions on use, or even withdrawal of a drug from the market. The reporting systems as they were originally configured had several significant shortcomings; there was little guidance to practitioners as to what should be reported; there was inconsistent reporting across the territories in which the drug was being sold; and within the pharmaceutical companies there was often poor information on the number of units prescribed globally and hence there was no reliable denominator with which to judge whether there was a change in the incidence of a particular event over time.

Unsurprisingly, the science of pharmacovigilance has developed beyond recognition from its humble origins, due to a combination of legislation, globalization and technological advancement. Adverse events deemed to be serious (for which there is an internationally recognized definition) are required to be reported to Sponsors and regulators on an expedited basis if they are unexpected for that product, and the Sponsor maintains a lifetime database of all safety reports, regardless of origin, from which reports are submitted to regulatory authorities on an annual basis. A common language for adverse events has been adopted (MedDRA), which provides terminology allowing adverse events to be categorized and collated. Estimates of past and current incidence (based on sales) and trend analyses are made to evaluate whether the incidence of any particular event is changing. The level of detail supporting each report has increased over time to allow for covariate analyses, for example to assess the impact of a particular concomitant medication or disease state, and it is not unusual for follow-up information requests to be made on a particular reported event up to its conclusion. Not surprisingly, the Clinical Safety or Pharmacovigilance departments within companies developing and marketing drugs have grown proportionately in numbers and sophistication, to process the enhanced information flow.

As mentioned earlier, risk management has been embedded in the drug approval process in the last decade or so, complementing the established methods for monitoring the safety of marketed products (FDA, 2005b). Although differing in form between the EU and the USA, the aims of risk planning remain similar. The applicant is required to assess the benefit–risk balance of its products, based on the available preclinical and clinical data, and propose methods for monitoring the risk side once the product is marketed. The risks can be established for the product i.e. already known the safety database or theoretically based on the mechanism of action of the drug or the disease state. Some risks may arise from the presence of concomitant diseases, which may have been excluded from the clinical trial protocols used for registration, but which may be expected to be encountered once the drug is marketed. The risk plan will describe these risks and how they will be specifically addressed, with a description of how the effectiveness of the monitoring procedure will be assessed. The proactive approach to risk management benefits all sides as it provides an opportunity for early intervention in the event of unexpected safety findings, before more serious damage is done.

2.6 Conclusion and Future Outlook

Psychiatric drug discovery and development has had some remarkable successes over the past 60 years or so. A large number of medicines have been delivered and entered clinical practice providing benefit to patients and carers. However, despite the abundant armamentarium of pharmacological therapies there is still a strong need for more effective treatments, particularly with improved efficacy in highly debilitating diseases such as schizophrenia (e.g. for negative symptoms and cognitive deficits). Despite growing effort and commitment in this area, a quantum breakthrough has been elusive with many costly failures provoking disinvestment and questions regarding how best to conduct psychiatric drug discovery. This chapter describes in some detail the current challenges and various processes involved in the discovery and development of new psychiatric drugs. Knowledge garnered from the Human Genome Project together with the continuing technological revolution in molecular biology, and in automation and information technology has accelerated an evolutionary change in the execution and operational management of drug discovery in all areas. The authors have considerable and varied experience, and have provided a comprehensive coverage of all aspects of the topic including factors that we hope will facilitate future progress and success. We have drawn from personal drug discovery experience in psychiatric drug discovery to provide updated information with relevant case illustrations (e.g. asenapine and AUT00206 for schizophrenia). One key message is the critical importance of translational science, in animal and human studies, based on availability of reliable biomarkers (for drug target engagement, proof of mechanism, patient stratification and efficacy prediction) to enable evidence-based assessment of confidence in the drug target and drug candidate. For this to happen, the traditional 'me too' compound-based approach will have to be replaced by a more rational genetic risk factor-linked and molecular pathology-driven drug discovery paradigm.

Pharma cannot do this alone and require the support of many other stakeholders with a common interest, in particular, academic (clinical and non-clinical) research groups, patients and their support groups, and government regulatory agencies. Some academic groups of course are now engaging in drug discovery with funding provided by the Research Councils but require collaboration with Pharma and larger investment for full development work. Strengthening of such collaborations and partnerships as well as mutual trust is critical for future success. As we described here, issues of reproducibility of scientific results, incorporation of both sexes/gender in preclinical studies and publication of negative data need to be tackled. Building high confidence in all aspects of the process is what will ultimately improve the probability of success in the future and so provide better therapeutics and quality of life for patients and carers. Indeed, the authors believe that the stage is set for a renaissance in psychiatric drug discovery and development. It is hoped that this chapter will serve to inform and update clinicians and researchers alike and provoke some thoughtful consideration as well as being a useful source of information relevant to both practice and science.

References

Ayhan Y, Pletnikov M (2016). Contributions to understanding the causes and treatment of schizophrenia. In T Abel, T Nickl-Jockshatt, eds., *The Neurobiology of Schizophrenia 1*. Cambridge, MA: Academic Press.

Bale TL, Epperson CN (2017). Sex as a biological variable: who, what, when, why, and how. *Neuropsychopharmacology*, 42, 386–396.

Banzi R, Geraldi C, Bertele V, Garattini S (2017). Conditional approval of medicines by EMA. *BMJ*, 357, j2062.

Barnes SA, Sawiak SJ, Caprioli D, et al. (2014). Impaired limbic cortico-striatal structure and sustained visual attention in a rodent model of schizophrenia. *Int J Neuropsychopharmacol*, 18(2), 1–12.

Baroni A, Castellanos FX (2015). Stimulants, cognition and ADHD. *Curr Opin Behav Sci*, 4, 109–114.

Belzung C, Lemoine M (2011). Criteria of validity for animal models of psychiatric disorders: focus on anxiety disorders and depression. *Biol Mood Anxiety Disord*, 1(1), 9.

Bespalov A, Steckler T, Altevogt B, et al. (2016). Failed trials for central nervous system disorders do not necessarily invalidate preclinical models and drug targets. *Nat Rev Drug Discov*, 15, 516.

Bhakta SG, Young JW (2017). The 5 choice continuous performance test (5C-CPT): a novel tool to assess cognitive control across species. *J Neurosci Methods*, 292, 53–60.

Birnbaum R, Weinberger DR (2017). Genetic insights into the neurodevelopmental origins of schizophrenia. *Nature Rev Neuorsci*, 18: 727–740. doi:10.1038/nrn.2017.125.

Bishop KM (2017). Progress and promise of antisense oligonucleotide therapeutics for central nervous system diseases. *Neuropharmacology*, 120, 56–62.

Borsook D, Becerra L, Fava M (2013). Use of functional imaging across clinical phases in CNS drug development. *Transl Psychiatry*, 3(7), e282. doi:10.1038/tp.2013.43.

Buchanan RW, Panagides J, Zhao J, et al. (2012). Asenapine versus olanzapine in people with persistent negative symptoms of schizophrenia. *J Clin Psychopharmacol*, 32, 36–45.

Bugarski-Kirola D, Blaettler T, Arango C, et al. (2017). Bitopertin in negative symptoms of schizophrenia – results from the phase III FlashLyte and DayLyte studies. *Biol Psychiatry*, 82, 8–16.

Cacabelos R, Torrellas C, Fernández-Novoa L, López-Muñoz F (2016). Histamine and immune biomarkers in CNS disorders. *Mediators Inflamm*, 2016, 1924603. doi:10.1155/2016/1924603.

Cadinu D, Grayson B, Podda G, et al. (2018). NMDA receptor antagonist rodent models for cognition in schizophrenia and identification of novel drug treatments, an update. *Neuropharmacology*, 142, 41–62. doi:10.1016/j.neuropharm.2017.11.045.

Cahill L (2014). Equal not equal the same: sex differences in the human brain. *Cerebrum*, 2014, 5.

Caron J, Rochoy M, Gaboriau L, Gautier S (2016). The history of pharmacovigilance. *Thérapie*, 71, 129–134.

Catafau AM, Bullich S (2013). Molecular imaging PET and SPECT approaches for improving productivity of antipsychotic drug discovery and development. *Curr Med Chem*, 20(3), 378–388.

Chandra S, Siraj S, Wong DKY (2017). Recent advances in biosensing for neurotransmitters and disease biomarkers using microelectrodes. *ChemElectroChem*, 4, 822–833. doi:10.1002/celc.201600810.

Chaudhry IB, Husain N, ur Rahman R, et al. (2015). A randomised double-blind placebo-controlled 12-week feasibility trial of methotrexate added to treatment as usual in early schizophrenia: study protocol for a randomised controlled trial. *Trials*, 16, 9.

Chen X, Broeyer F, de Kam M, et al. (2017). Pharmacodynamic response profiles of anxiolytic and sedative drugs. *Br J Clin Pharmacol*, 83(5), 1028–1038.

Choudhury SR, Hudry E, Maguire CA, et al. (2017). Viral vectors for therapy of neurologic diseases. *Neuropharmacology*, 120, 63–80.

Clayton JA (2017). Studying both sexes: a guiding principle for biomedicine. *FASEB J*, 30(2), 519–524.

Clayton JA, Collins FS (2014). Policy: NIH to balance sex in cell and animal studies. *Nature*, 509, 282–283.

Clementz BA, Sweeney JA, Hamm JP, et al. (2016). Identification of distinct psychosis biotypes using brain-based biomarkers. *Am J Psychiatry*, 173, 373–384.

Cook D, Brown D, Alexander R, et al. (2014). Lessons learned from the fate of AstraZeneca's drug pipeline: a five-dimensional framework. *Nat Rev Drug Discov*, 13, 419–431.

Cuthbert BN (2015). Research domain criteria: toward future psychiatric nosologies. *Dialogues Clin Neurosci*, 17(1), 89–97.

Dolgin E (2014). Drug discoverers chart path to tackling data irreproducibility. *Nat Rev Drug Discov*, 13(12), 875–876.

Dolgos H, Trusheim M, Gross D, et al. (2016). Translational Medicine Guide transforms drug development processes: the recent Merck experience. *Drug Discov Today*, 21, 517–526.

Downing AM, Kinon BJ, Millen BA, et al. (2014). A double-blind, placebo-controlled comparator study of LY2140023 monohydrate in patients with schizophrenia. *BMC Psychiatry*, 14, 351–363.

Doyle OM, De Simoni S, Schwarz AJ, et al. (2013). Quantifying the attenuation of the ketamine pharmacological magnetic resonance imaging response in humans: a validation using antipsychotic and glutamatergic agents. *J Pharmacol Exp Ther*, 354(1), 151–160.

Erickson MA, Ruffle A, Gold JM (2016). A meta-analysis of mismatch negativity in schizophrenia: from clinical risk to disease specificity and progression. *Biol Psychiatry*, 79(12), 980–987.

European Medicines Agency (2014). EMA/CHMP/539931/2014. Draft guidance on the clinical investigation of medicines for the treatment of Alzheimer's disease and other dementias.

European Medicines Agency (2016). EMA/CHMP/458101/2016. Guideline on the qualification and reporting of physiologically based pharmacokinetic modelling and simulation: consultation document.

European Medicines Agency (2018). EMEA/CHMP/SWP/28367/07 Rev 1. Guideline on strategies to identify and mitigate risks for first-in-human clinical trials with investigational medicinal products.

Evans BJ (2012). The ethics of postmarketing observational studies of drug safety under section 505(o)(3) of the Food, Drug, and Cosmetic Act. *Am J Law Med*, 38(4), 577–606.

FDA (2005a). Estimating the Maximum Safe Starting Dose in Initial Clinical Trials for Therapeutics in Adult Healthy Volunteers: Guidance for Industry. Center for Drug Evaluation and Research (CDER). Available at: www.fda.gov/drugs/guidances-drugs/all-guidances-drugs (last accessed 19.8.19).

FDA (2005b). Development and Use of Risk Minimization Action Plans: Guidance for Industry. Available at: www.fda.gov/drugs/guidances-drugs/all-guidances-drugs (last accessed 19.8.19).

FDA (2018). Physiologically Based Pharmacokinetic Analyses – Format and Content: Guidance for Industry. Center for Drug Evaluation and Research (CDER). Available at: www.fda.gov/drugs/guidances-drugs/all-guidances-drugs (last accessed 19.8.19).

Fineberg NA, Haddad PM, Carpenter L, et al. (2013). The size, burden and cost of the brain in the UK. *J Psychopharmacol*, 27(9), 761–770.

Finnema S, Eid T, Dhaher R, et al. (2016). 11C-UCB-J as a biomarker for synaptic density – an *in vivo/in vitro* validation study. *J Nucl Med*, 57(Suppl 2), 1800.

Foley C, Corvin A, Nakagome S (2017). Genetics of schizophrenia: ready to translate? *Curr Psychiatry Rep*, 19(9), 61.

Fosgerau K, Hoffmann T (2015). Peptide therapeutics: current status and future directions. *Drug Discov Today*, 20, 122–128.

French JA, Krauss GL, Kasteleijn D, DiVentura BD, Bagiella E (2014). Effects of marketed antiepileptic drugs and placebo in the human photosensitivity screening protocol. *Neurotherapeutics*, 11(2), 412–418.

Freskgård PO, Urich E (2017). Antibody therapies in CNS diseases. *Neuropharmacology*, 120, 38–55.

Frye SV, Arkin MR, Arrowsmith CH, et al. (2015). Tackling reproducibility in academic preclinical drug discovery. *Nat Rev Drug Discov*, 14(11), 733–734.

Garden GA, Campbell BM (2016). Glial biomarkers in human central nervous system disease. *Glia*, 64(10), 1755–1771.

Gashaw I, Ellinghaus P, Sommer A, Asadullah K (2012). What makes a good drug target? *Drug Discov Today*, 17 Suppl, S24–S30.

Geerts H, Spiros A, Roberts P (2017). Phosphodiesterase 10 inhibitors in clinical development for CNS disorders. *Expert Rev Neurother*, 17, 553–560.

Girgis RR, Ciarleglio A, Choo T, et al. (2018). Randomized double-blind, placebo-controlled clinical trial of tocilizumab, an interleukin-6 receptor antibody, for residual symptoms in schizophrenia. *Neuropsychopharmacology*, 43, 1317–1323.

Goetghebeur PJD, Dias R (2014). The attentional set-shifting test paradigm in rats for the screening of novel pro-cognitive compounds with relevance for cognitive deficits in schizophrenia. *Curr Pharm Des*, 20, 5060–5068.

Grabowski HG, Hansen RW (2014). Costs of developing a new drug. Tufts Center for the Study of Drug Development. Available at: http://csdd.tufts.edu (last accessed 20.10.19).

Grünberger J, Saletu B, Linzmayer L, Stöhr H (1985). Determination of pharmacokinetics and pharmacodynamics of amisulpride by pharmaco-EEG and psychometry. In P Pichot, P Berner, R Wolf, K Thau, eds., *Psychiatry the State of the Art.* Boston, MA: Springer, pp. 681–686.

Harrison RK (2016). Phase II and phase III failures: 2013–2015. *Nat Rev Drug Discov*, 15, 817–818.

Heekeren K, Daumann J, Neukirch A, et al. (2008). Mismatch negativity generation in the human 5HT2A agonist and NMDA antagonist model of psychosis. *Psychopharmacology (Berl)*, 199, 77–88.

Hendrie C, Pickles A (2013). The failure of the antidepressant drug discovery process is systemic. *J Psychopharmacol*, 27(5), 407–416.

Herrero JF, Laird JM, López-García JA (2000). Wind-up of spinal cord neurones and pain sensation: much ado about something? *Prog Neurobiol*, 61(2), 169–203.

Herrmann WM, Fichte K, Itil TM, Kubicki ST (1979). Acute efficacy of 20 psychotropic drugs on human EEG power spectrum variables shown by multivariate and univariate statistics. In B Saletu, P Berner, L Hollister, eds., *Neuropsychopharmacology: Proceedings of the 11th Congress of the Collegium Internationale Neuro-Psychopharmacologicum, Vienna 1978.* Oxford: Pergamon Press, pp. 371–382.

Hutson PH, Clark JA, Cross AJ (2017). CNS target identification and validation: avoiding the valley of death or naive optimism? *Ann Rev Pharmacol Toxicol*, 57, 171–187.

Insel T, Cuthbert B, Garvey M, et al. (2010). Research domain criteria (RDoC): toward a new classification framework for research on mental disorders. *Am J Psychiatry*, 167(7), 748–751.

Jentsch JD, Roth RH (1999). The neuropsychopharmacology of phencyclidine: from NMDA receptor hypofunction to the dopamine hypothesis of schizophrenia. *Neuropsychopharmacology*, 20, 201–225.

Jones HM, Rowland-Yo K (2013). Basic concepts in PBPK modelling in drug discovery and development. *Pharmacometrics Syst Pharmacol*, 2, e63.

Jones HM, Mayawala K, Poulin P (2013). Dose selection based on physiologically based pharmacokinetic (PBPK) approaches. *AAPS J*, 15(2), 377–387.

Kas MJ, Penninx B, Sommer B, et al. (2019). A quantitative approach to neuropsychiatry: the why and the how. *Neurosci Biobehav Rev*, 97, 3–9.

Keefe RS, Bilder RM, Davis SM, et al.; CATIE Investigators; Neurocognitive Working Group (2007). Neurocognitive effects of antipsychotic medications in patients with chronic schizophrenia in the CATIE Trial. *Arch Gen Psychiatry*, 64(6), 633–647.

Keshavan MS, Lawler AN, Nasrallah HA, Tandon R (2017). New drug developments in psychosis: challenges, opportunities and strategies. *Prog Neurobiol*, 152, 3–20.

Kesselheim AS (2010). Innovation and the Orphan Drug Act,1983–2009: regulatory and clinical characteristics of approved orphan drugs. In MJ Field, TF Boat, eds., *Rare Disease and Orphan Products: Accelerating Research and Development.* Washington, DC: National Academies Press, Appendix B.

Khoury C, Duque R, Freiberg M (2015). Trial design and market access implications: outcomes from comparator choice. *Value Health*, 18(7), A723.

Kola I (2008). The state of innovation in drug development. *Clin Pharmacol Ther*, 83, 227–230.

Kothur K, Wienholt L, Brilot F, Dale RC (2016). CSF cytokines/chemokines as biomarkers in neuroinflammatory CNS disorders: a systematic review. *Cytokine*, 77, 227–237.

Knuesel I, Chicha L, Britschgi M, et al. (2014). Maternal immune activation and abnormal brain development across CNS disorders. *Nat Rev Neurol*, 10, 643–660.

Leger M, Neill JC (2016). A systematic review comparing sex differences in cognitive function in schizophrenia and in rodent models for schizophrenia, implications for improved therapeutic strategies. *Neurosci Biobehav Rev*, 68, 979–1000.

Leger M, Alvaro G, Large C, Harte MK, Neill JC (2015). AUT6, a novel Kv3 channel modulator, reverses cognitive and neurobiological dysfunction in a rat model of relevance to schizophrenia symptomatology. *Eur Neuropsychopharmacol*, 25, S480.

Marder SR (2006). The NIMH-MATRICS project for developing cognition-enhancing agents for schizophrenia. *Dialogues Clin Neurosci*, 8(1), 109–113.

Marsh S (2015). Investigation of the neuronal marker N-acetylaspartate as a potential biomarker for neurological diseases. Unpublished PhD thesis, University of Manchester.

Marson FAL, Bertuzzo CS, Ribeiro JD (2017). Personalized or precision medicine? The example of cystic fibrosis. *Front Pharmacol*, 8, 390.

Matthews H, Hanison J, Nirmalan N (2016). 'Omics'-informed drug and biomarker discovery: opportunities, challenges and future perspectives. *Proteomes*, 4(3), 28.

Matthews PM, Rabiner EA, Passchier J, Gunn RN (2012). Positron emission tomography molecular imaging for drug development. *Br J Clin Pharmacol*, 73(2), 175–186.

Millan MJ, Goodwin GM, Meyer-Lindenberg A, Ove Ögren S (2015). Learning from the past and looking to the future: emerging perspectives for improving the treatment of psychiatric disorders. *Eur Neuropsychopharmacol*, 25(5), 599–656.

Möller HJ, Czobor P (2015). Pharmacological treatment of negative symptoms in schizophrenia. *Eur Arch Psychiatry Clin Neurosci*, 265, 567–578.

Moran PM (2016). Behavioral phenotypes of genetic models: contributions to understanding the causes and treatment of schizophrenia. In T Abel, T Nickl-Jockshatt, eds., *The Neurobiology of Schizophrenia 1*. Cambridge, MA: Academic Press, pp. 383–396.

Morgan P, Van Der Graaf PH, Arrowsmith J, et al. (2012). Can the flow of medicines be improved? Fundamental pharmacokinetic and pharmacological principles toward improving Phase II survival. *Drug Discov Today*, 17, 419–424.

Munafò M, Neill JC (2016). Null is beautiful: on the importance of publishing null results. *J Psychopharmacol*, 30(7), 585.

Neill JC, Kulkarni J (eds.) (2011). Biological basis of sex differences in psychopharmacology. *Current Topics in Behavioral Neurosciences*, Vol. 8 (series editors: C Marsden, B Ellenbroek, M Geyer). Heidelberg: Springer-Verlag, pp. v–vii.

Neill JC, Barnes S, Cook S, et al. (2010). Animal models of cognitive dysfunction and negative symptoms of schizophrenia: focus on NMDA receptor antagonism. *Pharmacol Ther*, 128(3), 419–432.

Neill JC, Harte MK, Haddad PM, Lydall ES, Dwyer DM (2014). Acute and chronic effects of NMDA receptor antagonists in rodents, relevance to negative symptoms of schizophrenia: a translational link to humans. *Eur Neuropsychopharmacol*, 24, 822–835.

Németh B, Laszlovsky I, Czobor P, et al. (2017). Cariprazine versus risperidone monotherapy for treatment of predominant negative symptoms in patients with schizophrenia: a randomised, double-blind, controlled trial. *Lancet*, 389(10074), 1103–1113. doi:10.1016/S0140-6736(17)30060-0.

Newhouse PA, Conley AC, Key AP (2017). Exploring novel cognitive and electrophysiological markers of target engagement in Phase 1 and 2 studies of putative cholinergic cognitive enhancers. *Alzheimers Dement*, 13(7), P1255–P1256. https://doi.org/10.1016/J.JALZ.2017.06.1870.

Nielsch U, Fuhrmann U, Jaroch S (2016). New approaches to drug discovery. *Handb Exp Pharmacol*, 232, v–vi.

Nutt DJ, Stahl S, Blier B, et al. (2017). Inverse agonists – what do they mean for psychiatry? *Eur Neuropsychopharmacol*, 27(1), 87–90. http://dx.doi.org/10.1016/j.euroneuro.2016.11.013.

Olesen AE, Andresen T, Staahl C, Drewes AM (2012). Human experimental pain models for assessing the therapeutic efficacy of analgesic drugs. *Pharmacol Rev*, 64(3), 722–779.

Pak C, Danko T, Zhang Y, et al. (2015). Human neuropsychiatric disease modeling using conditional deletion reveals synaptic transmission defects caused by heterozygous mutations in *NRXN1*. *Cell Stem Cell*, 17(3), 316–328.

Picton TW (1992). The P300 wave of the human event-related potential. *J Clin Neurophysiol*, 9(4), 456–479.

Plosker GL, Deeks ED (2016). Asenapine: a review in schizophrenia. *CNS Drugs*, 30(7), 655–666.

Pompili M, Verzura C, Trovini G, et al. (2017) Lurasidone: efficacy and safety in the treatment of psychotic and mood disorders. *Expert Opin Drug Saf*, 26, 1–9.

Potkin SG, Cohen M, Panagides J (2007). Efficacy and tolerability of asenapine in acute schizophrenia: a placebo- and risperidone-controlled trial. *J Clin Psychiatry*, 68(10), 1492–1500.

Potkin SG, Phiri P, Szegedi A, et al. (2013). Long-term effects of asenapine or olanzapine in patients with persistent negative symptoms of schizophrenia: a pooled analysis. *Schizophr Res*, 150, 442–449.

Pringle A, Harmer CJ (2015). The effects of drugs on human models of emotional processing: an account of antidepressant drug treatment. *Dialogues Clin Neurosci*, 17(4), 477–487.

Prinz F, Schlange T, Asadullah K (2011). Believe it or not: how much can we rely on published data on potential drug targets? *Nat Rev Drug Discov*, 10(9), 712.

Rao P, Benito E, Fischer A (2013). MicroRNAs as biomarkers for CNS disease. *Front Mol Neurosci*, 26(6), 39.

Rekowski J, Köllmann C, Bornkamp B, Ickstadt K, Scherag A (2017). Phase II dose-response trials: a simulation study to compare analysis method performance under design considerations. *J Biopharm Stat*, 21, 1–17.

Reynolds GP, Neill JC (2016). Modelling the cognitive and neuropathological features of schizophrenia with phencyclidine. *J Psychopharmacol*, 30(11), 1141–1144.

Sahli ZT, Tarazi FI (2018). Pimavanserin: novel pharmacotherapy for Parkinson's disease psychosis. *Expert Opin Drug Discov*, 13(1), 103–110.

Sanacora G, Frye MA, McDonald W, et al.; American Psychiatric Association (APA) Council of Research Task Force on Novel Biomarkers and Treatments (2017). A consensus statement on the use of ketamine in the treatment of mood disorders. *JAMA Psychiatry*, 74, 399–405.

Sanchez C, Asin KE, Artigas F (2015). Vortioxetine, a novel antidepressant with multimodal activity: review of preclinical and clinical data. *Pharmacol Ther*, 145, 43–57.

Scarff JR (2017). The prospects of cariprazine in the treatment of schizophrenia. *Ther Adv Psychopharmacol*, 7(11), 237–239.

Schizophrenia Working Group of the Psychiatric Genomics C (2014). Biological insights from 108 schizophrenia-associated genetic loci. *Nature*, 511(7510), 421–427.

Schmidt R (1988). Dose-finding studies in clinical drug development. *Eur J Clin Pharmacol*, 34(1), 15–19.

Seshadri M, Banerjee D, Viswanath B, et al. (2017). Cellular models to study schizophrenia: a systematic review. *Asian J Psychiatr*, 25, 46–53.

Shahid M, Walker GB, Zorn SH, Wong EH (2009). Asenapine: a novel psychopharmacologic agent with a unique human receptor signature. *J Psychopharmacol*, 23(1), 65–73.

Shannon RJ, Carpenter KLH, Guilfoyle MR, Helmy A, Hutchinson PJ (2013). Cerebral microdialysis in clinical studies of drugs: pharmacokinetic applications. *J Pharmacokinet Pharmacodyn*, 40(3), 343–358.

Singh I, Morgan C, Curran V, et al. (2017). Ketamine treatment for depression: opportunities for clinical innovation and ethical foresight. *Lancet Psychiatry*, 4, 419–426.

Sirven JI (2010). New uses for older drugs: the tales of aspirin, thalidomide, and gabapentin. *Mayo Clin Proc*, 85(6), 508–511.

Snyder PJ, Bednar MM, Cromer JR, Maruff P (2005). Reversal of scopolamine-induced deficits with a single dose of donepezil, an acetylcholinesterase inhibitor. *Alzheimers Dement*, 1(2), 126–135.

Soliman MA, Aboharb F, Zeltner N, Studer L (2017). Pluripotent stem cells in neuropsychiatric disorders. *Mol Psychiatry*, 22(9), 1241–1249.

Staahl C, Drewes AM (2004). Experimental human pain models: a review of standardised methods for preclinical testing of analgesics. *Basic Clin Pharmacol Toxicol*, 95(3), 97–111.

Suntharalingam G, Perry MR, Ward S, et al. (2006). Cytokine storm in a Phase 1 trial of the anti-CD28 monoclonal antibody TGN1412. *N Engl J Med*, 355, 1018–1028.

Takano A (2010). The application of PET technique for the development and evaluation of novel antipsychotics. *Curr Pharm Des*, 16(3), 371–377.

Talpos JC (2017). Symptomatic thinking: the current state of Phase III and IV clinical trials for cognition in schizophrenia. *Drug Discov Today*, 22, 1017–1026.

Tarazi FI, Neill JC (2013). The preclinical profile of asenapine: clinical relevance for the treatment of schizophrenia and bipolar mania. *Expert Opin Drug Discov*, 8(1), 93–103.

Tarazi FI, Shahid M (2009). Asenapine maleate: a new drug for the treatment of schizophrenia and bipolar mania. *Drugs Today (Barc)*, 45, 865–876.

Turner MA, Catapano M, Hirschfeld S, Giaquinto C; Global Research in Paediatrics (2014). Paediatric drug development: the impact of evolving regulations. *Adv Drug Deliv Rev*, 73, 2–13.

Waring MJ, Arrowsmith J, Leach AR, et al. (2015). An analysis of the attrition of drug candidates from four major pharmaceutical companies. *Nat Rev Drug Discov*, 14, 475–486.

Wen Z, Christian KM, Song H, Ming GL (2016). Modeling psychiatric disorders with patient-derived iPSCs. *Curr Opin Neurobiol*, 36, 118–127.

Wilkinson ST, Sanacora G (2019). A new generation of antidepressants: an update on the pharmaceutical pipeline for novel and rapid-acting therapeutics in mood disorders based on glutamate/GABA neurotransmitter systems. *Drug Discov Today*, 24, 606–615.

Willner P (1984). The validity of animal models of depression. *Psychopharmacology*, 83, 1–16.

Wong DF, Tauscher J, Gründer G (2008). The role of imaging in proof of concept for CNS drug discovery and development. *Neuropsychopharmacology*, 34, 187–203.

Yener GG, Basar E (2013). Brain oscillations as biomarkers in neuropsychiatric disorders: following an interactive panel discussion and synopsis. In E Basar, C Basar-Erogu, A Ozerden, PM Rossini, GG Yener, eds., *Applications of Brain Oscillations in Neuropsychiatric Diseases*, Vol. 62. Elsevier, pp. 343–363.

Yuen ES, Sims JR (2014). How predictive are photosensitive epilepsy models as proof of principle trials for epilepsy? *Seizure*, 23(6), 490–493.

Zhang H, Cohen AE (2017). Optogenetic approaches to drug discovery in neuroscience and beyond. *Trends Biotechnol*, 35(7), 625–639.

Zheng W, Thorne N, McKew JC (2013). Phenotypic screens as a renewed approach for drug discovery. *Drug Discov Today*, 18(21–22), 1067–1073.

Zohar J, Stahl S, Moller HJ, et al. (2015). A review of the current nomenclature for psychotropic agents and an introduction to the Neuroscience-based Nomenclature. *Eur Neuropsychopharmacol*, 25(12), 2318–2325.

Chapter

3 Neurotransmission and Mechanisms of Drug Action

Brian E. Leonard

3.1 Introduction

This chapter falls into three broad sections. The first considers basic principles and information regarding neurons, the nerve impulse and neurotransmission. The second section considers the principle neurotransmitters in the brain: acetylcholine, the catecholamines, dopamine, serotonin (5-hydroxytryptamine (5-HT)), histamine and the amino acid neurotransmitters. The final section reviews minor neurotransmitters, namely neuropeptides, purine neurotransmitters, prostaglandins, neurosteroids, gaseous transmitters and endocannabinoids. It is not possible for this chapter to provide a comprehensive and in-depth view of neurotransmission. This is a rapidly advancing field and those wishing to obtain a more extensive account should consult the numerous reviews and monographs. However, the main areas of the subject are covered, and this will provide a basis for the reader to appreciate the succeeding chapters of this book.

The concept of chemical transmission in the nervous system arose in the early years of the twentieth century when it was discovered that the functioning of the autonomic nervous system was largely dependent on the secretion of acetylcholine and noradrenaline from the parasympathetic and sympathetic nerves, respectively. The physiologist Sherrington proposed that nerve cells communicated with one another, and with any other type of adjacent cell, by liberating the neurotransmitter into the space, or *synapse*, in the immediate vicinity of the nerve ending. He believed that transmission across the synaptic cleft was unidirectional and, unlike conduction down the nerve fibre, was delayed by some milliseconds because of the time it took the transmitter to diffuse across the synapse and activate a specific neurotransmitter receptor on the cell membrane.

While it was generally assumed that the brain also contained acetylcholine and noradrenaline as transmitters, it was only in the early 1950s that experimental evidence accumulated that there were also many other types of transmitter in the brain. The indoleamine neurotransmitter 5-HT, or serotonin, which is now recognized as an important component of mental function, was first studied by Erspamer in Italy and by Page in the United States in enterochromaffin tissue and platelets, respectively. It was left to Gaddum and colleagues in Edinburgh to show that 5-HT was present in the mammalian brain where it may have neurotransmitter properties.

The potential importance of 5-HT to psychopharmacology arose when Woolley and Shaw in the United States suggested that lysergic acid diethylamide (LSD) owed its potent hallucinogenic properties to its ability to interfere in some way with brain 5-HT, the similarity in chemical structure of these molecules suggesting that they might compete for a common receptor site on the neuronal membrane.

3.2 Basic Principles

3.2.1 The Neuron

It has been estimated that there are several hundred billion neurons that comprise the mammalian brain which, together with their surrounding glial cells, form a unique network of connections which are ultimately responsible for all thoughts and actions. While the glial cells may play a critical role in brain development, their main function in the mature brain is to maintain the structure and metabolic homeostasis of the neurons which they surround. A typical neuron consists of a cell body and an axonal projection through which information in the form of an action potential passes from the cell body to the axonal terminal (Figure 3.1). Information is received by the cell body via a complex array of dendrites which make contact with adjacent neurons.

The structural complexity and the number of dendritic processes vary according to the type of nerve cell and its physiological function. For example, the granule cells in the dentate gyrus of the hippocampus (a region of the brain which plays a role in short-term memory) receives and integrates information from up to 10 000 other cells in the vicinity.

The majority of the inputs to the granule cells are excitatory, each of which provides a small depolarizing current to the membrane of the cell body. The point of contact between the axonal projection from the neuron and an adjacent cell is termed the synapse, which under the electron microscope appears as a swelling at the end of the axon. Most synapses are excitatory and are usually located along the dendritic branches of the neuron. The contributions of the individual excitatory synapses are additive and, as a result, when an excitatory stimulus occurs a wave of depolarizing current travels down the axon to stimulate the adjacent cell body. However, some synapses are inhibitory, usually fewer in number and strategically located near the cell body. These synapses, when activated, inhibit the effects of any excitatory currents which may travel down the dendritic processes and thereby block their actions on the neuron.

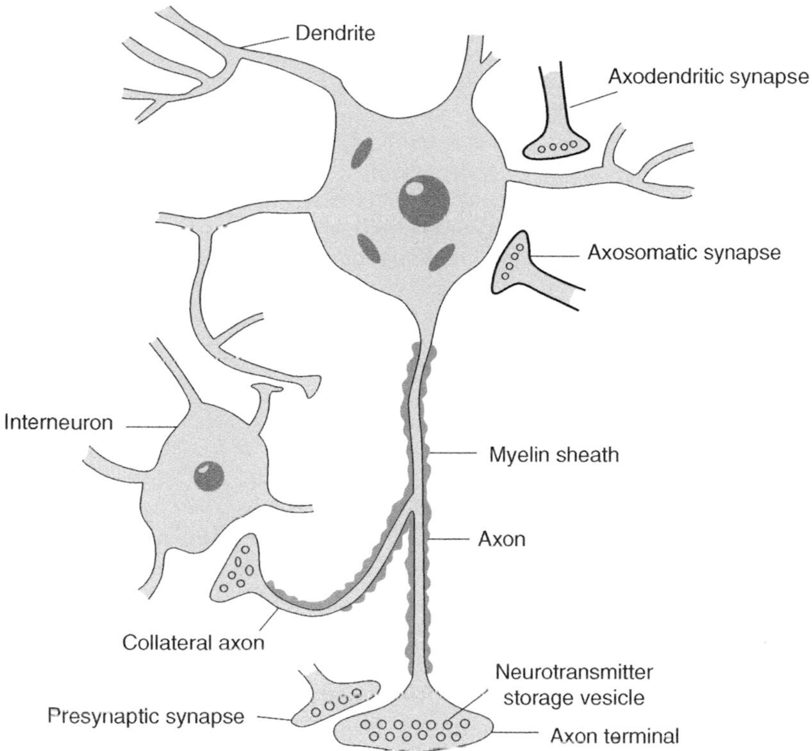

Figure 3.1 Diagram of a single neuron illustrating the contacts with surrounding neurons and with an adjacent interneuron. Whereas the neuron can release either excitatory or inhibitory neurotransmitters depending on its function and position in the brain, the interneuron is primarily inhibitory as its major neurotransmitter is gamma-aminobutyric acid (GABA).

3.2.2 The Nerve Impulse

Action potentials are the means whereby information is passed from one neuron to an adjacent neuron. The balance between the excitatory and inhibitory impulses determines how many action potentials will reach the axonal terminal and, by releasing a specific type of neurotransmitter from the terminal, influence the adjacent neuron. Thus, in summary, chemical information in the form of small neurotransmitter molecules released from axonal terminals is responsible for changing the membrane potential at their synaptic junctions which may occur on the dendrites or directly on the cell body. The action potential then passes down the axon to initiate the release of the neurotransmitter from the axonal terminal and thereby pass information on to any adjacent neurons.

The interaction between neurons is primarily by chemical transmission involving the release of neurotransmitter from the axon terminal. Box 3.1 summarizes criteria that should be fulfilled for a substance to be considered a neurotransmitter though there are exceptions. The activity of the individual neurons is influenced by adjacent neurons that, in the brain, form a neuronal network. This interneuronal communication is affected by synapses from adjacent neurons on the axon terminal, from the interneurons on the

Box 3.1 Criteria that must be fulfilled for a substance to be considered as a transmitter

- It should be present in a nerve terminal and in the vicinity of the area of the brain where it is thought to act.
- It should be released from the nerve terminal, generally by a calcium-dependent process, following stimulation of the nerve.
- The enzymes concerned in its synthesis and metabolism should be present in the nerve ending, or in the proximity of the nerve ending.
- It should produce a physiological response following its release by activating a postsynaptic receptor site. Such changes should be identical to those seen following the local application of the transmitter (e.g. by micro-ionophoresis).
- Its effects should be selectively blocked by a specific antagonist and mimicked by a specific agonist.

* These criteria should be regarded as general guidelines, not specific rules.

dendrites and from the axosomatic synapses, as the cell body. These synaptic contacts may be excitatory or inhibitory and thereby modulate the release of the neurotransmitter from the axon terminal. In the brain, the interneurons are mainly inhibitory and are therefore GABAergic. The nature of the receptor on the axon, dendrite or cell body is determined by the characteristic of the adjacent neuron. For example, 5-HT_{1A} receptors on the cell body acutely inhibit the axonal firing of a serotonergic neuron. Following the chronic administration of a serotonin reuptake inhibitor[1] (e.g. fluoxetine) and the inhibition of the serotonin transporter on the nerve terminal, serotonin accumulates in the synapse and dendrites. Serotonin then desensitizes the axosomatic inhibitory 5-HT_{1A} receptors, thereby facilitating the increased release of the neurotransmitter from the axonal terminal.

A summary of the main neurotransmitters and neuromodulators that have been identified in the mammalian brain is given in Table 3.1. The term neuromodulator is applied to those substances that may be released with a transmitter but which do not produce a direct effect on a receptor; a neuromodulator seems to work by modifying the responsiveness of the receptor to the transmitter.

The metabolic unity of the neuron requires that the same transmitter is released at all its synapses. This is known as Dale's Law (or principle), which Sir Henry Dale proposed in 1935. Dale's Law only applies to the presynaptic portion of the neuron, not the postsynaptic effects which the transmitter may have on other target neurons. For example, acetylcholine released at motor neuron terminals has an excitatory action at the motor neuron junction, whereas the same transmitter released at vagal nerve terminals has an inhibitory action on the heart; this is because the postsynaptic receptors are different, some are excitatory and some inhibitory. In addition to the diversity of action of a single transmitter released from a neuron, it has become well established that among invertebrates up to four different transmitters can occur in the same neuron.

In the vertebrate there is also increasing evidence from the seminal studies of Höckfelt and colleagues in Stockholm that some neurons in the central nervous system can also contain more than one transmitter. Such neurons appear to contain a peptide

[1] Serotonin reuptake inhibitor (SERT) is the Neuroscience-based Nomenclature term for a group of drugs that includes the selective serotonin reuptake inhibitors (SSRIs).

Table 3.1 Some of the neurotransmitters and neuromodulators that have been identified in the mammalian brain

Transmitter/ modulator	Distribution in the brain	Physiological effect	Involvement in disease
Noradrenaline	Most regions: long axons project from pons and brainstem	α_1-adrenoceptors – inhibitory β_1-adrenoceptors – inhibitory β_2-adrenoceptors – excitatory	Depression Mania
Dopamine	Most regions: short, medium and long axonal projections	D_1/D_5 receptors – stimulatory D_2 receptors – inhibitory D_3/D_4 receptors – ?	Schizophrenia Mania?
Serotonin	Most regions: project from pons and brainstem	5-HT_{1A} receptors – inhibitory 5-HT_2 receptors – ? 5-HT_3 receptors – ?	Depression Schizophrenia? Anxiety
Acetylcholine	Most regions: long and short axonal projections from basal forebrain	M_1 receptors – excitatory M_2 receptors – inhibitory N receptors – excitatory	Dementias Mania?
Adrenaline	Midbrain and brain	Possibly same as for noradrenaline	Depression?
GABA	Supraspinal interneurons	A-receptors – hyperpolarize membranes (inhibitory) B-receptors – inhibitory	Anxiety Seizures, epilepsy
Glycine	Spinal interneurons; modulates NMDA amino acid receptors in brain	Hyperpolarize membranes Strych-sensitive receptors – inhibitory Strych-insensitive receptors – excitatory	Seizures? Learning and memory Seizures?
Glutamate and aspartate	Long neurons	Quisqualate – depolarizes membranes NMDA – depolarizes membranes Kainate – depolarizes membranes	Seizures Schizophrenia?

Substances with a neuromodulatory effect on brain neurotransmitters by direct actions of specific receptors that modify the actions of the transmitters listed include: prostaglandins, adenosine, enkephalins, substance P, cholecystokinin, endorphins, endogenous benzodiazepine receptor ligands and possibly histamine. NMDA, *N*-methyl-D-aspartate; Strych, Strychnine.

within monoamine-containing terminals. Peptide transmitters (usually referred to as neuropeptides) are contained in specific types of storage vesicles. Thus, Dale's Law has to be modified to allow for the presence of neuropeptides in amine-containing nerve terminals, whose function is to act as a neuromodulator of the amine when it acts on the postsynaptic receptor.

3.2.3 Neurotransmitter Receptor Mechanisms

3.2.3.1 Role of Ion Channels in Nerve Conduction

Ion channels are large proteins which form pores through the neuronal membrane. The precise structure and function of the ion channels depend on their physiological function and distribution along the dendrites and cell body. These include specialized neurotransmitter-sensitive receptor channels. In addition, some ion channels are activated by specific metal ions such as sodium or calcium. The structure of the voltage-dependent sodium channel has been shown to consist of a complex protein with both a hydrophilic and a hydrophobic domain, the former domain occurring within the neuronal membrane while the latter domain occurs both inside and outside the neuronal membrane (Figure 3.2).

Four regions containing the hydrophilic units are arranged in the membrane in the form of a pore, with two units forming the remaining sides of the pore. This allows the sodium ions to pass in a regulated manner as the diameter of the pore, and the negative electrical charges on the amino acids which comprise the proteins lining the pore, determines the selectivity of the ion channel for sodium.

Advances in molecular biology have shown that the deoxyribonucleic acid (DNA) sequences which code for the proteins that make up the ion channels can enable the

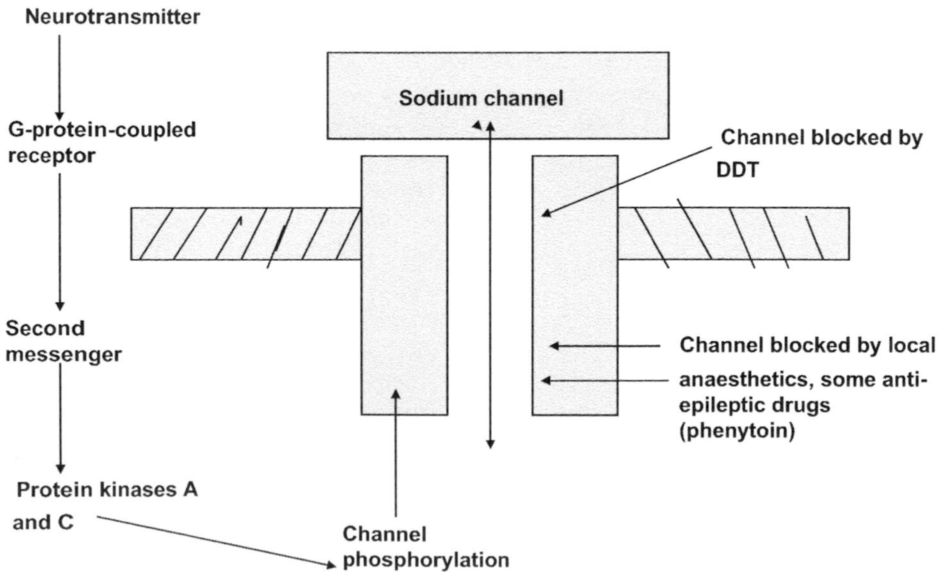

Figure 3.2 Diagram of a voltage-gated sodium channel. The movement of sodium ions through the channel is controlled by metabotropic receptors which are linked to G-proteins in the neuronal membrane. The opening of the ion channel follows the neurotransmitter-activated G-protein complex which, by a cascade of secondary messengers (such as cAMP and cGMP) and the protein kinases, leads to the phosphorylation of the sodium channel. This opens the channel to permit the repolarization of the neuron. The diagram also indicates how some drugs and toxins can close the channel by direct action and thereby inactivate it. Apart from some antiepileptic drugs, this is not a frequent action of psychotropic drugs.

protein structure to be modified by point mutations. By changing the structure of the protein by even a single amino acid it is now apparent that the properties of the ion channel also change, resulting, for example, in the opening and closing of the channel for longer or shorter periods of time or in carrying larger or smaller currents. As a consequence of molecular biological studies, it is now recognized that most ion channels of importance in neurotransmission are composed of three to five protein subunits. Their identification and characterization have now made it possible to map their location on specific neurons and to correlate their location with their specific function.

There are two major types of receptor which are activated by neurotransmitters. These are the ionotropic and metabotropic receptors. The former receptor type is illustrated by the amino acid neurotransmitter receptors for glutamate, gamma-aminobutyric acid (GABA) and glycine, and the acetylcholine receptors of the nicotinic type. These are examples of fast transmitters in that they rapidly open and close the ionic channels in the neuronal membrane. Peptides are often co-localized with these fast transmitters but act more slowly and modulate the excitatory or inhibitory actions of the fast transmitters. By contrast to the amino acid transmitters, the biogenic amine transmitters such as noradrenaline, dopamine and serotonin, and the non-amine transmitter acetylcholine, acting on the muscarinic type of receptor, activate metabotropic receptors. These receptors are linked to intracellular second messenger systems by means of G (guanosine triphosphate-dependent) proteins. These comprise the slow transmitters because of the relatively long time period required for their physiological response to occur. It must be emphasized however that a number of metabotropic receptors have recently been identified that are activated by fast transmitters so that the rigid separation of these receptor types is somewhat blurred. Over 50 different types of neurotransmitter have so far been identified in the mammalian brain and these may be categorized according to their chemical structure.

3.2.3.2 Presynaptic Mechanisms

Another important mechanism whereby the release of a neurotransmitter may be altered is by presynaptic inhibition. Initially this mechanism was thought to be restricted to noradrenergic synapses, but it is now known to occur at GABAergic, dopaminergic and serotonergic terminals also. In brief, it has been shown that at noradrenergic synapses the release of noradrenaline may be reduced by high concentrations of the transmitter in the synaptic cleft. Conversely, some adrenoceptor antagonists, such as phenoxybenzamine, have been found to enhance the release of the amine. It is now known that the subclass of adrenoceptors responsible for this process of autoinhibition are distinct from the 11 adrenoceptors which are located on blood vessels, on secretory cells and in the brain. These autoinhibitory receptors, or α_2-adrenoceptors, can be identified by the use of specific agonists and antagonists, for example clonidine and idazoxan or yohimbine, respectively. Drugs acting as specific agonists or antagonists on α_1-adrenoceptors, for example the agonist methoxamine and the antagonist prazosin, do not affect noradrenaline release by this mechanism.

The inhibitory effect of α_2-adrenoceptor agonists on noradrenaline release involves a hyperpolarization of the presynaptic membranes by opening potassium ion channels.

The reduction in the release of noradrenaline following the administration of an α_2-adrenoceptor agonist is ultimately due to a reduction in the concentration of free cytosolic calcium, which is an essential component of the mechanism whereby the synaptic vesicles containing noradrenaline fuse to the synaptic membrane before their release.

3.2.3.3 Synaptic Transmission

Box 3.2 summarizes the stages of neurotransmission in the brain. The sequence of events that result in neurotransmission of information from one nerve cell to another across the synapses begins with a wave of depolarization which passes down the axon and results in the opening of the voltage-sensitive calcium channels in the axonal terminal. These channels are frequently concentrated in areas which correspond to the active sites of neurotransmitter release. A large (up to 100 μM) but brief rise in the calcium concentration within the nerve terminal triggers the movement of the synaptic vesicles, which contain the neurotransmitter, towards the synaptic membrane. By means of specific membrane-bound proteins (such as synaptobrevin from the neuronal membrane and synaptotagrin from the vesicular membrane) the vesicles fuse with the neuronal membrane and release their contents into the synaptic gap by a process of exocytosis. Once released of their contents, the vesicle membrane is reformed and recycled within the neuronal terminal. This process is completed once the vesicles have accumulated more neurotransmitter by means of an energy-dependent transporter on the vesicle membrane (Box 3.2).

The neurotransmitters diffuse across the synaptic cleft in a fraction of a millisecond where, on reaching the postsynaptic membrane on an adjacent neuron, they bind to specific receptor sites and trigger physiological responses.

There is evidence that a number of closely related phosphoproteins associated with the synaptic vesicles, called synapsins, are involved in the short-term regulation of neurotransmitter release. These proteins also appear to be involved in the regulation of synapse formation, which allows the nerve network to adapt to long-term passage of nerve impulses.

Experimental studies have shown that the release of a transmitter from a nerve terminal can be decreased or increased by a variety of other neurotransmitters. For example, stimulation of 5-HT receptors on noradrenergic terminals can lead to an enhanced release of noradrenaline. While the physiological importance of such

Box 3.2 Stages of neurotransmission in the brain

1. Action potential depolarizes the axonal terminal.
2. Depolarization produces opening of voltage-dependent calcium channels.
3. Calcium ions diffuse into the nerve terminal and bind with specific proteins on the vesicular and neuronal membranes.
4. Vesicles move towards the presynaptic membrane and fuse with it.
5. Neurotransmitter is released into the synaptic cleft by a process of exocytosis and activates receptors on adjacent neurons.
6. The postsynaptic receptors respond either rapidly (ionotropic type) or slowly (metabotropic type) depending on the nature of the neurotransmitter.

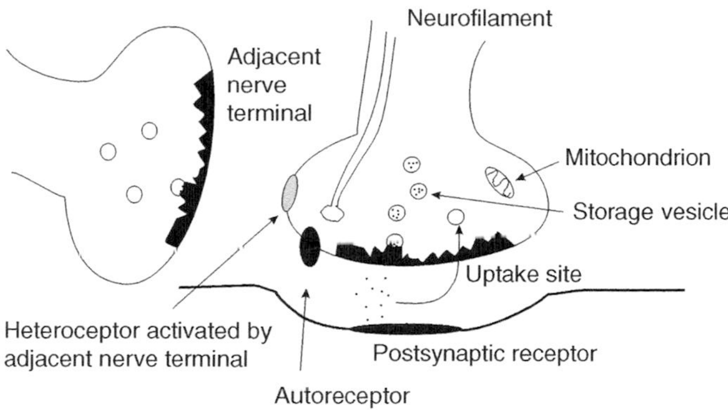

Figure 3.3 Relationship between pre- and postsynaptic receptors. Storage vesicles for the neurotransmitter are formed from the neurofilament network, which projects from the cell body to the nerve terminal. Following the reuptake of the transmitter by an energy-dependent, active transport process, the transmitter may be restored in empty vesicles or metabolized in the case of biogenic amines by monoamine oxidase. The enzyme is associated with mitochondria, which also may act as a source of energy in the form of adenosine triphosphate (ATP).

a mechanism is unclear, this could be a means whereby drugs could produce some of their effects. Such receptors have been termed heteroreceptors.

In addition to the physiological process of autoinhibition, another mechanism of presynaptic inhibition has been identified in the peripheral nervous system, although its precise relevance to the brain is unclear. In the dorsal horn of the spinal cord, for example, the axon terminal of a local neuron makes axo-axonal contact with a primary afferent excitatory input, which leads to a reduction in the neurotransmitter released. This is due to the local neuron partly depolarizing the nerve terminal, so that when the axon potential arrives, the change induced is diminished, thereby leading to a smaller quantity of transmitter being released. In the brain, it is possible that GABA can cause presynaptic inhibition in this way.

In summary, the release of a transmitter from its nerve terminal is not only dependent upon the passage of an action potential but also on the intersynaptic concentration of the transmitter and the modulatory effects of other neurotransmitters that act presynaptically on the nerve terminal. The interrelationship between these different processes is illustrated in Figure 3.3.

3.2.3.4 Postsynaptic Mechanisms

Neurotransmitters can either excite or inhibit the activity of a cell with which they are in contact. When an excitatory transmitter such as acetylcholine acting on a nicotinic receptor on a muscle or neuron, or an inhibitory transmitter such as GABA, is released from a nerve terminal it diffuses across the synaptic cleft to the postsynaptic membrane, where it activates the receptor site. Some receptors, such as the nicotinic receptor, are directly linked to sodium ion channels, so that when acetylcholine stimulates the nicotinic receptor, the ion channel opens to allow an exchange of sodium and potassium ions across the nerve membrane. Such receptors are called ionotropic receptors.

Acetylcholine can also have an inhibitory effect on the heart and this is because it acts on muscarinic receptors which work quite differently to ionotropic ones and are called metabotropic receptors. For example, the stimulation of β-adrenoceptors by noradrenaline results in the activation of adenylyl cyclase (also called adenylate cyclase) on the inner side of the nerve membrane. This enzyme catalyzes the breakdown of adenosine triphosphate (ATP) to the very labile, high-energy compound cyclic 3,5-adenosine monophosphate (cAMP). cAMP then activates a protein kinase which, by phosphorylating specific membrane proteins, opens an ion channel to cause an efflux of potassium and an influx of sodium ions. Many monoamine neurotransmitters are now thought to work by this receptor-linked second messenger system. In some cases, however, stimulation of the postsynaptic receptors can cause the inhibition of adenylyl cyclase activity. For example, D_2 dopamine receptors inhibit, while D_1 receptors stimulate, the activity of the cyclase. Such differences have been ascribed to the fact that the cyclase is linked to two distinct guanosine triphosphate (GTP) binding proteins in the cell membrane, termed G_1 and G_S. The former protein inhibits the cyclase, possibly by reducing the effects of the G_s protein which stimulates the cyclase. The relationship between the postsynaptic receptor and the second messenger system is illustrated in Figure 3.4.

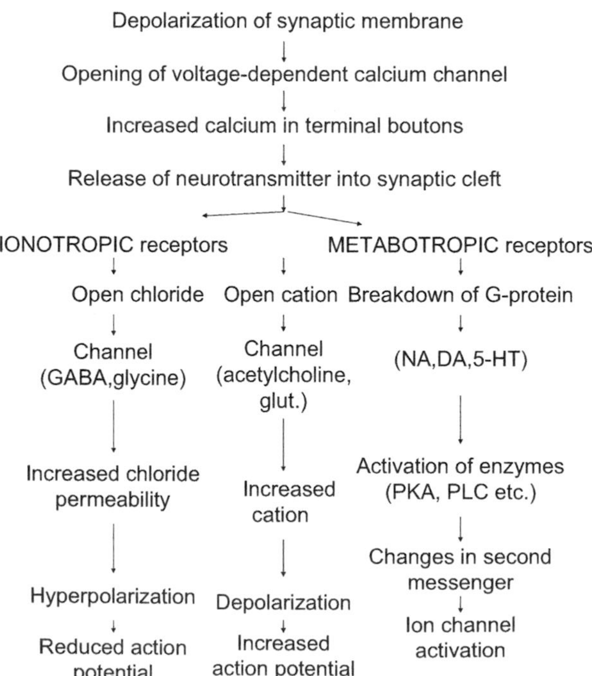

Figure 3.4 Slow and fast neurotransmitter receptors. Summary of the actions of some inhibitory and excitatory neurotransmitters on fast ionotropic receptors. The slow metabotropic receptors are activated by noradrenergic, dopaminergic and most types of serotonin receptors. Following the breakdown on the receptor-linked G-proteins, the metabotropic receptors cause a cascade of changes by activating enzymes such as phosphokinase A which initiate the synthesis of the high-energy second messengers such as cAMP and cGMP. These phosphorylate membrane proteins and thereby activate ion channels. Ionotropic receptors cause direct hyperpolarization (inhibitory transmitters) or depolarization (excitatory transmitters) by acting directly on the membrane-bound postsynaptic receptors.

Recently, there has been much interest in the possible role of the family of protein kinases which translate information from the second messenger to the membrane proteins. Many of these kinases are controlled by free calcium ions within the cell. It is now established that some serotonin (5-HT) receptors, for example, are linked via G-proteins to the phosphatidylinositol pathway which, by mobilizing membrane-bound diacylglycerol and free calcium ions, can activate a specific protein kinase C. This enzyme affects the concentration of calmodulin, a calcium sequestering protein that plays a key role in many intracellular processes. Box 3.3 summarizes the role of G-proteins in neurotransmission.

Structurally G-proteins are composed of three subunits termed α, β and γ. Of these, the α subunits are structurally diverse so that each member of the G-protein superfamily has a unique α subunit. Thus, the multiplicity of the α, and to a lesser extent the β and γ, subunits provides for the coupling of a variety of receptors to different second messenger systems. In this way, different receptor types are able to interact and regulate each other, thereby allowing for greater signal divergence, convergence or filtering than could be achieved solely on the basis of the receptor diversity.

The functional response of a nerve cell to a transmitter can change as a result of the receptor becoming sensitized or desensitized following a decrease or increase, respectively, in the concentration of the transmitter at the receptor site. Among those receptors that are directly coupled to ion channels, receptor desensitization is often rapid and pronounced. Most of the experimental evidence came initially from studies of the frog motor end plate where the desensitization of the nicotinic receptor caused by continuous short pulses of acetylcholine was associated with a slow conformational change in that the ion channel remained closed despite the fact that the transmitter was bound to the receptor surface. A similar mechanism has also been shown to occur in brain cells. For example, continuous exposure of β-adrenoceptors to an agonist such as noradrenaline decreases their function. It seems likely that the receptors are not lost but move into the cell membrane and are therefore no longer accessible to the transmitter.

The importance of the changes in receptor sensitivity to our understanding of the chronic effects of psychotropic drugs is discussed later. It must be emphasized that there is considerable integration and modulation between the various second messenger systems and these interactions lead to cross-talk between neurotransmitter systems.

Box 3.3 The role of G-proteins in neurotransmission

1. An excitatory neurotransmitter such as noradrenaline or serotonin acts on its receptor and activates the intermembrane G-protein by converting GDP to GTP, thereby linking the receptor to the second messenger system, usually adenylyl cyclase.
2. The second messenger, for example cAMP, then activates cAMP-dependent protein kinase which modulates the function of a broad range of membrane receptors, intracellular enzymes, ion channels and transcription factors.
3. An inhibitory neurotransmitter activates an inhibitory G-protein, thereby leading to a reduction in cAMP synthesis.
4. The termination of signal transduction results from the hydrolysis of GTP to GDP by GTPase, thereby returning the G-protein to its inactive form.

Such cross-talk between the second messenger systems may account for changes in the sensitivity of neurotransmitter receptors following prolonged stimulation by an agonist whereby a reduction in the receptor density is associated with a reduced physiological response (also termed receptor down-regulation).

In summary, neurotransmitters can control cellular events by two basic mechanisms. Firstly, they may be linked directly to sodium (e.g. acetylcholine acting on nicotinic receptors, or excitatory amino acids such as glutamate acting on glutamate receptors) or chloride (as exemplified by GABA) ion channels, thereby leading to the generation of fast excitatory postsynaptic potentials or inhibitory postsynaptic potentials, respectively. Secondly, the receptor may be linked to a second messenger system that mediates slower postsynaptic changes. These different mechanisms whereby neurotransmitters may change the activity of a postsynaptic membrane by fast, voltage-dependent mechanisms, or slower second messenger-mediated mechanisms, provide functional plasticity within the nervous system.

3.2.3.5 Co-transmission

During the mid-1970s, studies on such invertebrates as the mollusc *Aplysia* showed that at least four different types of transmitters could be liberated from the same nerve terminal. This was the first evidence that Dale's Law does not always apply. Extensive histochemical studies of the mammalian peripheral and central nervous systems followed, and it was shown that transmitters such as acetylcholine, noradrenaline and dopamine can coexist with such peptides as cholecystokinin, vasoactive intestinal peptide and gastrin-like peptides.

It is now evident that nerve terminals in the brain may contain different types of storage vesicles that store the peptide co-transmitters. Following their release, these peptides activate specific pre- or postsynaptic receptors, and thereby modulate the responsiveness of the membrane to the action of the traditional neurotransmitters such as acetylcholine or noradrenaline. In the mammalian and human brain, acetylcholine has been found to localize with vasoactive intestinal peptide; dopamine with cholecystokinin-like peptide, and 5-HT with substance P. In addition, there is increasing evidence that some peptides may act as neurotransmitters in their own right in the mammalian brain. These include the enkephalins, thyrotrophin-releasing hormone, angiotensin II, vasopressin, substance P, neurotensin, somatostatin and corticotrophin, among many others. With the advent of specific and sensitive immunocytochemical techniques, several more peptides are being added to this list every year. The similarities and differences between the peptide transmitters/co-transmitters and the 'classical' transmitters such as acetylcholine are summarized in Box 3.4. The peptide transmitters form the largest group of neurotransmitters in the mammalian brain, at least 40 different types having been identified so far. The mechanism governing their release differs from those of the non-peptide transmitters. Thus, peptides are stored in large, dense core vesicles which appear to require more prolonged and widespread diffusion of calcium into the nerve terminal before they can be released. In general, the peptide transmitters form part of the slow transmitter group as they activate metabotropic receptors. The neuropeptides will be discussed further later in this chapter.

3.2.3.6 An Overview of Neurotransmitter Receptors

The 1930s in the UK was probably best described as the Golden Age for classical pharmacology with the likes of Gaddum, Hill and Clark describing the quantitative

Box 3.4 Similarities and differences between the peptide transmitters/ co-transmitters

1. Both neurotransmitters and peptides show high specificity for their specific receptors.
2. Neurotransmitters produce physiological responses in nano- or micromolar (10^{-9} to 10^{-6}) concentrations, whereas peptides are active in picomolar (10^{-12}) concentrations.
3. Neurotransmitters bind to their receptors with high affinity but low potency, whereas peptides bind with very high affinity and high potency.
4. Neurotransmitters are synthesized at a moderate rate in the nerve terminal, whereas the rate of synthesis of peptides is probably very low.
5. Neurotransmitters are generally of low molecular weight (200 or below) whereas peptides are of intermediate molecular weight (1000 to 10 000 or occasionally more).

nature of the interaction of agonists and antagonists with specific receptors (mainly cholinergic and adrenergic) in isolated tissue preparations. In more recent times, with the development of molecular neurobiology and the identification of the protein structure of macromolecules, the precise nature of different classes of neurotransmitter receptors has been recognized. The technique of molecular cloning has enabled most types of receptors, for neurotransmitters and non-neurotransmitters, to be evaluated.

As a consequence of these advances, it is now recognized that all 'classical' neurotransmitters (such as the adrenergic, dopaminergic, serotonergic, GABAergic, glutamatergic, histaminergic) have multiple receptor targets. This is important for the functional expression of the neurotransmitters. Thus, a single, small neurotransmitter molecule can exert different effects on different regions of the brain depending on the type of receptor, and its component signalling system. Serotonin, for example, can initiate either fast or slow excitatory responses depending on whether it activates one of the different types of slow metabotropic (5-HT_{1A}, 5-HT_{2A} etc.) or the fast 5-HT_3 ionotropic receptor. Similarly, noradrenaline can induce excitatory or inhibitory responses by activating α_1- or α_2-adrenoceptors, respectively, both via G-proteins. In addition to the classified neurotransmitter receptors, there are also orphan receptors which include receptors on neuronal membranes and in the nucleus but for which specific ligands have so far not been identified. However, it is apparent that whereas the neurotransmitter receptors are found on neuronal membranes where they are accessible to the neurotransmitter following its release from the postsynaptic site, some steroids and the thyroid hormones activate specific receptors located intracellularly, particularly in the nucleus.

How can a receptor be defined? Not only is it essential for the macromolecule as a putative receptor to be capable of specifically binding the transmitter but it is also essential that the binding results in a functional response. This would usually be expressed in some form of biological response. In the laboratory, this process can be examined by measuring the changes in the second messenger signalling molecules (cAMP, cGMP, diacylglycerol etc.) which are produced in response of the receptor to the neurotransmitter or specific ligand. Alternatively, microelectrodes can be inserted into the cell and the electrophysiological changes in the cell, or tissue, recorded in response to the application of the ligand. The number and nature of the binding sites or the receptors can then be determined experimentally by means of the Scatchard plot analysis and its distribution determined by immunohistochemistry. The following lists the characteristics that a receptor should exhibit before it can be authenticated:

1. A dose–response curve for the binding of different concentrations of the ligand to the receptor should demonstrate *saturability*. Specific receptor binding of a neurotransmitter to a receptor for example should exhibit high affinity but low capacity. Conversely, non-specific binding of a ligand would be demonstrated by a low affinity but a high capacity.
2. It is essential to demonstrate the specificity of the binding by determining how the putative receptor behaves in the presence of different chemically similar agonists and antagonists. Complications can arise if the ligand exists in stereoisomeric states. In most cases, only the laevorotatory isomer should bind preferentially. It is also necessary to be aware that some ligands show a high affinity for glass and plastic surfaces! Ideally the specificity should be linked to the changes in the biological response.
3. The binding of the ligand should be *reversible* and removable from the receptor surface in chemically uncharged state. This is important to distinguish ligand–receptor from ligand–enzyme interactions.
4. Finally, the isolation and chemical identification of the receptor should be determined. Now, with microbiological techniques, the gene can also be isolated.

3.2.3.7 Signal Transduction Mechanisms

The neurotransmitter and hormonal receptors which translate the signals from the pre- to the postsynaptic membrane are of four major types (Box 3.5).

The most rapid transfer of information is due to the ionotropic receptors (also known as ligand-gated receptors) and exemplified by the *N*-methyl-D-aspartate (NMDA) glutamate receptor, the $GABA_A$ receptor and the $5\text{-}HT_3$ receptor. The essential features of the ionotropic receptor is a number of subunits arranged around a central pore, which, once the receptor has been activated by a ligand, opens to permit the passage of Na^+, K^+ and Ca^{++} ions (for an excitatory response) or Cl^- ions (for an inhibitory response). The NMDA and $5\text{-}HT_3$ receptors are examples of excitatory ionotropic types while the $GABA_A$ receptor is an example of an inhibitory type; as a consequence, the membranes are either depolarized or hyperpolarized, respectively.

Box 3.5 **Summary of the ways in which neurotransmitters activate the different types of receptors**

Type 1: Cell surface ionotropic receptors exemplified by nicotinic acetylcholine receptors, *N*-methyl-D-aspartate glutamate receptors, $GABA_A$ receptors and $5\text{-}HT_3$ receptors.

Type 2: Cell surface metabotropic receptors coupled to G-proteins. These are generally modulatory or enhancing signal transduction as exemplified by cholinergic, adrenergic, dopaminergic, serotonergic, metabotropic glutamatergic, opiate, peptidergic and some purinergic receptors.

Type 3: Steroids, thyroid, vitamin D are lipophilic and act on nuclear receptors where they bind to DNA and stimulate transcription via gene expression.

Type 4: The tyrosine kinase receptors are cell membrane bound and activated by insulin and numerous growth factors (e.g. brain-derived neurotrophic factor, nerve growth factor). With the ligand, the receptor dimerizes the kinase then autophosphorylates it.

The most frequent type of membrane-bound receptor for neurotransmitters is the metabotropic receptor. These are coupled to G-proteins and only respond relatively slowly to the actions of the transmitter (seconds to minutes). The metabotropic receptors consist of seven hydrophobic transmembrane domains linked to hydrophilic groups. Muscarinic cholinergic, adrenergic, dopaminergic, serotonergic, metabotropic glutamatergic, opiate, peptidergic and purinergic receptors are all of the metabotropic type.

The *G-proteins* comprise a large family of at least 22 different types of G-protein α subunits, 5 types of β subunit and 12 γ subunits. The G-proteins are classified into G_s, G_i, G_q and G_{12} groups which respond differently to the ligands activating the G-protein-linked metabotropic receptor. Thus, activation of the G_s subunit increases the activity of adenylyl cyclase, opens calcium channels and inhibits sodium channels. The G_i subunit inhibits adenylyl cyclase and closes calcium channels but opens potassium channels and activates cyclic 'guanosine' monophosphate (cGMP) phosphodiesterase and possibly phospholipase A_2. Phospholipase C acts on second messengers in many neurotransmitter processes and is the effector for the G_q protein. The involvement of the G_{12} protein in signalling mechanisms is presently unclear for a variety of intracellular proteins, thereby resulting in neuronal growth repair etc. The importance of the G-protein-coupled metabotropic receptors is demonstrated by the observation that about 50% of all clinically effective drugs modulate such receptors.

3.2.3.8 Changes in Receptor Function Following Chronic Activation

Under normal physiological conditions neurons are switched 'on' and 'off' according to need by a process of feedback inhibition. This is illustrated for the monoamine neurotransmitters in which a rise in the intersynaptic concentration of the transmitter results in the activation of the presynaptic autoreceptor that inhibits the rate-limiting enzyme that synthesizes the neurotransmitter.

Receptor desensitization is another mechanism whereby the activity of a neuron can be regulated. A rapid mechanism involves the phosphorylation of the receptor, a process occurring in seconds or at most minutes. A more sustained desensitization, taking minutes or even hours involves the movement of the receptor from the surface of the cell into the membrane by a process of endocytosis. In some cases, this can result in the irreversible down-regulation of the receptor. Sustained receptor desensitization can occur following the prolonged activation of the receptor by an agonist (*receptor down-regulation*) whereas, conversely, prolonged administration of an antagonist can lead to an increase (*up-regulation*) of the receptor on the neuronal membrane, thereby resulting in sensitization of the receptor. This is thought to occur to dopamine D_2 receptors following the chronic administration of typical antipsychotic drugs such as haloperidol.

3.3 Principle Neurotransmitters in the Brain

3.3.1 Acetylcholine

3.3.1.1 Synthesis and Metabolism

Acetylcholine has been implicated in learning and memory in all mammals, and the gross deficits in memory found in patients suffering from Alzheimer's disease have been ascribed to a defect in central cholinergic transmission. This transmitter has also been implicated in the altered mood states found in mania and depression, while many different classes of psychotropic drugs are known to have potent anticholinergic properties which undoubtedly have adverse consequences for brain function.

Acetylcholine is synthesized within the nerve terminal from choline (from both dietary and endogenous origins) and acetyl coenzyme A (acetyl CoA) by the enzyme choline acetyltransferase. Acetyl CoA is derived from glucose and other intermediates via the glycolytic pathway and ultimately the pyruvate oxidase system, while choline is selectively transported into the cholinergic nerve terminal by an active transport system. There are believed to be two main transport sites for choline, the high-affinity site being dependent on sodium ions and ATP and which is inhibited by membrane depolarization, while the low-affinity site operates by a process of passive diffusion and is therefore dependent on the intersynaptic concentration of choline. The uptake of choline by the high-affinity site controls the rate of acetylcholine synthesis, while the low-affinity site, which occurs predominantly in cell bodies, appears to be important for phospholipid synthesis. As the transport of choline by the active transport site is probably optimal, there seems little value in increasing the dietary intake of the precursor in an attempt to increase acetylcholine synthesis. This could be one of the reasons why feeding choline-rich diets (e.g. lecithin) to patients with Alzheimer's disease has been shown to be ineffective.

As with all the major transmitters, acetylcholine is stored in vesicles within the nerve terminal from which it is released by a calcium-dependent mechanism following the passage of a nerve impulse. The rate of release of acetylcholine is influenced by the M_2 autoreceptor which, on stimulation by acetylcholine, inhibits the release of the transmitter. The M_1 receptors are most abundant in the cortex, hippocampus and striatum and are involved in cognitive function and, via their presynaptic action, decrease the release of dopamine. The M_3 and M_4 receptors are widely expressed in the brain. The M_3 receptors inhibit dopamine release and enhance the synthesis of nitric oxide (NO); M_3 receptors also increase food intake. M_4 receptors function as autoreceptors and heteroreceptors that mediate inhibition of some neurotransmitter release in the brain but can facilitate dopamine release; M_4 receptors facilitate analgesia. M_5 receptors also facilitate dopamine release and augment drug-seeking behaviours and reward. There is also evidence that M_5 receptors are involved in the dilation of cerebral arteries and arterioles.

It is well established that acetylcholine can be catabolized by both *acetylcholinesterase* (AChE) and *butyrylcholinesterase* (BChE); these are also known as 'true' and 'pseudo' cholinesterase, respectively. Such enzymes may be differentiated by their specificity for different choline esters and by their susceptibility to different antagonists. They also differ in their anatomical distribution, with AChE being associated with nervous tissue while BChE is largely found in non-nervous tissue. In the brain there does not seem to be a good correlation between the distribution of cholinergic terminals and the presence of AChE, choline acetyltransferase having been found to be a better marker of such terminals. An assessment of cholinesterase activity can be made by examining red blood cells, which contain only AChE, and plasma, which contains only BChE. Of the anticholinesterases, the organophosphorus derivatives such as diisopropylfluorophosphonate are specific for BChE, while drugs such as ambenonium inhibit AChE. Most cholinesterase inhibitors inhibit the enzyme by acylating the esteratic site on the enzyme surface.

Physostigmine and neostigmine are examples of *reversible anticholinesterases* which are in clinical use. Both act in similar ways but they differ in terms of their lipophilicity, the former being able to penetrate the blood–brain barrier while the latter cannot. The main clinical use of these drugs is in the treatment of glaucoma and myasthenia gravis.

Irreversible anticholinesterases include the organophosphorus inhibitors and ambenonium, which irreversibly phosphorylate the esteratic site. Such drugs have few clinical uses but have been developed as insecticides and nerve gases. Besides blocking the muscarinic receptors with atropine sulphate in an attempt to reduce the toxic effects that result from an accumulation of acetylcholine, the only specific treatment for organophosphate poisoning would appear to be the administration of 2-pyridinealdoxime methiodide, which increases the rate of dissociation of the organophosphate from the esteratic site on the enzyme surface.

3.3.1.2 Anatomical Distribution of the Central Cholinergic System

The cholinergic pathways in the mammalian brain are extremely diffuse and arise from cell bodies located in the hindbrain and the midbrain. Of these areas, there has been considerable interest of late in the nucleus basalis magnocellularis of Meynert because this region appears to be particularly affected in some patients with familial Alzheimer's disease. As the projections from this area innervate the cortex, it has been speculated that a disruption of the cortical cholinergic system may be responsible for many of the clinical features of the illness.

3.3.1.3 Cholinergic Receptors

Sir Henry Dale noticed that the different esters of choline elicited responses in isolated organ preparations which were similar to those seen following the application of either of the natural substances muscarine (from poisonous toadstools) or nicotine. This led Dale to conclude that, in the appropriate organs, acetylcholine could act on either *muscarinic* or *nicotinic receptors*. Later it was found that the effects of muscarine and nicotine could be blocked by atropine and tubocurarine, respectively. Further studies showed that these receptors differed not only in their molecular structure but also in the ways in which they brought about their physiological responses once the receptor has been stimulated by an agonist. Thus, nicotinic receptors were found to be linked directly to an ion channel and their activation always caused a rapid increase in cellular permeability to sodium and potassium ions. Conversely, the responses to muscarinic receptor stimulation were slower and involved the activation of a second messenger system which was linked to the receptor by G-proteins.

3.3.1.3.1 Muscarinic Receptors

To date, five subtypes of these receptors have been cloned. Before this, studies relied on the pharmacological effects of the muscarinic antagonist pirenzepine which was shown to block the effect of several muscarinic agonists. These receptors were termed M_1 receptors to distinguish them from those receptors for which pirenzepine had only a low affinity and therefore failed to block the pharmacological response. These were termed M_2 receptors. More recently, M_3, M_4 and M_5 receptors have been identified which, like the M_1 and M_2 receptors, occur in the brain. The M_1 and M_3 receptors are located postsynaptically in the brain whereas the M_2 and M_4 receptors occur presynaptically where they act as inhibitory autoreceptors that inhibit the release of acetylcholine.

The M_2 and M_4 receptors are coupled to the inhibitory G_i protein which reduces the formation of cAMP within the neuron. By contrast, the M_1, M_3 and M_5 receptors are coupled to the stimulatory G_s protein which stimulates the intracellular hydrolysis of the phosphoinositide messenger within the neuron. Drugs are often used to dissect the function of receptors. This has been partially successful with the M receptors. Thus, the agonist and antagonist for the M_1 receptor can be exemplified by oxotremorine and pirenzepine, respectively. A specific M_2 antagonist is AF DX 116 while the antagonists for the M_3 receptors are illustrated by dimethylphenyl silafenidol and tiotropium.

The cholinergic system has the capacity to adapt to changes in the physiological environment of the brain. Thus, the density of the cholinergic receptors is increased by antagonists and decreased by agonists. The reduction in the density of the receptors is a result of their rapid internalization into the neuronal membrane (receptor sequestration) followed by their subsequent destruction. This phenomenon may have a bearing on the long-term loss of efficacy of cholinomimetic drugs and anticholinesterases which are currently used in the symptomatic treatment of Alzheimer's disease.

While it is widely believed that the relapse in the response to treatment is due to the continuing neurodegenerative changes in the brain which are unaffected by cholinomimetic drugs, it is also possible that such treatments could impair cholinergic function by causing an increased sequestration and destruction of muscarinic receptors. The possible detrimental effect of cholinergic agonists on memory is supported by the observation that the chronic administration of physostigmine or oxotremorine to rats decreases the number of muscarinic receptors and leads to an impairment of memory when the drugs are withdrawn. Conversely, chronic treatment with a cholinergic antagonist such as atropine increases the number of cholinergic receptors and leads to a memory improvement when the drug is withdrawn. Whether these effects in experimental animals are relevant to the clinical situation in which cholinomimetic agents are administered for several months is unknown. Although other transmitters such as noradrenaline, serotonin and glutamate are involved, there is now substantial evidence to suggest that muscarinic receptors play a key role in learning and memory. It is well established that muscarinic antagonists such as atropine and scopolamine impair memory and learning in man and that their effects can be reversed by anticholinesterases. Conversely, muscarinic agonists such as arecholine improve some aspects of learning and memory. However, cholinomimetic drugs such as carbachol which stimulate the inhibitory autoreceptors impair memory by blocking the release of acetylcholine in the hippocampus and cortex; the selective autoreceptor antagonist secoverine has the opposite effect.

3.3.1.3.2 Nicotinic Receptors

Following studies of the actions of specific agonists and antagonists on the nicotinic receptors from skeletal muscle and sympathetic ganglia, it was soon apparent that not all nicotinic receptors are the same. The heterogeneity of the nicotinic receptors was further revealed by the application of molecular cloning techniques. This has led to the classification of nicotinic receptors into N-m receptors and N-n receptors, the former being located in the neuromuscular junction, where activation causes end-plate depolarization and muscle contraction, while the latter are found in the autonomic ganglia (involved in ganglionic transmission), adrenal medulla (where activation causes catecholamine release) and in the brain, where their precise physiological importance is currently unclear. Of the specific antagonists that block these receptor subtypes, and which have clinical applications, tubocurarine and related neuromuscular blockers inhibit the N-m type receptor while the antihypertensive agent trimethaphan blocks the N-n receptor; an agonist for the N-n receptor is dimethylphenylpiperazinium (DMPP).

In contrast to the more numerous muscarinic receptors, much less is known about the function of nicotinic receptors in the brain. In addition to their distribution in the neuromuscular junction, ganglia and adrenal medulla, nicotinic receptors occur in a high density in the neocortex. Nicotinic receptors are of the ionotropic type which, on stimulation by acetylcholine, nicotine or related agonists, open to allow the passage of sodium ions into the neuron. There are structural differences between the peripheral and neuronal receptors, the former being pentamers composed of two α and one β, γ and δ subunits while the latter consist of groups of five single α and β subunits. It is now known that there are at least four variants of the α and two of the β subunits in the brain. In Alzheimer's disease it would appear that there is a selective reduction in the nicotinic receptors which contain the α_3 and α_4 subunits.

Unlike the muscarinic receptors, repeated exposure of the neuronal receptors to nicotine, both in vivo and in vitro, results in an increase in the number of receptors; similar changes are reported to occur after physostigmine is administered directly into the cerebral ventricles of rats. These changes in the density of the nicotinic receptors are accompanied by an increased release of acetylcholine. Following the chronic administration of physostigmine, however, a desensitization of the receptors occurs. Functionally, nicotinic receptors appear to be involved in memory formation; in clinical studies it has been shown that nicotine can reverse the effects of scopolamine on short-term working memory and both nicotine and arecholine have been shown to have positive, though modest effects on cognition in patients with Alzheimer's disease.

Activation of the nicotinic receptors by the natural agonist nicotine produces dose-dependent effects, low doses producing analgesia while higher doses (toxic) lead to tremor and seizures. The changes are linked to the release of other transmitters such as dopamine (the rewarding effect of nicotine) and other biogenic amines and excitatory amino acids. High doses of nicotine act directly on the medulla oblongata causing stimulation which if prolonged can cause depression and respiratory failure (nicotine poisoning).

3.3.2 The Catecholamines: An Overview

3.3.2.1 Synthesis and Metabolism

The catecholamines are monoamine neurotransmitters that contain a catechol group (benzene with two hydroxyl side groups next to each other) and a side-chain amine. The main members are noradrenaline, adrenaline and dopamine.

One of the first demonstrations of the central monoamine pathways in the mammalian brain was by a fluorescence technique in which thin sections of the animal brain were exposed to formaldehyde vapour which converted the amines to their corresponding fluorescent isoquinolines. The distribution of these compounds could then be visualized under the fluorescent microscope. Using this technique, it has been possible to map the distribution of the noradrenergic, dopaminergic and serotonergic pathways in the animal and human brain.

Much attention has been paid to the catecholamines noradrenaline and dopamine following the discovery that their depletion in the brain leads to profound mood changes and locomotor deficits. Thus, noradrenaline has been implicated in the mood changes associated with mania and depression, while an excess of dopamine has been implicated in schizophrenia and a deficit in Parkinson's disease.

Noradrenaline (also termed norepinephrine) is the main catecholamine in postganglionic sympathetic nerves and in the central nervous system; it is also released from the adrenal gland together with adrenaline. Recently, *adrenaline* has also been shown to be a transmitter in the hypothalamic region of the mammalian brain so, while the terms 'noradrenergic' and 'adrenergic' are presently used interchangeably, it is anticipated that they will be used with much more precision once the unique functions of adrenaline in the brain have been established.

The catecholamines are formed from the dietary amino acid precursors phenylalanine and tyrosine. Phenylalanine is converted to tyrosine, which is converted to L-dopa, which is converted to dopamine and finally this is converted to noradrenaline. The rate-limiting step in the synthesis of the catecholamines from tyrosine is tyrosine hydroxylase, so that any drug or substance which can reduce the activity of this enzyme, for example by reducing the concentration of the tetrahydropteridine cofactor, will reduce the rate of synthesis of the catecholamines. Under normal conditions tyrosine hydroxylase is maximally active, which implies that the rate of synthesis of the catecholamines is not in any way dependent on the dietary precursor tyrosine. Catecholamine synthesis may be reduced by *end product inhibition*. This is a process whereby catecholamine present in the synaptic cleft, for example as a result of excessive nerve stimulation, will reduce the affinity of the pteridine cofactor for tyrosine hydroxylase and thereby reduce synthesis of the transmitter. The experimental drug alpha-methyl-*para*-tyrosine inhibits the rate-limiting step by acting as a false substrate for the enzyme, the net result being a reduction in the catecholamine concentrations in both the central and peripheral nervous systems.

Drugs have been developed which specifically inhibit the L-aromatic amino acid decarboxylase step (L-dopa converted to dopamine) in catecholamine synthesis and thereby lead to a reduction in catecholamine concentration. Carbidopa and benserazide are examples of decarboxylase inhibitors which are used clinically to prevent the peripheral catabolism of L-dopa (levodopa) in patients being treated for Parkinsonism. As these drugs do not penetrate the blood–brain barrier they will prevent the peripheral decarboxylation of dopa so that it can enter the brain and be converted to dopamine by dopamine beta-oxidase (also called dopamine beta-hydroxylase).

Dopamine beta-oxidase inhibitors (the enzyme that catalyzes the conversion of dopamine to noradrenaline) are only of limited clinical use at the present time, probably due to their relative lack of specificity. Diethyldithiocarbamate and disulfiram are examples of drugs that inhibit dopamine beta-oxidase by acting as copper-chelating agents and thereby reducing the availability of the cofactor for this enzyme. Whether their clinical use in the treatment of alcoholism is in any way related to the reduction in brain catecholamine concentrations is uncertain. The main action of these drugs is to inhibit liver aldehyde dehydrogenase activity, thereby leading to an accumulation of acetaldehyde, and the onset of nausea and vomiting, should the patient drink alcohol.

Two enzymes are concerned in the metabolism of catecholamines, namely *monoamine oxidase (MAO)*, which occurs mainly intraneuronally, and *catechol-O-methyltransferase (COMT)*, which is restricted to the synaptic cleft. The process of oxidative deamination is the most important mechanism whereby all monoamines are inactivated (i.e. the catecholamines, 5-HT and the numerous trace amines such as phenylethylamine and tryptamine). MAO occurs in virtually all tissues, where it appears to be bound to the outer mitochondrial membrane. Whereas there are several specific and therapeutically useful MAO inhibitors (MAOIs), inhibitors of COMT have found less application. This is mainly due to the fact that at most only 10% of the monoamines released from the nerve terminal are catabolized by this enzyme. However, the COMT inhibitors entacapone and tolcapone have recently become available for the treatment of Parkinsonism.

3.3.2.2 Catecholamine Transporters

There are two main groups of monoamine transporters, namely the vesicular amine transporter (VMAT-2) and the neuronal membrane transporters for noradrenaline (NET) and dopamine (DAT).

The VMAT-2 transporter, located on intracellular amine storage vesicle membranes, is activated by pH and potential gradients that are established by ATP-dependent proton translocase. For each amine molecule transported, two H^+ ions are extruded. The alkaloid reserpine owes its pharmacological effects to its ability to block the VMAT-2 transporter, thereby contributing to the depletion of catecholamines from peripheral and central sympathetic nerve terminals. The VMAT-2 transporter has been cloned and consists of 12 transmembrane units. The neuronal membrane transporters are members of an extended family sharing common structural features (e.g. the 12 transmembrane helices) but they have a greater substrate specificity than the vesicular transporters. These transporters carry dopamine, noradrenaline, adrenaline and serotonin.

In addition to the neuronal transporters, there are also three extraneuronal transporters that transport a number of endogenous and exogenous substrates. The extraneuronal amine transporter (ENT, also termed uptake 2 transporter) is an organic cation transporter found in the brain cortex (and widely in non-nervous tissue such as the kidney and liver) and associated with the glia: the transporter has a greater affinity for adrenaline over noradrenaline and dopamine. The other organic cation transporters (OCT_1 and OCT_2) are not so widely distributed as ENT. Only OCT_2 has been detected in the brain, where it has been located in glial cells in dopamine-rich regions and some non-adrenergic areas of the brain. All three cation transporters can transport catecholamines in addition to a variety of organic acids and include serotonin, histamine and the trace amine spermine. The latter trace amines may have a neurotransmitter function in some vertebrates.

3.3.3 Noradrenaline

3.3.3.1 Physiological Functions of Central Noradrenergic Pathways

The main physiological functions of the noradrenergic system in the brain are in memory, alertness/vigilance, reinforcement, the regulation of the sleep–wake cycle, and as an important neurotransmitter in the stress/anxiety response. However, noradrenaline also plays a vital role in the control of cerebral blood flow and in brain metabolism. The central control of noradrenaline function by the locus coeruleus is reflected in the behavioural vigilance which increases in response to external environmental stimuli but is reduced in response to tonic vegetative behaviours.

3.3.3.2 Anatomy of the Central Noradrenergic System

This is not so diffusely distributed as the cholinergic system. In the lower brainstem, the neurons innervate the medulla oblongata and the dorsal vagal nucleus, which are thought to be important in the central control of blood pressure. Other projections arising from cell bodies in the medulla descend to the spinal cord where they are believed to be involved in the control of flexor muscles. However, the most important noradrenergic projections with regard to psychological functions arise from a dense collection of cells in the locus coeruleus and ascend from the brainstem to innervate the thalamus, dorsal hypothalamus, hippocampus and cortex. The ventral noradrenergic bundle occurs caudally and ventrally to the locus coeruleus and terminates in the hypothalamus and the subcortical limbic regions. The dorsal bundle arises from the locus coeruleus and innervates the cortex. Both the dorsal and ventral noradrenergic systems appear to be involved psychologically in drive and motivation, in mechanisms of reward and in rapid eye movement (REM) sleep. As such processes are severely deranged in the major affective disorders it is not unreasonable to speculate that the central noradrenergic system is defective in such disorders.

3.3.3.3 Regulation of the Noradrenergic Terminal

The storage vesicles are formed in the noradrenergic cell body and transported down the axon to the axon terminal. The amine content of the vesicles in the cell body is relatively low (10–100 μg per g vesicles) but in the terminal region the amine content is increased up to 30-fold. Under the electron microscope the terminal vesicle appears as the dense core granules.

Noradrenaline is synthesized from tyrosine by tyrosine hydroxylase. The rate of synthesis of noradrenaline by this enzyme is regulated by calcium ions and by feedback inhibition by noradrenaline: dopamine, the precursor of noradrenaline, can also reduce the activity of tyrosine hydroxylase. Tyrosine hydroxylase is also regulated by calcium ions and the nerve impulse.

The release of noradrenaline is regulated by autoreceptors. In addition to the α_2-adrenoceptor, β_2-adrenoceptors, nicotinic cholinergic receptors and angiotensin II receptors can also modulate noradrenaline release.

The metabolism of noradrenaline is controlled by MAO-A and COMT. Whereas MAO-A is mainly located intraneuronally and associated with the outer mitochondrial membrane, COMT is mainly extraneuronal. The major metabolites formed are normetanephrine (from COMT) and methoxyhydroxyphenylglycol (MHPG) from MAO-A + COMT.

3.3.4 Adrenaline

3.3.4.1 The Central Adrenergic System

It is only relatively recently that sensitive techniques (such as HPLC and GC-mass fragmentography) have been developed to demonstrate the presence of specific 'adrenergic', as distinct from noradrenergic, tracks in the mammalian brain. These are concentrated in three areas. Thus, the C1 neurons are co-located with the noradrenergic cells in the lateral tegmentum while the C2 neurons are associated with the noradrenergic neurons of the dorsal medulla. These adrenergic tracks project to the hypothalamus. The C3 adrenergic neurons occur on the midline region. Adrenergic pathways innervate the locus coeruleus, spinal cord and dorsal motor nucleus of the vagus. Despite the evidence of the presence of adrenergic pathways in the brain, precise information on their physiological role is presently uncertain. It has been suggested that adrenaline plays a role in the central control of blood pressure and, via its input to the hypothalamus, in neuroendocrine regulation.

3.3.4.2 Adrenergic Receptors

Ahlquist, in 1948, first proposed that adrenaline could produce its diverse physiological effects by acting on different populations of adrenoceptors, which he termed α and β receptors. This classification was based upon the relative selectivity of adrenaline for the α receptors and isoprenaline for the β receptors; drugs such as phentolamine were found to be specific antagonists of the α receptors, and propranolol for the β receptors.

3.3.4.2.1 Alpha-Adrenoceptors

It later became possible to separate these main groups of receptors further, into α_1 and α_2; based on the selectivity of the antagonists prazosin, the antihypertensive agent that blocks α_1-adrenoceptors, and yohimbine, which is an antagonist of α_2-adrenoceptors.

At one time it was thought that α_1-adrenoceptors were postsynaptic and the α_2 type were presynaptic and concerned with the inhibitory control of noradrenaline release. Indeed, novel antidepressants such as mianserin, and more recently the highly selective α_2-adrenoceptor antagonist idazoxan, or yohimbine, were thought to act by stimulating the release of noradrenaline from central noradrenergic synapses. It is now established, however, that the α_2-adrenoceptors also occur postsynaptically, and that their stimulation by such specific agonists as clonidine leads to a reduction in the activity of the vasomotor centre, thereby leading to a decrease in blood pressure. Conversely, the α_2-adrenoceptor antagonist yohimbine enhances noradrenaline release.

The α_1-adrenoceptors are excitatory in their action, while the α_2-adrenoceptors are inhibitory, these activities being related to the different types of second messengers or ion channels to which they are linked. These receptors hyperpolarize presynaptic membranes by opening potassium ion channels and thereby reduce noradrenaline release. Conversely, stimulation of α_1-adrenoceptors increases intracellular calcium via the phosphatidylinositol cycle, which causes the release of calcium from its intracellular stores; protein kinase C activity is increased as a result of the free calcium, which then brings about further changes in the membrane activity.

Both types of receptor occur in the brain as well as in vascular intestinal smooth muscle: α_1-adrenoceptors are found in the heart whereas α_2-adrenoceptors occur on the platelet membrane (stimulation induces aggregation) and nerve terminals (stimulation inhibits release of the transmitter). It is now recognized that there are several subtypes of α_1- and α_2-adrenoceptors, but their precise function is unclear. Table 3.2 presents a simplified summary of subtypes of adrenergic receptors.

3.3.4.2.2 Properties of Adrenoceptors

The adrenergic receptors are divided into three major classes according to their coupling to the G receptors. Thus, the α_1-adrenoceptors activate phospholipase C via the G_q

Table 3.2 Characteristics of subtypes of adrenergic receptors

Alpha$_1$	Alpha$_2$	Beta$_1$	Beta$_2$
Adrenergic –	[–] release	–	[+] release
Cholinergic –	[–] release	–	–
Brainstem –	[–] sympathetic Outflow	–	–
Second messenger			
[+] PLC [+] IT [+] DAG [+] Ca^{++}	[–] cAMP [–] Ca^{++} channels [+] K^{+} channels	[+] cAMP	[+] cAMP
Selective agonists			
Phenylephrine Methoxamine	Clonidine	Dobutamine	Salbutamol Terbutaline Clenbuterol
Selective antagonists			
Prazocin Doxazocin	Yohimbine Idozoxan	Atenolol Metoprolol	Butoxamine

Alpha$_1$-adrenoceptors are subdivided into α_{1A}, α_{1B}, α_{1C}, α_{1D}.
Alpha$_{1B}$- and α_{1C}-adrenoceptors are located in the brain.
Beta$_2$-adrenoceptors are subdivided into β_1, β_2 and β_3.
Beta$_1$-adrenoceptors are located in the brain.
DAG, diacylglycerol; IT, inositol triphosphate; PLC, phospholipase C.

receptor while the α_2-adrenoceptors, via the G_i receptor, activate potassium channels, decrease adenylyl cyclase and reduce the activity of calcium channels. Activation of the β-adrenoceptors increases adenylyl cyclase activity and L-type Ca^{++} channels via G_s receptors.

The α_1-adrenoceptors are involved in the control of calcium mobilization into vascular tissue and central neurons by stimulating phospholipases A, C and D. By contrast, the α_2-adrenoceptors are negatively linked to adenylyl cyclase via the G_i proteins. This protein is activated by GTP but inhibits the generation of cAMP by the catalytic unit. In peripheral nerves, the α_2-adrenoceptors are mainly on presynaptic terminals where they inhibit the impulse-dependent release of noradrenaline. Thus, the α_1-adrenoceptors have primarily an excitatory effect on central neurotransmission whereas the α_2-adrenoceptors have largely an inhibitory action.

3.3.4.2.3 Beta-Adrenoceptors

The β-adrenoceptors regulate many physiological actions including heart rate and contractility, smooth muscle relaxation, metabolism and postsynaptic changes in central sympathetic neurons. The β-adrenoceptors differ from the α-adrenoceptors in that prolonged stimulation leads to receptor desensitization of the receptor function. This process is associated with an uncoupling of the receptor from the adenylyl cyclase signalling pathway and by a decrease in the number of β-adrenoceptors on the outer neuronal membrane (down-regulation of the receptor!). Physiologically it is apparent that the β-adrenoceptors are primarily excitatory in their action.

So far three subtypes of β-adrenoceptors have been identified and cloned. They differ in their distribution, the β_1 type being found in the heart, the β_2 in the lung, smooth muscle, skeletal muscle and liver, while the β_3 type occurs in adipose tissue. There is evidence that β_2-adrenoceptors occur on the lymphocyte membrane also but the precise function there is unknown. The antihypertensive drugs propranolol and atenolol are clinically effective example of β-adrenoceptor antagonists while terbutaline and salbuterol are agonists.

All the β-adrenoceptor subtypes are linked to adenylyl cyclase as the second messenger system. It seems that both β_1- and β_2-adrenoceptor types occur in the brain and that their activation leads to excitatory effects. Of particular interest to the psychopharmacologist is the finding that chronic antidepressant treatment leads to a decrease in the functional responsiveness of the β-adrenoceptors in the brain, and in the density of these receptors on lymphocytes, which coincides with the time necessary for the therapeutic effects of the drug to manifest. Such changes have been ascribed to the drugs affecting activity of the G-proteins that couple the receptor to the cyclase subunit. The term 'down-regulation' of the β-adrenoceptor has been used to describe this phenomenon and was one of the first pieces of experimental evidence to suggest why there was a delay of several days, or even weeks, before the therapeutic effects of antidepressants became established.

3.3.5 Dopamine

The central dopaminergic system is considerably more complex than the noradrenergic system. This may reflect the greater density of dopamine-containing cells, which have been estimated to be 30–40 000 in number compared with 10 000 noradrenaline-containing cells. There are several dopamine-containing nuclei as well as specialized dopaminergic neurons localized within the retina and the olfactory bulb. The dopaminergic system within the mammalian brain can be divided according to the length of the efferent fibres into the intermediate and long length systems. The intermediate length systems include the tuberoinfundibular system, which projects from the arcuate and periventricular nuclei into the intermediate lobe of the pituitary and the median eminence. This system is responsible for the regulation of such hormones as prolactin. The interhypothalamic neurons send projections to the dorsal and posterior hypothalamus, the lateral septal nuclei and the medullary periventricular group, which are linked to the dorsal motor nucleus of the vagus; such projections may play a role in the effects of dopamine on the autonomic nervous system.

The *long length fibres* link the ventral tegmental and substantia nigra dopamine-containing cells with the neostriatum (mainly the caudate and the putamen), the limbic cortex (the medial prefrontal, cingulate and entorhinal areas) and with limbic structures such as the septum, nucleus accumbens, amygdaloid complex and piriform cortex. These projections are usually called the *mesocortical and mesolimbic dopaminergic systems*, respectively, and are functionally important in psychotic disorders and in the therapeutic effects of antipsychotic drugs. Conversely, changes in the functional activity of the dopaminergic cells, together with the GABAergic interneurons, are responsible for movement disorders such as Parkinson's and Huntingdon's disease.

3.3.5.1 Dopaminergic Pathways and Their Function

The dopaminergic pathways innervate several major regions of the brain which determine their functional importance. The *nigrostriatal system* has received particular attention because of its involvement in the control of cognition, emotion and motor pathways. For over 50 years, it has been realized that the nigrostriatal system is defective in patients with Parkinson's disease leading to the typical symptoms of bradykinesia, rigidity and tremor. However, the dopaminergic innervation of the limbic and cortical regions is also affected in Parkinson's disease. The symptoms of Parkinson's disease do not appear until approximately 80% of the dopaminergic neurons in the substantia nigra are lost.

The mesolimbic dopaminergic system, particularly from the ventral tegmental area to the nucleus accumbens is primarily involved in reward, attention and motivational behaviour. For this reason, the mesolimbic dopaminergic system is linked to addictive types of behaviour, by reinforcing and sensitizing the dopaminergic system to the addictive stimulus. In addition, in schizophrenia, there is evidence from imaging studies that the mesolimbic dopaminergic system is hyperactive in contrast to the mesocortical dopaminergic system, which is hypoactive.

Following the seminal research of Hornykiewicz and colleagues in Austria in the early 1960s into the role of the dysfunctional dopaminergic system in the causation of Parkinson's disease, until recently the primary emphasis has been placed on the mechanism whereby the loss of dopaminergic neurons in the basal ganglia causes the clinical characteristics of the disorder. It is now apparent that the basal ganglia function is to regulate the flow of information from the cortex to the motor neurons of the spinal cord. In addition to the dopaminergic neurons that innervate the areas of the basal ganglia, the interneurons that modulate the dopaminergic neurons of the striatum contain acetylcholine and neuropeptides such as substance P and dynorphin. Such interneurons have a slow modulatory effect on dopaminergic signalling.

The striatal neurons influence other brain regions via direct and indirect pathways. The direct striatal pathway projects to the substantia nigra reticulata and the globus pallidus interna, regions that relay information to the thalamus and thence to the cortex. The main neurotransmitter of the direct pathway is GABA, an inhibitory transmitter, so the net effect of the direct pathway is to increase the excitatory input to the cortex via the thalamus.

The indirect striatal pathway comprises neurons which connect to the globus pallidus externa which innervates the subthalamic nucleus; this pathway then connects to the substantia nigra and globus pallidus but whereas the first part of the indirect pathway is mediated by GABA, the final input to the substantia nigra/globus pallidus is mediated by the excitatory transmitter glutamate. The net effect of activation of the indirect pathway is to reduce the excitatory impact of the thalamus on the cortex.

In addition to the primary role dopamine plays in the basal ganglia, the dopamine D_1 and D_2 receptors are of primary importance. Thus, the striatal neurons that control the direct pathway are D_1 receptors while those controlling the indirect pathway are of the inhibitory D_2 type. Thus, under normal physiological conditions, dopamine released from the striatum activates the direct and reduces the indirect pathway. The depletion of dopamine in Parkinson's disease increases the inhibitory outflow from the substantia nigra/pars compacta to the thalamus and thereby reduces the excitatory influence on the cortex.

Knowledge of the non-dopaminergic neurotransmitters in the functioning of the basal ganglia could be important in the development of novel drug treatments for Parkinson's disease. Clearly, muscarinic receptor antagonists, such as benztropine and benzhexol, have been used clinically for many decades but their effects are, at best, modest. Future approaches may involve drugs that modify the GABAergic function. However, most of the recently introduced anti-Parkinson's main drugs are aimed at the dysfunctional dopaminergic system using dopamine agonists, such as pramipexole and ropinirole, COMT inhibitors (entacapone, tolcapone) or MAO-B inhibitors (rasagiline, selegiline). Dopamine is metabolized predominantly by MAO-B, hence the use of these specific inhibitors to preserve the neurotransmitter in patients with Parkinsonism.

The mesocortical dopaminergic system consists of the prefrontal and neocortex which are connected to subcortical limbic regions. The prefrontal cortex is particularly important in cognitive function with respect to attention, selecting the important stimuli, comparing the incoming stimuli to internal cues and in devising abstract concepts. This region of the brain is particularly highly developed in *Homo sapiens* and the dopaminergic pathway may be involved in short-term memory so it is perhaps not surprising to find that, in schizophrenia, this region of the brain (as indicated by glucose and oxygen utilization studies) is subfunctional. This may account for the negative and cognitive deficits which characterize the disorder. The reduction in the dopaminergic pathways in this region may contribute to the increased activity of the dopaminergic pathways in the mesolimbic system and be of importance in the pathology of attention deficit hyperactivity disorder (ADHD) and Tourette syndrome

The fourth important dopaminergic pathway links the hypothalamus and thalamus to the spinal pathways, sometimes termed the *diencephalic system* (or the tuberoinfundibular dopaminergic system). This pathway projects from the arcuate nucleus and periventricular nucleus of the hypothalamus to the median eminence. The main physiological function of this pathway is the control (inhibition) of prolactin secretion. Dopamine is released into the hypophyseal portal system, a system of blood vessels that connects the hypothalamus to the anterior pituitary. Dopamine diffuses out of the blood vessels and inhibits lactototroph cells in the pituitary and so reduces their release of prolactin. The tuberohypophyseal dopamine pathway also inhibits the secretion of the alpha melanocyte stimulating hormone and proopiomelanocortin-like peptides. The importance of this pathway becomes evident when the D_2 receptors at the posterior pituitary are blocked by antipsychotics, for example, haloperidol. The secretion of melanocyte stimulating hormone is increased, leading to increased melanin pigments in the skin when exposed to sunlight, and there is a disruption of gonadotrophin secretion associated with infertility.

An improvement in understanding the functional importance of the central dopaminergic system in psychiatric and neurological disorders has been derived from advances in imaging techniques. Positron emission tomography (PET) and single photon emission computed tomography (SPECT) studies, using radiotracers, have enabled presynaptic sites to be studied, including the dopamine transporters on neuronal terminals and storage vesicles (DAT and VMAT, respectively) and the key enzyme involved in dopamine synthesis. Similarly, postsynaptic sites can be labelled for the distribution of D_1

and D_2 receptor type and an estimate made of the dopamine release by determining the displacement of the radiolabel by endogenous dopamine. The properties and side effects of drugs acting on the dopaminergic pathways have assisted in the understanding of the function and changes in dopamine in health and disease.

3.3.5.2 Dopamine Receptors

Traditionally, two main families of dopamine receptors have been characterized in the mammalian brain, termed D_1 and D_2. However, within these families are different subtypes of receptor (see Table 3.3) and this will be discussed further later on. The D_1/D_2 subtyping largely arose in response to the finding that while all types of clinically useful antipsychotics inhibit dopaminergic transmission in the brain, there is a poor correlation between reduction in adenylyl cyclase activity, believed to be the second messenger linked to dopamine receptors, and the clinical potency of the drugs. This was particularly true for the butyrophenone series (e.g haloperidol) which are known to be potent antipsychotics and yet relatively poor at inhibiting adenylyl cyclase. Detailed studies of the binding of ^{3}H-labelled haloperidol to neuronal membranes showed that there was a much better correlation between this therapeutic potency of an antipsychotic and its ability to displace this ligand from the nerve membrane. This led to the discovery of two types of dopamine receptor that are both linked to adenylyl cyclase but whereas the D_1 receptor is positively linked (activates) to the cyclase, the D_2 receptor is negatively linked (inhibits). It was also shown that the D_1 receptor is approximately 15 times more sensitive to the action of dopamine than the D_2 receptor.

Five major subtypes of dopamine receptors have now been cloned. These are divided into two main groups, D_1 and D_2, respectively. The D_1 receptors consist of D_1 and D_5

Table 3.3 Key features of dopamine receptors

	Dopamine 1 group (D_1 and D_5)		Dopamine 2 group (D_{2s}, D_{2l}, D_3 and D_4)		
Second messengers	[+] cAMP		[–] cAMP		
	[+] PIP_2 hydrolysis		[+] K^+ currents		
	Ca^{++} mobilization		[–] voltage Ca^{++} currents		
	[+] PKC				
Agonist	Dihydrexidine		Quinpirole		
Antagonist	SCH 39166		(–) Sulpiride, raclopride		
Distribution in brain	D_1	D_5	D_2	D_3	D_4
Cortex (arousal, mood)	+++	–	++	–	+
Limbic (emotion, stereotypy)	+++	+	++	+	+
Striatum (prolactin)	+++	+	++	+	+
Hypothal./pituitary	–	–	++	+	–

PIP_2, phosphatidylinositol (4,5)-bisphosphate; PKC, protein kinase C.

types and are positively linked to the adenylyl cyclase second messenger system, while the D_2 group consists of the D_2, D_3 and D_4 receptors which are negatively linked to the adenylyl cyclase system. The D_1 receptors have been subdivided into the D_{1A} and D_{1B} types and are coded by genes located on chromosomes 5 and 4, respectively. Several selective antagonists of the D_1 receptors have been developed (for example SCH 31966, SCH 23390 and SKF 83959), none of which has so far been developed for therapeutic use.

Apomorphine is an agonist at both the D_1 and D_2 receptors. From the pathological viewpoint, a malfunction of the D_1 receptors has been implicated in the negative symptoms of schizophrenia but as there is a close interaction between these receptor types it is difficult to conclude whether the changes seen in schizophrenia are attributable to a primary decrease in D_1 receptor function or an increase in D_2 receptor function. The function of the D_5 receptors is unclear; these receptors, though widely distributed in the brain, are only present in a relatively low density in comparison to the other dopamine receptor types.

The D_2 receptor types, besides being subdivided into D_3 and D_4 types, are further divided into the D_2 long and D_2 short forms. D_2 antagonists, in addition to virtually all therapeutically active antipsychotics, also include such novel drugs as raclopride, eticlopride and spiperone while quinpirole is an example of a specific D_2 receptor agonist. The latter drugs are not available for therapeutic use. A malfunction of the D_2 receptors has been associated with psychosis, extrapyramidal side effects and hyperprolactinaemia.

There is still some controversy over the precise anatomical location of the dopamine receptor subtypes, but there is now evidence that the D_2 receptors are located presynaptically on the corticostriatal neurons and postsynaptically in the striatum and substantia nigra. Conversely, the D_1 receptors are found presynaptically on nigrostriatal neurons, and postsynaptically in the cortex. It is possible to differentiate these receptor types on the basis of their agonist and antagonist affinities. In addition to these two subtypes, there is also evidence that the release of dopamine is partially regulated by feedback inhibition operating via the dopamine autoreceptor. With the development of D_1 and D_2 agonists, however, emphasis has become centred on the pharmacological characteristics of the specific drug in order to determine whether an observed effect is mediated by D_1 or D_2 receptors. It is now apparent that dopamine receptors with the same pharmacological characteristics do not necessarily produce the same functional responses at the same receptor. For example, D_2 receptors are present in both the striatum and the nucleus accumbens but cause an inhibition of adenylyl cyclase only in the striatum. Furthermore, recent studies indicate that dopamine receptors can influence cellular activities through mechanisms other than adenylyl cyclase. These may include direct effects on potassium and calcium channels, as well as modulation of the phosphatidylinositol cycle. To complicate the picture further, D_1 and D_2 receptors have opposite effects on some behaviours (e.g. chewing in rats) but are synergistic in causing other behaviours (e.g. locomotor activity and some types of stereotypy). The precise clinical importance of these interactions is unclear.

The densities and functional activities of dopamine receptors have been shown to change in response to the brain. Abrupt withdrawal of an antipsychotic following its prolonged administration is frequently associated with tardive dyskinesia, a disorder which may be partly due to the sudden activation of supersensitive dopamine receptors. Despite the appeal of this hypothesis, it should be emphasized that many other factors, such as brain damage and prior exposure to tricyclic antidepressants, may also predispose patients to this condition.

Dopamine has been implicated in a number of psychiatric conditions of which schizophrenia and the affective disorders are the most widely established. With regard to the change in dopamine receptor activity in disease, there is some evidence from post-mortem studies that the density of D_2 receptors is increased in the mesocortical areas of the schizophrenic brain, and in putamen and caudate nucleus in antipsychotic-free patients. PET of schizophrenic patients has, however, failed to confirm these findings but several studies have found increased dopamine synthesis measured using ^{18}F-dopa uptake. There is also evidence that the link between the D_1 and D_2 receptors is defective in some patients with diseases in which the dopaminergic system might be involved. Thus, the well-known loss of dopaminergic function in patients with Parkinson's disease is associated with a compensatory rise in the density of postsynaptic D_1 and D_2 receptors. The long-term treatment of Parkinson's disease with L-dopa reduces the receptor density to normal (so-called receptor 'down-regulation'). Similarly, the densities of D_1 and D_2 receptors are reduced in the striata of patients with Huntington's chorea, as is the linkage between these receptors.

The human D_3 gene has produced two variants, D_3 and D_{3s}. So far there do not appear to be any selective agonists or antagonists of the D_3 receptor which enable the function of this receptor to be clearly distinguished from that of the D_2 receptor. The D_3 receptors are located in the ventral and limbic regions of the brain but absent from the dorsal striatum. This suggests that specific antagonists of the D_3 receptors may be effective antipsychotics but without causing extrapyramidal side effects. The D_4 receptor has eight polymorphic variants in the human. However, even though several specific antagonists of this receptor type have been developed and shown to have antipsychotic activity in animal models of schizophrenia, the clinical findings have been disappointing. Because of the high density of the D_4 receptors in the limbic cortex and hippocampus, but their absence from the motor regions of the brain, it was anticipated that such drugs have antipsychotic efficacy without the motor side effects. In support of this view, it has been shown that the atypical antipsychotic clozapine has a high affinity for the D_4 receptors; other studies have also indicated that many of the atypical, and some of the typical, antipsychotics have similar affinities for these receptors. In addition to the postsynaptic receptors, dopamine autoreceptors also exist on the nerve terminals, dendrites and cell bodies. Experimental studies have shown that stimulation of the autoreceptors in the somatodendritic region of the neuron slows the firing rate of the dopaminergic neuron while stimulation of the autoreceptors on the nerve terminal inhibits both the release and the synthesis of the neurotransmitter. Structurally, the autoreceptor appears to be of the D_2 type. While several experimental compounds have been developed that show a high affinity for autoreceptors, to date there is no convincing evidence for their therapeutic efficacy.

3.3.6 Serotonin (5-Hydroxytryptamine)

5-HT, together with noradrenaline, has long been implicated in the aetiology of depression. Indirect evidence has been obtained from the actions of drugs which can either precipitate or alleviate the symptoms of depression and from the analysis of body fluids from depressed patients. More recently, development of novel anxiolytic drugs which appear to act as specific agonists for a subpopulation of 5-HT receptors (the 5-HT_{1A} type) suggests that this amine may also play a role in anxiety. To add to the complexity of the role of 5-HT, there is evidence that impulsive behaviour, as exhibited by patients with obsessive-compulsive disorders and bulimia, may also involve an abnormality of the serotonergic system. Whether 5-HT is primarily involved in this disparate group of disorders or whether it functions to 'fine-tune' other neurotransmitters which are causally involved is presently unclear.

5-HT is an indoleamine transmitter which is synthesized within the nerve ending from the amino acid L-tryptophan. Tryptophan, which is obtained from dietary and endogenous sources, is unique among the amino acids concerned in neurotransmitter synthesis in that it is about 85% bound to plasma proteins. This means that it is only the unbound portion that can be taken up by the brain and is therefore available for 5-HT synthesis. The pathway that leads to the synthesis of 5-HT in the periphery (e.g. in platelets and the enterochromaffin cells of the gastrointestinal tract) or in the brain is relatively minor. In the periphery, tryptophan may be metabolized in the liver by tryptophan pyrolase via the *kynurenine* pathway which is activated by stress-induced glucocorticoids such as cortisol. Thus, natural or synthetic glucocortiocoids can induce an increase in the activity of the pathway and thereby increase the catabolism of plasma-free tryptophan. Other steroids, such as the oestrogens used in the contraceptive pill, can also induce pyrolase activity. This has been proposed as a mechanism whereby the contraceptive pill, particularly the high oestrogen type of pill which has now largely been withdrawn, may predispose some women to depression by reducing the availability of free tryptophan for brain 5-HT synthesis. Despite the plausible belief that the availability of plasma-free tryptophan determines the rate of brain 5-HT synthesis, it now seems unlikely that such an important central transmitter would be in any way dependent on the vagaries of diet to sustain its synthesis! Nevertheless, changes in liver tryptophan pyrolase activity, which may be brought about by endogenous steroids, insulin, changes in diet and by the circadian rhythm, may play a secondary role in regulating brain 5-HT synthesis. Furthermore, there is evidence that a tryptophan-deficient diet can precipitate depression in depressed patients who are in remission. Thus, when such patients are given a drink containing high concentrations of amino acids but which lacks tryptophan, a depressive episode rapidly occurs.

In recent years the tryptophan-kynurenine pathway has received considerable attention because of its link to inflammatory changes, particularly where they affect the brain. It is known that this pathway occurs widely in both the periphery and brain and is controlled by the enzyme indoleamine dioxygenase (IDO). Thus, when the liver tryptophan dioxygenase/pyrolase is activated by glucocorticoids due to stress associated with psychological trauma, depression, anxiety disorders etc., the macrophages and monocytes in the periphery, and the microglia in the brain are also activated to release pro-inflammatory mediators (cytokines, chemokines) which activate indoleamine dioxygenase. Activation of the tryptophan-kynurenine pathway thereby contributes to the decrease in the synthesis of 5-HT from tryptophan. In addition, some of the kynurenine intermediates from the pathway increase oxidative stress and also have neurotoxic properties which could contribute to neurodegenerative changes in the brain.

Free tryptophan is transported into the brain and nerve terminal by an active transport system which it shares with tyrosine and a number of other essential amino acids. On entering the nerve terminal, tryptophan is hydroxylated by tryptophan hydroxylase, which is the rate-limiting step in the synthesis of 5-HT. Tryptophan hydroxylase is not bound in the nerve terminal and optimal activity of the enzyme is only achieved in the presence of molecular oxygen and a pteridine cofactor. Unlike tyrosine hydroxylase, tryptophan hydroxylase is not usually saturated by its substrate. This implies that if the brain concentration rises then the rate of 5-HT synthesis will also increase. Conversely, the rate of 5-HT synthesis will decrease following the administration of experimental drugs such as *para*-chlorophenylalanine, a synthetic amino acid which irreversibly inhibits the enzyme. *Para*-chloramphetamine also inhibits the activity of this enzyme, but this experimental drug also increases 5-HT release and delays its reuptake, thereby leading to the appearance of the so-called 'serotonin syndrome', which in animals is associated with abnormal movements, body posture and temperature.

Following the synthesis of 5-hydroxytryptophan (5-HTP) by tryptophan hydroxylase, the enzyme aromatic amino acid decarboxylase (also known as 5-HTP, or DOPA, decarboxylase) then decarboxylates the amino acid to 5-HT. L-Aromatic amino acid decarboxylase is approximately 60% bound in the nerve terminal and requires pyridoxal phosphate as an essential enzyme. There is evidence that the compartmentalization of 5-HT in the nerve terminal is important in regulating its synthesis. It appears that 5-HT is synthesized in excess of normal physiological requirements and that some of the amine which is not immediately transported into the storage vesicle is metabolized by intraneuronal MAO. Another autoregulatory mechanism governing 5-HT synthesis relies on the rise in the intersynaptic concentration of the amine stimulating the autoreceptor of the nerve terminal.

5-HT is metabolized by the action of MAO by a process of oxidative deamination to yield 5-hydroxyindoleacetic acid (5-HIAA). In the *pineal gland*, 5-HT is *O*-methylated to form melatonin. The physiological importance of this transmitter in the regulation of the oestrous cycle in ferrets would appear to be established, and there is now substantial evidence that in man it drives the circadian rhythm which regulates the sleep–wake cycle, and endocrine, immune and neurotransmitter rhythmicity. The disturbance in the circadian rhythm is a common occurrence in depression, bipolar disorder and the anxiety disorders.

3.3.6.1 Synthesis and Release of Serotonin

Tryptophan is converted to 5-HT by the rate-limiting enzyme tryptophan hydroxylase (TrpOH'lase) followed by the aromatic amino acid decarboxylase (AADC). Once formed, serotonin is stored in vesicles by the action of the vesicular monoamine transporter. Like all monoamine neurotransmitters, serotonin is released into the synaptic cleft in the presence of calcium ions where it can activate postsynaptic serotonergic receptors. The rate of release of serotonin from the axonal terminal is controlled by the 5-HT$_{1B/1D}$ autoreceptor and also by the somatodendritic 5-HT$_{1A}$ receptors. The main mechanism for the termination of action of serotonin is by the uptake transporter on the presynaptic membrane.

3.3.6.2 Anatomical Distribution of Serotonin Pathways

Neurons containing 5-HT are restricted to clusters of cells around the midline of the pons and upper brainstem; this is known as the raphé area of the midbrain. In addition, according to studies of rat brain, cells containing 5-HT are located in the area postrema and in the caudal locus coeruleus, which forms an anatomical basis for a direct connection between the serotonergic and noradrenergic systems. The more caudal groups of cells in the raphé project largely to the medulla and the spinal cord, the latter projections being physiologically important in the regulation of pain perception at the level of the dorsal horn. Conversely, the more rostral cells of the dorsal and median raphé project to limbic structures such as the hippocampus and, in particular, to innervate extensively the cortex. Unlike the noradrenergic cortical projections, there does not appear to be an organized pattern of serotonergic terminals in the cortex. In general, it would appear that the noradrenergic and serotonergic systems are co-localized in most limbic areas of the brain, which may provide the anatomical basis for the major involvement of these transmitters in the affective disorders.

3.3.6.3 5-Hydroxytryptamine Receptors

Gaddum and Picarelli, in 1957, were the first investigators to provide evidence for the existence of two different types of 5-HT receptor in peripheral smooth muscle. These receptors were termed D (for dibenzyline, an α_1-adrenoceptor antagonist which also blocked 5-HT receptors) and M (for morphine, which blocked the contractile response mediated through the myenteric plexus in the intestinal wall). Studies undertaken in the 1980s revealed the existence of multiple binding sites for 5-HT. The 5-HT_D receptor was shown to have the characteristics of the 5-HT_2 receptor, while the M receptor has been shown to be identical to the 5-HT_3 receptor in the brain and gastrointestinal tract.

5-HT contributes to the regulation of a variety of psychological functions which include mood, arousal, attention, impulsivity, aggression, appetite, perception and cognition. In addition, serotonin plays a crucial role in regulating the sleep–wake cycle and in the control of brain maturation. It is therefore understandable that a dysfunction of sleep frequently occurs in schizophrenia, depression, alcoholism and in phobic stat. Undoubtedly, interest in the role of the serotonergic system in psychiatry has been stimulated by the therapeutic success of the selective serotonin reuptake inhibitors (SSRIs) which have proven to be effective in alleviating the symptoms of many of these disorders.

The complexity of the serotonergic system lies in the number of different serotonin receptors within the brain. These are classified into seven distinct types that are heterogeneously distributed in the brain, each with its specific physiological function (see Table 3.4). The function of the serotonin receptors is a reflection of their structure. Thus the 5-HT_3 receptors are ionotropic in nature whereas the remainder are metabotropic, coupled to specific G-proteins and share a common seven membrane domain structure. These receptors have been cloned and their physiological activity shown to be associated with the activation of either phospholipase C (5-HT_2 receptors) or adenylyl cyclase but they inhibit the function of this second messenger system. Although the precise physiological activity of the different serotonin receptors is still the subject of ongoing studies, links between specific receptor subtypes and their possible involvement in specific neurological and psychiatric disorders have been identified. For example, the antimigraine drug sumatriptan decreases headache by activating the inhibitory 5-HT_{1D} receptors located presynaptically on perivascular nerve fibres. This blocks the release of pain-causing neuropeptides and the conduction in the trigeminal vascular neurons.

With regard to the 5-HT_{1A} receptors, agonists such as buspirone and ipsapirone act as anxiolytics while the antidepressant effects of the SSRIs have been associated with an indirect reduction in the activity of the 5-HT_{1A} receptors. Conversely the sexual side-effects of the SSRIs are attributed to their indirect action on 5-HT_{2C} receptors which follows the enhanced serotonergic function. These receptors may also be involved in the regulation of food intake, which could help to explain the antibulimic action of the SSRIs.

Table 3.4 Serotonin receptor subtypes and their functions

	Signal transduction	Function	Location	Agonist	Antagonist
5-HT_{1A}	Inhibits AC	Autoreceptor	Raphé, hippocampus	Flesinoxan, buspirone	Pindolol, asenapine
5-HT_{1B} & 5-HT_{1D}	Inhibits AC	Autoreceptor; cerebral vasoconstriction	Substantia nigra cranial blood vessels	Eltoprazine, sumatriptan	Metergoline, methiothepin, ritanserin
5-HT_{1E}	Inhibits AC	?Memory	Cortex, striatum	Tryptamine	Methiothepin
5-HT_{2A}	Activates PLC	Platelet aggregation; neural excitation	Cortex, platelets, smooth muscle	α-methyl serotonin, LSD, bufotenin	Ketanserin, pimavanserin, asenapine
5-HT_{2B}	Activates PLC	Contraction	Stomach fundus cortex	α-methyl serotonin, LSD	Agomelatine, tegaserod, asenapine
5-HT_{2C}	Activates PLC	Depolarization via Ca^{++} channels	Choroid plexus medulla hippocampus	α-methyl serotonin	Metergoline, agomelatine, ketanserin
5-HT_{3}	Ligand-operated channel	Neuronal excitation	Area postrema	2-Methyl serotonin	Ondansetron, tropisetron granisetron
5-HT_{4}	Activates AC	Transmitter release	Hippocampus colliculi GI tract	Renzapride, mosapride	L-lysine, piboserod
5-HT_{5A}	Inhibits AC	Sleep	Hippocampus	Valerenic acid	Dimebolin, asenapine
5-HT_{6}	Activates AC	Cognitive enhancing	Striatum cortex	Carboxytryptamine	Clozapine, iloperidone
5-HT_{7}	Activates AC	Thermoregulation; sleep	Amygdala hypothalamus	LSD	Clozapine, asenapine

AC, adenylyl cyclase; PLC, phospholipase C.

Several different types of serotonin receptor (for example, 5-HT_{1A}, 5-HT_{2A}, 5-HT_{2C}, 5-$HT_{1B/1D}$) have been associated with the motor side effects of the SSRIs which may arise should these drugs be administered in conjunction with a MAOI. Agonists of 5-HT_{2A} receptors are drugs such as LSD and psilocybin which cause hallucinations through activating this receptor.

The 5-HT_3 receptor is an example of a non-selective cation channel receptor which is permeable to both sodium and potassium ions and, because both calcium and magnesium ions can modulate its activity, the 5-HT_3 receptor resembles the glutamate NMDA receptor. Antagonists of the 5-HT_3 receptor, such as ondansetron, are effective anti-emetics and are particularly useful when nausea is associated with the administration of cytotoxic drugs or some anaesthetic agents. However, they are ineffective against the nausea of motion sickness or that induced by apomorphine, suggesting that the 5-HT_3 receptors function at the level of the vomiting centre in the brain. In addition, there is evidence from experimental studies that these receptors are involved in anxiety and in cognition. 5-HT_3 antagonists have both anxiolytic and cognitive-enhancing properties but it still remains to be proven that such properties are therapeutically relevant.

The precise function of the 5-$HT_{4,5,6}$ and $_7$ receptors is less certain. All these receptors have been cloned and their distribution in the brain determined. There is some evidence that 5-HT_4 receptors act as heteroreceptors on cholinergic terminals and thereby modulate the release of acetylcholine. While the physiological role of the 5-$HT_{5,6}$ and $_7$ receptors is unclear, it is of interest to note that several atypical antipsychotics, such as clozapine, and several antidepressants have a good affinity for these receptors. There is also evidence that selective agonists and antagonists, such as zacopride, ergotamine, methysergide and LSD, have a high affinity for the 5-HT_4 and 5-HT_5 receptors but how these effects relate to their pharmacological actions is presently unknown.

Figure 3.5 summarizes the possible sites of action of different classes of psychotropic drugs on the serotonin receptors in the brain. Clearly, much remains to be learned about the distribution and functional activity of these receptor subtypes before their possible roles in mental illness can be elucidated.

3.3.7 Histamine

Histamine has been suspected of being a neurotransmitter in the brain for many decades but it is only in recent years that sensitive immunohistochemical techniques have been developed that clearly demonstrated its presence in the posterior hypothalamus. In retrospect, it is not surprising that histamine is a central neurotransmitter as antihistamines that have been used therapeutically for the treatment of allergies and conditions such as hay fever invariably cause sedation.

Histamine is synthesized in the brain from the amino acid histidine by the enzyme L-amino acid decarboxylase (L-AADC)) that is activated by the H_3 autoreceptor in conjunction with protein kinase A and Ca^{++}-dependent calmodulin. Once formed, histamine is transported into storage vesicles from which it is released in the presence of Ca^{++}. On release, histamine can activate postsynaptic H_1, H_2 and H_3 receptors and H_3 autoreceptors. The main metabolite formed by the action of histamine-*N*-methyltransferase is methylhistamine which can be further metabolized to imidazoleacetic acid by MAO which is located postsynaptically. However, in the mammalian

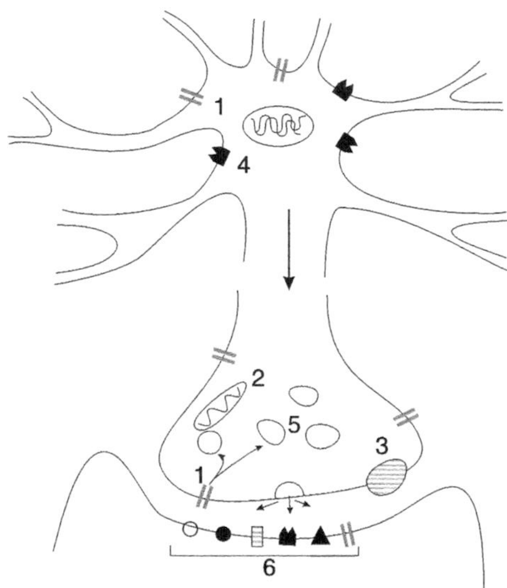

Figure 3.5 Sites of action of various types of psychotropic drugs on the cell body, neuronal terminal and synaptic sites in the brain. (1) Amine reuptake site, including the binding site for tricyclic antidepressants, where tricyclic antidepressants, SSRI antidepressants and dual action antidepressants (e.g. venlafaxine) act. (2) Monoamine oxidase, the site of action of MAOIs. (3) Autoreceptor, which, when activated by excessive amine concentration in the synaptic cleft, reduces the mobilization of calcium ions in the neuronal terminal and reduces the release of neurotransmitter from the terminal. (4) 5-HT_{1A} receptors located on the cell body. These are the site of action of novel anxiolytics such as buspirone. Stimulation of these receptors results in a reduction in the release of serotonin from the neuronal terminal. The 5-HT_{1A} receptors are desensitized following the chronic administration of SSRI antidepressants, thereby enhancing the release of serotonin. (5) Synaptic vesicles that store the biogenic amine neurotransmitter. On activation, the vesicles move to the terminal and in the presence of calcium ions fuse to the synaptic membrane and release their contents into the synaptic cleft. (6) Second messenger and tertiary messenger systems are linked to the array of postsynaptic receptors. Tertiary messengers link the second messenger signals (cAMP, cGMP etc.) to other enzymes (such as phosphokinases) that phosphorylate membrane proteins to open ion channels, activate gene transcription factors etc. On activation by the different types of neurotransmitters, the activation of these messengers results in the phosphorylation of the membrane-linked ion channels that results in the depolarization of the postsynaptic membrane. The tertiary messengers also activate the synthesis of nerve growth factors (e.g. brain-derived neurotrophic factor), leading to neuronal sprouting, repair and possibly synaptogenesis.

brain, the main metabolite is methylhistamine which is then oxidized by MAO-B to methylimidazoleacetic acid.

It is now possible to map the distribution of histamine neuronal tracks in the mammalian brain by studying the distribution of the decarboxylase which inhibits histamine synthesis. In addition, lesions of the main histaminergic tracts have validated the distribution of histamine tracts from the tuberomammillary nucleus in the posterior basal hypothalamus via the medial forebrain bundle to innervate the cortex, olfactory bulb, nucleus accumbens, thalamus, hippocampus and striatum. The tuberomammillary nucleus is also reactively innervated by catecholaminergic, serotonergic, peptidergic and glutamatergic neurons but the precise roles that the neurotransmitters play in the functioning of this region is presently unclear.

Histamine produces its physiological effects by activating three types of histamine receptors (H_1, H_2 and H_3). All are G-protein-linked receptors consisting of seven transmembrane domains. The physiological function of these three receptors are as follows:

- *H_1 receptors*: These are inositol phospholipid linked and initiate smooth muscle contraction, increased capillary permeability, hormone release and increased glycogenolysis in the brain. H_1 receptors are excitatory in nature. H_1 receptors are abundant in the cortex and stimulation of these is arousing and alerting and contributes to wakefulness.
- *H_2 receptors*: These are positively coupled to adenylyl cyclase via a G_s protein. The excitatory response of this receptor initiates smooth muscle relaxation, gastric acid secretion and positive chronotropic and inotropic effects on cardiac muscle. H_2 receptors also occur on immune cells where they exhibit inhibitory effects. Both H_2 and H_3 receptors occur in the cortex, caudate and putamen.
- *H_3 receptors*: This is a unique receptor as it acts as an autoreceptor, coupled to G_i proteins, and also as a heteroreceptor on multiple neurotransmitter terminals (serotonergic, aminergic, dopaminergic, cholinergic, peptidergic etc.) where it regulates the neurotransmitter release. Recently, an antagonist of the H_3 receptor has been licensed for the treatment of narcolepsy as it increases histamine release and so maintains daytime wakefulness. The H_3 receptor also has potential for exploitation in terms of novel drug development particularly in cognition and the regulation of food intake. An H_4 receptor has also been detected in peripheral tissues and on immune cells. It is thought to be involved in the regulation of immune function.

3.3.8 Amino Acid Neurotransmitters

Unlike for the 'classical' neurotransmitters such as acetylcholine and noradrenaline, it has not been possible to map the distribution of the amino acid transmitters in such detail in the mammalian brain. The reason is that the amino acids are in numerous metabolic pools in the brain and are not restricted to one particular type of neuron as occurs with the 'classical' transmitters. As an example, glutamate is involved in peptide and protein synthesis, in the detoxification of ammonia in the brain (by forming glutamine), in intermediary metabolism, as a precursor of the inhibitory transmitter GABA and as an important excitatory transmitter in its own right. While the evidence in favour of the amino acids glutamate, aspartate, glycine and GABA as transmitters is good, it is not yet possible to describe their anatomical distribution in detail.

With regard to the possible role of these neurotransmitters in psychiatric and neurological diseases, there is growing evidence that glutamate is causally involved in the brain damage that results from cerebral anoxia, for example following stroke and possibly epilepsy. Conversely, GABA deficiency has been implicated in anxiety states, epilepsy, Huntington's disease and Parkinsonism. The roles of the excitatory amino acid aspartate and the inhibitory transmitter glycine in diseases of the brain are uncertain.

There is a metabolic interrelationship between the amino acid transmitters glutamate, GABA and glycine. Glutamate and glycine synthesis are linked via the succinic acid component of the citric acid cycle. GABA, formed by the decarboxylation of glutamate, may also be metabolized to succinate via the 'GABA shunt'. Alpha-ketoglutarate acts as an intermediate between glutamate and glycine synthesis; the transfer of the -NH_2 group from glycine to alpha-ketoglutarate leads to the synthesis of glutamate and glyoxylate.

3.3.8.1 Aspartate and Glutamate

Aspartate and glutamate are the most abundant amino acids in the mammalian brain. While the precise role of aspartate in brain function is obscure, the importance of glutamate as an excitatory transmitter and as a precursor of GABA is well recognized. Despite the many roles which glutamate has been shown to play in intermediary metabolism and transmitter function, studies on the dentate gyrus of the hippocampal formation, where glutamate has been established as a transmitter, have shown that the synthesis of glutamate is regulated by feedback inhibition and by the concentration of its precursor glutamine. Thus, the neuronal regulation of glutamate synthesis would appear to be similar to that of the 'classical' transmitters. In the brain, there appears to be an inverse relationship between the concentration of glutamate and of GABA, apart from the context where both amino acids are present in low concentrations.

The glutamate pathways are widely distributed throughout the mammalian brain and are thought to influence more than 50% of the synapses. This may account for the importance of the transmitter in the majority of major psychiatric and neurological disorders.

Glutamate is synthesized in the nerve terminal from glutamine by glutaminase. Once released by a nerve impulse glutamate activates postsynaptic ionotropic (α-amino -3-hydroxy-5-methyl-4-isoxazolepropionic acid (AMPA), kainate, NMDA) and metabotropic (mGluR) receptors. Glutamate is then transported back into the nerve terminal by the excitatory amino acid transporter 2 and (primarily) into the adjacent neuroglia cell by the glial-type excitatory amino acid transporter. In the glia cell, glutamate is synthesized into glutamine and recycled back to the axonal terminal via the system A transporters on the glial and neuronal membranes. In addition to the postsynaptic metabotropic receptor, there is also a presynaptic metabotropic receptor that, on activation by glutamate, inhibits the synthesis of glutamate and its vesicular release.

3.3.8.2 Glycine

Glycine is structurally the simplest amino acid. There is evidence that it acts as an inhibitory transmitter in the hindbrain and spinal cord. The seizures that occur in response to strychnine poisoning are attributable to the convulsant-blocking glycine receptors in the spinal cord. Recent evidence also suggests that glycine can positively modulate the action of the excitatory transmitter glutamate on the major excitatory amino acid receptor complex in the brain, the NMDA receptor. The density of NMDA receptor sites is high in the cortex, amygdala and basal ganglia, areas of the brain which also have a relatively high concentration of glycine.

Two glycine transporters have been detected in the brain, GlyT-1 is located in the membrane of neuroglia while GlyT-2 is mainly associated with neurons. These transporters function in a similar manner to monoamine transporters and terminate the action of glycine on the inhibitory strychnine-sensitive glycine receptor. Glycine receptors play a major role in sensory processing and in motor control. They have also been implicated in pain perception and possibly in the pathological changes seen in autism.

In addition to its role as an inhibitory transmitter via the lower brainstem and spinal cord, glycine also activates a strychnine-insensitive site on the NMDA receptor. This leads to the enhancement of NMDA receptor function. It is suggested that the main action of glycine at the NMDA receptor is to increase the speed with which the NMDA receptors recover from glutamate desensitization, a state arising from prolonged receptor activation. The amino acid D-serine has a somewhat similar action in the NMDA receptor and occurs in glia cells as well as neurons. GlyT inhibitors are being developed as potential antipsychotics, due to their ability to enhance glutamate transmission which is reduced in schizophrenia.

3.3.8.3 Gamma-Aminobutyric Acid (GABA)

GABA is also present in very high concentrations in the mammalian brain, approximately 500 μg/g wet weight of brain being recorded for some regions. Thus, GABA is present in a concentration some 200–1000 times greater than neurotransmitters such as acetylcholine, noradrenaline and 5-HT.

GABA is one of the most widely distributed transmitters in the brain and it has been calculated that it occurs in over 40% of all synapses. Nevertheless, its distribution is quite heterogeneous, with the highest concentrations being present in the basal ganglia, followed by the hypothalamus, the periaqueductal grey matter and the hippocampus; approximately equal concentrations are present in the cortex, amygdala and thalamus.

GABA is present in storage vesicles in nerve terminals and also in the glia that are densely packed around nerve terminals, where they probably act as physical and metabolic 'buffers' for the nerve terminals. Following its release from the nerve terminal, the action of GABA may therefore be terminated either by being transported back into the nerve terminal by an active transport system or by being transported into the glia. GABA plays a major role in the interneurons throughout the brain.

The rate of synthesis of this transmitter is determined by glutamate decarboxylase, which synthesizes it from glutamate. A feedback inhibitory mechanism also seems to operate whereby an excess of GABA in the synaptic cleft triggers the GABA autoreceptor on the presynaptic terminal, leading to a reduction in transmitter release. Specific GABA-containing neurons have been identified as distinct pathways in the basal ganglia, namely in interneurons in the striatum, in the nigrostriatal pathway and in the pallidonigral pathway.

GABA is synthesized in GABA neurons from glutamate by the action of glutamate decarboxylase. This is a pyridoxal phosphate-dependent enzyme and can therefore be inhibited by hydrazides. GABA is released from the nerve ending in a calcium-dependent manner where it activates postsynaptic receptors. GABA is recycled by being transported back into the presynaptic terminal and restored in empty storage vesicles. GABA-T (GABA transaminase) transaminates GABA and thereby terminates its physiological action.

3.3.8.4 Amino Acid Receptors

There are two amino acid neurotransmitters, namely GABA and glutamate, which have been of major interest to the psychopharmacologist because of the potential therapeutic importance of their agonists and antagonists. The receptors upon which GABA and glutamate act to produce their effects differ from the 'classic' transmitter receptors in that they seem to exist as receptor complexes that contain sites for agonists, in addition to the amino acid transmitters; these sites, when occupied, modulate the responsiveness of the receptor to the amino acid. For example, the benzodiazepines have long been known to facilitate inhibitory transmission, and their therapeutic properties as anxiolytics and anticonvulsants are attributable to such an action. It is now apparent that benzodiazepines occupy a receptor site on the GABA receptor complex which enhances the responsiveness of the GABA receptor to the inhibitory action of GABA. Similarly, it has recently been shown that the inhibitory transmitter glycine can act on a strychnine-insensitive site on the NMDA receptor, and thereby modify its responsiveness to glutamate.

Knowledge of the mechanisms whereby the amino acid transmitters produce their effects has been valuable in the development of psychotropic drugs that may improve memory, reduce anxiety, or even counteract the effects of post-stroke hypoxia on brain cell survival. Some of these aspects are considered later.

3.3.8.5 GABA Receptors

The major amino acid neurotransmitters in the brain are GABA, an inhibitory transmitter, and glutamic acid, an excitatory transmitter. GABA is widely distributed in the mammalian brain and has been calculated to contribute to over 40% of the synapses in the cortex alone. While it is evident that a reduction in GABAergic activity is associated with seizures, and most anticonvulsant drugs either directly or indirectly facilitate GABAergic transmission, GABA also has a fundamental role in the brain by shaping, integrating and refining information transfer generated by the excitatory transmitters. Indeed, because of its wide anatomical distribution, GABA may be involved in such diverse functions due to its agonistic action on these receptors while phaclofen and gabazine are experimental drugs which act as antagonists.

There are three types of GABA receptor, A, B and C. Unlike the ionotropic $GABA_A$ receptors, the $GABA_B$ receptors are metabotropic and coupled via inhibitory G-proteins to adenylyl cyclase. Drugs that act on $GABA_A$ receptors are sedative (hypnotics) anaesthetics and anxiolytics. These are derivatives of valproic acid that not only inhibit the metabolism of GABA but may also act as antagonists of the GABA autoreceptor and thereby enhance the release of the neurotransmitter. GABA-uptake inhibitors have also been developed (for example, derivatives of nipecotic acid, guvacine) which also have anticonvulsant activity at least in experimental animals. Not only do the $GABA_B$ receptors inhibit the second messenger but they also modulate potassium and calcium channels in the neuronal membrane. $GABA_B$ receptors are widely distributed throughout the brain and in several peripheral organs. Their distribution differs from the $GABA_A$ receptors. In the cortex and several other brain regions, $GABA_B$ receptors occur on the terminals of both GABA and non-GABA neurons where they modulate neurotransmitter release.

Unlike drugs that act on $GABA_A$ receptors, $GABA_B$ receptor agonists have antinociceptive properties which may account for the efficacy of drugs like baclofen in the treatment of trigeminal neuralgia. Baclofen is a $GABA_B$ agonist also with therapeutic benefit for the treatment of spasticity. Experimental studies suggest that $GABA_B$ antagonists may also have antiepileptic activity.

$GABA_C$ receptors have only recently been identified and their function is still uncertain. There is evidence that, besides GABA, the GABA receptor agonists muscimol and isoguvacine have a high affinity for these receptors. A high density of $GABA_C$ receptors has been detected in the retina where they appear to be involved in the development of retinal rod cells. In the brain, there is evidence that $GABA_C$ receptors are concentrated in the superior colliculus where they have a disinhibitory role. There is also evidence that they play an important role in some aspects of neuroendocrine regulation both in the gastrointestinal tract and in the secretion of thyroid stimulating hormone.

The $GABA_A$ receptors have been cloned and the structures of some of the 10 subtypes of this receptor have been described. As these subtypes appear to be heterogeneously distributed throughout the brain, it may ultimately be possible to develop drugs that will affect only one specific species of $GABA_A$ receptor, thereby optimizing the therapeutic effect and reducing the possibility of non-specific side effects It seems likely that this will be an important area for psychotropic drug development in the near future. For example, the hypnotic zolpidem is selective for the α_1 subunit receptor subtype that mediates sedation. $GABA_A$ $\alpha_{2/3}$ selective agonists are being developed and tested in humans as non-sedative anxiolytic and antiepilepsy agents and may one day become established treatments.

The $GABA_A$ receptor is directly linked to chloride ion channels; activation of which results in an increase in the membrane permeability to chloride ions, and thereby the hyperpolarization of cell bodies. $GABA_A$ receptors are also found extrasynaptically where, following activation, they can depolarize neurons. The convulsant drug bicuculline acts as a specific antagonist of GABA on its receptor site, while the convulsant drug picrotoxin binds to an adjacent site on the $GABA_A$ receptor complex and directly decreases chloride ion flux; barbiturates have the opposite effect on the chloride channel and lock the channel open.

3.3.8.6 How Does the $GABA_A$ Receptor Work?

The inhibitory effect of GABA is mediated by the chloride ion channel (Figure 3.6). When the $GABA_A$ receptor is activated by GABA or a specific agonist such as muscimol, the frequency of opening of the channel is increased and the cell is hyperpolarized. Antagonists of the $GABA_A$ receptor include bicuculline, picrotoxin and gabazine, which block the receptor and cause seizures. Barbiturates, such as phenobarbitone, and possibly alcohol, facilitate the chloride ion influx, but these drugs increase the duration, rather than the frequency, of the channel opening. Recently, novel benzodiazepine receptor ligands have been produced which, like the typical benzodiazepines, increase the frequency of chloride channel opening. The cyclopyrrolone sedative/hypnotic zopiclone is an example of such a ligand. Some glucocorticoids are also known to have sedative effects which may be because they can activate specific steroid receptor facilitatory sites on the $GABA_A$ receptor. Benzodiazepine receptor agonists (which are also called positive allosteric modulators of $GABA_A$ receptors) have, depending on the dose administered, anxiolytic, anticonvulsant, sedative and amnestic properties. Benzodiazepine receptor drugs have also been developed which act as inverse agonists on the $GABA_A$ receptor. Such compounds have anxiogenic, promnestic and stimulant/convulsant properties. So far, these drugs have not been developed for clinical use but are of interest for their potential therapeutic value.

Naturally occurring inverse agonists called the β-carbolines have been isolated from human urine, but it now seems probable that these compounds are by-products of the extraction procedure. Thus, the benzodiazepine receptor is unique in that it has

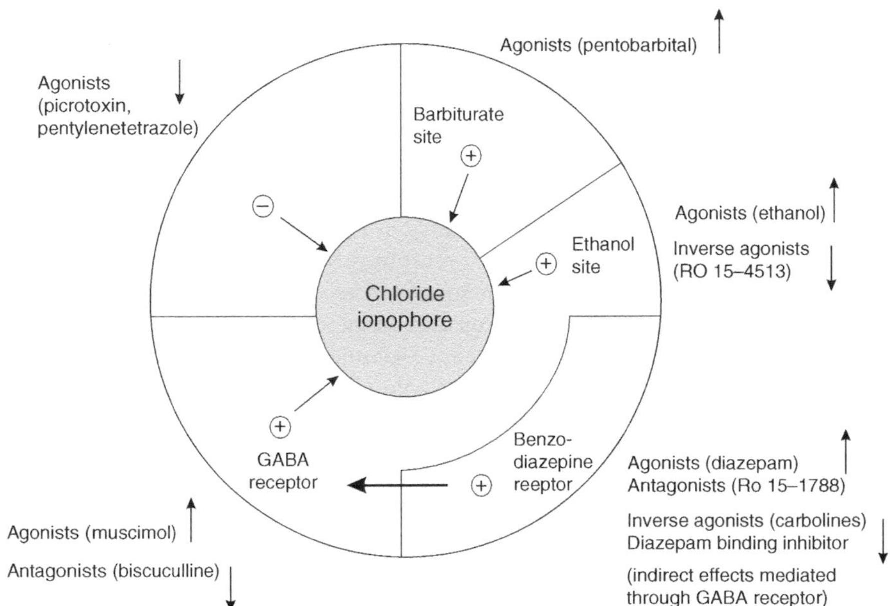

Figure 3.6 Diagrammatic representation of the GABA–benzodiazepine supramolecular complex. Compounds that increase inhibitory transmission may do so either by directly activating the GABA receptor site (e.g. muscimol) or by acting directly on the chloride ionophore (e.g. barbiturates). Benzodizepines (e.g. diazepam) enhance the sensitivity of the $GABA_A$ receptor to GABA. Compounds that decrease inhibitory transmission may do so by activating the picrotoxin site, which closes the chloride ionophore, or by blocking the $GABA_A$ receptor.

a bidirectional function. This may be of considerable importance in the design of benzodiazepine ligands which act as partial agonists. Such drugs may combine the efficacy of the conventional agents with a lack of unwanted side effects, such as sedation, amnesia and dependence. Partial inverse agonists have also been described. Such drugs appear to maintain the promnestic properties of the full inverse agonists without causing excessive stimulation and convulsions which can occur with full inverse agonists. The presence of a specific benzodiazepine site in the mammalian brain also raises the possibility that endogenous substances are present that modulate the activity of the site. While the precise identity of such natural ligands remains an enigma, there is evidence that substances such as tribulin, nephentin and the diazepam binding inhibitor could have a physiological and pathological function. There is also evidence that trace amounts of benzodiazepines (e.g. lorazepam) occur in human brain, human breast milk and also in many plants, including the potato. Such benzodiazepines have been found in post-mortem brains from the 1940s and 1950s before the clinical discovery of the benzodiazepine anxiolytics.

3.3.8.7 Excitatory Amino Acid Receptors: Glutamate Receptor

It has long been recognized that glutamic and aspartic acids occur in uniquely high concentrations in the mammalian brain and that they can cause excitation of nerve cells. However, these amino acids have only recently been identified as excitatory neurotransmitters because of the difficulty that arose in dissociating their transmitter from their metabolic role in the brain. For example, glutamate is an important component of brain proteins, peptides and a precursor of GABA. As a result of microdialysis and micro-iontophoretic techniques, in which the release and effect of local application could be demonstrated, and the synthesis and isolation of specific agonists for the different types of excitatory amino acid receptor (e.g. quisqualic, ibotenic and kainic acids), it is now generally accepted that glutamic and aspartic acids are excitatory transmitters in the mammalian brain.

Four main types of glutamate receptor have been identified and cloned. These are the ionotropic receptors (NMDA, AMPA and kainate types) and a group of metabotropic receptors of which eight types have been discovered. The AMPA and kainate receptors are involved in fast excitatory transmission whereas the NMDA receptors mediate slower excitatory responses and play a more complex role in mediating synaptic plasticity.

The ionotropic receptors have a pentameric structure. The most important of these, the NMDA receptors, are assembled from two subunits, NR_1 and NR_2, each of which can exist in different isoforms, thereby giving rise to structurally different glutamate receptors in the brain. The functional significance of these different receptor types is presently unclear. The subunits comprising the AMPA and kainate receptors, termed $mGlu_{1\text{-}7}$ and $KA_{1,2}$, are closely related.

The NMDA receptors are unique among the ligand-gated cation channel receptors in that they are permeable to calcium but blocked by magnesium, the latter acting at a specific receptor site within the ion channel (Figure 3.7). The purpose of the voltage-dependent magnesium blockade of the ion channel is to permit the summation of excitatory postsynaptic potentials. Once these have reached a critical point, the magnesium blockade of the ion channel is terminated and calcium enters the neuron to activate the calcium-dependent second messengers. Such a mechanism would appear to be particularly important for the induction of long-term potentiation, a process which underlies short-term memory formation in the hippocampus.

With regard to the action of psychotropic drugs on the NMDA receptors, there is evidence that one of the actions of the anticonvulsant lamotrigine is to modulate glutamatergic function, the antidementia drug memantine also has a similar action. Thus, the therapeutic efficacy of some of the newer drugs used to treat epilepsy and Alzheimer's disease owe their efficacy to their ability to modulate a dysfunctional glutamatergic system.

Some of the hallucinogens related to the dissociative anaesthetic ketamine, such as phencyclidine, block the ion channel of the NMDA receptor. Whether the hallucinogenic actions of phencyclidine are primarily due to this action is uncertain as the putative anticonvulsant dizocilpine (MK-801) is also an NMDA ion channel inhibitor but is not a notable hallucinogen. Presumably the ability of phencyclidine to enhance dopamine release, possibly by activating NMDA heteroreceptors on dopaminergic terminals, and also its action on sigma receptors which it shares with benzomorphan-like hallucinogens contribute to its hallucinogenic activity. It should be noted that ketamine also has unique properties as a fast-onset antidepressant, probably due to its combined actions by reducing the NMDA and increasing the activity of the AMPA receptors. There is experimental evidence that the increase in the AMPA receptor activity rapidly enhances synaptogenesis and restores damaged neuron contacts. This may be an explanation for the rapid (hours/days!) antidepressant action of ketamine.

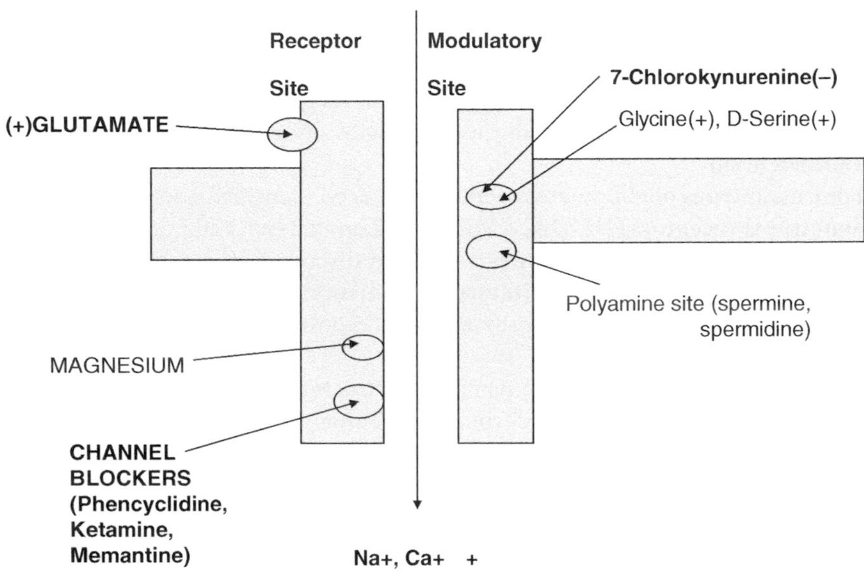

Figure 3.7 Diagram of NMDA glutamate receptor illustrating sites where neurotransmitters modulate the activity of the glutamate receptor. 1. To open the NMDA receptor channel, both glutamate and glycine are required. Glutamate acts on the receptor site while glycine occupies the adjacent modulatory site. Sodium and calcium ions move into the neuron following the opening of the channel. Magnesium ions block the channel unless it is in a depolarized state. Zinc ions can also regulate the opening of the channel. 2. The activity of the NMDA receptor is increased by excitatory amine acids (glutamate and aspartate) in the presence of glycine. 3. The specific sites on the modulatory site permit the ion channel to open (glycine, D-serine) or close (7-chlorokynurenine). The polyamines (spermine, spermidine) are neuromodulators that act on specific areas of the modulatory site. D-serine is released from astrocytes and enhances the channel opening by activating the glycine site.

3.3.8.8 The NMDA Receptor Complex

The NMDA receptor is a voltage-dependent ionotropic receptor (Figure 3.7). On activation, the magnesium ion that gates the ion channel is removed, allowing the influx of sodium and calcium ions. Potassium ions move down the concentration gradient as the counter ion. Zinc, like magnesium, also produces a voltage-dependent block of the ion channel.

The ion channel can be opened by glutamate activating the glutamate receptor, or by the activation of the modulatory sites, namely the glycine and polyamine sites. The glycine site can also be activated by D-serine and R(+) HA-966 (3-amino-1-hydroxypyrrolidone). Antagonists of the glycine site include 7-chlorokynurenine and 5,7-dichlorokynurenine; AP5 (2-amino 5-phosphopentanoic acid) is an antagonist of the glutamate receptor site. The NMDA ion channel is blocked by the dissociation anaesthetics phencyclidine and ketamine. The anticonvulsant dizocilpine (MK-801) is a partial antagonist of the phencyclidine site.

The NMDA receptor complex has been extensively characterized and its anatomical distribution in the brain determined. The NMDA receptor is analogous to the $GABA_A$ receptor in that it contains several binding sites, in addition to the glutamate site, whereby the movement of sodium and calcium ions into the nerve cell can be modulated. In addition to the glutamate and glycine sites on the NMDA receptor, there also exist polyamine sites which are activated by the naturally occurring polyamines spermine and spermidine. Specific divalent cation sites are also associated with the NMDA receptor, namely the voltage-dependent magnesium site and the inhibitory zinc site. In addition to the excitatory amino acids, the natural metabolite of brain tryptophan, quinolinic acid, which is the end product of the tryptophan-kynurenine pathway, can also act as an agonist of the NMDA receptor and may contribute to nerve cell death at high concentrations. Quinolinic acid has been implicated as an endogenous neurotoxin responsible for the neurodegenerative changes found in Alzheimer's disease and in elderly depressed patients.

Interest in the therapeutic potential of drugs acting on the NMDA receptor has risen with the discovery that epilepsy and related convulsive states may occur as a consequence of a sudden release of glutamate. Sustained seizures of the limbic system in animals result in brain damage that resembles the changes seen in glutamate toxicity. Similar changes are seen at autopsy in patients with intractable epilepsy. It has been shown that the non-competitive NMDA antagonists such as phencyclidine or ketamine can block glutamate-induced damage. The novel antiepileptic drug lamotrigine would also appear to act by this mechanism, in addition to its ability to block sodium channels, in common with many other types of antiepileptic drugs.

In addition to epilepsy, neuronal death due to the toxic effects of glutamate has also been implicated in cerebral ischaemia associated with multi-infarct dementia and possibly Alzheimer's disease. With the plethora of selective excitatory amino acid receptor antagonists currently undergoing development, some of which are already in clinical trials, one may expect definite advances in the drug treatment of neurodegenerative disorders in the near future.

3.3.8.9 Glutamate Metabotropic Receptors (mGluR)

In contrast to the ionotropic receptors, the metabotropic receptors are monomeric in structure and unique in that they show no structural similarity to the other G-protein-coupled neurotransmitter receptors. They are located both pre- and postsynaptically and there is experimental evidence that they are involved in synaptic modulation and excitotoxicity, functions which are also shared with the NMDA receptors. To date, no drugs have been developed for therapeutic use which are based on the modulation of these receptors, although there is clinical evidence that compounds modulating the $mGlu_{2/3}$ receptors may have antipsychotic activity despite lack of a direct antagonism of D_2 receptors. The mGluR are separated into three groups according to their molecular structure, signal transduction properties and pharmacological profile. The properties of these receptors are summarized in Table 3.5.

Clearly, advances in the development of drugs that specifically target the different subgroups of mGluR could be important for the development of a novel generation of drugs to treat neurological and major psychiatric disorders.

3.4 Minor Neurotransmitters and Neuromodulators in the Brain

3.4.1 Neuropeptides

Neuropeptides are now recognized as being important transmitters and modulators of neurotransmission in the mammalian brain. This is a major 'growth' area of neuroscience as many peptides, and non-peptide small molecules that are located in non-

Table 3.5 Properties of metabotropic glutamate receptors

Group	Receptor subtype	Actions
Group I	$mGlu_1$, $mGlu_5$	Promote long-term potentiation or long-term depression. Occur postsynaptically where they facilitate NMDA response and contribute to neural plasticity
Group II	$mGlu_2$, $mGlu_3$	These are presynaptic receptors which decrease neuronal excitability by inhibiting neurotransmitter release
Group III	$mGlu_4$, $mGlu_7$, $mGlu_8$	Occur presynaptically where they inhibit neurotransmitter release

nervous tissue such as the alimentary tract, are now found in the brain where they function as neuromodulators and/or co-transmitters of 'classical' neurotransmitters. The following pages present a summary of the main neuropeptides, purines, eicosanoids and steroids which contribute to central neurotransmitter function.

Sir Henry Dale, one of the important pioneers of British pharmacology in the 1930s, suggested that neurons only release one neurotransmitter. This formed the basis of 'Dale's Law'. However, in the past two decades or so it has become apparent that autonomic neurons can release more than one neurotransmitter, a 'classical' neurotransmitter such as acetylcholine or noradrenaline being released with a peptide. Indeed, it is now known that some neurons can release several different peptides in addition to the classical neurotransmitters. Such co-transmitters appear to act as modulators of the action of the classical neurotransmitter.

In the salivary gland, for example, the rate of release of acetylcholine and the co-transmitter *vasoactive intestinal peptide* (VIP) differ depending on the frequency of stimulation. Low-frequency stimulation results in the release of acetylcholine while the high-frequency stimulation primarily releases VIP. VIP is a potent vasodilator and thereby increases blood flow to the salivary gland, thereby aiding salivary secretion. In some sympathetic nerves, neuropeptide Y (NPY) coexists with noradrenaline where it is released by high-frequency stimulation and sensitizes smooth muscle to the effects of noradrenaline.

In recent years, attention has been directed to the role of neuropeptide co-transmitters in the brain. For example, the intestinal hormone *cholecystokinin* (CCK) coexists with dopamine and neurotensin in the substantia nigra and ventral-tegmental region and with substance P and serotonin in medullary neurons. Of the two types of CCK receptors, the CCK_2 receptor predominates in the brain. One of the physiological effects of CCK in the spinal cord is to act as an anti-opioid, thereby reducing the analgesic effects of opioids. Synthetic CCK_2 antagonists have anxiolytic effects in experimental models but so far the clinical evidence of such activity has been disappointing.

Corticotrophin-releasing hormone (CRH, also known as corticotrophin-releasing factor) is released from the hypothalamus in response to stress and activates the anterior pituitary gland to release adrenocorticotrophic hormone (ACTH). ACTH then acts on the adrenal cortex to stimulate the synthesis of glucocorticoids. The stress response is self-limiting when the elevated glucocorticoids activate the glucocorticoid receptors located in the hypothalamus. This is termed 'feedback' inhibition.

In addition to CRH acting as a stress hormone, it is now apparent that there is a network of CRH neurons in extra-hypothalamic sites in the brain (cortex, amygdala, forebrain, cerebellum) and in the locus coeruleus and raphé nucleus, areas associated with the noradrenaline and serotonin cell bodies, respectively.Thus, the stress response is linked to the activation of the hypothalamic–pituitary–adrenal (HPA) axis and to central noradrenergic and serotonergic function.

CRH activates CRH_1 and CRH_2 receptors and a soluble CRH binding protein. In the brain, CRH activates CRH_1 and $CRH_{2\alpha}$ receptors. CRH is also related to the urocortins. The CRH_1 receptor mediates anxiety-related behaviour and has been the subject of the target for potential non-benzodiazepine anxiolytics. Conversely, the CRH_2 receptor and CRH binding proteins appear to play a role in modulating anxiety behaviour. However, despite promising experimental studies showing that synthetic analogues of CRH have potential anxiolytic activity, so far the clinical data have been disappointing.

Galanin is an example of another gastrointestinal peptide that has been detected in the brain and the peripheral nervous system. Three specific galanin receptors have been identified which, when activated by galanin, inhibit post-sympathetic cellular functions; galanin also acts on presynaptic heteroreceptors to inhibit the release of other neurotransmitters and neuropeptides.

Galanin modulates pain responses in the spinal cord possibly by acting on the inhibitory GABAergic interneurons, NPY and enkephalins in the dorsal horn. Experimentally, galanin has been shown to reduce the effects of neuropathic pain. This suggests that non-peptide galanin agonists may be useful in the treatment of certain types of chronic pain. Of the three types of galanin receptors that have been investigated, antagonists of the $GalR_3$ receptor have been shown to exhibit antidepressant and anxiolytic-like activity in rodent models.

Neurotensin is yet another peptide of gastrointestinal location which occurs in the mammalian brain. In the brain, it is present in highest concentrations in the hypothalamus, the nucleus accumbens and septum; in the midbrain it is found as a co-transmitter with CCK and dopamine in the rodent brain, but not the human brain. Neurotensin produces its effects by activating the G-protein-linked NT_{S1} and NT_{S2} receptors. When administered intracerebrally to rodents, neurotensin elicits analgesia, hypothermia and anorexia. It also increases the sedative effects of barbiturates and ethanol and increases the release of growth hormone and prolactin. Recently, research has centred on the possible connection with the pathology of schizophrenia where the concentration of the peptide has been shown to be reduced in post-mortem brain material. In rodent models of schizophrenia, neurotensin produces behavioural effects similar to atypical antipsychotics. This suggests that non-peptide agonists of neurotensin may be useful as potential atypical antipsychotics.

3.4.1.1 Opioid Peptides

A major breakthrough in neuropeptide research occurred over 40 years ago with the discovery of leu- and met-enkephalin by Hughes and Kosterlitz in Aberdeen. Over 20 different opioid peptides are now known and classified according to the type of opioid receptor that they activate, namely the μ, δ, κ and orphanin-Q (ORL_1) or nociceptin

Table 3.6 Some principle opioid receptors and their peptides

	Receptor type		
Endogenous opioid peptide	**Mu**	**Delta**	**Kappa**
Met-enkephalin	++	+++	
Leu-enkephalin	++	+++	
Beta-endorphin	+++	+++	
Dynorphin A	++		+++
Dynorphin B	+	+	+++
Alpha-neoendorphin	+	+	+++

receptor. Table 3.6 summarizes some principle opioid peptides and the receptors they act on.

The more widely researched of these receptors and their ligands are the μ receptors that are activated by the opiate analgesics such as morphine, heroin, methadone etc. The natural peptides for these receptors are derived from the proopiomelanocortin (POMC) peptides from the intermediate lobe of the pituitary gland and the arcuate nucleus of the hypothalamus. Of these peptides, beta-endorphin is the most potent for its antinociceptive action. The tetrapeptides endomorphin 1 and 2 differ in their origin from the endorphins, are widely distributed in the central and peripheral nervous system and have a high affinity for the μ receptor. This accounts for the analgesic and rewarding properties of these and related ligands. The physiological effects of the μ, δ and κ receptors are summarized in Table 3.7.

3.4.1.2 Substance P and the Tachykinins

Substance P was first discovered in 1936 by von Euler and Gaddum from extracts from the intestine of the horse and the peptide sequence was finally elucidated by Leeman in 1970. Substance P is a undecapeptide member of the tachykinin family that activates three neurokinin receptors ($NK_{1, 2, 3}$). The tachykinins are so named because they initiate a fast contraction of smooth muscle.

Substance P has been the most widely studied tachykinin and is the preferred agonist of the NK_1 receptor. The peptide is present in small sensory nerves that project to the spinal cord. The type C fibres are important pain fibres that transmit pain from the spinal cord to the brain, thereby suggesting that substance P may act as a pain transmitter. However, non-peptide substance P antagonists have not had any proven beneficial effect in the treatment of arthritic or neuropathic pain or in migraine headache! In sensory nerves, substance P coexists with glutamate and the calcitonin gene-related peptide (CD-RP) and non-peptide antagonists of this pattern peptide have demonstrated antimigraine activity.

In higher centres of the brain, substance P has been shown to be involved in stress-induced anxiogenesis and NK_1 antagonists were developed for their possible anxiolytic/antidepressant activity (e.g. aprepitant). However, detailed controlled clinical trials could not replicate the initial promising finding. They are now shown to have therapeutic value counteracting chemotherapy-induced vomiting. Research into non-peptide antagonists of NK_2 and NK_3 receptors are continuing for possible anxiolytic/antidepressant and antipsychotic activity.

Table 3.7 Physiological effects of the μ, δ and κ receptors

Action	Receptor type	Physiological effect
Supraspinal, spinal analgesia	μ, δ, κ μ, δ, κ	Analgesia
Respiration	μ	Suppression
GI tract	μ, κ	Decreased transit
Psychotomimetic action	κ	Present
Appetite	μ, δ, κ	Increased
Sedation	μ, κ	Increased
Diuresis	κ	Increased
Hormone effects Prolactin	μ	Increased release
Growth hormone	μ? δ	Increased release
Neurotransmitter release		
Acetylcholine	μ	Inhibition
Dopamine	μ, δ	Inhibition

3.4.1.3 Vasopressin and Oxytocin

These nonapeptides are synthesized in the hypothalamus and are then translated to the posterior pituitary gland from which they are released into the circulation on demand. Like the CRH peptide, both oxytocin and arginine vasopressin (AVP) neurons occur in the brain where they activate specific receptors to produce their physiological response. Thus, AVP activates V_{1a}, V_{1b} and V_2 receptors while oxytocin activates a simple oxytocin (OT) receptor. These are all G-protein-linked receptors.

In the periphery, these neuropeptides have important physiological effects; AVP affects kidney (regulation of urine concentration) and cardiovascular function (vaso-constriction) while oxytocin is involved in parturition and lactation. In the brain, both AVP and oxytocin pay important roles in bonding behaviour between the mother and her infant and in parental care and protection. Recently, it has been shown that both peptides play important roles in maternal and romantic love (the 'love hormones') and that a disruption of these peptides may be involved in sexual dysfunction, in social aspects of autism and possibly social phobia. Such observations are leading to the development of non-peptide agonists of the OT receptor for the possible treatment of these conditions.

AVP in the brain acts at V_{1b} receptors which enhance the release of CRH and ACTH. This action of AVP is prominent in chronic stress where AVP is released from the posterior pituitary more readily than CRH and produces a more sustained release of ACTH than CRH. As the activation of the HPA axis is a common feature of anxiety and depression, such observations have led to the synthesis of non-peptide antagonists as potential anxiolytics and antidepressants. So far, the development of such compounds remains largely at the experimental stage as the initial clinical trials proved disappointing.

3.4.1.4 Other Diverse Neuropeptides with CNS Activity

Neuropeptide Y (NPY) is concentrated in the arcuate nucleus of the hypothalamus, a region of the brain concerned with feeding behaviour. Of the five receptor types activated by NPY, the Y_1 and Y_5 receptors appear to be the most important in mediating appetite.

The hypocretins (also known as orexins) A and B are also present in the hypothalamus where they also stimulate food intake by delaying satiety mechanisms. Antagonists of the orexin 1 receptor suppress food intake by increasing the onset of satiety. In addition, the orexins play a role in the control of sleep and wakefulness and synthetic derivatives could have therapeutic potential as hypnotic/sedatives. Recently, the first orexin antagonist, suvorexant, was licensed in the USA as a sleep-promoting drug.

3.4.2 Purine Neurotransmitters

While both ATP and adenosine were recognized as having potent effects on the cardiovascular system over 80 years ago, it has only recently been accepted that these, and related purines, act on specific purinergic receptors in the brain. It is now known that the purines activate four types of receptors (A_1, A_{2A}, A_{2B} and A_3) that, apart from the A_{2B} receptor, are widely distributed in the brain; the A_{2B} receptor appears to be primarily restricted to the striatum and nucleus accumbens. All the purinergic receptors are linked to G-proteins and, apart from the A_1 and A_3 receptor, activate adenylyl cyclase: the A_1 and A_3 receptors inhibit adenylyl cyclase. Thus, the purinergic receptors play an important role in central neurotransmission by various mechanisms such as the inhibition of calcium channels (A_1, A_{2A}), activating phospholipase C as an important second messenger (A_{2B}, A_3), increasing intracellular Ca^{++}(A_3). Activation of the A_1 receptor is particularly important as it inhibits release of all other neurotransmitters by hyperpolarizing the neurons. The A_1, A_{2A}, A_{2B} and A_3 receptors are also classified as P_1 receptors and separated from the P_{2X} and P_{2Y} receptors based on their differential affinity for alpha, beta, methylase ATP and 2-methylthio ATP, respectively. It is now apparent that in the brain, there is a family of P_{2X} receptors located in the cortex, hippocampus, hypothalamus and substantia nigra. The P_{2Y} receptor family also occur in the brain (striatum, nucleus accumbens, hippocampus and cerebellum) and are activated particularly by ADP.

Physiologically, adenosine promotes sleep and may be involved in the pathology of epilepsy. The stimulant effects of caffeine are directly attributable to the inhibition of adenosine receptors in the brain. In summary, it would appear that adenosine has such diverse effects on brain function by facilitating or inhibiting the release of many different types of neurotransmitters by acting on pre- and postsynaptic receptors. Of particular importance is the finding that adenosine regulates the NMDA/AMPA and metabotropic glutamate receptors, nicotinic cholinergic receptors and several neuropeptide receptors. Synthetic analogues of adenosine may be the basis for a new class of psychotropic drugs in the future.

3.4.3 Prostaglandins, Neurosteroids, Gaseous Transmitters and Endocannabinoids

Apart from the purines, all of the other neurotransmitters discussed in this chapter are 'classical' in the sense that they are synthesized within the neurons and released by a calcium-dependent mechanism from the nerve terminal following the passage of a nerve impulse. However, there are a number of substances which are now known to play an important role by modulating the intracellular responses to the classical neurotransmitters.

3.4.3.1 Prostaglandins

These lipid-soluble compounds (termed eicosanoids) are derived from the polyunsaturated fatty acid, arachidonic acid. The prostaglandins were first isolated from bull's semen (hence the name) in the 1930s and grouped into those compounds that were either soluble in ether (PGEs such as the ubiquitous PGE_2) and those that were soluble in phosphate (fosfat) buffer (PGF). The important breakthrough in understanding the physiological activity of the prostaglandins (particularly PGE_2) came with the discovery by Vane and colleagues in 1971 that non-steroidal anti-inflammatory drugs (NSAIDs) such as aspirin inhibited the cyclo-oxygenase (COX) 1 enzyme that synthesized the PGEs from arachidonic acid. Later, it was found that the brain contained a second COX enzyme (COX2) and more recently a third, COX3, that is possibly inhibited by paracetamol (in non-human brain tissue). The identification of the two main types of COX enzyme has been important therapeutically as COX1 occurs in the gastric mucosa where an inhibition by NSAIDs, gastric erosion and ulcers arise while COX2 is an enzyme that does not occur in the gastric mucosa and is induced by inflammation. This has led to the development of selective COX2 inhibitors for the treatment of inflammatory disorders (e.g. celecoxib), some of which have been withdrawn from use because of serious cardiovascular side effects.

As there is increasing evidence that chronic low-grade inflammation frequently occurs in depression and schizophrenia, celecoxib has been investigated for its possible beneficial effects in patients who are responding poorly to antidepressants or antipsychotics. Preliminary clinical trials have indicated that celecoxib can enhance the efficacy of standard drugs which are showing a minimal effect when administered alone. This is becoming an important area of interest for psychotropic drug development.

The prostaglandins are important neuromodulator compounds that are not stored but synthesized on demand. As neuromodulators, it is known that PGE_2 reduces noradrenaline release and has an anticonvulsant action against chemically induced seizures. PGE_2 plays an important role in neuroinflammation. It is raised in the cerebrospinal fluid of patients with major depression and also those with schizophrenia.

The main prostanoid receptors are EP_1, EP_2, EP_3 and EP_4. All are G-protein linked and activated by PGE_2. Several splice variants of the EP receptors have been discovered that can interfere with the signalling system of the prostanoids.

3.4.3.2 Neurosteroids

These steroids, exemplified by pregnenolone and dihydroepiandrosterone (DHEA) are synthesized from cholesterol by the oligodendroglioma, astrocytes and neurons in the brain. There are a number of neurosteroids formed in the brain from cholesterol (such as the allopregnenolones, progesterone) but the two most important neurosteroids are pregnenolone and DHEA, formed from pregnenolone. Unlike the adrenal steroids, the neurosteroids can act as *autocrines*, by modulating the cells in which they are synthesized, or as *paracrines* whereby they act locally near to the cells that synthesize them. These neurosteroids regulate the $GABA_A$ receptor and the NMDA receptor, the sulphated derivatives inhibiting the GABA receptor. By contrast, the allopregnenolone derivatives activate the $GABA_A$ receptor and induce anxiolytic, anticonvulsant and sedative effects.

There is pharmacological evidence that alcohol increases the concentrations of neurosteroids in the brain which may contribute to its sedative effects.

3.4.3.3 Receptors for Steroid and Thyroid Hormones

The receptors for steroid and thyroid hormones, vitamin D and retinoic acids differ from the ionotropic and metabotropic receptors by their location in the nucleus, not on the neuronal membrane. Thus, these ligands must penetrate the cell membrane and be transported to the cell nucleus where they bind to nuclear DNA and stimulate gene transcription. This is a relatively slow process and takes hours to days rather than minutes. These genomic effects of hormones are linked to the induction of enzymes involved in neurotransmitter function, in changes in the nature and position of receptors in the neuronal membrane and in the density of dendritic spikes. Such effects help to explain the neuropathological changes associated with hypercortisolaemia in major depression for example.

Similarly, steroids such as cortisol, unlike neurotransmitters, do not have membrane-bound receptors but, being lipophilic, easily diffuse through the neural cell wall, and bind to the intracellular glucocorticoid receptor (GR) to change its conformation. The activated receptor then enters the nucleus to induce nuclear translocation and the transcription of target genes.

In addition to the genomic effects of hormones, some steroid hormones, exemplified by the sex hormones progesterone, testosterone and oestrogens as well as adrenal steroids (so-called *neuroactive steroids*) modulate the $GABA_A$ receptor by activating specific steroid-sensitive sites on the receptor complex. These non-genomic effects result in sedative, anticonvulsant, anxiolytic and antidepressant-like activity. As these steroids can be synthesized in the mammalian brain, it is possible that they act as physiologically active *endocoids* and could play a role in modulating the symptoms of some psychiatric disorders.

3.4.3.4 Gaseous Neurotransmitters

3.4.3.4.1 Nitric Oxide (NO)

Nitric oxide (NO), the endothelium-derived relaxing factor, is synthesized from arginine by nitric oxide synthase (NOS). NOS exists in an inducible form (iNOS) that is induced by pro-inflammatory cytokines in macrophages and microglia, and a constituitive form (cNOS) that is activated by calcium and calmodulin. Neurons contain a third type of NOS (nNOS) that is activated by NMDA receptors. This enzyme is important in the second messenger cascade where it is activated by several kinases. NO is synthesized only when required as, being a gas, it cannot be stored in vesicles. Its physiological effects are therefore very brief and it is destroyed by reacting with haemoglobin and other iron-containing molecules in the tissues.

The primary action of NO is to stimulate soluble guanylyl cyclase and thereby increase the concentration of cGMP. This results in the phosphorylation of numerous cGMP-dependent kinases. NMDA glutamate receptors are activated by NO, an effect that would appear to be of neuroprotective importance when hypoxia occurs. NO is also involved in retrograde signalling and has many diverse effects on ion channels, transporters and metabolic enzymes. In short, NO plays a number of physiological roles both in the brain and in the periphery (example, the cardiovascular system).

3.4.3.4.2 Carbon Monoxide (CO)

This gaseous transmitter is synthesized by haem oxygenase contained within ageing erythrocytes. When haem is converted to the bile component biliverdin, carbon monoxide (CO) is eliminated. Of the three haem oxygenases that have been identified, haem oxygenase 2 is a constituitive enzyme in the hippocampus, cerebellum and olfactory bulbs.

Like NO, CO activates guanylyl cyclase and thereby increases cGMP. Both NO and CO may play a role in memory formation in the hippocampus. They differ in their durations of action; CO has a more prolonged action in initiating long-term potentiation in the hippocampus than NO.

3.4.3.4.3 Hydrogen Sulphide (H_2S)

Unlike NO and CO, it is only recently that hydrogen sulphide (H_2S) has been found in the mammalian brain where it is formed by the action of cystathione-β-synthase which is activated by glutamate. In vitro studies show that H_2S is involved in the facilitation of long-term potentiation. H_2S has been detected in micromolar concentrations in the brain where it may act as a retrograde transmitter following its release from postsynaptic sites. H_2S is synthesized from L-cysteine by cystathione-β-synthase following the activation of the ionotropic glutamate receptors (NMDA/AMPA) and the influx of calcium ions into the postsynaptic site. There is experimental evidence that H_2S is involved in the mechanism of long-term potentiation, the molecular basis of memory formation, in the hippocampus. In support of this, H_2S has been detected in micromolar concentrations in the hippocampus where it may act as a retrograde transmitter following its release from postsynaptic sites.

3.4.3.5 Endocannabinoids

Interest in the pharmacological properties of the cannabinoids goes back to antiquity but it is only relatively recently, within the past four decades, that a receptor was discovered in pig brain extracts that produced a similar response in isolated tissue preparations to tetrahydrocannabinoid (THC), the main active ingredient of cannabis resin. This fat-soluble molecule was found to be *N*-arachidonylethanolamine, now called anandamide (from 'ananda' meaning 'bliss' in Sanskrit). The endocannabinoids are part of a large family of lipid signalling molecules that include the prostaglandins and leukotrienes that are involved in inflammation. In addition to anandamide, other endocannabinoids with similar properties include 2-arachidonylglycerol and *N*-arichidonyldopamine.

Endocannabinoids such as anandamide are synthesized from membrane-bound arachidonic acid by phospholipase D; 2-arachidonylglycerol is synthesized by diacylglycerase lipase however. Like the gaseous neurotransmitters, anandamide is not stored in vesicles but is synthesized and released on demand. Activation of the glutamatergic system, with the increase in intraneuronal calcium, triggers the release of the transmitter. Once released, the endocannabinoids are rapidly catabolized by the intracellular enzyme fatty acid amide hydrolase (FAAH). This metabolizing enzyme occurs particularly in the brain regions containing cannabinoid (CB)-1 receptors. An endocannabinoid transporter carries the transmitter back into the presynaptic terminal. Physiologically, the endocannabinoids are involved in retrograde transmission whereby they induce long-term depression of presynaptic terminals following their release from the postsynaptic site. Cannabis receptor antagonists now exist, e.g. rimonabant.

The cannabinoids have long been known for their pleasurable and rewarding effects, hence their classification as drugs of abuse. More recently, natural and synthetic cannabinoids have been cited as possible trigger factors for schizophrenia and other major psychiatric disorders. They are also involved in the modulation of pain by their action at vanilloid receptor-1. Drugs acting on these receptors are now receiving attention for relieving intractable pain syndromes. The phenomenon of stress-induced analgesia would appear to be attributed to the rapid accumulation of anandamide particularly in the brainstem.

Basic References

Kelly JP (2010). *CNS Drug Development.* Chichester: Wiley.

Leonard BE (2003). *Fundamentals of Psychopharmacology.* Chichester: Wiley.

Rang HP, Ritter JM, Flower RT, Henderson G (eds.) (2016). *Rang and Dale's Pharmacology,* 8th ed. London: Elsevier.

Key Recent References for Further Reading

1. Principle Neurotransmitters in the Brain

Abrahamsson T, Chou CYC, Li SY, et al. (2017). Differential regulation and evoked spontaneous release by presynaptic NMDA receptors. *Neuron,* 96, 839–855.

Berger M, Gray JA, Roth BL (2009). The expanded biology of serotonin. *Ann Rev Med,* 60, 355–366.

Chandler CM, Overton JS, Rüedi-Bettschen D, Platt DM (2018). GABA receptor subtype mechanisms and abuse-related effects of ethanol: genetic and pharmacological evidence. *Handb Exp Pharmacol,* 248, 3–27. doi:10.1007/164_2017_80.

Chen XX, Zhang JH, Pan BH, et al. (2017). The atypical antipsychotic olanzapine causes weight gain by targeting 5HT2 receptors. *Life Sci,* 187, 64–73.

Cortes-Altamirano JL, Olmos-Hernandez A, Bonilla-Jaime H, et al. (2017). Review: $5HT_1$, $5HT_2$, $5HT_3$ and $5HT_7$ receptors and their role in the modulation of pain response in the central nervous system. *Curr Neuropharmacol,* 16, 210–221. doi:10.2174/1570159x1566617091 1121027.

Di Menna L, Joffe ME, Iacovelli L, et al. (2018). Functional partnership between mGlu3 and mGlu5 metabotropic glutamate receptors in the central nervous system. *Neuropharmacology,* 128, 301–313.

Doly S, Quentin E, Eddine R, et al. (2017). Serotonin 2B receptors in mesoaccumbens dopaminergic pathway regulate dopaminergic responses. *J Neurosci,* 37, 10372–10388.

Glasgow NG, Povysheva NV, Azoleifa AM, Johnson JW (2017). Memantine and ketamine differentially alter NMDA receptor desensitization. *J Neurosci,* 37, 9686–9704.

Huang X, Yang J, Yang S, et al. (2017). Role of tandospirone, a 5HT1A receptor partial agonist, in the treatment of CNS disorders and the underlying mechanisms. *Oncotarget,* 8, 102705–102720.

Kaushik V, Smith ST, Mikobi E, Kaji MA (2018). Acetylcholinesterase inhibitors: beneficial effects on co-morbidities in patients with Alzheimer's disease. *Am J Alzheimers Dis Other Dement,* 33, 73–85.

Li D-J, Fu H, Tong B, et al. (2018). Cholinergic anti-inflammatory pathway inhibits neointimal hyperplasia by suppressing inflammation and oxidative stress. *Redox Biol,* 15, 22–33.

Makera C, Dondio G, Braida D, et al. (2018). Effects of the antidepressant mirtazepine and zinc on nicotinic acetylcholine receptors. *Eur J Pharmacol,* 820, 265–273.

Niswender CM, Conn PJ (2010). Metabotropic glutamate receptors: physiology, pharmacology and disease. *Ann Rev Pharmacol Toxicol,* 50, 295–322.

Overden ES, McGregor NW, Emsley RA, Warnick L (2018). DNA methylation and antipsychotic treatment in schizophrenia: progress and future directions. *Prog Neuropsychopharmacol Biol Psychiatry*, 81, 38–49.

Palma E, Ruffolo G, Cifelli P, et al. (2017). Modulation of GABA-A receptors in the treatment of epilepsy. *Curr Pharm Des*, 23, 5563–5568. doi.2174/1381612823666170809100230.

Pytliak M, Vargova V, Mechirova V, Felsoci M (2011). Serotonin receptors – from molecular biology to clinical applications. *Physiol Rev*, 60, 15–25.

Viana GSDB, Xanvier CC, Costa RD, Neves KRT (2018). The monoaminergic pathways and inhibition of monoamine transporters interfere with the antidepressant-like behavior of ketamine. *IBRO Rep*, 4, 7–13.

Vizi ES, Lendvai B (1999). Modulatory role of presynaptic nicotinic receptors in synaptic and non synaptic chemical communication in the central nervous system. *Brain Res Rev*, 30, 219–235.

Williams DJ, Sidaway P, Cunnane TV, Brain KL (2011). Mechanisms involved in nicotinic acetylcholine receptor induced neurotransmitter release from sympathetic nerve terminals. *PLoS One*, 6, e29209. doi:1371/journal.pone 0029209.

Xiao X, Shang X, Zhai B, et al. (2018). Nicotine alleviates chronic stress induced anxiety in patients with Alzheimer's disease. *Neurochem Int*, 114, 58–70.

2. Minor Neurotransmitters and Neurotransmitter Modulators

Ahmadi-Soleimani SM, Azizi H, Gompf HS, Semnanian S (2017). Role of orexin type-1 receptors in the paragiganto-coerulear modulation of opioid withdrawal and tolerance; a site specific focus. *Neuropharmacology*, 126, 25–37.

Andrabi SS, Parvez S, Tabassum H (2017). Neurosteroids and ischaemic stroke: progesterone as a promising agent in reducing brain injury in ischemic stroke. *J Environ Pathol Toxicol Oncol*, 36, 191–205.

Balthazart J, Choleris E, Remage-Healey L (2018). Steroids and the brain: 50 years of research, conceptual shifts and the ascent of non-classical and membrane initiated actions. *Horm Behav*, 99, 1–8.

Bodnar RJ (2017). Endogenous opiates and behavior: 2015. *Peptides*, 88, 126–188.

D'Souza DC, Sewell RA, Ranganathan M (2009). Cannabis and psychosis/schizophrenia: human studies. *Eur Arch Psychiatry Clin Neurosci*, 259, 413–431.

Fantegrosse WE, Wilson CD, Berquist MD (2018). Pro-psychotic effects of synthetic cannabinoids: interactions with central dopamine, serotonin and glutamate receptors. *Drug Metab Rev*, 50, 65–78. doi:10.1080/03602532.2018.1428343.

Grund T, Goyon S, Li Y, et al. (2007). Neuropeptide S activates paraventricular oxytocin neurons to induce anxiolysis. *J Neurosci*, 37, 12214–12225.

Henry MS, Gendron L, Tremblay ME, Drolet G (2017). Enkephalins: endogenous analgesics with an emerging role in stress resilience. *Neural Plast*, 2017, 1546125.

Smith AS, Tabbaa M, Lei K, et al. (2016). Local oxytocin tempers anxiety by activating $GABA_A$ receptors in the hypothalamic paraventricular nucleus. *Psychoneuroendocrinology*, 63, 50–58.

Starwicz K, Finn DP (2017). Cannabinoids and pain: sites and mechanisms of action. *Adv Pharmacol*, 80, 437–475.

Chapter

4 Pharmacodynamics and Pharmacokinetics

Stuart Banham and David Taylor

4.1 Introduction

Pharmacokinetics refers to the effects the body has upon a consumed drug, by considering a variety of processes which a drug undergoes during its time within the body. In contrast, pharmacodynamics can be considered as the effects a drug has upon the body that has consumed it, by considering the drug's effects at its principal sites of action. Safe and effective therapeutic management of drugs for individual patients requires application of pharmacokinetic and pharmacodynamic principles to enhance efficacy and minimize toxicity. Chapter 5 (Pharmacogenomics and Psychopharmacology) provides a detailed review of the genes relevant for drug absorption, distribution, metabolism and excretion. As such, these issues are only dealt with briefly in this chapter.

4.2 Key Concepts in Pharmacokinetics

Pharmacokinetics can be broken down into four phases, each representing a different stage in the journey a medicine has through the body.

These stages are:

1. Absorption
2. Distribution
3. Metabolism
4. Excretion.

Individual drugs will have different pharmacokinetic properties and these will vary between different patients depending upon factors such as: age, genetic polymorphisms, co-administered drugs and co-morbid conditions. A practical understanding of the impact pharmacokinetics has upon drug therapy will allow clinicians to understand interpatient variations in response to drug therapy as well as to select appropriate drug dosage regimens.

The four phases of pharmacokinetics (absorption, distribution, metabolism and elimination) will determine the rise and fall in the plasma concentration of a drug after a dose is taken. Four key parameters that help describe this are C_{max}, T_{max}, half-life ($t_{½}$) and the area under the curve (AUC). C_{max} is the maximum plasma concentration that is reached. T_{max} is the time between administration of a dose and C_{max} being reached. $t_{½}$ is the time it takes for the plasma concentration to fall by half. The AUC after a single dose is proportional to the amount of drug in the plasma, i.e. the bioavailability. As such, the AUC can be used to determine the fraction of the administered dose that is absorbed. $t_{½}$ and the related issue of steady state are considered in more detail later in the chapter.

4.3 Absorption

4.3.1 Method of Administration

Before an administered dose of drug can have any effect it first needs to be absorbed, i.e. to enter the body. Within psychiatry the most frequently used route of administration is the oral route. Other routes of administration include: intramuscular (IM), intravenous (IV), inhaled and transdermal. The route of administration will affect the C_{max} and T_{max}. C_{max} will be higher and T_{max} shorter with inhaled and intravenous administration compared with oral or IM administration. An example of an inhaled drug in psychiatry is inhaled loxapine powder (Adavsuve) which is indicated for the rapid control of mild to moderate agitation in adults with bipolar disorder or schizophrenia. Loxapine is a dopamine receptor antagonist. The inhaled route of admission ensures a median time between administration and maximum plasma concentration (T_{max}) of 2 minutes (electronic Medicines Compendium, 2018a). An example of transdermal absorption is the use of a nicotine patch in smoking cessation. In emergency situations, where oral medication and psychosocial strategies are ineffective or not possible to employ, lorazepam and certain dopamine antagonists may be administered IM to help control severely agitated or disturbed behaviour. This is termed rapid tranquillisation (National Institute for Health and Care Excellence, NICE, 2015).

4.3.2 Oral Route of Administration

The majority of drugs used within psychiatry are administered via the oral route. Medications taken orally can be administered in different preparations, e.g. liquid formations, orodispersible tablets and slow-release tablets. Liquid formulations and orodispersible tablets can be of value where poor adherence is suspected (assuming medication taking can be supervised) or for patients who have difficulty swallowing tablets. Olanzapine, risperidone and mirtazapine are available as rapidly dissolving orodispersible tablets as well as conventional tablets.

The oral route is the safest, most convenient and economical as well as arguably having the greatest degree of patient acceptability. There are however disadvantages to the oral route of administration with some drugs due to:

- Limited absorption due to physical characteristics such as low water solubility.
- The drug irritating the gastric mucosa, leading to emesis or damage of the mucosa
- Destruction of drugs due to gastric enzymes or low pH of the stomach.
- Large first-pass metabolism in gut wall or liver reducing the amount that reaches the brain. Several drugs used in psychiatry, especially buprenorphine and asenapine, have to be taken in via the oral mucosa to minimize first-pass effects.

Additionally, the presence of food within the stomach can affect drug absorption, leading to either reduced or accelerated drug absorption. For most drugs in psychiatry this is not relevant but there are exceptions. For example, lurasidone (a dopamine receptor antagonist licensed in the UK for the treatment of schizophrenia) needs to be taken with food to ensure maximal absorption. In a food effect study, the mean C_{max} and AUC for lurasidone increased by approximately 2–3 times and 1.5–2 times, respectively, when lurasidone was taken with food compared with the levels observed when the drug was taken in the fasting state (electronic Medicines Compendium, 2018b). A final consideration with the oral route of administration is the need for patient cooperation, a factor which is sometimes difficult to ensure within psychiatry.

4.3.3 Rate of Absorption/Bioavailability

Solid dosage forms of pharmaceutical products include tablets (either immediate release or delayed/extended release) and capsules. Of these the most widespread formulation of solid dosage form is the disintegrating tablet. Following oral ingestion of a disintegrating tablet the active pharmaceutical ingredient (API) needs to dissolve in the stomach contents prior to absorption occurring. Tablet disintegration needs to occur prior to the dissolution of the API. Immediate-release tablets are designed to rapidly disintegrate and dissolve, within 2.5 to 10 minutes (Markl & Zeitler, 2017). With extended-release tablets a variety of mechanisms are employed within the design of the tablet to achieve slow and sustained dissolution or selective absorption of the API across the gastrointestinal tract.

The majority of drug absorption occurs within the small intestine due to the large surface area and permeability of membranes at this location. Drug absorption occurs largely by passive diffusion with a rate determined by the ionization and lipid solubility of the drug. Passive diffusion occurs across a concentration gradient from regions of high drug concentration (within the gastrointestinal fluids) to areas of low concentration (within the bloodstream). Drug molecules which are either strongly acidic (pKa (acid dissociation constant) <3) or strongly basic (pKa >10) have poor oral absorption due to being fully ionized within physiological solutions. Passive epithelial diffusion requires the drug molecules to be in a non-ionized state, to facilitate transfer across lipid membranes.

Active absorption occurs at specific sites within the small intestine and is limited to drugs sharing structural similarities with endogenous substances. Specific transporter proteins within the epithelial membrane can facilitate absorption against the underlying concentration gradient. For example, L-dopa is absorbed from the small intestine by the transporter protein that normally transports the amino acid phenylalanine.

Approximately 75% of an oral dose, from a disintegrating tablet (not modified release) is absorbed within 1 to 3 hours of oral administration. This approximate figure is influenced by several physiological or pharmaceutical factors. The main factors influencing rate of oral absorption are:

- tablet disintegration rate
- dissolution of active pharmaceutical ingredient
- gastrointestinal motility
- abdominal blood flow
- particle size and formulation
- physicochemical factors.

Oral bioavailability is the fraction of the administered dose which is absorbed into the systemic bloodstream. Factors which affect oral bioavailability can be divided into physiological, physiochemical and biopharmaceutical as these factors influence the fraction of oral dose absorbed, the fraction eliminated via gut wall metabolism and the fraction eliminated via first-pass hepatic metabolism. Poor oral bioavailability is one of the major causes of therapeutic variability between individuals (El-Kattan & Varma, 2012).

Following oral administration of a drug, cytochrome P450 enzymes located in the intestine and the liver may reduce the portion of the dose reaching the systemic circulation, and so reduce the oral bioavailability. This is termed first-pass metabolism. For about 40% of commonly used drugs the oral bioavailability is less than 50% because of limited oral absorption or first-pass metabolism.

4.3.4 Alternative Routes of Administration

Intravenous (IV) injection is one of the few routes of administration where bioavailability is 100%, i.e. the total administered dose reaches the systemic circulation. The peak drug concentration the tissues are exposed to depends upon the rate of injection. Direct access to the systemic circulation also ensures a rapid onset of activity when drugs are administered via IV administration. Other injectable routes of administration, such as IM or subcutaneous (SC) provide a more rapid onset of activity, compared with oral administration, but the rate of absorption varies considerably, depending upon the site of injection and local blood flow. Physiological factors which influence absorption from IM injection are:

- Diffusion through the tissue at the site of injection.
- Removal from the injection site by local blood flow.

Long-acting injectable formulations of antipsychotic drugs (depot injections) utilize chemical strategies to delay the absorption of active drug from the injection site. The strategies are:

- Formulation of the drug as a lipophilic ester dissolved in oil. The early antipsychotic depots, such as zuclopenthixol decanoate, are all esters of the parent first-generation antipsychotic combined with a long-chain fatty acid dissolved in an oily base such as coconut, sesame or a synthetic vegetable oil. Following injection, the ester gradually leaves the oil and is then hydrolysed liberating the parent antipsychotic.
- Formulation of the drug as an insoluble salt suspended in a liquid base. Other than risperidone long-acting injection, all the other long-acting injections available in the UK (i.e. paliperidone palmitate, olanzapine pamoate and aripiprazole long-acting injection) consist of insoluble crystals in an aqueous suspension. Over time the crystals gradually dissolve liberating the parent antipsychotic.
- Risperidone long-acting injection (RLAI) has a unique delivery system among current antipsychotic long-acting injections. The risperidone is encapsulated within biodegradable polymer microspheres. After injection the microspheres are slowly hydrolysed liberating the risperidone.

In summary, with all these strategies absorption is delayed by the active drug needing to be hydrolysed from the ester, insoluble salt or microsphere before absorption can take place.

4.4 Distribution

4.4.1 Volume of Distribution

Following absorption into the systemic circulation the dose of drug is distributed throughout the body's organ and tissue structures. Drug distribution results from the concentration of the drug reaching equilibrium between different compartments of the body. A consequence of distribution is a drop in the plasma concentration of the drug. Drug distribution is rarely uniform due to physical chemical properties, for example drug pH, lipid or water solubility or tissue binding properties, or physiological conditions, for example blood perfusion. This results in drug accumulation in specific organs or tissue structures. For psychiatric drugs, it is the concentration within the brain, the target tissue, that is relevant to their therapeutic effect.

The apparent volume of distribution is a theoretical calculation providing the size of a compartment which will account for the total amount of drug in the body if it were present in the same concentration as it were present in plasma. Drugs which are concentrated in specific body tissues, and are not evenly distributed throughout the body, will have a large volume of distribution, often exceeding the total body volume. For dopamine receptor antagonist drugs the volume of distribution usually varies between 10 and 50 L/kg. However, some antipsychotics show a low volume of distribution, such as sulpiride, clozapine or risperidone (2.6, 1.6 and 0.7 L/kg, respectively) (Patteet et al., 2012).

4.4.2 Single-Compartment Model

This is the simplest means by which the distribution of a drug throughout the body can be considered. In this model the body is a single compartment (or box) into which an IV bolus of drug is administered and is distributed instantly throughout the body. Elimination begins to occur immediately following the IV injection. This simplistic model is illustrated in Figure 4.1. It is rarely adequate to consider the complexity of drug distribution and so a two-compartment model is preferred.

4.4.3 Two-Compartment Model

Even though the body is composed of numerous tissue compartments into which a drug dose may distribute, for practical purposes a two-compartment model is used, with the plasma (central compartment) being one compartment and the tissues (peripheral compartment) being another single, separate compartment. Figure 4.2 shows distribution of an administered dose between the central and peripheral compartments. Following the administration of a dose of drug the initial high plasma concentration will fall rapidly due to distribution into tissues and elimination of the drug from the plasma compartment (α phase). Over time (often hours, but dependent upon the drug characteristics) an equilibrium will be reached between the plasma and tissue compartment, marking the point when distribution is complete. Following the completion of the distribution phase the plasma level falls more slowly, due to elimination of the drug from the plasma (β phase). If distribution is completed quickly (within minutes) then the α phase is not seen and

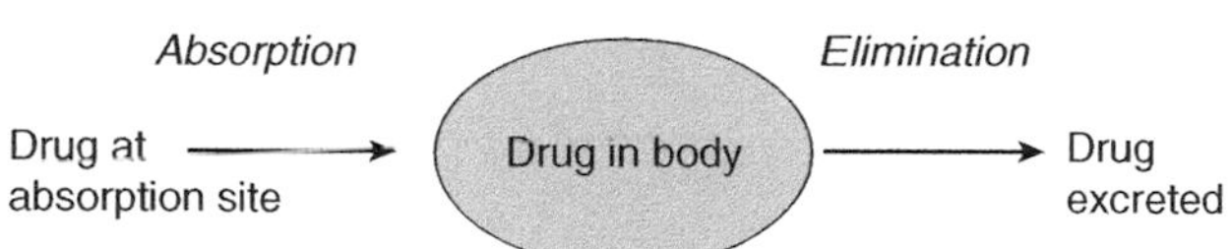

Figure 4.1 Simplified one-compartment model of drug handling.

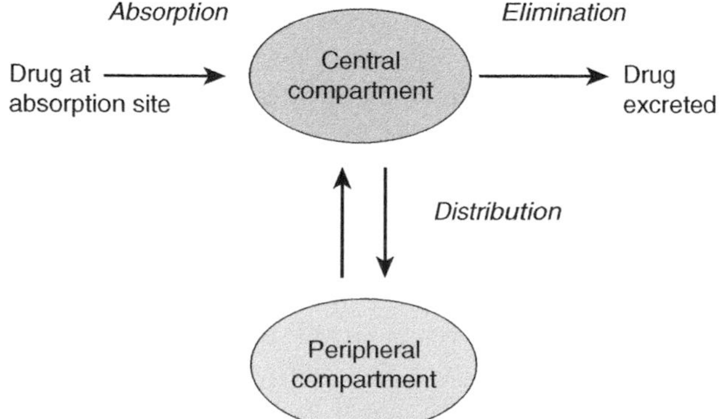

Figure 4.2 Two-compartment drug distribution model.

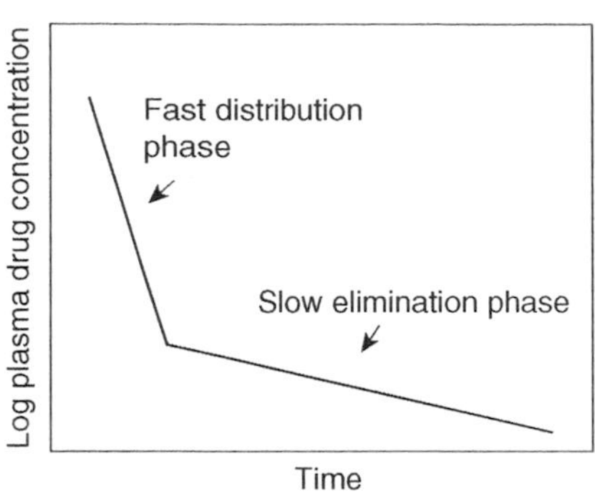

Figure 4.3 Drug disappearance from plasma, following single intravenous dose, in a two-compartment model.

the drug is said to follow a single-compartment model. The fall in plasma level following a single IV dose within a two-compartment model is shown in Figure 4.3. The practical consideration of a two-compartment model is that plasma drug samples, taken for monitoring purposes, need to be taken after the distribution phase is completed, otherwise erroneously high results will be received.

4.4.4 Protein Binding

Within the plasma a proportion of administered drug dose will exist in the free form (unbound) but a further proportion of drug will be reversibly bound to proteins contained within plasma, for example albumin, alpha-1 acid glycoprotein and lipoproteins. Only the unbound drug can passively diffuse to tissue sites where a pharmacological action can occur. Acidic drugs will predominantly bind to albumin, whereas basic drugs will bind more extensively to alpha-1 glycoprotein or lipoproteins.

Protein binding can have significant consequences as a potential for drug/drug interactions, where one drug will displace another drug from protein binding sites with a subsequent increase in free drug. Valproate is highly protein bound and has been reported to displace other drugs from protein binding, such as warfarin, and itself can be displaced by high doses of aspirin (Zhou et al., 2018). For most drugs the total plasma concentration required for a clinical effect is less than the total protein binding capacity, so the protein binding sites are far from saturated and the fraction of drug bound is independent of the drug concentration. For drugs where the total plasma concentration is much higher, and saturation of protein binding becomes a possibility, dose increases can have a disproportionate effect upon therapeutic activity as when protein binding becomes saturated a larger proportion of the drug is in the free, active state.

4.4.5 Blood–Brain Barrier

Distribution of an administered drug into the target tissues will frequently require the drug to penetrate a cellular barrier. Psychotropic drugs all need to penetrate the blood–brain barrier, a continuous layer of endothelial cells, joined by tight junctions, which surrounds the capillaries within the brain and separates circulating blood from the central nervous system (CNS). The blood–brain barrier restricts the exchange of solutes between the blood and cerebral extracellular fluid, protecting the brain against potentially harmful neurotoxins or infections.

In addition to forming a protective barrier preventing the influx of harmful substances, the blood–brain barrier also plays a role in CNS homeostasis, regulating the internal CNS biochemistry profile and maintaining neurotransmitters within the CNS. As the CNS and peripheral nervous system utilize the same neurotransmitters this function prevents 'cross-talk' between the different parts of the nervous system (Abbott et al., 2010).

Drugs can penetrate the blood–brain barrier by one of three mechanisms: simple diffusion, facilitated transport or receptor-mediated transport. For drugs to penetrate the blood–brain barrier via simple diffusion they must possess a sufficient lipid solubility to facilitate diffusion. This results in the majority of psychotropic drugs being lipid soluble and consequently requiring extensive hepatic metabolism to enable clearance from the body. It is worth remembering that the anterior pituitary gland is located outside of the blood–brain barrier (to facilitate its role in hormone regulation). A consequence of this is dopamine D_2 receptor-acting agents do not have to cross the blood–brain barrier to access dopamine receptors situated on pituitary cells and thereby interfere with the control of prolactin.

4.5 Metabolism

4.5.1 A Two-Stage Process

The principle routes of drug clearance from the body are either via the kidneys (in urine) or the liver (in bile). Clearance from both of these routes is promoted by increasing the aqueous solubility of the drug and this is achieved by a two-stage process within the liver. Metabolic reactions will frequently inactivate the drug, but some drug metabolites are pharmacologically active, sometimes even more so than the parent drug. Prodrugs are pharmacologically inactive, but metabolic enzymes convert the inactive parent drug into a pharmacologically active substrate. An example of this is codeine, which itself has minimal analgesic effect, but is metabolized by the cytochrome P450 2D6 (CYP2D6) enzyme to morphine. Individuals who have absent or low intrinsic CYP2D6 activity, or who are receiving drugs which inhibit this enzyme activity (e.g. fluoxetine) will receive limited analgesic effect from codeine. By contrast, those with particularly high CYP2D6 activity may experience signs of overdose including confusion and respiratory depression, which has been fatal in children. The Clinical Pharmacogenetics Implementation Consortium (CPIC) therefore recommends use of another analgesic in CYP2D6 poor metabolizers or ultrarapid metabolizers (see Chapter 5 for enzyme definitions).

Drug metabolism is a two-stage process, with Phase I reactions resulting in non-synthetic chemical modification, formation or cleavage of functional groups within the compound. Phase II reactions involve conjugation with an endogenous substance, e.g. glycine, sulphate or glucuronic acid, to form molecules which have greater aqueous solubility.

4.5.2 Cytochrome P450

Phase I drug metabolic reactions are mediated in the liver by cytochrome P450 enzymes (CYP). In addition to mediating drug metabolism CYP enzymes are important in the biosynthesis and degradation of endogenous compounds such as steroids, lipids and vitamins. Classification of CYP enzymes are based upon the similarity of their constituent amino acids and they are given a family number, a subfamily letter and a number for an individual enzyme. Drug metabolism is predominantly undertaken by CYP1, CYP2 and CYP3 enzyme families. The most important isoenzymes for psychotropic drugs are: CYP1A2, CYP2A6, CYP2B6, CYP2D6, CYP2C19, CYP2C9, CYP3A4/5 and CYP3A43.

Some drugs are substrates of specific cytochrome enzymes and others are blockers and some can induce the production of more cytochromes. These are illustrated in Table 4.1.

Table 4.1 Interactions of psychotropic drugs with cytochromes
The table summarizes predominant metabolic pathway. Some psychotropics listed will have other minor metabolic pathways involving alternative cytochrome enzymes. This is not a comprehensive list and an up-to-date formulary should be consulted when considering drug interactions.

Substrates	Inhibitors	Inducers
	CYP1A2	
Agomelatine	Fluvoxamine	Phenobarbital
Asenapine		
Clozapine		
Melatonin		
Olanzapine		
	CYP2B6	
Bupropion		
Methadone		
Nicotine		
Sertraline		
	CYP2C9	
Lamotrigine		
Valproic acid		
	CYP2D6	
Amitriptyline	Amitriptyline	
Amphetamines	Asenapine	
Aripiprazole	Bupropion	

Table 4.1 (cont.)

Substrates	Inhibitors	Inducers
Atomoxetine	Duloxetine	
Clomipramine	Fluoxetine	
Fluoxetine	Paroxetine	
Galantamine		
Iloperidone		
Imipramine		
Mianserin		
Nortriptyline		
Olanzapine		
Perphenazine		
Risperidone		
Trimipramine		
Venlafaxine		
Vortioxetine		
Zuclopenthixol		
	CYP3A4	
Alfentanil	Fluoxetine	Asenapine
Alprazolam	Paroxetine	Carbamazepine
Amitriptyline		Modafinil
Aripiprazole		Phenobarbital
Buprenorphine		Phenytoin
Buspirone		St John's wort
Carbamazepine		
Clonazepam		
Donepezil		
Dosulepin		
Fentanyl		
Fluoxetine		

Table 4.1 (cont.)

Substrates	Inhibitors	Inducers
Galantamine		
Lurasidone		
Methadone		
Midazolam		
Mirtazapine		
Nitrazepam		
Pimozide		
Quetiapine		
Reboxetine		
Sertindole		
Trazodone		
Zaleplon		
Ziprasidone		
Zolpidem		
Zopiclone		

From Taylor et al. (2018).

4.5.3 Cytochrome System Polymorphisms

The production of enzymes within the cytochrome system is controlled by specific genetic variants, or alleles, within the individual DNA, as well as other mechanisms of regulation of gene expression; see, for example, the epigenetic mechanisms of regulation of CYP3A enzymes described in Chapter 5. Genetic polymorphisms (or sequence variants) occur when distinct, different genetic alleles are present at the same locus (position on the DNA strand) within different individuals (Albert, 2011). Polymorphisms within alleles coding for enzyme production can explain large individual variability in drug metabolism, both in the liver and other sites including the brain, which might account for observed differences in drug efficacy and safety (Stingl & Viviani, 2015). For example, a recent meta-analysis investigated whether CYP2C19 polymorphisms predicted the efficacy and side effects in patients treated with citalopram or escitalopram (Fabbri et al., 2018). CYP2C19 phenotypes include poor metabolizers and extensive metabolizers. The analysis showed that CYP2C19 poor metabolizers had higher remission rates and greater symptom improvement compared to extensive metabolizers. In addition, poor metabolizers had more side-effects early on in treatment (Fabbri et al., 2018).

Table 4.2 Variations of CYP2D6 and CYP2C19 phenotypes according to ethnicity (approximate frequencies, %) (de Leon et al., 2006)

Phenotype	Caucasian	East Asians	African-Americans	North African and Middle Eastern	Mexican Americans
CYP2D6 PM	5–10	1	1–2	2	3
CYP2D6 UM	1–10	0–2	2	10–29	1
CYP2C19 PM	2–4	10–25	1–5	2	4

Approximately 25% of all prescribed drugs and 80% of antipsychotics and antidepressants are metabolized via CYP2D6 (Ingelman-Sundberg, 2004; Tiwari et al., 2009). A range of alleles can affect the enzymatic activity of CYP2D6 and, depending upon the combination present, individuals are classified as either: ultrarapid metabolizers (UM), extensive (or normal) metabolizers (EM) or poor metabolizers (PM) (Muller et al., 2013). The incidence of altered alleles, leading to PM status, is greatest amongst Caucasian ethnic groups and a lower frequency of these alleles amongst Asian, African and South American populations explains the lower incidence of poor metabolizers amongst these groups (Zanger & Schwab, 2013) (see Table 4.2). Similarly, ethnic variation in enzymatic activity can be shown for CYP2C19, responsible for metabolism of drugs including citalopram, escitalopram, amitriptyline and sertraline (Brandl et al., 2013). Chapter 5 provides more details on genetic polymorphism of CYP2D6.

4.5.4 Pharmacokinetic Drug Interactions

Drugs which alter the activity of cytochrome P450 enzymes, either by inhibiting or increasing their action, are a potential source of drug interactions. Drugs which inhibit P450 enzymes will increase the levels of drugs metabolized by those enzymes, possibly leading to toxic effects. An example of this is the inhibition of CYP2D6 by fluoxetine, leading to increased plasma levels of other drugs metabolized by this enzyme, resulting in increased side effects and possible toxicity, e.g. amitriptyline (see Table 4.1). Conversely, drugs which are enzyme inducers will lead to a reduced level of the substrate drug, resulting in possible therapeutic failure. Rifampicin, an antibiotic used in the treatment of tuberculosis, is a potent inducer of CYP3A4, an important enzyme in the metabolism of aripiprazole. Co-administration of aripiprazole with rifampicin, or other inducers of this enzyme (such as carbamazepine, phenytoin, phenobarbital, efavirenz, nevirapine or St John's wort) can lead to reduced plasma levels of aripiprazole and possible treatment failure. In general, drugs that are metabolized by more than one CYP are less likely to be associated with significant pharmacokinetic drug interactions. However, one important exception is clozapine, which is a substrate for three CYPs but can still develop excessive alterations in plasma levels when 1A2 enzyme levels are altered, e.g. induced by smoking.

4.6 Excretion

The process by which drugs leave the body is termed excretion. The principal site for drug excretion is the kidneys. Biliary excretion is important with some drugs where the glucuronide conjugate might be concentrated in bile and returned to the intestines. In the intestines the glucuronide conjugate can then be hydrolysed and the free drug becomes available for reabsorption. This enterohepatic circulation creates a reservoir of recirculating drug that can account for up to 20% of total drug available in the body, prolonging drug action. Enterohepatic circulation is an important consideration in the excretion of morphine.

Renal filtration accounts for the majority of drug clearance from the body. Within the kidneys, pores in the glomerular endothelium filter out approximately 20% of the plasma into the renal tubules. The majority of water and most electrolytes are either passively or actively reabsorbed from the renal tubules back into circulation. As most drug compounds are polar molecules (ionized) they are unable to diffuse back into the circulation and so are excreted in urine. Renal drug excretion reduces the older an individual is; when aged 80 years the renal clearance is about 50% of what it was when an individual was aged 30. Renal clearance is governed by the principles of transmembrane passage. Drugs bound to plasma proteins are not filtered, due to the large molecular size of the protein. Drugs, or their metabolites, in the unionized state will be readily reabsorbed from the renal tubule. The degree to which a drug or metabolite is ionized will be affected by the urine pH, which varies from 4.5 to 8.0. Drugs which are weak acids will be more readily reabsorbed in acidic urine, so if the pH of urine drops the excretion of acidic drugs will decrease. If the pH of urine increases then the renal excretion of weakly basic drugs will fall, due to an increased proportion being in the unionized form.

4.7 Half-Life and Related Issues

4.7.1 Half-Life ($t_{½}$)

Half-life is a term by which the longevity of a drug within the body can be expressed. It is defined as the length of time it takes for the level to fall by one-half (see Figure 4.4). For any given drug, population-based studies are used to record the expected elimination $t_{½}$. This expected elimination $t_{½}$ for a drug will be increased by factors such as age and any co-morbid medical conditions, especially those which impair hepatic function. Co-administered drugs can increase the elimination $t_{½}$ if they inhibit the action of CYP enzymatic pathways responsible for the drug's hepatic metabolism. Conversely, co-administered drugs which induce CYP enzymes will reduce the $t_{½}$. Enzymatic induction can take days or weeks to be seen as the process requires synthesis of new proteins. Enzymatic inhibition is a much more rapid process, with clinical effects being observed within hours of administering an inhibiting agent.

4.7.2 Steady State

Steady state refers to a position where the concentration of an administered drug has become as stable as it can be within the body following repeated dosing. It marks the point in time where the rate of absorption of a drug into plasma equals the rate of clearance. The time to reach a steady-state plasma level is related to the $t_{½}$ for the drug. With oral drugs there is always some variation around the mean concentration with a small elevation during the absorption phase which then falls into the so-called 'trough' phase. With depots then the plasma concentration at steady state can be very stable.

Table 4.3 Relationship between half-life and steady state

Number of half-lives	% of steady state
1	50
2	75
3	87.5
4	93.8
5	96.9
6	98.4
7	99.2

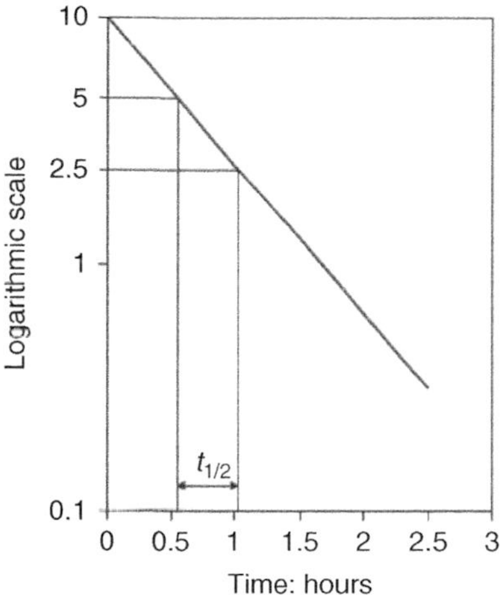

Figure 4.4 Plasma concentration against time after a single intravenous dose of a drug with a $t_{1/2}$ of 0.5 hours.

In most situations a drug is said to be in steady state when five half-lives have elapsed (Table 4.3). As the time to reach steady state is increased with drugs that have a long $t_{1/2}$ so the time before full effects (both therapeutic and adverse) are fully realized will be longer. With psychotropic drugs this is a particular concern with the administration of antipsychotic long-acting injections (depots), whose half-lives have been extended to between 7 and 28 days by the use of pharmaceutical formulation techniques previously described in the chapter.

4.7.3 Therapeutic Range

Some psychiatric drugs have a recognized therapeutic range of plasma concentrations, examples including lithium and clozapine. The therapeutic index (also referred to as the therapeutic ratio) is a comparison of the concentration of a drug that causes the therapeutic effect to the concentration that causes toxicity. Dugs with a low therapeutic index (i.e. toxic concentration is just a few multiples of the therapeutic one) usually require monitoring of their plasma concentration. The main such drug in psychiatry is lithium. Examples of drugs used in general medicine with a low therapeutic index include aminoglycosides, digoxin, phenytoin, rifampicin, theophylline and warfarin.

4.7.4 Loading Doses

For drugs which have a long $t_{½}$ the time to reach therapeutic target levels can be reduced using loading doses. With depot antipsychotics, or long-acting injections, the initial doses can be increased or the frequency between injections can be reduced. It is possible to calculate the dose required to produce a given plasma level if the $t_{½}$ and volume of distribution for a given drug is known. Standard initiation loading strategies are used to speed up the time to therapeutic plasma levels when commencing some psychiatric drugs including certain long-acting antipsychotic injections, e.g. paliperidone palmitate.

4.8 Pharmacokinetic Characteristics of Psychotropic Drugs

Most psychotropic drugs share a number of pharmacokinetic characteristics (Hiemke et al., 2011):

- Good absorption from the gastrointestinal tract with plasma concentrations reaching a maximum within 1–6 hours.
- Highly variable first-pass metabolism, with systemic bioavailability ranging from 5% to 90%.
- Fast distribution from plasma to the CNS with 2- to 40-fold greater levels in brain tissue than plasma.
- High apparent volumes of distribution (about 10–50 L/kg).
- Low trough plasma concentrations under steady state (approximately 0.1–500 ng/ml).
- Slow elimination from plasma, mainly by hepatic metabolism with half-lives ranging between 12 and 36 hours.
- Linear pharmacokinetics at therapeutic doses, meaning doubling the daily dose will result in doubling of plasma levels.
- Low renal excretion and low impact of renal insufficiency upon plasma drug levels
- Cytochrome P450 and UDP-glucuronosyltransferases as major metabolic enzyme systems.

Importantly, there are several key exceptions to the above general rules, which are worth noting (Hiemke et al., 2011):

- Venlafaxine, quetiapine and rivastigmine exhibit short elimination half-lives (approximately 2–10 hours).
- Aripiprazole and fluoxetine both have long elimination half-lives (72 hours for aripiprazole and 3–15 days for fluoxetine (including its active metabolite norfluoxetine).
- Amisulpride, sulpiride, lithium salts, memantine and gabapentin are mainly excreted renally and are poorly metabolized by the liver.
- Paroxetine exhibits non-linear pharmacokinetics due to the inhibition of its own metabolism by one of its metabolites.

- Clozapine may also inhibit its own metabolism but the clinical consequences of this are not clearly understood.

4.9 Therapeutic Drug Monitoring (TDM)

4.9.1 General Principles of TDM

Therapeutic drug monitoring (TDM) is the measurement of drug levels combined with the application of clinical interpretation to alter prescribing for individual patients. Most frequently this involves the measure of plasma drug levels and adjustment of prescribing for drugs with a narrow therapeutic index and a high degree of interpatient pharmacokinetic variability. The considerable interpatient variability of pharmacokinetic properties should not be underestimated. Differences between patients in the ability to absorb, distribute, metabolize and excrete drugs can produce greater than 20-fold variation in the plasma level resulting from identical drug doses. Application of TDM can result in optimal drug doses being prescribed for individual patients which will maximize the therapeutic benefits and minimize the risk of toxic effects. A further potential of TDM is the ability to improve cost-effectiveness of drug therapy.

A key assumption of TDM is that for the given drug there is an established relationship between blood levels and clinical effects such as therapeutic effects, adverse effects and toxicity. This assumption further requires a plasma concentration range for the drug with a minimum effectiveness drug plasma level and a maximum safe level (Hiemke, 2008). This range can be described by a range of terms such as: therapeutic index, therapeutic window, therapeutic reference range or optimal plasma concentration. The AGNP (Arbeitsgemeinschaft für Neuropsychopharmakologie und Pharmakopsychiatrie) consensus Guidelines on TDM uses the term therapeutic reference ranges and defines it as a range of medication concentrations with a lower limit below which a drug-induced therapeutic response is unlikely to occur and an upper limit above which tolerability decreases or above which it is relatively unlikely that therapeutic improvement will be further enhanced.

4.9.2 Indications for TDM in Psychiatry

Typical indications for measuring plasma concentrations of medication in psychiatry include:

- Dose optimization after initial prescription or dose change.
- Psychotropic agents with a narrow therapeutic index, for which TDM is mandatory (e.g. lithium).
- Suspected non-adherence to medication.
- Lack of clinical improvement following administration of recommended dose.
- Co-prescribing of drugs with known potential to interact with an established drug regimen.
- Patients with pharmacokinetically relevant co-morbidities (e.g. hepatic or renal impairment).
- Elderly patients (>65 years).
- Pregnant or breastfeeding patient.
- Non-response or relapse despite administration of adequate doses.

4.9.3 Practical Aspects for TDM in Psychiatry

Therapeutic drug monitoring should be requested when the result will provide an answer to a specific question, the result will be of little value if it is not clear what the question is. Frequently, a series of sample measurements will be required to answer a therapeutic question, for example to clarify whether poor therapeutic response is the result of poor medication adherence. The majority of TDM in psychiatry is based upon trough levels taken at steady-state pharmacokinetics. This will be achieved by blood samples being taken in the morning, prior to any morning doses being administered. Although usual TDM for lithium requires blood sampling 12 hours post-dose, rather than trough levels, blood sampling in the morning will typically be 12 hours after the previous night's dose, hence why once-daily lithium doses are administered at night. With most psychotropic drugs having elimination half-lives between 12 and 36 hours then steady-state pharmacokinetics will be reached approximately 3–8 days after commencing therapy or a change in dosage has occurred.

An integral part of TDM is the clinical decisions made in response to the plasma level results received. Decisions regarding increasing or reducing doses will be guided by whether the result is within, above or below the reference range for that drug. However, it is important to also consider the patient's presentation when interpreting plasma level results. The therapeutic reference range will have been derived from population-based studies, but individual patients might demonstrate a response which falls outside of this range. Some patients will demonstrate a therapeutic response, even though their plasma level is below the minimum threshold of the therapeutic reference range. Alternatively, some patients might present with pronounced side effects and still have a plasma level below the maximum threshold. It is worth remembering the general advice to treat the patient, rather than treat the level.

Table 4.4 provides details of therapeutic range, suggested sample timing and time to reach steady state for a range of frequently prescribed psychotropic drugs (Taylor et al., 2018).

4.10 Introduction to Pharmacodynamics

Pharmacodynamics is the study of the effect that an administered dose has upon the body. To completely understand the pharmacological action of a drug, both its desired effects and adverse effects, then the pharmacodynamic effects need to be considered. This involves considering the biochemical, physiological and molecular effects of the drug which will influence receptor binding or chemical interactions of the drug upon target proteins. Pharmacological response to an administered dose is dependent upon the drug binding to the target, as well as the concentration of drug at the target site. The following sections review key aspects of pharmacodynamics including protein targets for drug binding, drug–receptor interactions, drug–receptor affinity and efficacy, dose–response relationships, concept of tolerance and withdrawal reactions.

4.11 Protein Targets for Drug Binding

There are four main protein targets for drug activity within the body, each representing a different type of regulatory protein.

Table 4.4 Therapeutic drug monitoring criteria for common psychotropic agents

Drug	Target range	Sample timing	Time to steady state	Comments
Amisulpride	200–320 µg/L	Trough	3 days	
Aripiprazole	150–210 µg/L	Trough	15–16 days	
Carbamazepine	>7 mg/L	Trough	2 weeks	Carbamazepine induces own metabolism. Time to steady state dependent upon autoinduction
Clozapine	350–500 µg/L Upper limit of target range is ill-defined	Trough	2–3 days	
Lamotrigine	Not established, but suggest 2.5–15 mg/L	Trough	5 days Autoinduction thought to occur, time to steady state may be longer	Debate over utility of lamotrigine levels, particularly in bipolar disorder. Toxicity may be increased above 15 mg/L, but normally well tolerated
Lithium	0.6–1.0 mmol/L 0.4 mmol/L may be sufficient for some indications; >1.0 mmol/L required for mania	12 hours post-dose	5 days	Well-established therapeutic range, although largely derived from older data sources
Olanzapine	20–40 µg/L	12 hours post-dose	1 week oral 2 months for depot	
Paliperidone	20–60 µg/L (9-OH risperidone)	Trough	2–3 days oral 2 months depot	Therapeutic range same as for risperidone. Like risperidone, plasma level monitoring is not recommended

Table 4.4 (cont.)

Drug	Target range	Sample timing	Time to steady state	Comments
Phenytoin	10–20 mg/L	Trough	Variable	Follows zero order kinetics. Measurement of free (unbound) phenytoin levels more useful than total plasma level
Quetiapine	Around 50–100 µg/L	Trough	2–3 days	Therapeutic range not clearly defined. Plasma level monitoring is not recommended
Risperidone	20–60 µg/L (active moiety)	Trough	2–3 days oral 6–8 weeks depot	Plasma level monitoring is not recommended
Tricyclic Antidepressants	Nortriptyline 50–150 µg/L Amitriptyline 100–200 µg/L	Trough	2–3 days	Rarely used and dubious benefit. Use electrocardiogram to aid assessment of cardiotoxicity
Valproate	50–100 µg/L Epilepsy and bipolar	Trough	2–3 days	Some doubt over values of plasma levels in epilepsy and bipolar disorder. Adverse effects are more common when plasma level exceeds 125 µg/L

1. Receptors. Target molecules through which physiological mediators such as neurotransmitters produce their effects. Important examples for the action of psychotropic drugs include dopaminergic or serotonergic receptors within the brain. All currently available antipsychotics are dopamine D_2 receptor antagonists or dopamine D_2 receptor partial agonists.
2. Enzymes. Numerous drugs exert their pharmacological effect by inhibiting the action of enzymes. Within psychiatry this is often the inhibition of enzymes which deactivate target neurotransmitters, for example acetylcholinesterase inhibitors used in the treatment of dementias (see Chapter 14). Another example is the monoamine oxidase inhibitors (MAOIs), a class of antidepressant, that inhibit the breakdown of monoamine neurotransmitters (see Chapter 7).
3. Carrier molecules (transporter proteins). The physiological role of transporter proteins is to convey ions or small organic molecules across cell membranes. Transporter proteins within the presynaptic membrane of nerve cells facilitate the reuptake of neurotransmitters such as noradrenaline or serotonin. These are the principal target for many drugs used to treat depression including selective serotonin reuptake inhibitors (SSRIs) and serotonin and noradrenaline reuptake inhibitors (SNRIs).
4. Ion channels. An example of this protein type is the ligand-gated ion channels, where the incorporated receptor facilitates the opening of the ion channel under the influence of an agonist. The GABA (gamma-aminobutyric acid) receptor is an example of this type of receptor, with benzodiazepines targeting a distinct portion of the receptor complex and facilitating the opening of the channel by the inhibitory neurotransmitter GABA. Lithium is believed to exert its actions partly through antagonism of calcium channels.

A small number of centrally acting drugs exert their actions through mechanisms other than binding with the four protein targets listed above. For example, amphetamine causes release of noradrenaline and dopamine into the synaptic cleft while L-tryptophan is the precursor for 5-hydroxytryptamine (5-HT) and its administration leads to increased 5-HT synthesis.

4.12 Drug–Receptor Interactions

Drugs can have either an agonist or antagonist action when interacting with a target receptor. Drugs can bind to various sites on a receptor; the active site where the endogenous agonist binds (the orthosteric site), an allosteric site or a unique binding site that is not involved in the normal physiological regulation of the receptor's activity. When the binding of a drug to a receptor leads to activation of the receptor, meaning there is a tissue response caused by the action of the drug, it is referred to as an agonist. Alternatively, if a drug binds to a receptor and there is no tissue response it is referred to as an antagonist. In cases of antagonist binding to drug receptors this will prevent either drugs or endogenous substances from elucidating a tissue response. Antagonists are sometimes termed 'blockers', for example β-blockers and calcium channel blockers.

The ability of a drug to activate a receptor is not an absolute, all or nothing action, rather it is a graded response. Drugs which can produce a maximal response, that is, the largest response a tissue can give, are referred to as full agonists whereas drugs which only produce a partial tissue response are referred to as partial agonists. The difference between full agonists and partial agonists is accounted for by the difference between occupancy and response. Partial agonists might have a similar receptor occupancy as that of a full agonist, but at any given degree of occupancy the response seen is less with a partial agonist, such that even at 100% occupancy a partial agonist will not elucidate a full tissue response.

Most drugs have the ability to interact with multiple receptors, but they do have relative selectivity. Selectivity is the degree to which a drug acts upon a given receptor, or subtype, relative to others.

Antagonists can be competitive or less commonly non-competitive. A competitive antagonist competes with an endogenous agonist for the active site on a receptor. The antagonist can be displaced from the active site by the agonist. Consequently, high doses of the endogenous agonist can overcome the inhibitor and still exert a maximal effect. The degree of response that is achieved will depend on the relative doses and affinities of the agonist and competitive antagonist. Competitive antagonists can be used to reverse the effects of drugs that have already been consumed. Examples include flumazenil, which can reverse the effects of benzodiazepines, and naloxone, which is used to reverse overdose caused by opioid drugs such as heroin or morphine.

A non-competitive antagonist cannot be displaced from the receptor by an agonist and so the maximal effect of the agonist is reduced irrespective of its dose, i.e. the antagonism is insurmountable. Non-competitive inhibitors may bind to the active site or an allosteric site on a receptor. Non-competitive inhibitors can be reversible or irreversible. A reversible non-competitive antagonist can be removed from the receptor site whereas an irreversible non-competitive antagonist is permanently bound to the receptor. Phenelzine, a MAOI, is an example of an irreversible inhibitor; it binds irreversibly to the enzyme MAO. Re-establishing full function of MAO will only occur when new molecules of the enzyme are synthesized, and the inhibited molecules are broken down. This explains why drug interactions can still occur for several weeks after an irreversible MAOI such as phenelzine is stopped.

4.13 Drug–Receptor Affinity and Efficacy

The binding affinity of a drug refers to how strongly it binds to the receptor binding sites. Drugs with a high binding affinity will demonstrate strong intermolecular binding forces between the drug and the receptor, with the opposite being true for drugs with a low binding affinity. Frequently, high-affinity binding of a drug to a receptor will produce a higher degree of occupancy, so for a given drug concentration the proportion bound to the receptor will be greater for a drug with higher affinity than for a drug with lower binding affinity. Binding affinity is usually measured by the equilibrium dissociation constant (KD); the smaller the KD value, the greater the binding affinity of a drug for its target. The efficacy, or intrinsic activity, of a drug refers to how strongly it activates a receptor after binding to it.

4.14 Dose–Response Relationships

The response produced by a drug in a given physiological tissue can be graphically represented, with the drug dose or concentration plotted on the x-axis and the measured effect (as a proportion of the maximal effect) plotted on the y-axis. This representation

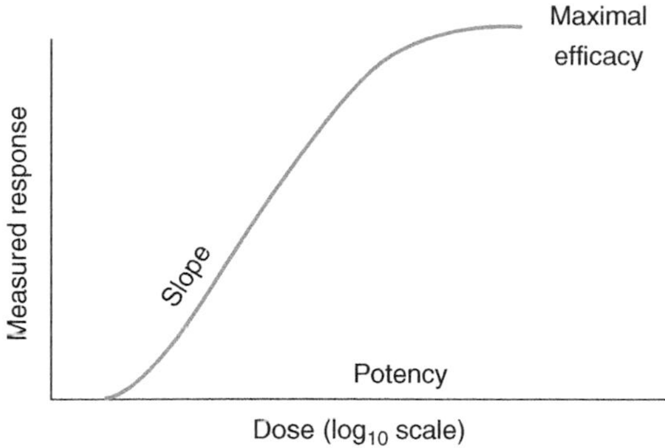

Figure 4.5 Theoretical dose–response curve.

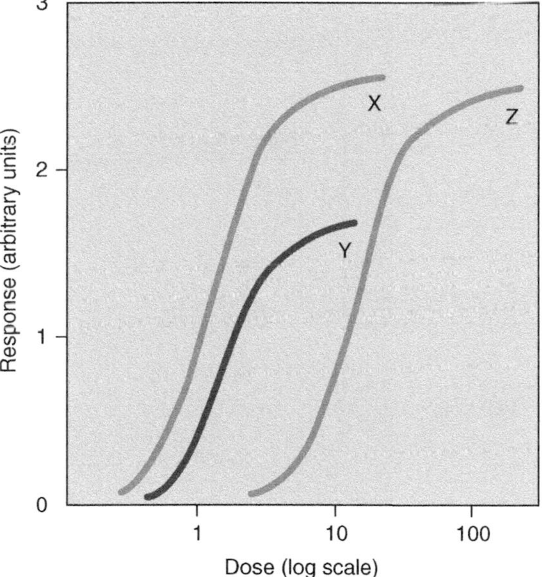

Figure 4.6 Comparison of dose–response curves.

will produce the dose–response relationship for a given drug independent of time. A theoretical example is given in Figure 4.5.

The position of the curve along the *x*-axis provides an indication of the drug's potency. More potent drugs will produce a response at lower concentrations resulting in a curve shifted towards the left-hand side, closer to the *y*-axis. For many drugs there is a maximal efficacy, or ceiling effect, where larger doses fail to produce a greater response. On the dose–response curve this effect is seen by a flattening, or plateau, of the curve. These differing effects can be seen in Figure 4.6.

In Figure 4.6 drug X has greater biological activity per dosing equivalent and is thus more potent than drug Y or Z. Drugs X and Z have equal efficacy, indicated by their maximal attainable response (ceiling effect). Drug Y is more potent than drug Z, but its maximal efficacy is lower.

Figures 4.5 and 4.6 are theoretical, illustrative examples. However, it is possible to produce similar graphs for psychotropic agents, based upon research-derived data. The

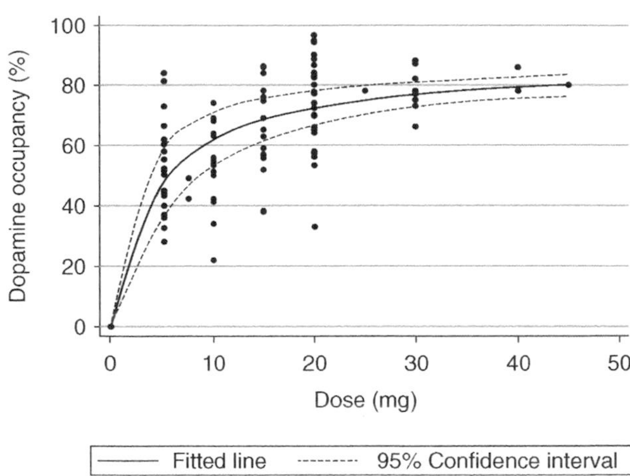

Figure 4.7 Striatal dopamine occupancy versus olanzapine dose (Bishara et al., 2013).

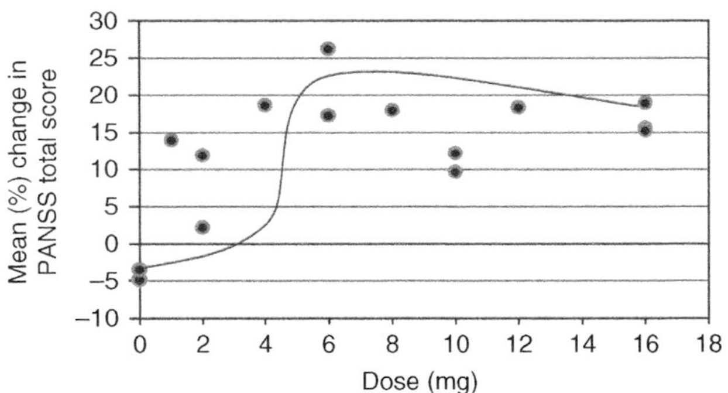

Figure 4.8 Mean percentage change in PANSS total score versus risperidone dose (1–16 mg).

study by Bishara et al. (2013) collected data from six papers exploring the relationship between olanzapine dose and striatal dopamine receptor occupancy using positron emission tomography. The dose–response curve is shown in Figure 4.7. Dopamine occupancy seems to reach the threshold for response (65%) at approximately olanzapine 12 mg daily. The model predicted the maximum dopamine receptor occupancy to be 87% and a dose of olanzapine 4 mg to achieve 50% of this.

Dose–response curves can also be used to assess the impact of higher doses on clinical measures, such as the Positive and Negative Symptom Score (PANSS). Figure 4.8 shows the mean change in PANSS score for a range of risperidone doses (Ezewuzie & Taylor, 2006). Data taken from three studies showed an increase in efficacy with risperidone doses up to 4 mg per day, with the effect plateauing, or even reducing when doses exceeded 6 mg per day.

4.15 Pharmacodynamic Drug Interactions

Pharmacodynamic drug interactions are where agents with similar neurotransmitter effects, or physiological actions, combine to produce an exaggerated response in an individual. In contrast to the pharmacokinetic drug interactions described above with pharmacodynamic drug interactions, the magnitude and duration of drug action remains unchanged but the sensitivity or responsiveness to a drug is altered by the interacting agent having an agonist or antagonist effect. Usually these effects occur at the receptor level when agents share the same neurotransmitter effects, but can also occur when agents produce similar physiological responses by differing neurotransmitter effects.

Examples of pharmacodynamic drug interactions in psychiatry include:

- Benzodiazepines and opioids, both agents cause generalized suppression of CNS activity which can lead to increased sedations and respiratory suppression when these agents are taken together.
- Alcohol and benzodiazepines, combined use leading to generalized CNS suppression and risk of increased sedation and respiratory suppression.
- SSRIs and 5-HT_1 receptor agonists (triptans), combined use can lead to serotonin syndrome, potentially fatal range of symptoms resulting from excess CNS serotonin activity.
- Gabapentin and opioids, combined use can lead to excess sedation and death.

4.16 Tolerance

Over time repeated interaction of a drug at a receptor can result in a diminished response. Instances where this occurs quickly (over a few minutes of repeated or continuous interaction) are referred to as desensitization or tachyphylaxis. Where there is a more gradual decrease in responsiveness to a drug, taking days or weeks to develop, this is referred to as tolerance. Receptor tolerance can occur via different mechanisms:

- Change in receptors.
- Rapid desensitization occurs at ion channels coupled to receptors, caused by a conformational change in the receptor resulting in tight binding of the agonist molecule without opening the ionic channel. A slower mechanism, phosphorylation of intracellular receptor regions, is an alternative mechanism by which ion channels become desensitized. Phosphorylation can cause desensitization of G-protein-coupled receptors.
- Loss of receptors.
- Prolonged exposure to agonists often results in a decreased number of receptors expressed on the cellular surface. Internalization, a process whereby receptors are taken into the cell via endocytosis, reduces the number of receptors available.
- Exhaustion of mediator stores.
- Depletion of an essential intermediate or final substance. Amphetamine works by releasing amines from nerve terminals. Repeated exposure to amphetamine will result in depletion of these amine stores and subsequent reduced pharmacological effect.
- Increased metabolic degradation of the drug.
- The physiological effects of a drug are gradually reduced over time if that drug induces its own metabolism by CYP hepatic enzymes. Carbamazepine induces the activity of CYP3A4 enzymes and is itself metabolized via this route. Over time doses of carbamazepine need to be increased in order to compensate for this effect and maintain a consistent plasma level of drug.
- Physiological adaption.

- The net physiological effects of a drug are reduced by increased activity in a competing neurotransmitter pathway, e.g. increased noradrenaline activity to compensate for alcohol sedation. If the drug is suddenly stopped and a withdrawal reaction is induced then the increased activity is unopposed, this can account for many withdrawal symptoms encountered (see next section).

4.17 Withdrawal Reactions

Withdrawal reactions are defined as a group of symptoms which occur on cessation or reduction of use of a psychoactive substance, which has been taken repeatedly, usually for a prolonged period or at high doses. Specific features of a withdrawal syndrome will depend upon the substance that has been taken, but some features common to many withdrawal syndromes include: sweating, nausea, agitation/anxiety or aching muscles. Symptoms of a withdrawal reaction may initially appear within a few hours of ceasing substance consumption and will be relieved by further substance use (World Health Organization, 1992). Withdrawal can be precipitated by giving a person dependent on an agonist a competitive antagonist to the receptor as in the case of naloxone with opioids and flumazenil with benzodiazepines.

The physiological mechanism that accounts for this withdrawal reaction is the body's response to the receptor-mediated mechanisms of tolerance. In situations where repeated administration of a drug has resulted in the development of tolerance the normal physiological processes will have become reduced. When the drug is abruptly withdrawn characteristic symptoms will be present until the normal level of physiological activity has been restored.

It is important to differentiate between withdrawal symptoms which are a physiological reaction to stopping or reducing a drug and a drug dependence syndrome. ICD-10 highlights that dependence is a '*cluster of physiological, behavioural, and cognitive phenomena in which the use of a substance or a class of substances takes on a much higher priority for a given individual than other behaviours that once had greater value*' (World Health Organization, 1992). Withdrawal symptoms are one criterion for dependence syndrome in ICD-10 but their presence alone is insufficient for diagnosis. DSM-5 eliminated the DSM-4 division of dependence and abuse and combined both disorders in a single category of substance use disorder (American Psychiatric Association, 2013). Withdrawal symptoms are one of 11 criteria for substance use disorder and at least two criteria are required for diagnosis. Many psychiatric drugs can cause withdrawal symptoms but usually without other features of dependence/ substance use disorder. Examples include antidepressants, antipsychotics and lithium.

Note also withdrawal reactions can be of two types (Nutt, 2003). Usually they are the return of symptoms previously suppressed by the drug, e.g. benzodiazepine withdrawal leading to anxiety. But in some cases, e.g. antidepressant and antipsychotic withdrawal, new symptoms can emerge that were never experienced before – these are called discontinuation reactions. With the SSRIs they can include feelings of electric shock down the spine or alterations in visual perception. With olanzapine insomnia may emerge. Their origins are unclear but presumably reflect adaptations in other systems, e.g. in the case of olanzapine an up-regulation of histamine receptors following chronic blockade by this drug.

4.18 Conclusions

The complex processes and effects which occur within pharmacokinetic and pharmacodynamic actions go some way in explaining the wide individual variation in response to drug therapy. Overall, it is important to consider the patient's response to therapy, and adjust any drug regimen accordingly, even if this response differs from that predicted by population norms.

References

Abbott J, Patabendige AAK, Dolman DEM, et al. (2010). Structure and function of the blood–brain barrier. *Neurobiol Dis*, 37(1), 13–25.

Albert PR (2011). What is a functional genetic polymorphism? Defining classes of functionality. *J Psychiatry Neurosci*, 36(6), 363–365.

American Psychiatric Association (2013). *Diagnostic and Statistical Manual of Mental Disorders*, 5th ed. Arlington, VA: American Psychiatric Association.

Bishara D, Olofinjana O, Sparshatt A, et al. (2013). Olanzapine: a systematic review and meta-regression of the relationships between dose, plasma concentration, receptor occupancy, and response. *J Clin Psychopharmacol*, 33(3), 329–335.

Brandl EJ, Tiwari AK, Zhou X, et al. (2013). Influence of CYP2D6 and CYP2C19 gene variants on antidepressant response in obsessive-compulsive disorder. *Pharmacogenomics J*, 14(2), 176–181.

de Leon J, Armstrong SC, Cozza KL (2006). Clinical guidelines for psychiatrists for the use of pharmacogenetic testing for CYP450 2D6 and CYP450 2C19. *Psychosomatics*, 47(1), 75–85.

electronic Medicines Compendium (2018a). Summary of Product Characteristics: Loxapine (Asasuve) 9.1 mg inhalation powder, pre-dispensed. Galen. Available at: www.medicines.org.uk/emc/medicine/32246 (last accessed 13.2.18).

electronic Medicines Compendium (2018b). Summary of Product Characteristics: Lurasidone (Latuda). Sunovion Pharmaceutical Ltd. Available at: www.medicines.org.uk/emc/product/3299/smpc (last accessed 13.2.18).

El-Kattan A, Varma M (2012). Oral absorption, intestinal metabolism and human oral bioavailability. In Topics on drug metabolism. InTech. Available at: www.intechopen.com/books/topics-on-drug-metabolism/oral-absorption-intestinal-metabolism-and-human-oral-bioavailability (last accessed 15.1.18).

Ezewuzie N, Taylor D (2006). Establishing a dose-response relationship for oral risperidone in relapsed schizophrenia. *J Psychopharmacol*, 20(1), 86–90.

Fabbri C, Tansey KE, Perlis RH, et al. (2018). Effect of cytochrome CYP2C19 metabolizing activity on antidepressant response and side effects: meta-analysis of data from genome-wide association studies. *Eur Neuropsychopharmacol*, 28(8), 945–954.

Hiemke C (2008). Clinical utility of drug measurement and pharmacokinetics – therapeutic drug monitoring in psychiatry. *Eur J Clin Pharmacol*, 64(2), 159–166.

Hiemke C, Baumann P, Bergemann N, et al. (2011). AGNP Consensus Guidelines for Therapeutic Drug Monitoring in Psychiatry: Update 2011. *Pharmacopsychiatry*, 44(6), 195–235.

Ingelman-Sundberg M (2004). Human drug metabolising cytochrome P450 enzymes: properties and polymorphisms. *Naunyn Schmiedebergs Arch Pharmacol*, 369(1), 89–104.

Markl D, Zeitler JA (2017). A review of disintegration mechanisms and measurement techniques. *Pharm Res*, 34(5), 890–917.

Muller DJ, Kekin I, Kao ACC, Brandl E (2013). Towards the implementation of CYP2D6 and CYP2C19 genotypes in clinical practice: update and report from a pharmacogenetic service clinic. *Int Rev Psychiatry*, 25(5), 554–571.

National Institute for Health and Care Excellence (NICE) (2015). *Violence and Aggression: Short-term management in mental health, health and community settings*. NICE Guideline [NG10]. London: National Institute for Health and Care

Excellence. Available at: http://nice.org.uk/guidance/ng10 (last accessed 13.2.18).

Nutt DJ (2003). Death and dependence: current controversies over the selective serotonin reuptake inhibitors. *J Psychopharmacol*, 17, 355–364.

Patteet L, Morrens M, Maudens KE, Niemegeers P, Sabbe B (2012). Therapeutic drug monitoring of common antipsychotics. *Ther Drug Monit*, 34(6), 629–651.

Stingl J, Viviani R (2015). Polymorphism in CYP2D6 and CYP2C19, members of the cytochrome P450 mixed-function oxidase system, in the metabolism of psychotropic drugs. *J Intern Med*, 277(2), 167–177.

Taylor D, Barnes TRE, Young AH (2018). *The Maudsley Prescribing Guidelines in Psychiatry*, 13th ed. Chichester: Wiley Blackwell.

Tiwari AK, Souza RP, Muller DJ (2009). Pharmacogenetics of anxiolytic drugs. *J Neural Transm (Vienna)*, 116(6), 667–677.

World Health Organization (1992). *The ICD-10 Classification of Mental and Behavioural Disorders: Clinical Descriptions and Diagnostic Guidelines*. Geneva: World Health Organization.

Zanger UM, Schwab M (2013). Cytochrome P450 enzymes in drug metabolism: regulation of gene expression, enzyme activities and impact of genetic variation. *Pharmacol Ther*, 138(1), 103–141.

Zhou C, Sui Y, Zhao W, et al. (2018). The critical interaction between valproate sodium and warfarin: case report and review. *BMC Pharmacol Toxicol*, 19, 60. doi 10.1186/s40360-018-0251-0.

Pharmacogenomics and Psychopharmacology

Diego L. Lapetina, Esther H. Yang, Beatriz C. Henriques and Katherine J. Aitchison

5.1 Introduction

While genome-wide association analysis and related multi-omic strategies have in recent years dominated the field of complex disorders including mental health and addictions, in pharmacogenomics, drug metabolizing enzymes show Mendelian patterns of inheritance with correspondingly large effect sizes. Consistent with this, genes encoding these enzymes make up the majority of the genes for which the strength of the association with clinical effect of psychiatric medications is sufficient to recommend clinical utility (Bousman et al., 2018). Moreover, such enzymes are expressed in the brain (Aitchison et al., 2010; Kalow & Tyndale, 1992). We herein provide a comprehensive review of the relevance of drug metabolizing enzyme and transporter genes to mental health and addictions.

Drug metabolism comprises Phase I (addition of a reactive group to the molecule) and Phase II (transfer of a polar group to the Phase I metabolite) (Xu et al., 2005). The term Phase III was introduced by Ishikawa (1992) for drug export by ATP binding cassette (ABC) efflux transporters. Later on, the uptake process by solute carrier proteins was referred to as the 'phase 0 transport' of drugs (Doring & Petzinger, 2014). Phase I comprises hydrolysis (by esterases, peptidases and amidases), oxidation (by cytochrome P450 enzymes, mixed function oxidases and monoxygenases) and reduction (by reductases). If not further metabolized by Phase II enzymes, the intermediate, reactive metabolites produced by such enzymes can interact with DNA or proteins causing deleterious effects to the organism (Xu et al., 2005). Phase II enzymes include *N*-acetyltransferases, sulfotransferases, uridine diphosphate (UDP)-glucuronosyltransferases (UGTs), glutathione *S*-transferases and epoxide hydrolases, which can either further activate the Phase I metabolite leading to further toxicity, or can conjugate hydrophilic moieties to the Phase I metabolites leading to the formation of more hydrophilic molecules that will be more easily excreted by the renal or biliary organs. Phase III transporters include not only ABC transporters such as multidrug resistance protein 1 (also known as P-glycoprotein (P-gp) and encoded by the *ABCB1* gene) but also organic anion transporting polypeptides (OATPs).

5.2 Phase I Metabolism

Reactions catalyzed by Phase I enzymes alter substrate hydrophobicity and include oxidation, reduction and hydrolysis. Outlined below are components particularly relevant to psychopharmacology.

5.2.1 Esterases

Esterases contribute to the metabolism of approximately 10% of all current therapeutic drugs containing ester, amide and thioester bonds (Fukami & Yokoi, 2012). Cholinesterases such as acetylcholinesterase (AChE) are members of the B-esterase family (Espinoza et al., 2016; Staudinger et al., 2010). The gene encoding AChE is on chromosome 7 (Massoulié et al., 1993). The enzyme is predominantly produced in the brain, muscle and erythrocytes. AChE regulates cholinergic neurotransmission by selectively and efficiently inactivating acetylcholine released from presynaptic cholinergic neurons in the brain, skeletal muscle and the autonomic nervous system (Hasin et al., 2005). Studies have shown that AChE accelerates the formation of amyloid plaques (Carvajal & Inestrosa, 2011). The first generation of medications for Alzheimer's disease was cholinesterase inhibitors, to which adverse drug reactions (ADRs) may occur (Grossberg, 2003). The rs2571598 polymorphism has been associated with plasma AChE levels in patients with multiple sclerosis (Reale et al., 2018), and other sources of variation have been noted: tissue-specific differential C-terminal splicing (resulting in the G1, G2 and G4 variants), as well as glycosylation (Grisaru et al., 1999; Saez-Valero et al., 1999).

5.2.2 Epoxide Hydrolases

Epoxide hydrolases are a family of enzymes responsible for transforming highly reactive epoxide molecules into less reactive and more soluble diols (El-Sherbeni & El-Kadi, 2014). Exons 2–9 of the gene (*EPHX1*) encoding microsomal epoxide hydrolase (mEH) are expressed, with exon 1 containing several promoters (Hartsfield et al., 1998; Hassett et al., 1994; Jackson et al., 1987; Skoda et al., 1988). The enzyme is expressed at highest levels in the liver, adrenal gland, lung, kidney and intestine (El-Sherbeni & El-Kadi, 2014; Oesch et al., 1977). *EPHX1* is highly polymorphic, with over 100 single nucleotide polymorphisms (SNPs) having been identified (Václavíková et al., 2015). The c.337 T>C mutation decreases enzyme activity by 40%, with the c.416 A>G mutation reducing enzymatic function by 25% (Caruso et al., 2014). Genetic variants in *EPHX1* have been associated with response to carbamazepine and warfarin (Caruso et al., 2014; Daci et al., 2015; Liu et al., 2015; Nakajima et al., 2005; Puranik et al., 2013), while alcohol dependence has been associated with the c.337 T>C and c.416 A>G mutations (Bhaskar et al., 2013).

5.2.3 Oxidoreductases

Oxidoreductase enzymes include the cytochrome P450 family and flavin monooxygenases. Drug and other xenobiotic metabolism occurs primarily in the liver; however, these enzymes are in fact widespread across multiple tissues (Aitchison et al., 2010). Cytochrome P450s are a large superfamily of enzymes usually bound to microsomal or to mitochondrial membranes. Their expression may be modulated by multiple different mechanisms, including competitive inhibition, non-competitive inhibition and induction (Chen et al., 2018; Hisaka et al., 2010; Pelkonen et al., 2008).

The classification of P450 enzymes (CYPs) was led for decades by the Cytochrome P450 Nomenclature Committee based at the Karolinska Institute (retained in archival form, henceforth abbreviated to CYP Database), and has more recently been transferred to the US-based PharmVar. By convention, P450 enzymes are designated by the letters CYP followed by an Arabic number indicating the CYP family (Cupp & Tracy, 1998). To cluster enzymes in the same family, they must contain a minimum of 40% amino acid sequence identity (e.g. the CYP1 and CYP2 families). The next layer of division is represented by the presence of a letter indicating the subfamily (e.g. CYP1A, CYP1B). Within a subfamily, enzymes share 55% amino acid identity. In the next layer, another Arabic numeral represents the individual gene, or isoform (e.g. CYP2C18, CYP2C19). (Consistent with the convention throughout human genetics, gene names are italicized, with corresponding protein names not being italicized.)

Polymorphism in the cytochrome P450 enzyme family has been extensively studied since the mid-1970s (Eichelbaum, 1984; Mahgoub et al., 1977). Initial observations resulted from noting individuals sensitive to the antihypertensive agent debrisoquine and to the antiarrhythmic agent sparteine (Johansson & Ingelman-Sundberg, 2011; Smith, 1986) led to sequencing efforts with identification of the first *CYP2D6* loss-of-function mutation (Gough et al., 1990; Hanioka et al., 1990; Kagimoto et al., 1990; Pinto & Dolan, 2011). Multiple mutations in P450s relevant to mental health and addictions have subsequently been identified, with the frequency of such varying by ethnicity (Aitchison et al., 2000c).

Mutations can reduce enzyme stability, or enzyme-substrate affinity, or generate mutations such as splice site variants leading to lack of functional protein (Ingelman-Sundberg, 2004a, 2004b). Increased enzyme activity (ultrarapid metabolizers), on the other hand, may be linked to gene duplication or multiplication or to enhancer SNPs (Johansson et al., 1993; Sim et al., 2006; Wang et al., 2014, 2015). P450 mutations can be classified in two different manners, in standard genetic terms (loss or gain of function) or pharmacologically in terms of enzyme function (poor, intermediate, normal or ultrarapid metabolizers) (van der Weide & Steijns, 1999). Loss-of-function mutations reduce drug clearance, consequently increasing plasma concentration, while gain-of-function variants do the reverse and hence reduce the concentration (Zanger & Schwab, 2013). Many CYPs have four distinct phenotypes: poor, intermediate, normal and ultrarapid, while some CYPs have an additional fifth phenotype, 'rapid' (Blake et al., 2013). CYPs relevant to psychiatry are outlined in Figure 5.1.

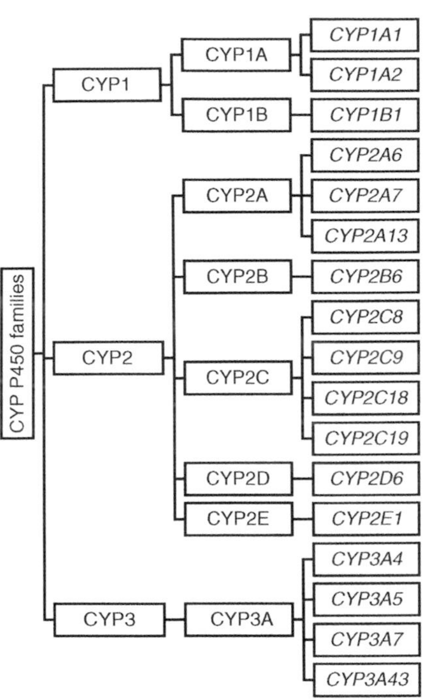

Figure 5.1 Cytochrome P450s relevant to psychiatry: three families (CYP1, CYP2 and CYP3), eight subfamilies (CYP1A, CYP1B, CYP2A, CYP2B, CYP2C, CYP2D, CYP2E and CYP3A) and 17 isoforms.

5.2.3.1 The CYP1 Family

The CYP1 family includes CYP1A and CYP1B, with the CYP1A subfamily genes (*CYP1A1* and *CYP1A2*) being located on chromosome 15, and sharing a high degree of sequence homology. They contain aryl hydrocarbon receptor binding elements known as xenobiotic responsive elements in their shared promoter region (the genes are in a head-to-head configuration). CYP1A2 is inducible by various dietary substances, drugs and toxins, including cruciferous vegetables (*Cruciferae*, including broccoli, cauliflower, brussel sprouts, cabbage, watercress and radishes), heterocyclic amines (produced in meat browned at high temperatures), polycyclic aromatic hydrocarbons (e.g. 3-methylcholanthrene), and heterocyclic aromatic hydrocarbons (such as 2,3,7,8-tetrachlorodibenzo-p-dioxin), caffeine, products of combustion such as cigarette or cannabis smoke, paracetamol, omeprazole, primaquine and carbamezepine (Aitchison et al., 2000a; Arici & Özhan, 2017; Dobrinas et al., 2011; Ghotbi et al., 2007; Parker et al., 1998; Rost et al., 1994; Yoshinari et al., 2008). Brussels sprouts can in fact induce multiple enzymes (CYP1A1, CYP1A2, CYP1B1, epoxide hydrolase, UGT1A1, thioredoxin reductase, and haem oxygenase in the lungs (Robbins et al., 2011)) and the effect of cruciferous vegetables on amine metabolism may be of substantial duration (Murray et al., 2001). CYP1A2 may be inhibited by lutein (in leafy green vegetables (Le Marchand et al., 1997)), apiaceous vegetables (parsnips, celery, dill, parsley (Lampe et al., 2000)), grapefruit juice (Fuhr et al., 1993), oestrogens (Abernethy & Todd, 1985; Knutti et al., 1981; Le Marchand et al., 1997; Rietveld et al., 1984; Vistisen et al., 1992), quinolone antibiotics (Fuhr et al., 1992), fluvoxamine (Brøsen et al., 1993) and, in smokers, heavy ethanol consumption (Rizzo et al., 1997).

This enzyme plays a major role in the metabolism of many commonly used drugs, including analgesics (e.g. paracetamol), antipsychotics (chlorpromazine, trifluoperazine, clozapine, olanzapine), antidepressants including tertiary amine tricyclic antidepressants (TCAs; amitriptyline, imipramine and clomipramine) as well as some selective serotonin reuptake inhibitors (such as fluvoxamine), zopiclone, tacrine, xanthines (caffeine, theophylline, aminophylline), anti-inflammatories and cardiovascular agents (e.g. lignocaine) (Aitchison et al., 2000b; Imaoka & Funae, 1990; Lobo et al., 2008; Turpeinen et al., 2009; Zanger & Schwab, 2013). It is also involved in the metabolism of the neurotoxin 1-methyl-4-phenyl-1,2,3,6-tetrahydropyridine (MPTP), which produces a Parkinsonian syndrome in man (Coleman et al., 1996), and in the activation of arylamines and heterocyclic amines implicated in the genesis of colon and bladder cancer (Boobis et al., 1994; Eaton et al., 1995; Hammons et al., 1997; McManus et al., 1990).

Given that smoking increases *CYP1A2* expression, this is particularly relevant for psychiatric patients, many of whom are smokers (Aitchison et al., 2000b; Dobrinas et al., 2011; Fiore et al., 1995; Ghotbi et al., 2007; Nakajima et al., 1999). To date, studies have detected several polymorphisms in *CYP1A2*, but no gene copy number variants (Browning et al., 2010; Jiang et al., 2005). Of note, the *CYP1A2*6* allele containing the c.1291 C>T (previously known as the c.5090 C>T) mutation creates an Arg431Trp amino acid substitution resulting in a non-functional enzyme (Zhou et al., 2004). Other SNPs in *CYP1A2* have been implicated in caffeine metabolism, smoking inducibility and in olanzapine serum concentration reduction. The *CYP1A2*1C* has a promoter mutation (-3860 G>A) that has been associated with reduced caffeine metabolism and reduced inducibility by smoking in Japanese (Nakajima et al., 1999); a rodent model of reduced CYP1A2 activity indicates that people with this variant could experience more ADRs to clozapine (Aitchison et al., 2000b). Conversely, individuals with the *CYP1A2*1F* allele with the -163C>A SNP have higher levels of caffeine metabolism and a 22% decrease in olanzapine serum concentration (Cornelis et al., 2006; Laika et al., 2010).

5.2.3.2 The CYP2 Family

Several *CYP2* gene clusters are found on different chromosomes (Sezutsu et al., 2013; Zanger & Schwab, 2013). The CYP2A subfamily includes *CYP2A6* and *CYP2A13* (Hoffman et al., 2001; Zanger & Schwab, 2013). While CYP2A6 is mainly expressed in the liver, accounting for approximately 4% of total hepatic P450 content (Haberl et al., 2005; Shimada et al., 1994), CYP2A13 is expressed at a low level in the respiratory tract (Leclerc et al., 2011; Raunio & Rahnasto-Rilla, 2012). First identified as the enzyme responsible for coumarin 7-hydroxylation, it is also the major nicotine C-oxidase (Fuhr et al., 2007; Mwenifumbo et al., 2007; Pelkonen et al., 2000; Raunio & Rahnasto-Rilla, 2012). It contributes to the metabolism of valproic acid, promazine and disulfiram, as well as to the metabolism of fadrozole, halothane, osigamone, methoxyflurane and pilocarpine and activates precarcinogens (such as aflatoxin B1 and *N*-nitrosodiethylamine) (Crespi et al., 1990; Gonzalez & Gelboin, 1994; Komatsu et al., 2000; Murai et al., 2009; Oscarson et al., 1998; Yamazaki et al., 1992). Of note, this is a highly polymorphic gene, with many mutations known to affect CYP2A6 enzymatic activity including gene deletion, duplication or conversion events, multiple nucleotide insertions/deletions and SNPs. The frequency of such varies by ethnicity, with

Caucasians being the least affected by loss-of-function mutations (~9%) and Asians the most affected (~50%) (di Iulio et al., 2009; Nakajima et al., 2006). *CYP2A6*2* and *CYP2A6*4* are common alleles conferring an enzymatic loss of function. The *CYP2A6*2* allele encodes an enzyme with a Leu160His substitution, which yields an inactive enzyme (in a vaccinia virus-based expression system) and affects 1–5% of the Caucasian population (Tanner et al., 2017). The *CYP2A6*4* allele represents a complete gene deletion (its various subtypes, such as *CYP2A6*4A* and *CYP2A6*4H*, representing slightly different genomic mechanisms, or cross-over junctions, for creation of the gene deletion) and is found particularly in Asians and Blacks (e.g. *CYP2A6*4A* has a 20% frequency in Asians). There are also variants associated with reduced enzyme activity, such as *CYP2A6*9*. Loss or reduction in CYP2A6 enzymatic function may result in reduced treatment efficacy of relevant drugs, with atypical metabolite formation (e.g. switching from coumarin 7-hydroxylation to 3-hydroxylation) (Fujita & Sasaki, 2007; Hadidi et al., 1997; Komatsu et al., 2000).

The *CYP2B* subfamily comprising *CYP2B6* and a pseudogene (*CYP2B7P*) is strongly modulated by phenobarbital (Nelson et al., 2004). CYP2B6 is expressed in the liver, accounting for ~1% of total P450 content (Ward et al., 2003), with expression levels varying up to 300-fold between individuals (Desta et al., 2007; Hofmann et al., 2008; Lamba et al., 2003; Lang et al., 2001; Ohtsuki et al., 2012; Wang & Tompkins, 2008). Consistent with this, over 38 different allelic combinations of SNPs in *CYP2B6* (leading to amino acid changes) have been identified (Fuhr et al., 2007; Klein et al., 2005; Lamba et al., 2003; Lang et al., 2001, 2004; Zanger et al., 2007; Zukunft et al., 2005). The most common allele is *CYP2B6*6*, with a frequency of 15–60% across different ethnicities (being particularly common in Blacks); this has c.516G>A and c.785A>G variants, which lead to amino acid substitutions Gln172His and Lys262Arg, associated with a 50–75% decrement in enzyme activity (Hofmann et al., 2008; Lang et al., 2001; Tsuchiya et al., 2004; Zanger & Klein, 2013). Individuals homozygous for *CYP2B6*6* show increased plasma concentration of relevant drugs and are hence more susceptible to ADRs (Haas et al., 2004; King & Aberg, 2008; Lubomirov et al., 2011; Ribaudo et al., 2006; Yimer et al., 2012; Zanger & Klein, 2013; Zanger et al., 2007). *CYP2B6*4* is present in 2–6% of the population and has higher activity towards substrates such as bupropion and nicotine (Hesse et al., 2004; Johnstone et al., 2006; Kirchheiner et al., 2003; Lang et al., 2001; Rotger et al., 2007). The allele *CYP2B6*18* with 21011 T>C (old, or c.983T>C in the new nomenclature) in the gene resulting in an Ile328Thr substitution is found particularly in those from African countries such as Ghana.

The CYP2C subfamily contains four genes – *CYP2C8, CYP2C9, CYP2C18* and *CYP2C19* – forming a ~390 kb cluster at chromosome 10q24 (Goldstein & de Morais, 1994; Nelson et al., 2004). Sharing a high degree of DNA and protein homology, they are responsible for metabolizing partially overlapping subsets of drugs (Coller et al., 2002; Koukouritaki et al., 2004; Naraharisetti et al., 2010; Ohtsuki et al., 2012; Rettie & Jones, 2005). While mainly produced in the liver, accounting for approximately 20% of hepatic P450 content (Shimada et al., 1994), they are also found in other organs (Aitchison et al., 2010). CYP2C9 is the most abundant, followed by CYP2C19 and CYP2C8. These contribute to the metabolism of 40% of prescribed drugs, including several for which therapeutic drug monitoring (TDM) is indicated (Shimada et al., 1994). In terms of psychotropics, substrates for CYP2C19 include selective serotonin reuptake inhibitors (SSRIs), tricyclics, diazepam, propranolol and phenytoin. CYP2C18 lies distal to

CYP2C19 on chromosome 10, is 85.7% homologous to CYP2C19 and shows similar substrate specificity in regard to diazepam (Jung et al., 1997) and phenytoin (Bajpai et al., 1996; Mamiya et al., 1998b). Interestingly, co-segregation of poor metabolizer (PM) mutations of CYP2C19 and CYP2C18 has been described (Mamiya et al., 1998a), indicating that CYP2C18 may not be able to take over from CYP2C19 in individuals deficient in CYP2C19.

CYP2C9 contributes to the metabolism of phenytoin. It is also relevant to many other medications commonly prescribed to those with chronic mental health conditions and accompanying physical comorbidities: fluvastatin, warfarin, antidiabetic agents (such as tolbutamide, glimepiride and nateglinide), angiotensin II blockers (losartan, valsartan, candesartan and irbesartan) and non-steroidal anti-inflammatory drugs (NSAIDs) including COX2 inhibitors (e.g. celecoxib) (Michaels & Wang, 2014). The most common reduced function variants are *CYP2C9*2* (R144C) and *CYP2C9*3* (I359L) in Caucasians, which have been studied in relation to the metabolism of drugs with a narrow therapeutic index, such as warfarin, phenytoin and tolbutamide (Lee et al., 2002). In vitro analyses indicate that the protein encoded by the *CYP2C9*2* allele has a substrate-dependent 30–50% reduction in enzyme activity, while that encoded by *CYP2C9*3* has an approximately 95% reduction in (*S*)-warfarin clearance. Individuals who have two reduced function alleles have a higher probability to develop ADRs such as hypoglycaemia, gastrointestinal bleeding from NSAIDs and serious bleeding on warfarin (Holstein et al., 2005). In a genome-wide association study of warfarin response, a previously identified marker in *CYP2C9* was genotyped separately in addition to the array-based genomic analysis and identified as the top signal (Takeuchi et al., 2009). Subsequent predictive modelling including a target of the drug (*VKORC1*) as well as *CYP2C9* has been conducted (Eriksson & Wadelius, 2012); the Food and Drug Administration (FDA) label for warfarin includes recommendations for dosage based on *CYP2C9* genotype.

CYP2C19 is found not only in the liver but also extrahepatically (Aitchison et al., 2010). Psychotropic substrates of this enzyme include tertiary amine tricylics (e.g. amitriptyline, imipramine and clomipramine), SSRIs (fluoxetine, sertraline, paroxetine, citalopram, escitalopram), diazepam and its metabolite desmethyldiazepam, and moclobemide (Roh et al., 1996), as well as clozapine, olanzapine, propranolol and phenytoin to lesser extents. The above-mentioned SSRIs also inhibit CYP2C19. Other substrates of this enzyme include the anticoagulant clopidogrel, proton pump inhibitors (omeprazole and pantoprazole), proguanil, voriconazole, nelfinavir, thalidomide and cyclophosphamide (Desta et al., 2002). The CYP Database describes 35 allelic variants of the gene, of which *CYP2C19*2-*8* are the most common loss-of-function (PM) alleles.

There is substantial interethnic variation in the incidence of PMs of CYP2C19, being 2–5% in Caucasians, 2% in Saudi Arabians, 4% in Black Zimbabweans, 5% in Ethiopians, 13% in Koreans, 15–17% in Chinese, 21% in Indians and 18–23% in Japanese (Aitchison et al., 2000c). Indeed, when the square root of the PM phenotypic frequency (equal to the frequency of PM *CYP2C19* alleles) is plotted versus longitude, an increase in this value versus longitude may be seen, with an increment in the value occurring between Saudi Arabia and Bombay (Saeed & Mayet, 2013).

The most common PM allele is *CYP2C19*2* (a c.G681A substitution in exon 5, which creates an aberrant splice site) (de Morais et al., 1994), accounting for 86% of Caucasian PM and 69–87% of East Asian alleles. The second most common PM allele is *CYP2C19*3* (a c.G636A mutation in exon 4, which creates a premature stop codon); this comprises

13–31% of PM East Asian alleles and 1.5% Caucasian. A third variant, *CYP2C19*4* (an A→G mutation in the initiation codon, or c.1A>G), accounts for 3% of Caucasian PM alleles. *CYP2C19*5* (a c.C1297T mutation in exon 9 which results in an Arg433Trp change in the haem binding region) accounts for 1.5% of Caucasian PM alleles and is rare in East Asians. *CYP2C19*6* (a c.G395A base substitution resulting in an Arg132Gln coding change in exon 3) and *CYP2C19*7* (a GT→GA mutation in the donor splice site of intron 5 at c.819 +2) each account for a further 1.5% of Caucasian PM alleles. *CYP2C19*8* (a c.T358C substitution resulting in a Trp120Arg change in exon 3) is a less common PM allele. The products of *CYP2C19*6* and *CYP2C19*8* show reduced catalytic activity (2% and 9% of wild-type S-mephenytoin hydroxylase activity, respectively); the others described above are associated with failure to express active CYP2C19. *CYP2C19*2A* and *CYP2C19*3* have both been identified in an Ethiopian population and found to account for all the PM alleles in the 114 individuals studied (Persson et al., 1996).

The clearance of diazepam is significantly lower in CYP2C19 PMs than extensive metabolizers (NMs) (Bertilsson, 1995). Owing to the relatively high frequency of PMs in East Asians, there is a greater frequency of individuals carrying one PM allele (i.e. heterozygous PMs), and therefore the mean clearance is lower in Chinese compared to Caucasians. Consistent with this, 'many Hong Kong physicians routinely prescribe smaller diazepam doses for Chinese than for white Caucasians' (Kumana et al., 1987). The main variant responsible for this effect is the G681A, which has a gene-dosage association effect on diazepam clearance (Qin et al., 1999). Dose adjustment by *CYP2C19* genotype has been published for amitriptyline, citalopram, clorimipramine, imipramine, moclobemide and trimipramine (Kirchheiner et al., 2001), while CYP2C19 PMs show a significantly higher efficacy for triple therapy for *Helicobacter pylori* (proton pump inhibitor, clarithromycin and amoxicillin) (Klotz, 2006, 2009).

The *CYP2D* cluster comprises *CYP2D6*, with two pseudogenes, *CYP2D7* and *CYP2D8* (Yasukochi & Satta, 2011). CYP2D6 accounts for 1.5% of hepatic microsomal P450 content (Michaels & Wang, 2014), and is involved in the metabolism of the majority of psychotropics (Bertilsson et al., 2002). It is also found in multiple other organs including the brain (Aitchison et al., 2010; Niznik et al., 1990; Siegle et al., 2001), and has been linked to neurotransmitter synthesis (Niwa et al., 2017; Yu et al., 2003). The *CYP2D6* gene is highly polymorphic; with over 110 different alleles identified (Kertesz et al., 2007), it is the most extensively studied genetically variable drug metabolizing enzyme (Bertilsson et al., 2002; Del Tredici et al., 2018). There is marked variation in the distribution of such allelic variants by ethnicity (Aitchison et al., 2000c). For example, while the *CYP2D6*4* (previously known as g.1847G>A), genomic location on NG_008376.3 1847G>A (Gough et al., 1990; Hanioka et al., 1990; Kagimoto et al., 1990), allele has a frequency of 19% in Caucasians (approximately 70–90% of all the PM alleles) (Aitchison et al., 1999), the frequency of this allele in Africans is 6% and approximately 1% in South Asians (Aitchison et al., 2000c; Mammen et al., 2018). *CYP2D6*5* is the second most common frequent PM allele in Caucasians (allele frequency 2–2.5%) (Aitchison et al., 1999), representing a complete deletion of the gene and occurs at a frequency of 5.3%, 2.9% and 2.9% in Africans, Hispanic and Asians, respectively (Bradford, 2002; Del Tredici et al., 2018). The *CYP2D6*10* allele is characterized by C188T and G4268C base substitutions in exons 1 and 9 that result in Pro34Ser and Ser486Thr amino acid substitutions (Sakuyama et al., 2008; Yokota et al., 1993), which are associated with reduced enzymatic activity (Johansson et al., 1994). The allele frequency is high in East Asians at 0.43 (43%) (Aitchison et al., 2000c; Mammen et al., 2018), and has been associated with some ADRs, such as tardive dyskinesia (Ohmori et al., 1998; Puangpetch et al., 2016). A similar decrease in enzymatic activity is observed for the *CYP2D6*17* allele (Masimirembwa et al., 1996; Oscarson et al., 1997), found predominantly in Africans, with a frequency of 34% in Zimbabwe, 28% in Ghana, 17% in Tanzania and 9% in Ethiopia (Bertilsson et al., 2002). In Caucasians, the most common reduced activity (IM) allele is the *CYP2D6*41*, with an intronic 2989G>A (genomic position on NG_008376.3 7189G>A) substitution that leads to a splicing defect (Hicks et al., 2013, 2016; Raimundo et al., 2000, 2004; Rau et al., 2006; Toscano et al., 2006; Wang et al., 2014). At the opposite end of the enzyme activity spectrum, the most common ultrarapid metabolizer (UM) allelic variants have extra functional copies of the *CYP2D6* gene in tandem on the chromosome, occurring at a frequency of 0.9–4% in Caucasians (Aitchison et al., 1999; Johansson et al., 1993), with a less common mechanism for increased enzyme activity being a SNP associated with enhancer activity (Wang et al., 2015). Such individuals were first identified by their having much lower concentrations than expected of TCAs such as clomipramine (Bertilsson et al., 1993b; Roberts et al., 2004). The prevalence of *CYP2D6* gene duplication or multiplication events is up to 29% in Ethiopians (Aklillu et al., 1996).

The resultant diversity in *CYP2D6* phenotype has clinical implications: individuals with two PM alleles have no functional enzyme, are known as PMs and are more prone to ADRs for drugs with a narrow therapeutic window (Steimer et al., 2004, 2005), and UMs may also show more ADRs, such as tardive dyskinesia (Koola et al., 2014) or symptoms of morphine overdose on codeine (Crews et al., 2014), owing to enhanced formation of toxic metabolites (Pinto & Dolan, 2011). Variation in *CYP2D6* is highly relevant to psychiatry: for most (18) antidepressants and antipsychotics, there are clinical guidelines that state that pharmacogenomic information for *CYP2D6* could or should be used in prescribing (Bousman et al., 2019). A review with modelling found that for antidepressants metabolized by CYP2D6, NMs would require at least double the dose required by PMs, while a cost analysis associated PM status with not only higher ADRs but also more dropouts from treatment (Kirchheiner et al., 2004).

For *CYP2E1*, a relatively small number of allelic variants have been identified, such as *CYP2E1*2*, which is associated with reduced enzyme activity (Hu et al., 1997; Mittal et al., 2015). This enzyme is produced primarily in the liver, and is responsible for metabolizing ethanol, paracetamol and other substances such as acetone. Gene transcription is induced by ethanol consumption (at a moderate alcohol level producing a rapid and reversible increase).

5.2.3.3 The CYP3 Family

The CYP3 family comprises the *CYP3A* subfamily of four genes – *CYP3A4*, *CYP3A5*, *CYP3A7* and *CYP3A43* – and two pseudogenes. CYP3A4 is usually the most abundant, although CYP3A5 and CYP3A4 often share substrate specificity and in those deficient in CYP3A4, CYP3A5 and other members of the CYP3A family become more important. Total CYP3A activity is the sum of the activity of all CYP3As, which are responsible for metabolizing approximately 50% of all clinically relevant drugs (Bu, 2006; Guengerich, 1999), as well as endogenous and exogenous steroids. They are found mainly in the liver, with lower concentrations in the intestine, respiratory tract, brain, lung and kidney (Shimada et al., 1994). In the intestine, they play a significant role in the first-pass metabolism of orally administered drugs. The high sequence similarity between the enzymes leads to the similar substrate specificity. There is substantial interindividual and interethnic variation in CYP3A enzyme activity, partly owing to genetic polymorphism and in addition, marked effects of inducers and inhibitors. CYP3A inducers (such as rifampicin, carbamazepine or phenytoin) can greatly decrease plasma levels of other substrates. Conversely, the administration of CYP3A inhibitors (e.g. ketoconazole) can increase the plasma concentration of other CYP3A substrates, increasing ADRs or even toxicity.

For some drugs in some individuals, inhibition/induction effects at the level of the intestine may be more important than those occurring at the hepatic level. Indeed, efflux transporters such as P-gp present on the apical intestinal membrane can increase exposure to CYP3A enzymes by prolonging transit time across the enterocyte (Wacher et al., 2001). Interestingly, there is overlap between substrates and inhibitors of CYP3A enzymes and P-gp (Bruyere et al., 2010).

CYP3A4 is the most abundant CYP3A isoform in the liver and intestine (Nebert & Russell, 2002). Up to 40-fold interindividual variation in activity is seen (Lamba et al., 2002); however, unlike the distribution of enzymes strongly under genetic control (such as CYP2D6), the distribution is unimodal. Some functional polymorphisms, such as *CYP3A4*22*, have been identified in East Asians (who have a lower CYP3A activity) (Okubo et al., 2013). A mutation that leads to a premature stop codon, *CYP3A4*26*, has been identified (Werk et al., 2014), and recent screening of over 1000 Han Chinese for mutations in *CYP3A4* found seven novel exonic variants (*CYP3A4*28-*34*) (Hu et al., 2017).

Midazolam clearance or an erythromycin breath test may be used to measure the activity of the enzyme in vivo (Goh et al., 2002). Alfentanil is demethylated by CYP3A4; pupillary response after alfentanil administration may also be used as a measure of CYP3A4 metabolic activity (Baririan et al., 2005; Klees et al., 2005). Other in vivo probes of CYP3A activity include: alprazolam (4-hydroxylation), triazolam (1-hydroxylation), cortisol (6-β hydroxylation), dextromethorphan (N-demethylation), diazepam (N-demethylation), nifedipine (oxidation), terfenadine (C-hydroxylation) and testosterone (6-β hydroxylation) (Jurica & Sulcova, 2012). Ketoconazole and itraconazole are potent CYP3A4 inhibitors (Jurica & Sulcova, 2012). Owing to the presence of multiple substrate binding domains within CYP3A4, it is in fact recommended to use at least two structurally unrelated probe substrates; crystal structures show that multiple substrate/inhibitor molecules may be simultaneously bound (Ekroos & Sjogren, 2006; Foti et al., 2010; Khan et al., 2002; Korzekwa et al., 1998; Schrag & Wienkers, 2001; Tucker et al., 2001).

The major mechanisms for the regulation of CYP3A expression in fact appear to be epigenetic rather than genetic, including DNA methylation (Dannenberg & Edenberg, 2006), histone acetylation and miRNA-mediated mechanisms. In regard to the second, histone acetylation in the 5' region of CYP3A4 occurs in response to the pregnane X receptor (PXR) agonist rifampicin (Xie et al., 2009), and also in the promoter region of the constitutive androstane receptor (CAR) in response to dexamethasone (Assenat et al., 2004), the latter indirectly affecting *CYP3A* gene expression. Hepatocyte nuclear factor 4α also participates in the regulation of the gene expression of PXR and in CAR-mediated xenobiotic induction of CYP3A4 (Tirona et al., 2003). In regard to miRNA-mediated mechanisms, miR-27b binds to the 3' untranslated region (UTR) of CYP3A4 (Pan et al., 2009), miR-148a binds to the 3' UTR of the PXR (Takagi et al., 2008) and the vitamin D receptor (VDR, also an indirect modulator of CYP3A) may be down-regulated by miR-27b (Li et al., 2015). Target genes of the PXR are *CYP3A4*, *MDR1*, *CYP2B6*, members of UGT superfamily, MRP3 and OATP2 transporters in multiple cell types (Klaassen & Slitt, 2005; Tolson & Wang, 2010). Of note, PXR activation regulates P-gp expression at the blood–brain barrier (Bauer et al., 2004). The PXR is also known as the steroid and xenobiotic receptor (SXR); tamoxifen activates both *CYP3A4* and *MDR1* gene expression in breast cancer cells through the PXR/SXR (Nagaoka et al., 2006). PXR, CAR and VDR are part of a family of nuclear receptors that also includes RXR, FXR, LXR and PPARα, which together participate in the complex coordinated regulation of transcription of drug metabolizing enzyme and transporter genes (Czekaj, 2000; Czekaj & Skowronek, 2012). Genetic variants in nuclear receptors contribute to interindividual variance in response to CYP3A-metabolized medications (Lamba & Schuetz, 2008).

The *CYP3A5*3* (6986A>G, NM_000777.4:c.219-237A>G) and *CYP3A5*6* (14690G>A) alleles are both alternative splice site mutations resulting in non-functional truncated proteins, and are responsible for CYP3A5 being more frequently expressed in those of African descent (60%) compared to Caucasians (33%) (Kuehl et al., 2001). Functional effects of combined CYP3A4 and CYP3A5 enzyme deficiency may be marked (Werk et al., 2014).

While *CYP3A7* is mainly found in embryonic, fetal and newborn liver, it may persist; it metabolizes dehydroepiandrosterone and its sulfate. A promoter variant, *CYP3A7*1C*, has been associated with persistent CYP3A7 expression in adults and with lower levels of dehydroepiandrosterone sulfate in women with polycystic ovary syndrome (Goodarzi et al., 2008).

Although *CYP3A43* represents a relatively low proportion of total CYP3A hepatic content, variants have been identified and analyzed for association with clearance with antipsychotics. There is a frameshift mutation (c.74delA from the sequence start or c.-30delA from the ATG start, rs61469810) leading to a premature stop codon, a missense mutation (c.1018C>G/P340A, rs680055) and other silent/non-functional mutations. In an analysis of CYP3A43 markers available on a particular array (the Affymetrix 500 K), an association between increased olanzapine clearance and rs472660 AA genotype in the Clinical Antipsychotic Trials of Intervention Effectiveness (CATIE) sample was found (Bigos et al., 2011). The A allele is more frequent in those of African descent; after accounting for *CYP3A43* genotype, race was no longer a significant predictor of olanzapine clearance.

5.2.3.4 Flavin-Containing Monooxygenases

There are six human flavin-containing monooxygenase genes (Krueger et al., 2002), encoding enzymes FMO1-5 (the sixth gene is a pseudogene). FMO substrates include chlorpromazine, trifluoperazine, prochlorperazine, promazine, promethazine and other phenothiazines (Lomri et al., 1993), imipramine, desipramine, clomipramine, moclobemide, amphetamine, methamphetamine, olanzapine, clozapine, tamoxifen, ketoconazole and ranitidine (Beedham, 1997; Foti & Dalvie, 2016; Motika et al., 2007).

FMO1 is expressed in fetal liver and in adult kidney and intestine (Yeung et al., 2000). Lower quantities are found in other organs such as the ovaries, testis, adrenal gland and bladder. Substrates include psychotropics mentioned above, nicotine, disulfiram and pesticides (Phillips & Shephard, 2017). A promoter SNP (characterizing the *FMO1*6* allele) has a frequency of 30%, 13% and 11% in Hispanics, those of African descent and Europeans, and appears to account for some of the variability in FMO1 expression.

Flavin-containing monooxygenase 2 (FMO2) is expressed in the lungs. The majority of Caucasians and Asians are homozygous for a non-functional allele: *FMO2**2A (a C>T mutation at position 1414 that results in a premature stop codon). The wild-type (*FMO2*1)* allele is found in African-Americans (26%), Puerto Ricans (7%) and Mexicans (2%) (Furnes et al., 2003; Whetstine et al., 2000). In some populations in Africa, the frequency approaches 50% (Veeramah et al., 2008). While the functional allele increases the risk of pulmonary toxicity for chemicals containing thioureas, it also protects against toxicity caused by organophosphate insecticides (Veeramah et al., 2008). It can metabolize drugs including nicotine, trifluoperazine and prochlorperazine (Krueger & Williams, 2005) and is responsible for activating antitubercular drugs. FMO2 expression is regulated by hormones including gonadal hormones (and possibly corticosteroroids – a glucocorticoid responsive element has been found in the 5′ flanking region of the rabbit *FMO2* gene).

Flavin-containing monooxygenase 3 (FMO3) is present mainly in the liver, with lower concentrations in the lung, kidney, small intestine and brain (Chen et al., 2016). Substrates include chlorpromazine, imipramine, clozapine, nicotine, amphetamine and methamphetamine. Multiple SNPs have been identified in the *FMO3* gene, which at least partly explain the interindividual and interethnic protein concentration variability (Cashman & Zhang, 2002; Krueger et al., 2002). These lead to amino acid substitutions or absence of functional protein, and are associated with the autosomal recessive hereditary condition of trimethylaminuria and mild forms thereof (Mackay et al., 2011). Trimethylaminuria may be associated with various neuropsychiatric presentations, ranging from anxiety and depression to suicidality, paranoia, addiction (Ayesh et al., 1993) and seizures (McConnell et al., 1997). Reduction in conversion of trimethylamine to trimethylamine x-oxide by FMO3 leads to trimethylamine being found not only in the urine but also in sweat, saliva, breath and vaginal secretions. One such variant (Glu158Lys or E158K) may be associated with mild trimethylaminuria and potentially greater neurotoxicity of amphetamine and methamphetamine (which are metabolized to a greater extent to hydroxylamine metabolites by the E158K compared to the wild-type enzyme) (Motika et al., 2007). FMO3 activity is affected by hormones (trimethylaminuria can be worse in women, especially after puberty, after taking oral contraceptives and at the time of the menstrual cycle or perimenopause), dietary content (choline, lecithin, tyramine) and intestinal bacterial growth (reducing trimethylamine *N*-oxide to trimethylamine). Brussel sprout consumption leads to inhibition of FMO3 and can worsen trimethylaminuria (Motika et al., 2007). For individuals deficient in FMO3, supplementation with folate and riboflavin is indicated (Motika et al., 2007). Choline and lecithin are found in: egg yolk, liver, kidney, legumes, soybeans, peas, shellfish and salt-water fish. The enzyme is subject to competitive inhibition effects (e.g. by chlorpromazine and imipramine) (Adali et al., 1998). Methimazole is a potent inhibitor of both FMO1 and FMO3. Recent publications have shown that *N*-oxidation of nicotine mediated by FMO1 and FMO3 occurs in the brain, and, moreover, that functional variation in FMO3 (rs2266780, E308G) is associated with nicotine dependence (Teitelbaum et al., 2018).

5.3 Phase II Metabolism

Phase II enzymes may be divided into type I conjugation, in which an activated conjugating agent combines with the substrate to yield a conjugated product through the addition of functional motifs (e.g. acetate, sulfate, glucuronate or glutathione, consequently increasing the xenobiotic polarity and hydrophilicity), and type II conjugation, in which the substrate is activated and then combined with a moiety such as a methyl group or amino acid (Jančová & Šiller, 2012).

5.3.1 Type I Conjugation

The *NAT1* and *NAT2* genes encode cytosolic enzymes expressed in the liver and intestine, with NAT1 showing additional wider tissue distribution (Sim et al., 2007, 2014; Windmill et al., 2000). NAT1 is expressed in fetal and neonatal tissue, while NAT2 is not expressed until about a year later (Pacifici et al., 1986; Pariente-Khayat et al., 1991). Substrates of NAT1 include caffeine (Jančová & Šiller, 2012). The substrate specificity of NAT1 and NAT2 overlaps. Moreover, the genetic variants in one are linked to those in another; these enzymes may therefore act in a concerted fashion to 'cox and box' against evolutionary selection pressures with mutually compensatory mechanisms.

Glutathione *S*-transferases are relevant not only to drug metabolism, but also to detoxification of reactive intermediates such as those formed by catecholamine peroxidation (aminochrome, dopachrome, adrenochrome) in the defence against oxidative stress (Jančová & Šiller, 2012).

Uridine diphosphate (UDP)-glucuronosyltransferases (UGTs), located mainly on the luminal membrane of the endoplasmic reticulum, act in concert with the cytochrome P450 enzymes present on the cytosolic surface (Ishii et al., 2007; Ouzzine et al., 1999), and are expressed in the brain as well as the liver and intestine (Ouzzine et al., 2014; Wu et al., 2011). Some glucuronidated products are less active, others, such as morphine-6-glucuronide, are pharmacologically active (Gong et al., 1991). UGT substrates of relevance to neuropsychiatry include: valproic acid, lamotrigine, ethanol, oxazepam, apomorphine, morphine, serotonin and dopamine. Drugs of relevance to psychiatry that undergo glucuronidation include valproic acid and lamotrigine; in addition, there are endogenous substrates such as serotonin and dopamine (Ouzzine et al., 2014). In the brain, UGTs are found in the endothelial cells and astrocytes of the blood–brain barrier, as well as in the pituitary, pineal, neuro-olfactory tissue and circumventricular organ (Ouzzine et al., 2014).

The human sulfotransferase superfamily of enzymes contains at least 13 members, with partially overlapping substrate specificities and tissue distributions (Riches et al., 2009). While sulfo-conjugation generally reduces biological activity, some sulfo-conjugates are active. For example, pregnenolone sulfate blocks the activation of $GABA_A$ receptors (Majewska et al., 1988) and is a positive allosteric modulator of the NMDA receptor (Wu et al., 1991)

5.3.2 Type II Conjugation

Many endogenous and exogenous compounds can undergo *N*-, *O*-, *S*- or arsenic-methylation (Feng et al., 2010). The cofactor required is *S*-adenosylmethionine, formed from ATP and L-methionine. Catechol-*O*-methyltransferase (COMT) is a magnesium-dependent enzyme (Axelrod, 1957) which plays a key role in the modulation of catechol-dependent functions such as cognition, cardiovascular function and pain processing. COMT is involved in the inactivation of catecholamine neurotransmitters (dopamine, noradrenaline), catechol oestrogens and other catechol drugs such as L-dopa (Weinshilboum et al., 1999). There are two forms of COMT: a cytoplasmic soluble form (S-COMT) and a membrane-bound form (MB-COMT), located on the cytosolic side of the rough endoplasmic reticulum. S-COMT is found in the liver, intestine and kidney (Taskinen et al., 2003), whereas the MB-COMT is more highly expressed in the central nervous system (Tunbridge et al., 2006). The *COMT* Val158Met (rs4680) polymorphism has been associated with a variety of relevant phenotypes including cognition (Goldman et al., 2009), pain tolerance (Goldman, 2014) and age of onset of psychosis after adolescent cannabis consumption (Caspi et al., 2005; Lodhi et al., 2017).

5.4 Phase III Metabolism

The last step in drug processing is the export of compounds away from the interior of cells in an energy-dependent manner. During this phase, the metabolized molecules are transported by the ATP binding cassette (ABC) superfamily, which use energy (ATP) to transport substances out of the cell against a concentration gradient in multiple different organs including the brain (Doring & Petzinger, 2014).

ABCB1 (previously called *MDR1*) was the first member to be cloned (Riordan et al., 1985; Roninson et al., 1986; Ueda et al., 1987), with the encoded protein (P-gp) being called multidrug resistance protein owing to the observation that it was overexpressed in tumour cells with resistance to multiple chemotherapeutic agents.

P-gp substrates include many psychotropic drugs (e.g. amitriptyline, chlorpromazine, olanzapine, desipramine, citalopram, paroxetine, venlafaxine, diazepam, lamotrigine, carbamazepine, phenytoin) (Aller et al., 2009; de Klerk et al., 2013; O'Brien et al., 2012; Palleria et al., 2013; Uhr et al., 2008). There is overlapping substrate specificity with other ABC transporters. It is expressed on the apical membrane of the intestine from the duodenum to the rectum, being co-regulated with CYP3A4 in the duodenum and jejunum and co-regulated with CYP3A5 in the rectum and sigmoid colon (Cascorbi, 2011; Fromm & Kim, 2011; Ufer et al., 2008; von Richter et al., 2004). P-gp shares substrate specificity with CYP3A4, and both are modulated by St John's wort (Johne et al., 1999), amongst other drugs. High-affinity substrates such as verapamil also act as inhibitors: the inhibition of P-gp at the blood–brain barrier by verapamil leads to central nervous system effects of loperamide (an antidiarrhoeal agent that does not usually have such effects) (Elsinga et al., 2004).

In the liver, P-gp levels vary 50-fold. Although more than 100 mutations in the coding sequence have been identified, with at least some (such as c.3435C>T, rs1045642) apparently affecting protein expression, the combined effect of the mutations identified to date does not adequately account for the variation in expression levels. The frequency of the c.2677G>T/A variant in exon 21 (rs2032582, encoding Ala893Ser/Thr in the eighth transmembrane domain) varies by ethnic group (e.g. being 0.46, 0.44 and 0.10 for the G, T and A alleles, respectively, in those from the Pacific Rim and 0.56, 0.39 and 0.04 in Hispanics); genotyping may be efficiently conducted using a TaqMan assay. The G (or C on the complementary strand) allele has been associated with remission on antidepressants that are P-gp substrates (citalopram, paroxetine, amitriptyline and venlafaxine)

(Uhr et al., 2008), and with serotonergic side effects to SSRIs (de Klerk et al., 2013), while the T allele has been associated with susceptibility to increase in fasting blood glucose level for patients on olanzapine (Kuzman et al., 2011).

The c.3435C>T (rs1045642) mutation is synonymous; it has been hypothesized that a rare tRNA being required for the synonymous amino acid may slow down co-translational folding. Additionally, it is in linkage disequilibrium with rs2032582 (and hence also varies in frequency by ethnic group, the T allele increasing in frequency from African to Asian to Caucasian), and so clinical associations identified may in fact relate to effects of rs2032582. Patients with the c.2677GG or c.3435CC genotype have been found to have lower dose-corrected clozapine levels than heterozygotes or TT carriers (Consoli et al., 2009; Jaquenoud Sirot et al., 2009). Additionally, c.3435CC patients needed higher daily doses of clozapine (246 ± 142 mg/day) compared with T carriers to achieve the same clinical benefit (Consoli et al., 2009). In another study, increase in body mass index after 3 and 12 months of clozapine treatment was greater in *ABCB1* rs1045642 T carriers than in those of CC genotype, which after adjusting for age and gender was significant only in the men. Similarly, a significant increase in diastolic blood pressure was found in the men. The combination of *ABCB1* rs1045642 TT and *ABCC1* rs212090 AA genotypes was associated with increased clozapine and norclozapine levels (Piatkov et al., 2017). It has been suggested that, analagous to combination drugs for HIV therapy (using a P-gp inhibitor such as ritonavir with another drug such as lopinavir), modulation of P-gp be employed in treatment-resistant schizophrenia (Hoosain et al., 2015).

5.5 Pharmacogenomics Applied to Psychiatry

In psychiatry, 40–60% of first time prescribed psychiatric medications (antipsychotics, antidepressants or mood stabilizers) either fail to work or cannot be tolerated (Correll et al., 2015). The current method for prescribing relies on physician judgement and a therapeutic trial; pharmacogenomics could be a game-changer. Barriers to uptake include standardization of data interpretation (Altman et al., 2013; Bousman & Hopwood, 2016; Bousman et al., 2018; de Leon, 2009). To address this, a 2009 collaboration between PharmGKB and the Pharmacogenomics Research Network created the Clinical Pharmacogenetics Implementation Consortium (CPIC) (Relling & Klein, 2011), to provide clinical guidelines regarding the interpretation of pharmacogenetic testing. CPIC guidelines have four levels describing gene–drug pairs (Table 5.1) (Caudle et al., 2016).

In order to allocate an association level, a literature review is conducted, with the results being presented to the CPIC writing committee, classifying the evidence as 'high' (evidence includes consistent results from well-designed, well-conducted studies), 'moderate' (evidence is sufficient to determine effects, but the strength of the evidence is limited by the number, quality or consistency of the individual studies; generalizability to routine practice; or indirect nature of the evidence) or 'weak' (evidence is insufficient to assess the effects on health outcomes because of limited number or power of studies, important flaws in their design or conduct, gaps in the chain of evidence or lack of information) (Caudle et al., 2014). Therapeutic recommendations are graded as: strong, where 'the evidence is high quality and the desirable effects clearly outweigh the undesirable effects'; moderate, in which 'there is a close or uncertain balance' as to whether the evidence is high quality and the desirable clearly outweigh the undesirable effects; and

Table 5.1 Clinical Pharmacogenetics Implementation Consortium (CPIC) level definitions for gene–drug pairs

CPIC Level	Clinical Context	Level of Evidence	Strength of Recommendation
A	Genetic information should be used to change prescribing of affected drug.	Preponderance of evidence is high or moderate in favour of changing prescribing	At least one moderate or strong action (change in prescribing) recommended.
B	Genetic information could be used to change prescribing of the affected drug because alternative therapies/dosing are extremely likely to be as effective and as safe as non-genetically based dosing.	Preponderance of evidence is weak with little conflicting data	At least one optional action (change in prescribing) is recommended.
C	There are published studies at varying levels of evidence, some with mechanistic rationale, but no prescribing actions are recommended because (a) dosing based on genetics makes no convincing difference or (b) alternatives are unclear, possibly less effective, more toxic or otherwise impractical or (c) few published studies or mostly weak evidence and clinical actions are unclear. Most important for genes that are subject of other CPIC guidelines or genes that are commonly included in clinical or DTC tests.	Evidence levels can vary	No prescribing actions are recommended.
D	There are few published studies, clinical actions are unclear, little mechanistic basis, mostly weak evidence or substantial conflicting data. If the genes are not widely tested for clinically, evaluations are not needed.	Evidence levels can vary	No prescribing actions are recommended.

Table 5.2 Mental health medications: Clinical Pharmacogenetics Implementation Consortium (CPIC) evidence levels, pharmacogenomic FDA label and associated genes

Drug	CPIC level	PGx on FDA label	Gene
Amitriptyline	A	Actionable PGx	*CYP2D6*
Fluvoxamine	A	Actionable PGx	*CYP2D6*
Nortriptyline	A	Actionable PGx	*CYP2D6*
Paroxetine	A	Informative PGx	*CYP2D6*
Aripiprazole & Brexipiprazole	B	Actionable PGx	*CYP2D6*
Atomoxetine	B	Actionable PGx	*CYP2D6*
Clomipramine	B	Actionable PGx	*CYP2D6*
Doxepin	B	Actionable PGx	*CYP2D6* & *CYP2C19*
Imipramine	B	Actionable PGx	*CYP2D6*
Pimozide	B	Genetic testing required	*CYP2D6*
Protriptyline	B	Actionable PGx	*CYP2D6*
Trimipramine	B	Actionable PGx	*CYP2D6*
Vortioxetine	B	Actionable PGx	*CYP2D6*
Perphenazine	B/C	Actionable PGx	*CYP2D6*
Citalopram & Escitalopram	A	Actionable PGx	*CYP2C19*
Carbamazepine	A	Genetic testing required	*HLA-B*1502*
Desipramine	B	Actionable PGx	*CYP2D6*
Valproic acid	B	Genetic testing required	*POLG*
Venlafaxine	B	Actionable PGx	*CYP2D6*

optional, in which the desirable effects of pharmacogenetic-based dosing are closely balanced with undesirable effects and there is room for differences in opinion as to the need for the recommended course of action (Caudle et al., 2014). Guidelines currently focus on gene–drug pairs for which at least one of the prescribing recommendations is actionable (level A or B) (Table 5.2).

The rest of this section provides details of pharmacogenomics relevant to the clinical use of a range of psychiatric drugs. This is not a comprehensive review but rather a series of examples to illustrate major applicable principles.

5.5.1 Mood Stabilizers

There is substantial interindividual variation in response to treatment with mood stabilizers, and severe ADRs may occur (Murru et al., 2015; Pisanu et al., 2016; Tang & Pinsky, 2015). The current CPIC gene–drug pair list includes three mood stabilizers carbamazepine, oxcarbazepine and valproic acid (Drozda et al., 2014; Saruwatari et al., 2010), with guidelines being available for the first two (Phillips et al., 2018; Relling et al., 2011).

Carbamazepine and oxcarbazepine are aromatic anticonvulsants structurally related to TCAs approved for treatment of epilepsy, trigeminal neuralgia and bipolar disorder (Phillips et al., 2018). The clinical utility of TDM for anticonvulsants is well established. Both drugs share dose- or concentration-dependent (type A) ADRs including dizziness, ataxia, nystagmus. Type B ADRs (idiosyncratic, not predictable from the pharmacology) are more severe, some potentially lethal, and include osteoporosis, liver injury, aplastic anaemia and Stevens–Johnson syndrome/toxic epidermal necrolysis (SJS/TEN).

Genetic variants with an actionable level of association with carbamazepine and oxcarbazepine are *HLA-B*15:02, HLA-A*31:01* and *SCN1A* (Phillips et al., 2018; Relling & Klein, 2011). The association between the *HLA-B*15:02* allele and carbamazepine-induced SJS/TEN is in Asians (Ferrell & McLeod, 2008; Stern & Divito, 2017). The initial report (in Han Chinese in 2004) found that *HLA-B*15:02* genotyping reduced the frequency of the potentially lethal SJS/TEN to zero per cent (Chung et al., 2004). The *HLA-B*15:02* allele frequency is highest in East Asia (up to approximately 15%) although recent data suggest *HLA-B*15:02* testing should no longer be restricted to Asians (Fang et al., 2019). The *HLA-A*31:01* allele (Fan et al., 2017) also varies by ethnicity, being up to 15% in most Asian and Caucasian groups and relatively infrequent in those of African descent. This variant has been primarily linked with maculopapular exanthema, an ADR with eosinophilia and systemic symptoms (Mushiroda et al., 2018; Sukasem et al., 2018), and to a lesser extent than *HLA-B*15:02* SJS/TEN.

Other genes associated with carbamazepine response are *SCN1A* (a sodium channel α-subunit) and *EPHX1*. Polymorphisms in *SCN1A* (c.603-91G>A, otherwise known as IVS5-91 or rs3812718, AA genotype) and *EPHX1* (c.337T>C, CC genotype) have been associated with lower plasma carbamazepine concentrations when compared to patients carrying non-mutant alleles (Daci et al., 2015).

Valproic acid is a branched short-chain fatty acid derived from the naturally occurring valeric acid. Valproic acid increases the levels of gamma-aminobutyric acid (GABA) in the brain by inhibiting the catabolism and increasing the synthesis of GABA, blocks voltage-gated ion channels (particularly calcium and sodium) and also acts as an inhibitor of histone deacetylase enzymes including HDAC1. Genetic factors are associated with differential efficacy and ADRs (Fricke-Galindo et al., 2018; Kasperavičiūte & Sisodiya, 2009; Löscher et al., 2009). Metabolism is in the liver via CYP-mediated oxidation (including CYP2A6, CYP2B6 and CYP2C9), glucuronidation (mediated by UGT1A3, UGT1A4, UGT1A6, UGT1A7, UGT1A8, UGT1A9, UGT1A10 and UGT1A15) and mitochondrial reactions including conjugation with glutathione and oxidation by mEH (Ghodke-Puranik et al., 2013; Johannessen & Landmark, 2010).

ADRs associated with valproic acid include hepatotoxicity, mitochondrial toxicity, teratogenicity, and potentially fatal hyperammonaemic encephalopathy among others (Johannessen & Landmark, 2010; Singh et al., 2015). Valproic acid is contraindicated in patients with disorders secondary to mutations in DNA polymerase gamma (*POLG*), which conducts replication of human mitochondrial DNA. Patients with POLG-related disorders are at elevated risk of fatal hyperammonaemic encephalopathy. Symptoms suggestive of this type of condition include unexplained encephalopathy, refractory epilepsy (focal, myoclonic), status epilepticus at presentation, developmental delays, psychomotor regression, axonal sensorimotor neuropathy, myopathy cerebellar ataxia, ophthalmoplegia or complicated migraine with occipital aura. The onset of such may vary from childhood to late adulthood. It is therefore contraindicated in children with clinical suspicion of a hereditary mitochondrial disorder, while in those over two years of age with suggestive symptoms, valproate should be used only after other anticonvulsants have failed and with monitoring of liver function (liver function tests, clotting and clinical evaluation).

5.5.2 Antipsychotics

5.5.2.1 Perphenazine

Perphenazine is a phenothiazine antipsychotic that undergoes substantial first-pass hepatic Phase I and II metabolism, and as a result, owing to the polymorphic variation in multiple Phase I enzymes, its serum concentrations vary very widely in treated patients; for example, 30-fold in CYP2D6 NMs (Linnet & Wiborg, 1996). Initial studies in the 1980s showed that after four to five weeks, clinical improvement was associated with plasma perphenazine concentrations above 2 nmol/L, while extrapyramidal side-effects occurred mainly at plasma concentrations above 3 nmol/L (Hansen, 1981; Hansen & Larsen, 1983; Hansen et al., 1982). In a subsequent larger study of more than 200 patients, a slightly wider therapeutic range (2–6 nmol/L) was suggested (Hansen & Larsen, 1985).

The main active metabolite, 7-hydroxyperphenazine (having 70% and 50% of the antagonism of perphenazine at dopamine D_2 and at α_1/α_2-adrenoceptors, respectively) (Hals et al., 1986), is formed in a reaction catalyzed by CYP2D6, with other metabolites including *N*-dealkylated perphenazine (formed by CYP2D6, CYP1A2, CYP3A4 and CYP2C8, CYP2C9, CYP2C18 and CYP2C19) and perphenazine sulfoxide (Dahl-Puustinen et al., 1989; Olesen & Linnet, 2000). At steady state, the concentration of *N*-dealkylated perphenazine is approximately three times that of perphenazine, while that of perphenazine sulfoxide is in the same range as the parent drug (Hansen et al., 1979). *N*-dealkylperphenazine has a higher in vitro affinity for 5-HT2A receptors than for D2 receptors, while perphenazine and 7-hydroxyperphenazine both have a higher affinity for D2 receptors than for 5-HT2A receptors (Sweet et al., 2000). Minor metabolic pathways may include *N*-oxidation and direct glucuronidation (Huang & Kurland, 1964; van Kempen, 1971). At therapeutically relevant concentrations of perphenazine, as indicated by the effect of ketoconazole inhibition, CYP3A4 accounts for about 40% of the *N*-dealkylation, with CYP isoforms 1A2, 2C19 and 2D6 contributing 20–25% (as measured by inhibition using furafylline, fluvoxamine or quinidine, respectively) (Olesen & Linnet, 2000).

Both the maximum concentration and the drug clearance have been related to CYP2D6 activity. Specifically, the peak serum concentration and the area under the curve (AUC) of perphenazine for CYP2D6 PMs is about three and four times, respectively, that of NMs in single-dose kinetics (Dahl-Puustinen et al., 1989), its disposition co-segregates with debrisoquine hydroxylation (Bertilsson et al., 1993a), and at steady state, the median concentration-to-dose ratio of perphenazine in CYP2D6 PMs is about twice that of CYP2D6 NMs, with patients on concomitant inhibitors showing a median concentration in between that of the above two groups (Linnet & Wiborg, 1996). For one CYP2D6 PM, the initial concentration was very high and could potentially have been avoided had *CYP2D6* genotyping been available to the prescriber. Jerling et al. (1996) conducted a study on patients during continuous treatment and *CYP2D6* genotype was shown to significantly predict the oral clearance of perphenazine (patients with two *CYP2D6* PM alleles having a significantly lower clearance than heterozygote PMs or NMs).

It would therefore be expected that in individuals deficient in CYP2D6 or on potent CYP2D6 inhibitors, higher perphenazine concentrations would be found and hence more adverse effects, while in CYP2D6 UMs, lower concentrations would be seen, with less adverse effects and potentially a lower therapeutic efficacy unless overcome by titration of the medication according to clinical response. Consistent with this, paroxetine, a potent CYP2D6 inhibitor, increases the AUC of perphenazine sevenfold in NMs, which is associated with increased sedation, extrapyramidal symptoms and worse psychomotor performance (Ozdemir et al., 1997). In elderly patients with dementia, although low-dose perphenazine (0.05–0.1 mg/kg/day) appears to have equal efficacy for CYP2D6 PMs and NMs, PMs have significantly more adverse effects (primarily extrapyramidal and sedation) early in treatment, with these effects becoming similar between genotypic groups by day 17 of treatment (Pollock et al., 1995).

A single-dose kinetic study in non-smoking healthy male Chinese-Canadian volunteers reported a 2.9-fold higher AUC and C_{max} for perphenazine in individuals homozygous for the intermediate metabolizer (IM) *CYP2D6*10* allele compared to *CYP2D6*10* heterozygotes grouped together with those negative for *CYP2D6*10* and the other *CYP2D6* allele genotyped, *CYP2D6*5* (Ozdemir et al., 2007). Prolactin levels were elevated in rank order of genotypic group: *CYP2D6*10/*10>CYP2D6*10/*1>CYP2D6*1/*1*. When prolactin AUC was normalized for perphenazine AUC (AUC ratio), the *CYP2D6*10/*10* individuals showed the lowest prolactin response per unit perphenazine AUC, the *CYP2D6*1/*10* individuals showed the greatest variance AUC ratio and those negative for *CYP2D6*10* and *CYP2D6*5* showed a greater AUC ratio than the *CYP2D6*10* homozygotes. Although this was hypothesized to be related to the formation of serotonin from 5-methoxytryptamine, it could also be related to the formation of dopamine from m- and p-tyramine (Niwa et al., 2018), specifically, that in the *CYP2D6*10* homozygotes, there would be a lower rate of formation of dopamine and hence less intrinsic inhibition of prolactin secretion (the total prolactin concentration reflecting both intrinsic dopamine effect at pituitary lactotroph dopamine D_2 receptors and antagonism at the same receptors by the medication). In a follow-up study in this sample, both *CYP2D6* and dopamine D_2 receptor (*DRD2*) genotypes were independent predictors of prolactin levels (the *DRD2* Taq1A A1/A1 genotypic group showing higher 2-hour prolactin elevation) (Aklillu et al., 2007).

In summary, there are data to support clinical utility of genotyping for *CYP2D6* IM and PM alleles, while studies with more comprehensive *CYP2D6* genotyping, including for UM variants, could be undertaken. As with other medications, combining drug metabolizing enzyme and receptor genetics leads to ability to predict a greater proportion of the variance in clinical response.

5.5.2.2 Pimozide

Pimozide is a diphenylbutylpiperidine antipsychotic that has been used since 1984 to treat Tourette syndrome (Pringsheim & Marras, 2009), and also to treat psychotic disorders (particularly delusional disorder). However, its use has been limited owing to a specific ADR: prolongation of the QT interval on the electrocardiogram, which is associated with risk for torsade de pointes (a type of ventricular fibrillation that is associated with sudden cardiac death) (Fulop et al., 1987). Indeed, cases of sudden cardiac death have been reported in patients on pimozide (Committee on Safety of Medicines-Medicines Control Agency, 1995; Flockhart et al., 2000). In an isolated rabbit heart, this effect was shown to be attributable to pimozide itself, not to metabolites thereof (Flockhart et al., 2000); this is owing to a direct effect of the drug on potassium channels encoded by the human ether-a-go-go-related gene (*HERG*, otherwise known as *KCNH2*), which are responsible for the delayed repolarization current in the heart. Of note, the effect has been shown to be concentration dependent (Drolet et al., 2001), tending to occur with greater likelihood at doses above 5 mg.

TDM as well as a baseline and follow-up ECGs are therefore standard practice with pimozide, and it is clearly important to determine which cytochromes might contribute to pimozide's concentration profile (peak, variability over time and steady state). Initial in vitro analyses showed that the formation of the major metabolite of pimozide, 1,3-dihydro-1-(4-piperidinyl)-2H-benzimidazol-2-one (DHPBI), by *N*-dealkylation was dependent primarily on CYP3A4, with a lesser contribution by CYP1A2 (Desta et al., 1998). Although the above report did not conclude that CYP2D6 played a significant role in pimozide metabolism, it is possible that the conclusion from this in vitro analysis was affected by pimozide being a potent CYP2D6 inhibitor and therefore inhibiting its own metabolism by CYP2D6 in the microsomal assays.

Case reports of interactions between pimozide and CYP2D6 inhibitors such as paroxetine and fluoxetine (Ahmed et al., 1993; Horrigan & Barnhill, 1994), as well as investigation of differential interaction with clarithromycin (an inhibitor of CYP3A in the liver and gut) by CYP2D6 status led to recognition that CYP2D6 was in fact a major contributor to the in vivo pharmacokinetics of pimozide (Desta et al., 1998). Although Desta et al. (1999) reported that plasma concentrations of pimozide 'trended' (non-significantly) higher in CYP2D6 PMs relative to NMs (and in women relative to men), close examination of their data shows that this might have been owing to limited sample size (five PMs and seven NMs) and hence relatively large and unequal degrees of variance in the data and a parametric statistical test being used (1-tailed t test); the AUC in the PMs was in fact nearly three times that of NMs (245 ± 340 ng/ml/h versus 97 ± 41 ng/ml/h). The effect of a single dose of 6 mg on the QT interval corrected for heart rate was measured over time, which showed the greatest increase within the first 20 hours, with NMs in fact showing a higher increase (by nearly 20 ms), followed by a rapid reduction from 20 to 50 hours, and then a subsequent increase at approximately 60–100 hours. The late-onset elevation was more marked in CYP2D6 PMs, women and clarithromycin-treated individuals, and also appeared to be more sustained than the early increase. Although, owing to the more sustained nature, the late-onset elevation may be more relevant to clinically significant QT prolongation, the early peak in NMs warrants further investigation in UMs (none present in this study). In CYP2D6 PMs, the half-life increased from 29 ± 18 hours to 36 ± 19 hours, while in NMs, the corresponding values were 17 ± 7 and 23 ± 10 hours. For all subjects with relevant data, the pimozide-induced QTc interval changes coincided well with the concentration–time course of pimozide. Of note, the prescription of CYP3A inhibitors, such as valproate, is now contraindicated with pimozide.

In the above study, interestingly, pimozide rapidly increased plasma prolactin concentration, the maximum increase occurring 4 hours post-dose, with a sharp reduction thereafter, and concentrations nonetheless at 96 hours post-dose (with no measurable serum concentrations) being at 72% and 140% of baseline values in the placebo- and clarithromycin-treated groups (Desta et al., 1998). The persistent prolactin elevation at 96 hours may indicate persistent pharmacodynamic (such as high dopamine D_2 affinity and a low dissociation constant) and neuroendocrine effects and is consistent with initial persistence of symptom control when patients are non-compliant, with relapse occurring later than would be expected from pharmacokinetic calculations.

In single-dose analysis, co-administration of sertraline and pimozide resulted in statistically significant increases of 35% and 37% in pimozide maximal concentration and AUC, respectively; however, this did not result in a clinically significant (>15%) increase in QT interval. Sertraline is a weak inducer of hepatic microsomal enzymes, and has weak (defined as an inhibition constant (Ki) >50 μM) to moderate (Ki between 1 and 50 μM) inhibitory effects on CYP enzymes 2D6 and 3A4 (Hemeryck & Belpaire, 2002; Sproule et al., 1997). Perhaps the induction of CYP3A, followed by inhibition of the same, and inhibition of CYP2D6 was responsible for the overall reduction in pimozide concentration.

In a study of TDM data from 86 patients on pimozide who were genotyped for the *CYP3A4*22* allele (van der Weide & van der Weide, 2015), an association between *CYP3A4* genotype and concentration dose of pimozide was found (explaining about 5% of the variance in the same, dose explaining 15% to 20% of the variance). Genotyping for *CYP2D6* alleles **3, *4, *5, *6, *9, *10, *41* and gene multiplication was also undertaken, and although not reaching statistical significance (likely owing to subgroup sizes: 7 PMs, 40 NMs, 2 UMs), the mean concentration-to-dose ratio in CYP2D6 PMs was double that of NMs, and that in CYP2D6 UMs was 40% that of NMs. IMs were in this analysis relatively similar to NMs, although this may be owing to the inclusion of PM/NM genotype in this phenotypic group.

Simulated steady-state pharmacokinetic profiling of pimozide in CYP2D6 PMs, IMs and NMs (based on single-dose data submitted to the FDA) led to specification in the FDA label in 2011 that CYP2D6 PMs should not be prescribed more than 4 mg (approximating to 0.05 mg/kg/day, which was therefore set as the maximum dose for paediatric CYP2D6 PMs), the maximum recommended dose in CYP2D6 NMs being 10 mg (or 0.2 mg/kg/day in children) (Rogers et al., 2012). In the simulated data, 4 mg/day in CYP2D6 PMs was the maximum dose that would not result in plasma concentrations in excess of those observed in CYP2D6 NMs receiving 10 mg/day. The simulated half-life was about 61 hours in CYP2D6 PMs and 31 hours in the NMs; note that these values are approximately double those reported in the single-dose study by Desta and colleagues (1998; 29 ± 18 hours in PMs and 17 ± 7 hours in NMs) (Desta et al., 1998).

The dosing guidance for pimozide is commence at 0.05 mg/kg (Preskorn, 2012), preferably taken once daily at bedtime. If the patient is a known CYP2D6 NM and is not on a substantial CYP2D6 inhibitor, the dose may be increased every third day to a maximum of 0.2 mg/kg/day, not to exceed a maximum of 10 mg/day. If the CYP2D6 status is not known, then *CYP2D6* genotyping should be done before deciding to increase the dose above 0.05 mg/kg/day, which is the maximum dose for anyone who is a CYP2D6 PM either because of genetics or because of the co-administration of a substantial CYP2D6 inhibitor. Substantial CYP2D6 inhibitors include paroxetine, fluoxetine and bupropion. For example, at doses of 20 mg daily, paroxetine will convert 60% of CYP2D6 NMs to PMs, while at 40 mg daily, 95% will be phenocopied to PMs (Preskorn, 2003). Phenoconversion to CYP2D6 PM status is apparently six times more common than genetically determined CYP2D6 PM status (Preskorn, 2012, 2013). Of note, a long-acting injectable form of pimozide is available; this would not be subject to first-pass metabolism, and therefore might be substantially less CYP3A dependent than the oral form.

Given that CYP3A represents 70% and 30% of the total CYP450 in the intestine and the liver, respectively (Kolars et al., 1994; Shimada et al., 1994), first-pass metabolism of pimozide will include metabolism in the gut as well as in the liver. Of note, after oral administration, it is more than 50% absorbed. Such metabolism will be subject to the influence of gut microbiota, diet and other factors including hormones (CYP3A4 being subject to regulation by the pregnane X and androstane receptors, microRNAs and other epigenetic mechanisms) (Lamba et al., 2005; Pan et al., 2009). CYP3A lies on chromosome 7q2.1 in a cluster of *CYP3A* genes that also includes *CYP3A5*, *CYP3A7* and *CYP3A43*; some medications are metabolized by more than one member of the *CYP3A* gene family, whereas, for others, their metabolism is more specific to a particular enzyme.

Of note, the drug label does not currently include dosing recommendations for CYP2D6 UMs; further research including genotyping *CYP2D6* for the full range of common functional variants including UMs should be done not only for this medication but also for the many others for which CYP2D6 plays a significant role in the metabolism. The potential effect of CYP3A inhibition on QT interval for individuals who are CYP2D6 UMs is at present unknown.

Given the association of sudden cardiac death on pimozide with co-prescription with CYP3A4 inhibitors as well as with CYP2D6 inhibitors, it could be suggested that *CYP3A4* genotyping as well as *CYP2D6* genotyping should be recommended. The reason that *CYP3A4* genotyping has not yet made it to clinical guidelines is likely because there is a less clear genotype–phenotype relationship with CYP3A4 than with CYP2D6, the functional genotypes that have been identified to date accounting for a lower proportion of the variance than is the case for functional variants in CYP2D6; however, relevant knowledge of this and related enzymes (e.g. CYP3A5, CYP3A43) has been accumulating. An alternative is to conduct CYP3A4 phenotyping, with a probe drug such as nifedipine. Theoretically, it is possible to estimate the activity of multiple CYPs simultaneously (de Andrés et al., 2014); however, accurate estimation would require the patient not only to be medication-free, but also to abstain from all dietary substances and supplements that affect CYP activity – a situation rarely likely to be feasible in psychiatry.

Pimozide is not the only predominantly CYP3A-metabolized medication for which there has been shown to be a concentration-dependent QT prolongation: this also occurs with, for example, terfenadine, which like pimozide, also shows an increased risk of this ADR with concomitant CYP3A inhibitors (e.g. erythromycin or ketoconazole) (Woosley et al., 1993). Quetiapine and lurasidone are metabolized mainly by CYP3A. *CYP3A4*22* genotype is relevant for quetiapine, which has been associated with sudden cardiac death (product label, and reviewed in Aronow & Shamliyan, 2018). Both of these atypical antipsychotics could be predicted to show an increased risk of prolongation of the QT interval with CYP3A inhibitors, which, by analogy with the effects seen with pimozide, might also be more marked in those with deficiencies in other relevant CYPs (e.g. CYP2D6 PMs).

5.5.2.3 Aripiprazole

Aripiprazole is a third-generation antipsychotic (which was the first serotonin-dopamine stabilizer). In Europe, licensed indications are schizophrenia in patients aged 15 years or over, bipolar I disorder in adults (for moderate to severe manic episodes and to prevent new manic episodes in those who have predominantly manic episodes and whose manic episodes have responded to aripiprazole in the past) and for up to 12 weeks of moderate to severe manic episodes in bipolar I disorder in adolescents aged at least 13 years (Koskinen et al., 2010). Other licensed indications include adjunctive treatment of major depressive disorder; it is also used in Tourette syndrome, and for irritability in autism spectrum disorder (Mailman & Murthy, 2010). Kirschbaum and colleagues measured global therapeutic efficacy (using the Clinical Global Impressions Scale, item 2) versus aripiprazole and dehydroaripiprazole serum concentrations, and reported a 68% response rate in those with concentrations of 150–300 ng/ml of aripiprazole, a 57% and 50% response rate with concentrations less than 150 ng/ml or above 300 ng/ml, respectively (Kirschbaum et al., 2008). The most recent TDM has 'recommended' (level 2 evidence) for aripiprazole by the interdisciplinary TDM group of the Arbeitsgemeinschaft für Neuropsychopharmakologie und Pharmakopsychiatrie (AGNP), with a therapeutic range of 100–350 ng/ml for aripiprazole, or 150–500 ng/ml for aripiprazole and dehydroaripiprazole (Hiemke et al., 2018).

Unless administered in a long-acting injectable form, aripiprazole undergoes substantial first-pass metabolism in the liver. In vitro studies show that CYP3A4 and CYP2D6 enzymes conduct dehydrogenation and hydroxylation of aripiprazole, with CYP3A4 additionally catalyzing *N*-dealkylation. Although a substrate for these enzymes, it does not appear to inhibit the activity of these enzymes (in clinical studies, 10–30 mg/day doses of aripiprazole had no significant effect on CYP2D6 or CYP3A4 activity as indexed by dextromethorphan) (Hjorthoj et al., 2015). Additionally, it does not appear to be a clinically significant inhibitor of CYP2C9, CYP2C19 or CYP1A2 (Hjorthoj et al., 2015), and as it is not a substrate for CYP1A enzymes, no dose adjustment is required for smokers.

The dehydroaripiprazole metabolite has a similar affinity to aripiprazole for dopamine D2 receptors and is therefore thought to contribute to the overall efficacy; at steady state it represents about 40% of the aripiprazole plasma concentration (AUC) (Hjorthoj et al., 2015) after oral administration or 29–33% after administration in the form of the long-acting injectable (LAI) Abilify Maintena. Both aripiprazole and dehydroaripiprazole are highly plasma protein bound, mainly to albumin (reviewed in DeLeon et al., 2004). The mean elimination half-life is about 75 hours for oral aripiprazole, but in CYP2D6 PMs, the mean half-life is about 146 hours (Hjorthoj et al., 2015). In a single-dose pharmacokinetic study in Japanese, the half-life of oral aripiprazole in CYP2D6 IMs (75.2 hours) was significantly longer than that in CYP2D6 NMs (45.8 hours), and the systemic clearance of IM is approximately 60% that of NM subjects, with the maximum concentration being the same in IMs as in NMs (Kubo et al., 2007). At steady state, PMs have a significantly lower concentration-to-dose ratio than NMs, while in one report, IMs did not appear to differ (van der Weide & van der Weide, 2015). However, van der Weide et al. included in their IM group individuals who were heterozygous normal metabolizers (NM/PM genotype). In another report (Hendset et al., 2014), median serum concentrations were 1.6-fold or 1.8-fold higher in individuals of CYP2D6 PM/IM or IM/IM genotype, respectively, than in those who were heterozygous NMs. There are recommended dose adjustments for aripiprazole in patients who are known CYP2D6 PMs, with the FDA recommending administration of half of the usual dose, and the Dutch Pharmacogenetics Working Group guidelines stating that the maximum daily dose should be reduced to 10 mg/day. Given that at a dose as low as 3 mg, D_2 receptor occupancy is already maximal, and the recommendation by consensus guidelines of doses of aripiprazole lower than those used in the initial marketing phase of the drug (Aitchison et al., 2009), it may well be recommendable to start at the lowest dose (2 mg) and go no higher than 5 mg in CYP2D6 PMs. Similarly, for IMs, the Japanese data would suggest that a cautious dosing in the 2–5 mg range might well be appropriate.

There are also recommended dose adjustments for patients taking concomitant CYP2D6 inhibitors, CYP3A4 inhibitors and/or CYP3A4 inducers (Hjorthoj et al., 2015). Metoprolol, a CYP2D6 inhibitor, results in a 40% higher aripiprazole concentration (Kirschbaum et al., 2008). Quinidine, a potent CYP2D6 inhibitor, increases aripiprazole AUC by 107% (C_{max} is unchanged), while decreasing the AUC and C_{max} of dehydroaripiprazole by 32% and 47%, respectively. Co-administration of paroxetine decreases the clearance of aripiprazole by 58% and 23% in CYP2D6 NMs and IMs (Azuma et al., 2012). The recommendation is therefore that aripiprazole dose should be reduced to approximately one-half of its prescribed dose when there is concomitant administration with quinidine, paroxetine or other strong inhibitors of CYP2D6, such as fluoxetine. A potent inhibitor of CYP3A4 (ketoconazole) increases aripiprazole AUC and C_{max} by 63% and 37%, respectively, and increases the AUC and C_{max} of dehydroaripiprazole by 77% and 43%. The concomitant administration of itraconazole 100 mg, another potent CYP3A inhibitor, reduces the clearance of aripiprazole by approximately 30% and 50% in CYP2D6 NMs and IMs, respectively (Kubo et al., 2005). When concomitant administration of potent CYP3A inhibitors (e.g. ketoconazole, itraconazole, HIV protease inhibitors) with aripiprazole occurs, aripiprazole dose should therefore be reduced to approximately one-half of its prescribed dose. Weak inhibitors of CYP3A4 (e.g. diltiazem) or CYP2D6 (e.g. escitalopram) are likely to produce only modest increases in plasma aripiprazole concentrations.

For patients receiving a combination of inhibitors at both CYP3A4 and CYP2D6 (e.g. a strong CYP3A4 inhibitor and a moderate CYP2D6 inhibitor, or a moderate CYP3A4 inhibitor with a moderate CYP2D6 inhibitor), the dosing may be reduced to one-quarter (25%) of the usual dose initially and then titrated up according to clinical response (US National Library of Medicine, 2016). In CYP2D6 PMs, concomitant use of strong CYP3A4 inhibitors may result in higher plasma concentrations of aripiprazole compared with that in CYP2D6 NMs. When considering concomitant administration of ketoconazole or other strong CYP3A4 inhibitors with aripiprazole, potential benefits should therefore outweigh the potential risks.

Following concomitant administration of carbamazepine, a strong inducer of CYP3A4, the geometric means of C_{max} and AUC for aripiprazole were 68% and 73% lower, respectively, compared to when aripiprazole (30 mg) was administered alone. Similarly, for dehydroaripiprazole, the geometric means of C_{max} and AUC after carbamazepine co-administration were 69% and 71% lower, respectively. The recommendation is therefore that aripiprazole dose should be doubled over one to two weeks when concomitant administration occurs with carbamazepine. Concomitant administration of oxcarbazepine (structurally similar to carbamazepine and also a CYP3A4 inducer) reduces both aripiprazole and dehydroaripiprazole concentration-to-dose ratio. Specifically, with 1200 mg/day oxcarbazepine (resulting in a serum oxcarbazepine concentration towards the upper end of the therapeutic range at 31 mg/ml), a reduction of 68% and 50% in aripiprazole and dehydroaripiprazole concentration-to-dose ratios, respectively, was estimated. Concomitant administration with other CYP3A inducers (e.g. St John's wort, rifampicin or phenytoin) may be expected to have similar effects. When the co-administered CYP3A4 inducer is withdrawn, aripiprazole dosage should be reduced to the original level over one to two weeks (US National Library of Medicine, 2016).

When administered concomitantly with valproate, lithium or lamotrigine, there is no clinically important change in concentration of these mood stabilizers (Hjorthoj et al., 2015). However, there is the potential for induction of serotonin syndrome when lithium is used in combination with a pro-serotonergic agent (Sobanski et al., 1997). The particularly high serum levels of paroxetine reported by Sobanski and collegues may indicate that the individual had reduced activity of the enzymes mainly responsible for paroxetine metabolism (CYP2D6 and CYP3A4) (Jornil et al., 2010; Sobanski et al., 1997), and was then particularly susceptible to the inhibitory effect of paroxetine on its own metabolism by CYP2D6. By analogy, it is possible that caution should be exerted in regard to lithium add-on, or to the addition of antidepressants that may inhibit CYP2D6 or CYP3A enzymes, especially in ethnic groups with higher likelihood of already having reduced activity of CYP2D6 or CYP3A4 (such as East Asians).

In regard to effects on other enzymes, it has been noted that both aripiprazole and one of its metabolites, 2,3-(dichlorophenyl) piperazine (2,3-DCPP), inhibit 7-dehydrocholesterol reductase (DHCR7), the enzyme that converts 7-dehydrocholesterol to cholesterol (Genaro-Mattos et al., 2018; Kim et al., 2016; Korade et al., 2010, 2016). As cholesterol is of critical importance to brain development and mutations in DHCR7 result in a neurodevelopmental condition (Smith–Lemli–Opitz syndrome), administration of DHCR7 inhibitors during the first trimester of pregnancy is associated with increased rates of fetal malformations, intrauterine death and spontaneous abortions (Boland & Tatonetti, 2016). Aripiprazole should therefore be contraindicated during the first trimester of pregnancy; indeed, the Summary of Product Characteristics states 'this medicinal product should not be used in pregnancy unless the expected benefit clearly justifies the potential risk to the foetus'. As the most crucial period for neural tube development is in fact the first six weeks of gestation, when many women do not even realize they are pregnant, a discussion of whether the woman is sexually active and methods of contraception may be advisable for every woman on aripiprazole in reproductive years.

For the LAI, in a multiple-dose study, the mean terminal-phase elimination half-life was 29.9 days with the 300 mg dose and 46.5 days with the 400 mg dose (Mallikaarjun et al., 2013). Data regarding differential half-life of the LAI by *CYP2D6* genotype and/or CYP3A activity are not available. Aripiprazole lauroxil is a prodrug that undergoes bioactivation by hydroxylation, and can be administered once every six weeks, and is similarly lacking pharmacogenetic data thus far.

5.5.3 Antidepressants

The first TCA, imipramine, was derived from a phenothiazine and found to produce marked clinical improvement without serious side effects in 500 patients with severe depression (Hillhouse & Porter, 2015; Kuhn, 1958). Although TCAs are still used to treat depression (American Psychiatric Association, 2010), the treatment of pain (e.g. neuropathic or cancer-associated) is now their more common therapeutic use (Baltenberger et al., 2015; Laird et al., 2008; Watson, 2000).

Fluoxetine was approved by the FDA in 1987 and was the first SSRI to enter widespread use (Wong et al., 1974, 1975). SSRIs are now widely used in the treatment of depression, and amongst them, escitalopram has the highest affinity for the serotonin transporter (Owens et al., 2001).

TCAs and SSRIs both undergo first-pass metabolism in the liver, with the cytochrome P450 enzymes playing a prominent role in this. The cytochromes involved include CYP2D6, CYP2C19, CYP2C18, the CYP3A family, CYP1A2, CYP2C9 and CYP2B6, with the first two enzymes having a higher affinity for most antidepressants than the rest of the enzymes (Brøsen, 1993; Jann & Cohen, 2000; Koyama et al., 1997).

Tricyclics include tertiary and secondary amines, with the latter being formed by *N*-demethylation of the former in a reaction catalyzed by CYP2C19 among other enzymes. CYP2D6 conducts hydroxylation of both the tertiary and secondary amines, with CYP2C19 making a low-affinity contribution to the hydroxylation reactions (reviewed in Aitchison, 2003). For example, imipramine (a tertiary amine) is demethylated to desipramine (a secondary amine) by CYP2C19, as well as by CYP1A2 and the CYP3A family, and both imipramine and desipramine are 2-hydroxylated by CYP2D6 (Spina et al., 1997). Consistent with this, steady-state concentrations of desipramine and nortriptyline have been associated with CYP2D6 activity (Bertilsson & Aberg-Wistedt, 1983; Nordin et al., 1985), and the 2-hydroxylation of imipramine co-segregated with CYP2D6 phenotype and genotype in a Danish family study (Madsen et al., 1996). In Chinese, the *CYP2D6*10* allele affects plasma levels of nortriptyline in a dose-dependent manner, with heterozygous individuals showing higher nortriptyline concentrations than homozygous wild type, and **10* homozygotes showing the highest concentrations (Yue et al., 1998). Dalén and collegues showed that following a single oral dose of 25 mg nortriptyline to Caucasian volunteers known to have 0, 1, 2, 3 and 13 functional copies of the *CYP2D6* gene, the concentration of nortriptyline was inversely related to the number of gene copies, while the concentration of 10-hydroxynortriptyline was directly related (Dalen et al., 1998). Morita et al. (2000) showed that the number of mutant *CYP2D6* alleles accounted for 41% of the variance in logarithm_{10} (nortriptyline level corrected for dose and body weight). Koyama et al. (1996) studied imipramine and desipramine concentrations in relation to CYP2C19 enzyme activity, and showed that the mean *N*-demethylation index was significantly less in individuals deficient in CYP2C19 (Koyama et al., 1996). Secondary amine TCAs inhibit CYP2D6 slightly more potently than tertiary amine TCAs (for example, estimated Ki values for amitriptyline, imipramine, nortriptyline and desipramine are 31.0, 28.6, 7.9 and 12.5 μM, respectively) (Shin et al., 2002) with doxepin and clomipramine also showing clinically significant CYP2D6 inhibition (Kertesz et al., 2007; Manrique-Garcia et al., 2016). Tertiary amines (e.g. amitriptyline, imipramine) also inhibit CYP2C19 (estimated Ki of 37.7 and 56.8 μM, respectively), while the secondary amines show negligible CYP2C19 inhibition activity (Shin et al., 2002).

TCAs inhibit presynaptic noradrenaline reuptake via the noradrenaline transporter, presynaptic serotonin reuptake via the serotonin transporter, and in addition are antagonists at the following receptors: α_1- and α_2-adrenoceptors, muscarinic receptors and histamine H_1 receptors (Cusack et al., 1994; Owens et al., 1997; Sanchez & Hyttel, 1999; Vaishnavi et al., 2004). Tertiary amine tricyclics have a greater affinity for the serotonin transporter than secondary amine tricyclics, with the latter being relatively selective for the noradrenaline transporter (Owens, 1996). Some of the above effects may be related to specific metabolites (e.g. *N*-methyl quaternary ammonium derivatives of amitriptyline, doxepin and imipramine are antagonists at both central nervous system and cardiac muscarinic receptors) (Ehlert et al., 1990).

SSRIs (e.g. paroxetine and fluoxetine) are also metabolized at least partly by CYP2D6 (Brøsen, 1993). The initial step in paroxetine metabolism is demethylenation, which includes a high-affinity saturable process conducted by CYP2D6, with 25% of the conversion in CYP2D6 NMs being attributable to a low-affinity process that is CYP2D6 independent (Bloomer et al., 1992). Further metabolism of paroxetine by conjugation results in glucuronide and sulphate conjugated metabolites, which are renally excreted (Haddock et al., 1989). Paroxetine is also a potent competitive inhibitor of CYP2D6 (Bourin et al., 2001); Lam and colleagues (2002) described a subject with at least three functional *CYP2D6* genes who had an undetectable concentration of paroxetine. In diabetic neuropathy, paroxetine has an analgesic effect, with optimal response at plasma concentrations greater than 300–400 nmol/L (Sindrup et al., 1990, 1991). Fluoxetine is also a relatively potent inhibitor of CYP2D6, and more lastingly so, because of its longer half-life (Liston et al., 2002).

The primary route of metabolism for citalopram (racemic mixture of the *R*- and *S*-enantiomers of citalopram) and escitalopram (*S*-citalopram) is *N*-demethylation by CYP2C19, CYP2D6 and CYP3A4 (Kobayashi et al., 1997; Rochat et al., 1997; Sindrup et al., 1993; von Moltke et al., 2001), with approximate relative contributions at low concentrations of citalopram estimated at 34% for CYP3A, 36% for CYP2C19 and 30% for CYP2D6. For *S*-citalopram alone, taking into account the relative hepatic abundance of the different CYPs, the contributions to net intrinsic clearance have been estimated as 37% for CYP2C19, 28% for CYP2D6 and 35% for CYP3A4 (von Moltke et al., 2001). CYP2D6 then conducts the *N*-demethylation of *N*-desmethylescitalopram to *N*-didesmethylescitalopram (von Moltke et al., 2001). Both of these, as well as fluoxetine and sertraline also all inhibit CYP2C19 (Bertilsson & Dahl, 1996), while fluvoxamine is also a potent CYP1A2 inhibitor (Christensen et al., 2002). Metabolites may also inhibit enzymes, for example, citalopram and *R*- or *S*-desmethylcitalopram are only weak inhibitors of CYP2C19, while *R*- and *S*-didesmethylcitalopram are moderate inhibitors, with mean IC_{50} values of 18.7 and 12.1 μM, respectively. *S*-citalopram and *S*-desmethylcitalopram are weak inhibitors of CYP2D6 (IC_{50} = 70–80 μM), with *R*-desmethylcitalopram showing stronger inhibition at this enzyme (IC_{50} 25.5 ± 2.1 μM) (von Moltke et al., 2001).

SSRIs were designed to be more selective for the serotonin than the noradrenaline transporter and are, indeed, 20- to 1500-fold more selective for inhibiting serotonin over noradrenaline. They do not stimulate the release of serotonin or noradrenaline presynaptically (Rothman et al., 2001) and have weak or no direct pharmacological action at postsynaptic serotonin receptors (e.g. 5-HT_{1A}, 5-HT_{2A} and 5-HT_{2c}) (Owens et al., 1997; Sanchez & Hyttel, 1999; Thomas et al., 1987). They also have minimal binding affinity for other postsynaptic receptors (adrenergic α_1, α_2 and β, histamine H_1, muscarinic and dopamine D_2 receptors) (Owens et al., 1997; Thomas et al., 1987). Therefore, their efficacy and adverse effect profile are largely related to serotonergic effects.

Several studies support the existence of a concentration–effect relationship for TCAs and/or their active metabolites (Gram et al., 1984; Perry et al., 1987; Preskorn & Jerkovich, 1990; Sjöqvist et al., 1980; Ziegler et al., 1977). An early study linked high concentrations of nortriptyline with not only adverse effects, but also with decreased antidepressant effect (Asberg et al., 1971). Subsequent reports have described concentration-dependent side effects in individuals deficient in CYP2D6 treated with usual doses of TCAs due to the accumulation of the parent drug and/or active metabolites (Balant-Gorgia et al., 1989; Bertilsson et al., 1981; Sjöqvist & Bertilsson, 1984). It has been reported that at comparable doses of TCA, Black patients, who have a higher frequency of *CYP2D6* IM alleles, achieve higher levels of TCAs than Caucasians, and also have a faster rate of recovery from a depressive episode (Raskin & Crook, 1975; Rudorfer & Robins, 1982; Ziegler & Biggs, 1977). A higher frequency of inactivating *CYP2D6* alleles has been found amongst patients with a history of an adverse reaction to TCAs and relevant SSRIs (Chen et al., 1996), while a prospective study found that CYP2D6 PMs attained the highest levels of desipramine and had adverse effects necessitating dose reduction (Spina et al., 1997). In a study including patients on TCAs, a trend towards an inverse correlation between the frequency of adverse drug events and number of functional *CYP2D6* genes was found (Chou et al., 2003). Combined steady-state amitriptyline and nortriptyline concentrations have been associated with *CYP2D6* functional gene dosage (where 0 = PM, 0.5 = IM, 1 = NM) (Steimer et al., 2004). Increased side effects to amitriptyline (correlating with nortriptyline concentration) have been reported for individuals with only one functional *CYP2D6* allele compared to those with two functional alleles, with the lowest risk being observed for those with two functional *CYP2D6* alleles and at least one *CYP2C19* PM allele, and the highest risk being seen in those with two functional *CYP2C19* alleles and at least one *CYP2D6* PM allele (Steimer et al., 2005).

Herrlin et al. (2003) investigated the pharmacokinetics of the enantiomers of citalopram and its metabolites in relation to CYP2C19 and CYP2D6 enzyme activity and found that an individual who was deficient in both enzymes stopped taking citalopram after five days due to severe adverse effects and had a very long citalopram half-life of 95 hours. Rudberg et al. (2007) reported a lower escitalopram serum concentration in patients homozygous for the *CYP2C19*17* allele compared with wild-type (*CYP2C19*1/*1*) patients. We have previously reported an association between *CYP2C19* genotype and logarithm mean steady-state escitalopram concentration-to-dose ratio, with individuals of *CYP2C19*17/*17* genotype having a significantly lower log-transformed ratio ($p = 0.0001$) than CYP2C19 NMs, and those homozygous for a PM allele having a significantly higher ratio than NMs (Huezo-Diaz et al., 2012), covarying for *CYP2D6* genotype as this also had an effect on the ratio (CYP2D6 IM/PM genotype individuals showing a higher mean escitalopram concentration than CYP2D6 NM). In a meta-analysis of the *CYP2C19* variants defining the *CYP2C19*2* PM and *CYP2C19*17* UM alleles from four samples treated with citalopram or escitalopram (GENDEP, STAR*D, GenPod and PGRN-AMPS), PM/PM individuals had higher symptom improvement and higher remission rates compared to NM/NMs, while at weeks 2–4, PM/PMs showed higher risk of gastrointestinal, neurological and sexual side effects (Fabbri et al., 2018).

5.6 Conclusions

Many genetic variants in drug metabolizing enzymes and transporters have been shown to be relevant in psychiatry. Associations between these and response to many medications used in psychiatry are strong enough for genotyping to be recommended to accompany prescribing. While various companies have developed assays, consistency in technology and the interpretation thereof currently limits uptake. What the field now requires is a concerted approach to develop a consensus marker panel using robust reproducible technologies, reference samples for all functional variants, and standardized interpretation and reporting algorithms. Pharmacogenomically informed mental health care has the potential to not only reduce ADRs but also greatly improve treatment pathways and therefore enhance uptake and compliance, and hence quality of life not only of those affected but, given the high prevalence of common disorders such as depression, by a 'ripple effect', society as a whole.

References

Abernethy DR, Todd EL (1985). Impairment of caffeine clearance by chronic use of low-dose oestrogen-containing oral contraceptives. *Eur J Clin Pharmacol*, 28(4), 425–428.

Adali O, Carver GC, Philpot RM (1998). Modulation of human flavin-containing monooxygenase 3 activity by tricyclic antidepressants and other agents: importance of residue 428. *Arch Biochem Biophys*, 358(1), 92–97. doi:10.1006/abbi.1998.0835.

Ahmed I, Dagincourt PG, Miller LG, Shader RI (1993). Possible interaction between fluoxetine and pimozide causing sinus bradycardia. *Can J Psychiatry*, 38(1), 62–63.

Aitchison KJ (2003). Pharmacogenetic studies of CYP2D6, CYP2C19, and CYP1A2, and investigation of their role in clinical response to antipsychotics and antidepressants. Unpublished PhD thesis, King's College London.

Aitchison KJ, Munro J, Wright P, et al. (1999). Failure to respond to treatment with typical antipsychotics is not associated with CYP2D6 ultrarapid hydroxylation. *Br J Clin Pharmacol*, 48(3), 388–394.

Aitchison KJ, Gonzalez FJ, Quattrochi LC, et al. (2000a). Identification of novel polymorphisms in the 5' flanking region of CYP1A2, characterization of interethnic variability, and investigation of their functional significance. *Pharmacogenetics*, 10(8), 695–704.

Aitchison KJ, Jann MW, Zhao JH, et al. (2000b). Clozapine pharmacokinetics and pharmacodynamics studied with Cyp1A2-null mice. *J Psychopharmacol*, 14(4), 353–359. doi:10.1177/026988110001400403.

Aitchison KJ, Jordan BD, Sharma T (2000c). The relevance of ethnic influences on pharmacogenetics to the treatment of psychosis. *Drug Metabol Drug Interact*, 16(1), 15–38.

Aitchison KJ, Bienroth M, Cookson J, et al. (2009). A UK consensus on the administration of aripiprazole for the treatment of mania. *J Psychopharmacol*, 23(3), 231–240. doi:10.1177/0269881108098820.

Aitchison KJ, Datla K, Rooprai H, Fernando J, Dexter D (2010). Regional distribution of clomipramine and desmethylclomipramine in rat brain and peripheral organs on chronic clomipramine administration. *J Psychopharmacol*, 24(8), 1261–1268. doi:10.1177/0269881109105789.

Aklillu E, Persson I, Bertilsson L, et al. (1996). Frequent distribution of ultrarapid metabolizers of debrisoquine in an Ethiopian population carrying duplicated and multiduplicated functional CYP2D6 alleles. *J Pharmacol Exp Ther*, 278(1), 441–446.

Aklillu E, Kalow W, Endrenyi L, et al. (2007). CYP2D6 and DRD2 genes differentially impact pharmacodynamic sensitivity and time course of prolactin response to perphenazine. *Pharmacogenet Genomics*, 17(11), 989–993. doi:10.1097/FPC.0b013e3282f01aa3.

Aller SG, Yu J, Ward A, et al. (2009). Structure of P-glycoprotein reveals a molecular basis for poly-specific drug binding. *Science*, 323(5922), 1718–1722. doi:10.1126/science.1168750.

Altman RB, Whirl-Carrillo M, Klein TE (2013). Challenges in the pharmacogenomic annotation of whole genomes. *Clin Pharmacol Ther*, 94(2), 211–213. doi:10.1038/clpt.2013.111.

American Psychiatric Association (2010). *Practice Guideline for the Treatment of Patients with Major Depressive Disorder*, 3rd ed. Available at: https://psychiatryonline.org/guidelines (last accessed 5.12.18).

Arici M, Özhan G (2017). The genetic profiles of CYP1A1, CYP1A2 and CYP2E1 enzymes as susceptibility factor in xenobiotic toxicity in

Turkish population. *Saudi Pharm J*, 25(2), 294–297. doi:10.1016/j.jsps.2016.06.001.

Aronow WS, Shamliyan TA (2018). Effects of atypical antipsychotic drugs on QT interval in patients with mental disorders. *Ann Transl Med*, 6(8), 147. doi:10.21037/atm.2018.03.17.

Asberg M, Crönholm B, Sjöqvist F, Tuck D (1971). Relationship between plasma level and therapeutic effect of nortriptyline. *Br Med J*, 3(5770), 331–334.

Assenat E, Gerbal-Chaloin S, Larrey D, et al. (2004). Interleukin 1beta inhibits CAR-induced expression of hepatic genes involved in drug and bilirubin clearance. *Hepatology*, 40(4), 951–960. doi:10.1002/hep.20387.

Axelrod J (1957). O-Methylation of epinephrine and other catechols in vitro and in vivo. *Science*, 126(3270), 400–401. doi:10.1126/science.126.3270.400.

Ayesh R, Mitchell SC, Zhang A, Smith RL (1993). The fish odour syndrome: biochemical, familial, and clinical aspects. *BMJ*, 307(6905), 655–657.

Azuma J, Hasunuma T, Kubo M, et al. (2012). The relationship between clinical pharmacokinetics of aripiprazole and CYP2D6 genetic polymorphism: effects of CYP enzyme inhibition by coadministration of paroxetine or fluvoxamine. *Eur J Clin Pharmacol*, 68(1), 29–37.

Bajpai M, Roskos LK, Shen DD, Levy RH (1996). Roles of cytochrome P4502C9 and cytochrome P4502C19 in the stereoselective metabolism of phenytoin to its major metabolite. *Drug Metab Dispos*, 24(12), 1401–1403.

Balant-Gorgia AE, Balant LP, Garrone G (1989). High blood concentrations of imipramine or clomipramine and therapeutic failure: a case report study using drug monitoring data. *Ther Drug Monit*, 11(4), 415–420.

Baltenberger EP, Buterbaugh WM, Martin BS, Thomas CJ (2015). Review of antidepressants in the treatment of neuropathic pain. *Ment Health Clin*, 5(3), 123–133.

Baririan N, Horsmans Y, Desager JP, et al. (2005). Alfentanil-induced miosis clearance as a liver CYP3A4 and 3A5 activity measure in healthy volunteers: improvement of experimental conditions. *J Clin Pharmacol*, 45(12), 1434–1441. doi:10.1177/0091270005282629.

Bauer B, Hartz AM, Fricker G, Miller DS (2004). Pregnane X receptor up-regulation of P-glycoprotein expression and transport function at the blood-brain barrier. *Mol Pharmacol*, 66(3), 413–419. doi:10.1124/mol.66.3.

Beedham C (1997). The role of non-P450 enzymes in drug oxidation. *Pharm World Sci*, 19(6), 255–263.

Bertilsson L (1995). Geographical/interracial differences in polymorphic drug oxidation. Current state of knowledge of cytochromes P450 (CYP) 2D6 and 2C19. *Clin Pharmacokinet*, 29(3), 192–209. doi:10.2165/00003088-199529030-00005.

Bertilsson L, Aberg-Wistedt A (1983). The debrisoquine hydroxylation test predicts steady-state plasma levels of desipramine. *Br J Clin Pharmacol*, 15(3), 388–390.

Bertilsson L, Dahl ML (1996). Polymorphic drug oxidation – relevance to the treatment of psychiatric disorders. *CNS Drugs*, 5(3), 200–223. doi:10.2165/00023210-199605030-00006.

Bertilsson L, Mellstrom B, Sjokvist F, Martenson B, Asberg M (1981). Slow hydroxylation of nortriptyline and concomitant poor debrisoquine hydroxylation: clinical implications. *Lancet*, 1(8219), 560–561.

Bertilsson L, Dahl ML, Ekqvist B, Llerena A (1993a). Disposition of the neuroleptics perphenazine, zuclopenthixol, and haloperidol cosegregates with polymorphic debrisoquine hydroxylation. *Psychopharmacol Ser*, 10, 230–237.

Bertilsson L, Dahl ML, Sjoqvist F, et al. (1993b). Molecular basis for rational megaprescribing in ultrarapid hydroxylators of debrisoquine. *Lancet*, 341(8836), 63.

Bertilsson L, Dahl ML, Dalen P, Al-Shurbaji A (2002). Molecular genetics of CYP2D6: clinical relevance with focus on psychotropic drugs. *Br J Clin Pharmacol*, 53(2), 111–122.

Bhaskar LV, Thangaraj K, Patel M, et al. (2013). EPHX1 gene polymorphisms in alcohol dependence and their distribution among the Indian populations. *Am J Drug Alcohol Abuse*, 39(1), 16–22. doi:10.3109/00952990.2011.643991.

Bigos KL, Bies RR, Pollock BG, et al. (2011). Genetic variation in CYP3A43 explains racial difference in olanzapine clearance. *Mol Psychiatry*, 16(6), 620–625. doi:10.1038/mp.2011.38.

Blake CM, Kharasch ED, Schwab M, Nagele P (2013). A meta-analysis of CYP2D6 metabolizer phenotype and metoprolol pharmacokinetics. *Clin Pharmacol Ther*, 94(3), 394–399. doi:10.1038/clpt.2013.96.

Bloomer JC, Woods FR, Haddock RE, Lennard MS, Tucker GT (1992). The role of cytochrome P4502D6 in the metabolism of paroxetine by human liver microsomes. *Br J Clin Pharmacol*, 33(5), 521–523.

Boland MR, Tatonetti NP (2016). Investigation of 7-dehydrocholesterol reductase pathway to elucidate off-target prenatal effects of pharmaceuticals: a systematic review. *Pharmacogenomics J*, 16(5), 411–429. doi:10.1038/tpj.2016.48.

Boobis AR, Lynch AM, Murray S, et al. (1994). CYP1A2-catalyzed conversion of dietary heterocyclic amines to their proximate carcinogens is their major route of metabolism in humans. *Cancer Res*, 54(1), 89–94.

Bourin M, Chue P, Guillon Y (2001). Paroxetine: a review. *CNS Drug Rev*, 7(1), 25–47.

Bousman CA, Hopwood M (2016). Commercial pharmacogenetic-based decision-support tools in psychiatry. *Lancet Psychiatry*, 3(6), 585–590. doi:10.1016/S2215-0366(16)00017-1.

Bousman C, Allen J, Eyre HA (2018). Pharmacogenetic tests in psychiatry. *Am J Psychiatry*, 175(2), 189. doi:10.1176/appi.ajp.2017.17101086.

Bousman C, Maruf AA, Muller DJ (2019). Towards the integration of pharmacogenetics in psychiatry: a minimum, evidence-based genetic testing panel. *Curr Opin Psychiatry*, 32(1), 7–15. doi:10.1097/YCO.0000000000000465.

Bradford LD (2002). CYP2D6 allele frequency in European Caucasians, Asians, Africans and their descendants. *Pharmacogenomics*, 3(2), 229–243. doi:10.1517/14622416.3.2.229.

Brøsen K (1993). The pharmacogenetics of the selective serotonin reuptake inhibitors. *Clin Investig*, 71(12), 1002–1009.

Brøsen K, Skjelbo E, Rasmussen BB, Poulsen HE, Loft S (1993). Fluvoxamine is a potent inhibitor of cytochrome P4501A2. *Biochem Pharmacol*, 45(6), 1211–1214.

Browning SL, Tarekegn A, Bekele E, Bradman N, Thomas MG (2010). CYP1A2 is more variable than previously thought: a genomic biography of the gene behind the human drug-metabolizing enzyme. *Pharmacogenet Genomics*, 20(11), 647–664. doi:10.1097/FPC.0b013e32833e90eb.

Bruyere A, Decleves X, Bouzom F, et al. (2010). Effect of variations in the amounts of P-glycoprotein (ABCB1), BCRP (ABCG2) and CYP3A4 along the human small intestine on PBPK models for predicting intestinal first pass. *Mol Pharm*, 7(5), 1596–1607. doi:10.1021/mp100015x.

Bu HZ (2006). A literature review of enzyme kinetic parameters for CYP3A4-mediated metabolic reactions of 113 drugs in human liver microsomes: structure-kinetics relationship assessment. *Curr Drug Metab*, 7(3), 231–249.

Caruso A, Bellia C, Pivetti A, et al. (2014). Effects of EPHX1 and CYP3A4 polymorphisms on carbamazepine metabolism in epileptic patients. *Pharmgenomics Pers Med*, 7, 117–120. doi:10.2147/PGPM.S55548.

Carvajal FJ, Inestrosa NC (2011). Interactions of AChE with Aβ aggregates in Alzheimer's brain: therapeutic relevance of IDN 5706. *Front Mol Neurosci*, 4, 19. doi:10.3389/fnmol.2011.00019.

Cascorbi I (2011). P-glycoprotein: tissue distribution, substrates, and functional consequences of genetic variations. *Handb Exp Pharmacol*, 201, 261–283. doi:10.1007/978-3-642-14541-4_6.

Cashman JR, Zhang J (2002). Interindividual differences of human flavin-containing monooxygenase 3: genetic polymorphisms and functional variation. *Drug Metab Dispos*, 30(10), 1043–1052.

Caspi A, Moffitt TE, Cannon M, et al. (2005). Moderation of the effect of adolescent-onset cannabis use on adult psychosis by a functional polymorphism in the catechol-O-methyltransferase gene: longitudinal evidence of a gene X environment interaction. *Biol Psychiatry*, 57(10), 1117–1127. doi:10.1016/j.biopsych.2005.01.026.

Caudle KE, Klein TE, Hoffman JM, et al. (2014). Incorporation of pharmacogenomics into routine clinical practice: the Clinical Pharmacogenetics Implementation Consortium (CPIC) guideline development process. *Curr Drug Metab*, 15(2), 209–217.

Caudle KE, Gammal RS, Whirl-Carrillo M, et al. (2016). Evidence and resources to implement pharmacogenetic knowledge for precision medicine. *Am J Health Syst Pharm*, 73(23), 1977–1985. doi:10.2146/ajhp150977.

Chen J-T, Wei L, Chen T-L, Huang C-J, Chen R-M (2018). Regulation of cytochrome P450 gene expression by ketamine: a review. *Expert Opin Drug Metab Toxicol*, 14(7), 709–720.

Chen S, Chou WH, Blouin RA, et al. (1996). The cytochrome P450 2D6 (CYP2D6) enzyme polymorphism: screening costs and influence on clinical outcomes in psychiatry. *Clin Pharmacol Ther*, 60(5), 522–534. doi:10.1016/S0009-9236(96)90148-4.

Chen Y, Zane NR, Thakker DR, Wang MZ (2016). Quantification of flavin-containing monooxygenases 1, 3, and 5 in human liver microsomes by UPLC-MRM-based targeted quantitative proteomics and its application to the study of ontogeny. *Drug Metab Dispos*, 44(7), 975–983. doi:10.1124/dmd.115.067538.

Chou WH, Yan FX, Robbins-Weilert DK, et al. (2003). Comparison of two CYP2D6 genotyping methods and assessment of genotype-phenotype relationships. *Clin Chem*, 49(4), 542–551.

Christensen M, Tybring G, Mihara K, et al. (2002). Low daily 10-mg and 20-mg doses of fluvoxamine inhibit the metabolism of both caffeine (cytochrome P4501A2) and omeprazole (cytochrome P4502C19). *Clin Pharmacol Ther*, 71(3), 141–152. doi:10.1067/mcp.2002.121788.

Chung WH, Hung SI, Hong HS, et al. (2004). Medical genetics: a marker for Stevens-Johnson syndrome. *Nature*, 428(6982), 486. doi:10.1038/428486a.

Coleman T, Ellis SW, Martin IJ, Lennard MS, Tucker GT (1996). 1-Methyl-4-phenyl-1,2,3,6-tetrahydropyridine (MPTP) is N-demethylated by cytochromes P450 2D6, 1A2 and 3A4 – implications for susceptibility to Parkinson's disease. *J Pharmacol Exp Ther*, 277(2), 685–690.

Coller JK, Krebsfaenger N, Klein K, et al. (2002). The influence of CYP2B6, CYP2C9 and CYP2D6 genotypes on the formation of the potent antioestrogen Z-4-hydroxy-tamoxifen in human liver. *Br J Clin Pharmacol*, 54(2), 157–167. doi:10.1046/j.1365-2125.2002.01614.x.

Committee on Safety of Medicines-Medicines Control Agency (1995). Cardiac arrhythmias with pimozide (Orap). *Curr Probl Pharmacovigilance*, 21, 1.

Consoli G, Lastella M, Ciapparelli A, et al. (2009). ABCB1 polymorphisms are associated with clozapine plasma levels in psychotic patients. *Pharmacogenomics*, 10(8), 1267–1276. doi:10.2217/pgs.09.51.

Cornelis MC, El-Sohemy A, Kabagambe EK, Campos H (2006). Coffee, CYP1A2 genotype, and risk of myocardial infarction. *JAMA*, 295 (10), 1135–1141. doi:10.1001/jama.295.10.1135.

Correll CU, Detraux J, De Lepeleire J, De Hert M (2015). Effects of antipsychotics, antidepressants and mood stabilizers on risk for physical diseases in people with schizophrenia, depression and bipolar disorder. *World Psychiatry*, 14(2), 119–136. doi:10.1002/wps.20204.

Crespi CL, Penman BW, Leakey JAE, et al. (1990). Human cytochrome P450IIA3: cDNA sequence role of the enzyme in the metabolic activation of promutagens comparison to nitrosamine activation by human cytochrome P450IIE1. *Carcinogenesis*, 11(8), 1293–1300.

Crews KR, Gaedigk A, Dunnenberger HM, et al; Clinical Pharmacogenetics Implementation Consortium. (2014). Clinical Pharmacogenetics Implementation Consortium guidelines for cytochrome P450 2D6 genotype and codeine therapy: 2014 update. *Clin Pharmacol Ther*, 95(4), 376–382. doi:10.1038/clpt.2013.254.

Cupp MJ, Tracy TS (1998). Cytochrome P450: new nomenclature and clinical implications. *Am Fam Physician*, 57(1), 107–116.

Cusack B, Nelson A, Richelson E (1994). Binding of antidepressants to human brain receptors: focus on newer generation compounds. *Psychopharmacology (Berl)*, 114(4), 559–565.

Czekaj P (2000). Phenobarbital-induced expression of cytochrome P450 genes. *Acta Biochim Pol*, 47(4), 1093–1105.

Czekaj P, Skowronek R (2012). Transcription factors potentially involved in regulation of cytochrome P450 gene expression. In J Paxton, ed., *Topics on Drug Metabolism*. Croatia: InTech, pp. 171–190.

Daci A, Beretta G, Vllasaliu D, et al. (2015). Polymorphic variants of SCN1A and EPHX1 influence plasma carbamazepine concentration, metabolism and pharmacoresistance in a population of Kosovar Albanian epileptic patients. *PLoS One*, 10(11), e0142408. doi:10.1371/journal.pone.0142408.

Dahl-Puustinen M-L, Lidén A, Alm C, Nordin C, Bertilsson L (1989). Disposition of perphenazine is related to polymorphic debrisoquin hydroxylation in human beings. *Clin Pharmacol Ther*, 46(1), 78–81.

Dalen P, Dahl ML, Bernal Ruiz ML, Nordin J, Bertilsson L (1998). 10-Hydroxylation of nortriptyline in white persons with 0, 1, 2, 3, and 13 functional CYP2D6 genes. *Clin Pharmacol Ther*, 63(4), 444–452. doi:10.1016/S0009-9236(98)90040-6.

Dannenberg LO, Edenberg HJ (2006). Epigenetics of gene expression in human hepatoma cells: expression profiling the response to inhibition of DNA methylation and histone deacetylation. *BMC Genomics*, 7, 181. doi:10.1186/1471-2164-7-181.

de Andrés F, Sosa-Macías M, Llerena A (2014). A rapid and simple LC-MS/MS method for the simultaneous evaluation of CYP1A2, CYP2C9, CYP2C19, CYP2D6 and CYP3A4 hydroxylation capacity. *Bioanalysis*, 6(5), 683–696. doi:10.4155/bio.14.20.

de Klerk OL, Nolte IM, Bet PM, et al. (2013). ABCB1 gene variants influence tolerance to selective serotonin reuptake inhibitors in a large sample of Dutch cases with major depressive disorder. *Pharmacogenomics J*, 13(4), 349–353. doi:10.1038/tpj.2012.16.

de Leon J (2009). The future (or lack of future) of personalized prescription in psychiatry. *Pharmacol Res*, 59(2), 81–89. doi:10.1016/j.phrs.2008.10.002.

de Morais SM, Wilkinson GR, Blaisdell J, et al. (1994). The major genetic defect responsible for the polymorphism of S-mephenytoin metabolism in humans. *J Biol Chem*, 269(22), 15419–15422.

Del Tredici AL, Malhotra A, Dedek M, et al. (2018). Frequency of CYP2D6 alleles including structural variants in the United States. *Front Pharmacol*, 9, 305. doi:10.3389/fphar.2018.00305.

DeLeon A, Patel NC, Crismon ML (2004). Aripiprazole: a comprehensive review of its pharmacology, clinical efficacy, and tolerability. *Clin Ther*, 26(5), 649–666.

Desta Z, Kerbusch T, Soukhova N, et al. (1998). Identification and characterization of human cytochrome P450 isoforms interacting with pimozide. *J Pharmacol Exp Ther*, 285(2), 428–437.

Desta Z, Kerbusch T, Flockhart DA (1999). Effect of clarithromycin on the pharmacokinetics and pharmacodynamics of pimozide in healthy poor and extensive metabolizers of cytochrome P450 2D6 (CYP2D6). *Clin Pharmacol Ther*, 65(1), 10–20. https://doi.org/10.1016/S0009-9236(99)70117-7.

Desta Z, Zhao X, Shin JG, Flockhart DA (2002). Clinical significance of the cytochrome P450 2C19 genetic polymorphism. *Clin Pharmacokinet*, 41(12), 913–958. doi:10.2165/00003088-200241120-00002.

Desta Z, Saussele T, Ward B, et al. (2007). Impact of CYP2B6 polymorphism on hepatic efavirenz metabolism in vitro. *Pharmacogenomics*, 8(6), 547–558. doi:10.2217/14622416.8.6.547.

di Iulio J, Fayet A, Arab-Alameddine M, et al.; Swiss HIV Cohort Study (2009). In vivo analysis of efavirenz metabolism in individuals with impaired CYP2A6 function. *Pharmacogenet Genomics*, 19(4), 300–309. doi:10.1097/FPC.0b013e328328d577.

Dobrinas M, Cornuz J, Oneda B, et al. (2011). Impact of smoking, smoking cessation, and genetic polymorphisms on CYP1A2 activity and inducibility. *Clin Pharmacol Ther*, 90(1), 117–125. doi:10.1038/clpt.2011.70.

Doring B, Petzinger E (2014). Phase 0 and phase III transport in various organs: combined concept of phases in xenobiotic transport and metabolism. *Drug Metab Rev*, 46(3), 261–282. doi:10.3109/03602532.2014.882353.

Drolet B, Rousseau G, Daleau P, et al. (2001). Pimozide (Orap) prolongs cardiac repolarization by blocking the rapid component of the delayed rectifier potassium current in native cardiac myocytes. *J Cardiovasc Pharmacol Ther*, 6(3), 255–260. doi:10.1177/107424840100600306.

Drozda K, Müller DJ, Bishop JR (2014). Pharmacogenomic testing for neuropsychiatric drugs: current status of drug labeling, guidelines for using genetic information, and test options. *Pharmacotherapy*, 34(2), 166–184. doi:10.1002/phar.1398.

Eaton DL, Gallagher EP, Bammler TK, Kunze KL (1995). Role of cytochrome P4501A2 in chemical carcinogenesis: implications for human variability in expression and enzyme activity. *Pharmacogenetics*, 5(5), 259–274.

Ehlert FJ, Delen FM, Yun SH, Liem HA (1990). The interaction of amitriptyline, doxepin, imipramine and their N-methyl quaternary ammonium derivatives with subtypes of muscarinic receptors in brain and heart. *J Pharmacol Exp Ther*, 253(1), 13–19.

Eichelbaum M (1984). Polymorphic drug oxidation in humans. *Fed Proc*, 43(8), 2298–2302.

Ekroos M, Sjogren T (2006). Structural basis for ligand promiscuity in cytochrome P450 3A4. *Proc Natl Acad Sci U S A*, 103(37), 13682–13687. doi:10.1073/pnas.0603236103.

El-Sherbeni AA, El-Kadi AO (2014). The role of epoxide hydrolases in health and disease. *Arch Toxicol*, 88(11), 2013–2032. doi:10.1007/s00204-014-1371-y.

Elsinga PH, Hendrikse NH, Bart J, Vaalburg W, van Waarde A (2004). PET studies on P-glycoprotein function in the blood-brain barrier: how it affects uptake and binding of drugs within the CNS. *Curr Pharm Des*, 10(13), 1493–1503.

Eriksson N, Wadelius M (2012). Prediction of warfarin dose: why, when and how? *Pharmacogenomics*, 13(4), 429–440. doi:10.2217/pgs.11.184.

Espinoza M, Rivero Osimani V, Sánchez V, Rosenbaum E, Guiñazú N. (2016). B-esterase determination and organophosphate insecticide inhibitory effects in JEG-3 trophoblasts. *Toxicol In Vitro*, 32, 190–197. doi:10.1016/j.tiv.2016.01.001.

Fabbri C, Tansey KE, Perlis RH, et al. (2018). Effect of cytochrome CYP2C19 metabolizing activity on antidepressant response and side effects: meta-analysis of data from genome-wide association studies. *Eur Neuropsychopharmacol*, 28(8), 945–954. doi:10.1016/j.euroneuro.2018.05.009.

Fan WL, Shiao MS, Hui RC, et al. (2017). HLA association with drug-induced adverse reactions. *J Immunol Res*, 2017, 3186328. doi:10.1155/2017/3186328.

Fang H, Xu X, Kaur K, et al. (2019). A screening test for *HLA-B(*)15:02* in a large United States patient cohort identifies broader risk of carbamazepine-induced adverse events. *Front Pharmacol* 10, 149.

Feng J, Sun J, Wang MZ, et al. (2010). Compilation of a comprehensive gene panel for systematic assessment of genes that govern an individual's drug responses. *Pharmacogenomics*, 11(10), 1403–1425. doi:10.2217/pgs.10.99.

Ferrell PB, McLeod HL (2008). Carbamazepine, HLA-B*1502 and risk of Stevens-Johnson syndrome and toxic epidermal necrolysis: US FDA recommendations. *Pharmacogenomics*, 9(10), 1543–1546. doi:10.2217/14622416.9.10.1543.

Fiore MC, Jorenby DE, Schensky AE, et al. (1995). Smoking status as the new vital sign: effect on assessment and intervention in patients who smoke. *Mayo Clin Proc*, 70(3), 209–213. doi:10.1016/S0025-6196(11)64939-2.

Flockhart DA, Drici MD, Kerbusch T, et al. (2000). Studies on the mechanism of a fatal clarithromycin-pimozide interaction in a patient with Tourette syndrome. *J Clin Psychopharmacol*, 20(3), 317–324.

Foti RS, Dalvie DK (2016). Cytochrome P450 and non-cytochrome P450 oxidative metabolism: contributions to the pharmacokinetics, safety, and efficacy of xenobiotics. *Drug Metab Dispos*, 44(8), 1229–1245. doi:10.1124/dmd.116.071753.

Foti RS, Wienkers LC, Wahlstrom JL (2010). Application of cytochrome P450 drug interaction screening in drug discovery. *Comb Chem High Throughput Screen*, 13(2), 145–158.

Fricke-Galindo I, LLerena A, Jung-Cook H, López-López M (2018). Carbamazepine adverse drug reactions. *Expert Rev Clin Pharmacol*, 11(7), 705–718. doi:10.1080/17512433.2018.1486707.

Fromm MF, Kim RB (2011). *Drug Transporters: Handbook of Experimental Pharmacology v. 201*. Available at: http://dx.doi.org/10.1007/978-3-642-14541-4 (last accessed 5.12.18).

Fuhr U, Anders EM, Mahr G, Sorgel F, Staib AH (1992). Inhibitory potency of quinolone antibacterial agents against cytochrome P450IA2 activity in vivo and in vitro. *Antimicrob Agents Chemother*, 36(5), 942–948.

Fuhr U, Klittich K, Staib AH (1993). Inhibitory effect of grapefruit juice and its bitter principal, naringenin, on CYP1A2 dependent metabolism of caffeine in man. *Br J Clin Pharmacol*, 35(4), 431–436.

Fuhr U, Jetter A, Kirchheiner J (2007). Appropriate phenotyping procedures for drug metabolizing enzymes and transporters in humans and their simultaneous use in the 'cocktail' approach. *Clin Pharmacol Ther*, 81, 270–283.

Fujita K, Sasaki Y (2007). Pharmacogenomics in drug-metabolizing enzymes catalyzing anticancer drugs for personalized cancer chemotherapy. *Curr Drug Metab*, 8(6), 554–562.

Fukami T, Yokoi T (2012). The emerging role of human esterases. *Drug Metab Pharmacokinet*, 27(5), 466–477.

Fulop G, Phillips RA, Shapiro AK, et al. (1987). ECG changes during haloperidol and pimozide treatment of Tourette's disorder. *Am J Psychiatry*, 144(5), 673–675. doi:10.1176/ajp.144.5.673.

Furnes B, Feng J, Sommer SS, Schlenk D (2003). Identification of novel variants of the flavin-containing monooxygenase gene family in African Americans. *Drug Metab Dispos*, 31(2), 187–193.

Genaro-Mattos TC, Tallman KA, Allen LB, et al. (2018). Dichlorophenyl piperazines, including a recently-approved atypical antipsychotic, are potent inhibitors of DHCR7, the last enzyme in cholesterol biosynthesis. *Toxicol Appl Pharmacol*, 349, 21–28. doi:10.1016/j.taap.2018.04.029.

Ghodke-Puranik Y, Thorn CF, Lamba JK, et al. (2013). Valproic acid pathway: pharmacokinetics and pharmacodynamics. *Pharmacogenet Genomics*, 23(4), 236–241. doi:10.1097/FPC.0b013e32835ea0b2.

Ghotbi R, Christensen M, Roh HK, et al. (2007). Comparisons of CYP1A2 genetic polymorphisms, enzyme activity and the genotype-phenotype relationship in Swedes and Koreans. *Eur J Clin Pharmacol*, 63(6), 537–546. doi:10.1007/s00228-007-0288-2.

Goh BC, Lee SC, Wang LZ, et al. (2002). Explaining interindividual variability of docetaxel pharmacokinetics and pharmacodynamics in Asians through phenotyping and genotyping strategies. *J Clin Oncol*, 20(17), 3683–3690. doi:10.1200/JCO.2002.01.025.

Goldman D (2014). Roles of COMT, NPY and GCH1 in acute and chronic pain/stress response. *Mol Pain*, 10(Suppl 1), O5. doi:10.1186/1744-8069-10-S1-O5.

Goldman D, Weinberger DR, Malhotra AK, Goldberg TE (2009). The role of COMT Val158Met in cognition. *Biol Psychiatry*, 65(1), e1–e2; author reply e3–e4. doi:10.1016/j.biopsych.2008.07.032.

Goldstein JA, de Morais SM (1994). Biochemistry and molecular biology of the human CYP2C subfamily. *Pharmacogenetics*, 4(6), 285–299.

Gong QL, Hedner T, Hedner J, Bjorkman R, Nordberg G (1991). Antinociceptive and ventilatory effects of the morphine metabolites: morphine-6-glucuronide and morphine-3-glucuronide. *Eur J Pharmacol*, 193(1), 47–56.

Gonzalez FJ, Gelboin HV (1994). Role of human cytochromes P450 in the metabolic activation of chemical carcinogens and toxins. *Drug Metab Rev*, 26(1–2), 165–183.

Goodarzi MO, Xu N, Azziz R (2008). Association of CYP3A7*1C and serum dehydroepiandrosterone sulfate levels in women with polycystic ovary syndrome. *J Clin Endocrinol Metab*, 93(7), 2909–2912. doi:10.1210/jc.2008-0403.

Gough AC, Miles JS, Spurr NK, et al. (1990). Identification of the primary gene defect at the cytochrome P450 CYP2D locus. *Nature*, 347(6295), 773 776. doi:10.1038/347773a0.

Gram LF, Kragh-Sorensen P, Kristensen CB, et al. (1984). Plasma level monitoring of antidepressants: theoretical basis and clinical application. *Adv Biochem Psychopharmacol*, 39, 399–411.

Grisaru D, Sternfeld M, Eldor A, Glick D, Soreq H (1999). Structural roles of acetylcholinesterase variants in biology and pathology. *Eur J Biochem*, 264(3), 672–686.

Grossberg GT (2003). Cholinesterase inhibitors for the treatment of Alzheimer's disease: getting on and staying on. *Curr Ther Res Clin Exp*, 64(4), 216–235. doi:10.1016/S0011-393X(03)00059-6.

Guengerich FP (1999). Cytochrome P-450 3A4: regulation and role in drug metabolism. *Annu Rev Pharmacol Toxicol*, 39, 1–17. doi:10.1146/annurev.pharmtox.39.1.1.

Haas DW, Ribaudo HJ, Kim RB, et al. (2004). Pharmacogenetics of efavirenz and central nervous system side effects: an Adult AIDS Clinical Trials Group study. *AIDS*, 18(18), 2391–2400.

Haberl M, Anwald B, Klein K, et al. (2005). Three haplotypes associated with CYP2A6 phenotypes in Caucasians. *Pharmacogenet Genomics*, 15(9), 609–624.

Haddock RE, Johnson AM, Langley PF, et al. (1989). Metabolic pathway of paroxetine in animals and man and the comparative pharmacological properties of its metabolites. *Acta Psychiatr Scand*, 80(S350), 24–26.

Hadidi H, Zahlsen K, Idle JR, Cholerton S (1997). A single amino acid substitution (Leu160His) in cytochrome P450 CYP2A6 causes switching from 7-hydroxylation to 3-hydroxylation of coumarin. *Food Chem Toxicol*, 35(9), 903–907.

Hals P-A, Hall H, Dahl SG (1986). Phenothiazine drug metabolites: dopamine D2 receptor, α1-and α2-adrenoceptor binding. *Eur J Pharmacol*, 125(3), 373–381.

Hammons GJ, Milton D, Stepps K, et al. (1997). Metabolism of carcinogenic heterocyclic and aromatic amines by recombinant human cytochrome P450 enzymes. *Carcinogenesis*, 18(4), 851–854.

Hanioka N, Kimura S, Meyer UA, Gonzalez FJ (1990). The human CYP2D locus associated with a common genetic defect in drug oxidation: a G1934-A base change in intron 3 of a mutant CYP2D6 allele results in an aberrant 3' splice recognition site. *Am J Hum Genet*, 47(6), 994–1001.

Hansen LB (1981). The clinical significance of measuring perphenazine in plasma during oral antipsychotic treatment. In E Usdin, SG Dahl, LF Gram, O Lingjærde, eds., *Clinical Pharmacology in Psychiatry – Neuroleptic and Antidepressant Research*. London: Macmillan, pp. 211–216.

Hansen LB, Larsen NE (1983). Plasma levels of perphenazine related to clinical effect and extrapyramidal side-effects. In LF Gram, E Usdin, SG Dahl, et al., eds., *Clinical Pharmacology in Psychiatry – Bridging the Experimental-Therapeutic Gap*. London: Macmillan, pp. 175–181.

Hansen LB, Larsen NE (1985). Therapeutic advantages of monitoring plasma concentrations of perphenazine in clinical practice. *Psychopharmacology (Berl)*, 87(1), 16–19.

Hansen LB, Elley J, Christensen TR, et al. (1979). Plasma levels of perphenazine and its major metabolites during simultaneous treatment with anticholinergic drugs. *Br J Clin Pharmacol*, 7(1), 75–80.

Hansen LB, Larsen NE, Gulmann, N. (1982). Dose-response relationships of perphenazine in the treatment of acute psychoses. *Psychopharmacology (Berl)*, 78(2), 112–115.

Hartsfield JK Jr, Sutcliffe MJ, Everett ET, et al. (1998). Assignment1 of microsomal epoxide hydrolase (EPHX1) to human chromosome 1q42.1 by in situ hybridization. *Cytogenet Cell Genet*, 83(1–2), 44–45. doi:10.1159/000015164.

Hasin Y, Avidan N, Bercovich D, et al. (2005). Analysis of genetic polymorphisms in acetylcholinesterase as reflected in different populations. *Curr Alzheimer Res*, 2(2), 207–218.

Hassett C, Robinson KB, Beck NB, Omiecinski CJ (1994). The human microsomal epoxide hydrolase gene (EPHX1): complete nucleotide sequence and structural characterization. *Genomics*, 23(2), 433–442. doi:10.1006/geno.1994.1520.

Hemeryck A, Belpaire FM (2002). Selective serotonin reuptake inhibitors and cytochrome P-450 mediated drug-drug interactions: an update. *Curr Drug Metab*, 3(1), 13–37.

Hendset M, Molden E, Knape M, Hermann M (2014). Serum concentrations of risperidone and aripiprazole in subgroups encoding CYP2D6 intermediate metabolizer phenotype. *Ther Drug Monit*, 36(1), 80–85. doi:10.1097/FTD.0000000000000018.

Herrlin K, Yasui-Furukori N, Tybring G, et al. (2003). Metabolism of citalopram enantiomers in CYP2C19/CYP2D6 phenotyped panels of healthy Swedes. *Br J Clin Pharmacol*, 56(4), 415–421.

Hesse LM, He P, Krishnaswamy S, et al. (2004). Pharmacogenetic determinants of interindividual variability in bupropion hydroxylation by cytochrome P450 2B6 in human liver microsomes. *Pharmacogenetics*, 14(4), 225–238.

Hicks JK, Swen JJ, Thorn CF, et al. (2013). Clinical Pharmacogenetics Implementation Consortium guideline for CYP2D6 and CYP2C19 genotypes and dosing of tricyclic antidepressants. *Clin Pharmacol Ther*, 93(5), 402–408. doi:10.1038/clpt.2013.2.

Hicks JK, Sangkuhl K, Swen JJ, et al. (2016). Clinical pharmacogenetics implementation consortium guideline (CPIC) for CYP2D6 and CYP2C19 genotypes and dosing of tricyclic antidepressants: 2016 update. *Clin Pharmacol Ther*, 102(1), 37–44. doi:10.1002/cpt.597.

Hiemke C, Bergemann N, Clement HW, et al. (2018). Consensus Guidelines for Therapeutic Drug Monitoring in Neuropsychopharmacology: Update 2017. *Pharmacopsychiatry*, 51(1–2), e1. doi:10.1055/s-0037-1600991.

Hillhouse TM, Porter JH (2015). A brief history of the development of antidepressant drugs: from monoamines to glutamate. *Exp Clin Psychopharmacol*, 23(1), 1–21. doi:10.1037/a0038550.

Hisaka A, Ohno Y, Yamamoto T, Suzuki H (2010). Prediction of pharmacokinetic drug-drug interaction caused by changes in cytochrome P450 activity using in vivo information. *Pharmacol Ther*, 125(2), 230–248. doi:10.1016/j.pharmthera.2009.10.011.

Hjorthoj C, Ostergaard MLD, Benros ME, et al. (2015). Association between alcohol and substance use disorders and all-cause and cause-specific mortality in schizophrenia, bipolar disorder, and unipolar depression: a nationwide, prospective, register-based study. *Lancet Psychiatry*, 2(9), 801–808. doi:10.1016/S2215-0366(15)00207-2.

Hoffman SM, Nelson DR, Keeney DS (2001). Organization, structure and evolution of the CYP2 gene cluster on human chromosome 19. *Pharmacogenetics*, 11(8), 687–698.

Hofmann MH, Blievernicht JK, Klein K, et al. (2008). Aberrant splicing caused by single nucleotide polymorphism c.516G>T [Q172H], a marker of CYP2B6*6, is responsible for decreased expression and activity of CYP2B6 in liver. *J Pharmacol Exp Ther*, 325(1), 284–292. doi:10.1124/jpet.107.133306.

Holstein A, Plaschke A, Ptak M, et al. (2005). Association between CYP2C9 slow metabolizer genotypes and severe hypoglycaemia on medication with sulphonylurea hypoglycaemic agents. *Br J Clin Pharmacol*, 60(1), 103–106. doi:10.1111/j.1365-2125.2005.02379.x.

Hoosain FG, Choonara YE, Tomar LK, et al. (2015). Bypassing P-glycoprotein drug efflux mechanisms: possible applications in pharmacoresistant schizophrenia therapy. *Biomed Res Int*, 2015, 484963. doi:10.1155/2015/484963.

Horrigan JP, Barnhill LJ (1994). Paroxetine-pimozide drug interaction. *J Am Acad Child Adolesc Psychiatry*, 33(7), 1060–1061. doi:10.1097/00004583-199409000-00022.

Hu GX, Dai DP, Wang H, et al. (2017). Systematic screening for CYP3A4 genetic polymorphisms in a Han Chinese population. *Pharmacogenomics*, 18(4), 369–379. doi:10.2217/pgs-2016-0179.

Hu Y, Oscarson M, Johansson I, et al. (1997). Genetic polymorphism of human CYP2E1: characterization of two variant alleles. *Mol Pharmacol*, 51(3), 370–376.

Huang C, Kurland AA (1964). Perphenazine (trilafon) metabolism in psychotic patients. *Arch Gen Psychiatry*, 10(6), 639–646.

Huezo-Diaz P, Perroud N, Spencer EP, et al. (2012). CYP2C19 genotype predicts steady state escitalopram concentration in GENDEP. *J Psychopharmacol*, 26(3), 398–407. doi:10.1177/0269881111414451.

Imaoka S, Funae Y (1990). Purification and characterization of rat pulmonary cytochrome P-450. *J Biochem*, 108(1), 33–36.

Ingelman-Sundberg M (2004a). Human drug metabolising cytochrome P450 enzymes: properties and polymorphisms. *Naunyn Schmiedebergs Arch Pharmacol*, 369(1), 89–104. doi:10.1007/s00210-003-0819-z.

Ingelman-Sundberg M (2004b). Pharmacogenetics of cytochrome P450 and its applications in drug therapy: the past, present and future. *Trends Pharmacol Sci*, 25(4), 193–200. doi:10.1016/j.tips.2004.02.007.

Ishii Y, Iwanaga M, Nishimura Y, et al. (2007). Protein-protein interactions between rat hepatic cytochromes P450 (P450s) and UDP-glucuronosyltransferases (UGTs): evidence for the functionally active UGT in P450-UGT complex. *Drug Metab Pharmacokinet*, 22(5), 367–376.

Ishikawa T (1992). The ATP-dependent glutathione S-conjugate export pump. *Trends Biochem Sci*, 17(11), 463–468.

Jackson MR, Craft JA, Burchell, B (1987). Nucleotide and deduced amino acid sequence of human liver microsomal epoxide hydrolase. *Nucleic Acids Res*, 15(17), 7188.

Jančová P, Šiller M (2012). Phase II drug metabolism. In J Paxton, ed., *Topics on Drug Metabolism*. Croatia: InTech, pp. 35–60.

Jann MW, Cohen LJ (2000). The influence of ethnicity and antidepressant pharmacogenetics in the treatment of depression. *Drug Metabol Drug Interact*, 16(1), 39–67.

Jaquenoud Sirot E, Knezevic B, Morena GP, et al. (2009). ABCB1 and cytochrome P450 polymorphisms: clinical pharmacogenetics of clozapine. *J Clin Psychopharmacol*, 29(4), 319–326. doi:10.1097/JCP.0b013e3181acc372.

Jerling M, Dahl ML, Aberg-Wistedt A, et al. (1996). The CYP2D6 genotype predicts the oral clearance of the neuroleptic agents perphenazine and zuclopenthixol. *Clin Pharmacol Ther*, 59(4), 423–428. doi:10.1016/S0009-9236(96)90111-3.

Jiang Z, Dalton TP, Jin L, et al. (2005). Toward the evaluation of function in genetic variability: characterizing human SNP frequencies and establishing BAC-transgenic mice carrying the human CYP1A1_CYP1A2 locus. *Hum Mutat*, 25(2), 196–206. doi:10.1002/humu.20134.

Johannessen SI, Landmark CJ (2010). Antiepileptic drug interactions – principles and clinical implications. *Curr Neuropharmacol*, 8(3), 254–267. doi:10.2174/157015910792246254.

Johansson I, Ingelman-Sundberg M (2011). Genetic polymorphism and toxicology – with emphasis on cytochrome p450. *Toxicol Sci*, 120(1), 1–13. doi:10.1093/toxsci/kfq374.

Johansson I, Lundqvist E, Bertilsson L, et al. (1993). Inherited amplification of an active gene in the cytochrome P450 CYP2D locus as a cause of ultrarapid metabolism of debrisoquine. *Proc Natl Acad Sci U S A*, 90(24), 11825–11829.

Johansson I, Oscarson M, Yue QY, et al. (1994). Genetic-analysis of the Chinese cytochrome P4502d locus – characterization of variant Cyp2d6 genes present in subjects with diminished capacity for debrisoquine hydroxylation. *Mol Pharmacol*, 46(3), 452–459.

Johne A, Brockmoller J, Bauer S, et al. (1999). Pharmacokinetic interaction of digoxin with an herbal extract from St John's wort (*Hypericum perforatum*). *Clin Pharmacol Ther*, 66(4), 338–345. doi:10.1053/cp.1999.v66.a101944.

Johnstone E, Benowitz N, Cargill A, et al. (2006). Determinants of the rate of nicotine metabolism and effects on smoking behavior. *Clin Pharmacol Ther*, 80(4), 319–330. doi:10.1016/j.clpt.2006.06.011.

Jornil J, Jensen KG, Larsen F, Linnet K (2010). Identification of cytochrome P450 isoforms involved in the metabolism of paroxetine and estimation of their importance for human paroxetine metabolism using a population-based simulator. *Drug Metab Dispos*, 38(3), 376–385. doi:10.1124/dmd.109.030551.

Jung F, Richardson TH, Raucy JL, Johnson EF (1997). Diazepam metabolism by cDNA-expressed human 2C P450s: identification of P4502C18 and P4502C19 as low K(M) diazepam N-demethylases. *Drug Metab Dispos*, 25(2), 133–139.

Jurica J, Sulcova A (2012). Determination of cytochrome P450 metabolic activity using selective markers. In J Paxton, ed., *Topics on Drug Metabolism*. Croatia: InTech, pp. 191–220.

Kagimoto M, Heim M, Kagimoto K, Zeugin T, Meyer UA (1990). Multiple mutations of the human cytochrome P450IID6 gene (CYP2D6) in poor metabolizers of debrisoquine. Study of the functional significance of individual mutations by expression of chimeric genes. *J Biol Chem*, 265(28), 17209–17214.

Kalow W, Tyndale R (1992). Debrisoquine/sparteine monooxygenase and other P450s in brain. In W Kalow, ed., *Pharmacogenetics of Drug Metabolism*. Oxford: Pergamon Press, pp. 649–656.

Kasperavičiūte D, Sisodiya SM (2009). Epilepsy pharmacogenetics. *Pharmacogenomics*, 10(5), 817–836. doi:10.2217/pgs.09.34.

Kertesz SG, Pletcher MJ, Safford M, et al. (2007). Illicit drug use in young adults and subsequent decline in general health: the Coronary Artery Risk Development in Young Adults (CARDIA) study. *Drug Alcohol Depend*, 88(2–3), 224–233. doi:10.1016/j.drugalcdep.2006.10.017.

Khan KK, He YQ, Domanski TL, Halpert JR (2002). Midazolam oxidation by cytochrome P450 3A4 and active-site mutants: an evaluation of multiple binding sites and of the metabolic pathway that leads to enzyme inactivation. *Mol Pharmacol*, 61(3), 495–506.

Kim HY, Korade Z, Tallman KA, et al. (2016). Inhibitors of 7-dehydrocholesterol reductase: screening of a collection of pharmacologically active compounds in Neuro2a cells. *Chem Res Toxicol*, 29(5), 892–900. doi:10.1021/acs.chemrestox.6b00054.

King J, Aberg JA (2008). Clinical impact of patient population differences and genomic variation in efavirenz therapy. *AIDS*, 22(14), 1709–1717. doi:10.1097/QAD.0b013e32830163ad.

Kirchheiner J, Brøsen K, Dahl ML, et al. (2001). CYP2D6 and CYP2C19 genotype-based dose recommendations for antidepressants: a first step towards subpopulation-specific dosages. *Acta Psychiatr Scand*, 104(3), 173–192.

Kirchheiner J, Klein C, Meineke I, et al. (2003). Bupropion and 4-OH-bupropion pharmacokinetics in relation to genetic polymorphisms in CYP2B6. *Pharmacogenetics*, 13(10), 619–626. doi:10.1097/01.fpc.0000054125.14659.d0.

Kirchheiner J, Nickchen K, Bauer M, et al. (2004). Pharmacogenetics of antidepressants and antipsychotics: the contribution of allelic variations to the phenotype of drug response. *Mol Psychiatry*, 9(5), 442–473. doi:10.1038/sj.mp.4001494.

Kirschbaum KM, Müller MJ, Malevani J, et al. (2008). Serum levels of aripiprazole and dehydroaripiprazole, clinical response and side effects. *World J Biol Psychiatry*, 9(3), 212–218. doi:10.1080/15622970701361255.

Klaassen CD, Slitt AL (2005). Regulation of hepatic transporters by xenobiotic receptors. *Curr Drug Metab*, 6(4), 309–328.

Klees TM, Sheffels P, Dale O, Kharasch ED (2005). Metabolism of alfentanil by cytochrome P4503A (CYP3A) enzymes. *Drug Metab Dispos*, 33(3), 303–311. doi:10.1124/dmd.104.002709.

Klein K, Lang T, Saussele T, et al. (2005). Genetic variability of CYP2B6 in populations of African and Asian origin: allele frequencies, novel functional variants, and possible implications for anti-HIV therapy with efavirenz. *Pharmacogenet Genomics*, 15(12), 861–873.

Klotz U (2006). Clinical impact of CYP2C19 polymorphism on the action of proton pump inhibitors: a review of a special problem. *Int J Clin Pharmacol Ther*, 44(7), 297–302.

Klotz U (2009). Pharmacokinetics and drug metabolism in the elderly. *Drug Metab Rev*, 41(2), 67–76.

Knutti R, Rothweiler H, Schlatter C (1981). Effect of pregnancy on the pharmacokinetics of caffeine. *Eur J Clin Pharmacol*, 21(2), 121–126.

Kobayashi K, Chiba K, Yagi T, et al. (1997). Identification of cytochrome P450 isoforms involved in citalopram N-demethylation by human liver microsomes. *J Pharmacol Exp Ther*, 280(2), 927–933.

Kolars JC, Lown KS, Schmiedlin-Ren P, et al. (1994). CYP3A gene expression in human gut epithelium. *Pharmacogenetics*, 4(5), 247–259.

Komatsu T, Yamazaki H, Shimada N, Nakajima M, Yokoi, T. (2000). Roles of cytochromes P450 1A2, 2A6, and 2C8 in 5-fluorouracil formation from tegafur, an anticancer prodrug, in human liver microsomes. *Drug Metab Dispos*, 28(12), 1457–1463.

Koola MM, Tsapakis EM, Wright P, et al. (2014). Association of tardive dyskinesia with variation in CYP2D6: is there a role for active metabolites? *J Psychopharmacol*, 28(7), 665–670. doi:10.1177/0269881114523861.

Korade Z, Xu L, Shelton R, Porter NA (2010). Biological activities of 7-dehydrocholesterol-derived oxysterols: implications for Smith-Lemli-Opitz syndrome. *J Lipid Res*, 51(11), 3259–3269.

Korade Z, Kim HY, Tallman KA, et al. (2016). The effect of small molecules on sterol homeostasis: measuring 7-dehydrocholesterol in Dhcr7-deficient Neuro2a cells and human fibroblasts. *J Med Chem*, 59(3), 1102–1115. doi:10.1021/acs.jmedchem.5b01696.

Korzekwa KR, Krishnamachary N, Shou M, et al. (1998). Evaluation of atypical cytochrome P450 kinetics with two-substrate models: evidence that multiple substrates can simultaneously bind to cytochrome P450 active sites. *Biochemistry*, 37(12), 4137–4147. doi:10.1021/bi9715627.

Koskinen J, Lohonen J, Koponen H, Isohanni M, Miettunen J (2010). Rate of cannabis use disorders in clinical samples of patients with schizophrenia: a meta-analysis. *Schizophr Bull*, 36(6), 1115–1130. doi:10.1093/schbul/sbp031.

Koukouritaki SB, Manro JR, Marsh SA, et al. (2004). Developmental expression of human hepatic CYP2C9 and CYP2C19. *J Pharmacol Exp Ther*, 308(3), 965–974. doi:10.1124/jpet.103.060137.

Koyama E, Tanaka T, Chiba K, et al. (1996). Steady-state plasma concentrations of imipramine and desipramine in relation to S-mephenytoin 4'-hydroxylation status in Japanese depressive patients. *J Clin Psychopharmacol*, 16(4), 286–293.

Koyama E, Chiba K, Tani M, Ishizaki T (1997). Reappraisal of human CYP isoforms involved in imipramine N-demethylation and 2-hydroxylation: a study using microsomes obtained from putative extensive and poor metabolizers of S-mephenytoin and eleven recombinant human CYPs. *J Pharmacol Exp Ther*, 281(3), 1199–1210.

Krueger SK, Williams DE (2005). Mammalian flavin-containing monooxygenases: structure/function, genetic polymorphisms and role in drug metabolism. *Pharmacol Ther*, 106(3), 357–387. doi:10.1016/j.pharmthera.2005.01.001.

Krueger SK, Williams DE, Yueh MF, et al. (2002). Genetic polymorphisms of flavin-containing monooxygenase (FMO). *Drug Metab Rev*, 34(3), 523–532. doi:10.1081/DMR-120005653.

Kubo M, Koue T, Inaba A, et al. (2005). Influence of itraconazole co-administration and CYP2D6 genotype on the pharmacokinetics of the new antipsychotic ARIPIPRAZOLE. *Drug Metab Pharmacokinet*, 20(1), 55–64.

Kubo M, Koue T, Maune H, Fukuda T, Azuma, J (2007). Pharmacokinetics of aripiprazole, a new antipsychotic, following oral dosing in healthy adult Japanese volunteers: influence of CYP2D6 polymorphism. *Drug Metab Pharmacokinet*, 22(5), 358–366.

Kuehl P, Zhang J, Lin Y, et al. (2001). Sequence diversity in CYP3A promoters and characterization of the genetic basis of polymorphic CYP3A5 expression. *Nat Genet*, 27(4), 383–391. doi:10.1038/86882.

Kuhn R (1958). The treatment of depressive states with G 22355 (imipramine hydrochloride). *Am J Psychiatry*, 115(5), 459–464. doi:10.1176/ajp.115.5.459.

Kumana CR, Lauder IJ, Chan M, Ko W, Lin HJ (1987). Differences in diazepam pharmacokinetics in Chinese and white Caucasians – relation to body lipid stores. *Eur J Clin Pharmacol*, 32(2), 211–215.

Kuzman MR, Medved V, Bozina N, et al. (2011). Association study of MDR1 and 5-HT2C genetic polymorphisms and antipsychotic-induced metabolic disturbances in female patients with schizophrenia. *Pharmacogenomics J*, 11(1), 35–44. doi:10.1038/tpj.2010.7.

Laika B, Leucht S, Heres S, Schneider H, Steimer W (2010). Pharmacogenetics and olanzapine treatment: CYP1A2*1F and serotonergic polymorphisms influence therapeutic outcome. *Pharmacogenomics J*, 10(1), 20–29. doi:10.1038/tpj.2009.32.

Laird B, Colvin L, Fallon M (2008). Management of cancer pain: basic principles and neuropathic cancer pain. *Eur J Cancer*, 44(8), 1078–1082. doi:10.1016/j.ejca.2008.03.022.

Lam YW, Gaedigk A, Ereshefsky L, Alfaro CL, Simpson J (2002). CYP2D6 inhibition by selective serotonin reuptake inhibitors: analysis of achievable steady-state plasma concentrations and the effect of ultrarapid metabolism at CYP2D6. *Pharmacotherapy*, 22(8), 1001–1006.

Lamba J, Schuetz E (2008). Genetic variants of xenobiotic receptors and their implications in drug metabolism and pharmacogenetics. In W Xie, ed., *Nuclear Receptors in Drug Metabolism*. Hoboken: John Wiley & Sons, pp. 241–273.

Lamba JK, Lin YS, Schuetz EG, Thummel KE (2002). Genetic contribution to variable human CYP3A-mediated metabolism. *Adv Drug Deliv Rev*, 54(10), 1271–1294.

Lamba J, Lamba V, Schuetz E (2005). Genetic variants of PXR (NR1I2) and CAR (NR1I3) and their implications in drug metabolism and pharmacogenetics. *Curr Drug Metab*, 6(4), 369–383.

Lamba V, Lamba J, Yasuda K, et al. (2003). Hepatic CYP2B6 expression: gender and ethnic differences and relationship to CYP2B6 genotype and CAR (constitutive androstane receptor) expression. *J Pharmacol Exp Ther*, 307(3), 906–922. doi:10.1124/jpet.103.054866.

Lampe JW, King IB, Li S, et al. (2000). Brassica vegetables increase and apiaceous vegetables decrease cytochrome P450 1A2 activity in humans: changes in caffeine metabolite ratios in response to controlled vegetable diets. *Carcinogenesis*, 21(6), 1157–1162.

Lang T, Klein K, Fischer J, et al. (2001). Extensive genetic polymorphism in the human CYP2B6 gene with impact on expression and function in human liver. *Pharmacogenetics*, 11(5), 399–415.

Lang T, Klein K, Richter T, et al. (2004). Multiple novel nonsynonymous CYP2B6 gene polymorphisms in Caucasians: demonstration of phenotypic null alleles. *J Pharmacol Exp Ther*, 311(1), 34–43. doi:10.1124/jpet.104.068973.

Le Marchand L, Franke AA, Custer L, Wilkens LR, Cooney RV (1997). Lifestyle and nutritional correlates of cytochrome CYP1A2 activity: inverse associations with plasma lutein and alpha-tocopherol. *Pharmacogenetics*, 7(1), 11–19.

Leclerc J, Courcot-Ngoubo Ngangue E, Cauffiez C, et al. (2011). Xenobiotic metabolism and disposition in human lung: transcript profiling in non-tumoral and tumoral tissues. *Biochimie*, 93(6), 1012–1027. doi:10.1016/j.biochi.2011.02.012.

Lee CR, Goldstein JA, Pieper JA (2002). Cytochrome P450 2C9 polymorphisms: a comprehensive review of the in-vitro and human data. *Pharmacogenetics*, 12(3), 251–263.

Li F, Zhang A, Shi Y, Ma Y, Du Y (2015). 1alpha,25-Dihydroxyvitamin D3 prevents the differentiation of human lung fibroblasts via microRNA-27b targeting the vitamin D receptor. *Int J Mol Med*, 36(4), 967–974. doi:10.3892/ijmm.2015.2318.

Linnet K, Wiborg O (1996). Steady-state serum concentrations of the neuroleptic perphenazine in relation to CYP2D6 genetic polymorphism. *Clin Pharmacol Ther*, 60(1), 41–47. doi:10.1016/S0009-9236(96)90165-4.

Liston HL, DeVane CL, Boulton DW, et al. (2002). Differential time course of cytochrome P450 2D6 enzyme inhibition by fluoxetine, sertraline, and paroxetine in healthy volunteers. *J Clin Psychopharmacol*, 22(2), 169–173.

Liu HQ, Zhang CP, Zhang CZ, Liu XC, Liu ZJ (2015). Influence of two common polymorphisms in the EPHX1 gene on warfarin maintenance dosage: a meta-analysis. *Biomed Res Int*, 2015, 564149. doi:10.1155/2015/564149.

Lobo ED, Bergstrom RF, Reddy S, et al. (2008). In vitro and in vivo evaluations of cytochrome P450 1A2 interactions with duloxetine. *Clin Pharmacokinet*, 47(3), 191–202. doi:10.2165/00003088-200847030-00005.

Lodhi RJ, Wang Y, Rossolatos D, et al. (2017). Investigation of the COMT Val158Met variant association with age of onset of psychosis, adjusting for cannabis use. *Brain Behav*, 7(11), e00850. doi:10.1002/brb3.850.

Lomri N, Yang Z, Cashman JR (1993). Expression in *Escherichia coli* of the flavin-containing monooxygenase D (form II) from adult human liver: determination of a distinct tertiary amine substrate specificity. *Chem Res Toxicol*, 6(4), 425–429.

Löscher W, Klotz U, Zimprich F, Schmidt D (2009). The clinical impact of pharmacogenetics on the treatment of epilepsy. *Epilepsia*, 50(1), 1–23. doi:10.1111/j.1528-1167.2008.01716.x.

Lubomirov R, Colombo S, di Iulio J, et al.; Swiss, HIV Consortium Study (2011). Association of pharmacogenetic markers with premature discontinuation of first-line anti-HIV therapy: an observational cohort study. *J Infect Dis*, 203(2), 246–257. doi:10.1093/infdis/jiq043.

Mackay RJ, McEntyre CJ, Henderson C, Lever M, George PM (2011). Trimethylaminuria: causes and diagnosis of a socially distressing condition. *Clin Biochem Rev*, 32(1), 33–43.

Madsen H, Hansen TS, Brøsen K (1996). Imipramine metabolism in relation to the sparteine oxidation polymorphism – a family study. *Pharmacogenetics*, 6(6), 513–519.

Mahgoub A, Idle JR, Dring LG, Lancaster R, Smith RL (1977). Polymorphic hydroxylation of debrisoquine in man. *Lancet*, 2(8038), 584–586.

Mailman RB, Murthy V (2010). Third generation antipsychotic drugs: partial agonism or receptor functional selectivity? *Curr Pharm Des*, 16(5), 488–501.

Majewska MD, Mienville JM, Vicini S (1988). Neurosteroid pregnenolone sulfate antagonizes electrophysiological responses to GABA in neurons. *Neurosci Lett*, 90(3), 279–284.

Mallikaarjun S, Kane JM, Bricmont P, et al. (2013). Pharmacokinetics, tolerability and safety of aripiprazole once-monthly in adult schizophrenia: an open-label, parallel-arm, multiple-dose study. *Schizophr Res*, 150(1), 281–288. doi:10.1016/j.schres.2013.06.041.

Mamiya K, Ieiri I, Miyahara S, et al. (1998a). Association of polymorphisms in the cytochrome P450 (CYP) 2C19 and 2C18 genes in Japanese epileptic patients. *Pharmacogenetics*, 8(1), 87–90.

Mamiya K, Ieiri I, Shimamoto J, et al. (1998b). The effects of genetic polymorphisms of CYP2C9 and CYP2C19 on phenytoin metabolism in Japanese adult patients with epilepsy: studies in stereoselective hydroxylation and population pharmacokinetics. *Epilepsia*, 39(12), 1317–1323.

Mammen G, Rueda S, Roerecke M, et al. (2018). Association of cannabis with long-term clinical symptoms in anxiety and mood disorders: a systematic review of prospective studies. *J Clin Psychiatry*, 79(4), pii: 17r11839. doi:10.4088/JCP.17r11839.

Manrique-Garcia E, de Leon AP, Dalman C, Andreasson S, Allebeck P (2016). Cannabis, psychosis, and mortality: a cohort study of 50,373 Swedish men. *Am J Psychiatry*, 173(8), 790–798. doi:10.1176/appi.ajp.2016.14050637.

Masimirembwa C, Persson I, Bertilsson L, Hasler J, Ingelman-Sundberg M (1996). A novel mutant variant of the CYP2D6 gene (CYP2D6*17) common in a black African population: association with diminished debrisoquine hydroxylase activity. *Br J Clin Pharmacol*, 42(6), 713–719.

Massoulié J, Pezzementi L, Bon S, Krejci E, Vallette FM (1993). Molecular and cellular biology of cholinesterases. *Prog Neurobiol*, 41(1), 31–91.

McConnell HW, Mitchell SC, Smith RL, Brewster M (1997). Trimethylaminuria associated with seizures and behavioural disturbance: a case report. *Seizure*, 6(4), 317–321.

McManus ME, Burgess WM, Veronese ME, et al. (1990). Metabolism of 2-acetylaminofluorene and benzo(a)pyrene and activation of food-derived heterocyclic amine mutagens by human cytochromes P-450. *Cancer Res*, 50(11), 3367–3376.

Michaels S, Wang MZ (2014). The revised human liver cytochrome P450 'Pie': absolute protein quantification of CYP4F and CYP3A enzymes using targeted quantitative proteomics. *Drug Metab Dispos*, 42(8), 1241–1251. doi:10.1124/dmd.114.058040.

Mittal B, Tulsyan S, Kumar S, Mittal RD, Agarwal G (2015). Cytochrome P450 in cancer susceptibility and treatment. *Adv Clin Chem*, 71, 77–139.

Morita S, Shimoda K, Someya T, et al. (2000). Steady-state plasma levels of nortriptyline and its hydroxylated metabolites in Japanese patients: impact of CYP2D6 genotype on the hydroxylation of nortriptyline. *J Clin Psychopharmacol*, 20(2), 141–149.

Motika MS, Zhang J, Cashman JR (2007). Flavin-containing monooxygenase 3 and human disease. *Expert Opin Drug Metab Toxicol*, 3(6), 831–845. doi:10.1517/17425255.3.6.831.

Murai K, Yamazaki H, Nakagawa K, Kawai R, Kamataki T (2009). Deactivation of anti-cancer drug letrozole to a carbinol metabolite by polymorphic cytochrome P450 2A6 in human liver microsomes. *Xenobiotica*, 39(11), 795–802. doi:10.3109/00498250903171395.

Murray GI, Melvin WT, Greenlee WF, Burke MD (2001). Regulation, function, and tissue-specific expression of cytochrome P450 CYP1B1. *Annu Rev Pharmacol Toxicol*, 41, 297–316. doi:10.1146/annurev.pharmtox.41.1.297.

Murru A, Popovic D, Pacchiarotti I, et al. (2015). Management of adverse effects of mood stabilizers. *Curr Psychiatry Rep*, 17(8), 603. doi:10.1007/s11920-015-0603-z.

Mushiroda T, Takahashi Y, Onuma T, et al. (2018). Association of HLA-A*31:01 screening with the incidence of carbamazepine-induced cutaneous adverse reactions in a Japanese population. *JAMA Neurol*, 75(7), 842–849. doi:10.1001/jamaneurol.2018.0278.

Mwenifumbo JC, Sellers EM, Tyndale RF (2007). Nicotine metabolism and CYP2A6 activity in a population of black African descent: impact of gender and light smoking. *Drug Alcohol Depend*, 89(1), 24–33. doi:10.1016/j.drugalcdep.2006.11.012.

Nagaoka R, Iwasaki T, Rokutanda N, et al. (2006). Tamoxifen activates CYP3A4 and MDR1 genes through steroid and xenobiotic receptor in breast cancer cells. *Endocrine*, 30(3), 261–268. doi:10.1007/s12020-006-0003-6.

Nakajima M, Yokoi T, Mizutani M, et al. (1999). Genetic polymorphism in the 5'-flanking region of human CYP1A2 gene: effect on the CYP1A2 inducibility in humans. *J Biochem*, 125(4), 803–808.

Nakajima M, Fukami T, Yamanaka H, et al. (2006). Comprehensive evaluation of variability in nicotine metabolism and CYP2A6 polymorphic alleles in four ethnic populations. *Clin Pharmacol Ther*, 80(3), 282–297. doi:10.1016/j.clpt.2006.05.012.

Nakajima Y, Saito Y, Shiseki K, et al. (2005). Haplotype structures of EPHX1 and their effects on the metabolism of carbamazepine-10,11-epoxide in Japanese epileptic patients. *Eur J Clin Pharmacol*, 61(1), 25–34. doi:10.1007/s00228-004-0878-1.

Naraharisetti SB, Lin YS, Rieder MJ, et al. (2010). Human liver expression of CYP2C8: gender, age, and genotype effects. *Drug Metab Dispos*, 38(6), 889–893. doi:10.1124/dmd.109.031542.

Nebert DW, Russell DW (2002). Clinical importance of the cytochromes P450. *Lancet*, 360(9340), 1155–1162. doi:10.1016/S0140-6736(02)11203-7.

Nelson DR, Zeldin DC, Hoffman SM, et al. (2004). Comparison of cytochrome P450 (CYP) genes from the mouse and human genomes, including nomenclature recommendations for genes, pseudogenes and alternative-splice variants. *Pharmacogenetics*, 14(1), 1–18.

Niwa T, Shizuku M, Yamano K (2017). Effect of genetic polymorphism on the inhibition of dopamine formation from p-tyramine catalyzed by brain cytochrome P450 2D6. *Arch Biochem Biophys*, 620, 23–27. doi:10.1016/j.abb.2017.03.009.

Niwa T, Yanai M, Matsumoto M, Shizuku M (2018). Effect of cytochrome P450 (CYP) 2D6 genetic polymorphism on the inhibitory action of antidepressants on CYP2D6-mediated dopamine formation from p-tyramine. *J Pharm Pharm Sci*, 21(1), 135–142. doi:10.18433/jpps29673.

Niznik HB, Tyndale RF, Sallee FR, et al. (1990). The dopamine transporter and cytochrome P45OIID1 (debrisoquine 4-hydroxylase) in brain: resolution and identification of two distinct [3H]GBR-12935 binding proteins. *Arch Biochem Biophys*, 276(2), 424–432.

Nordin C, Siwers B, Benitez J, Bertilsson L (1985). Plasma concentrations of nortriptyline and its 10-hydroxy metabolite in depressed patients – relationship to the debrisoquine hydroxylation metabolic ratio. *Br J Clin Pharmacol*, 19(6), 832–835.

O'Brien FE, Dinan TG, Griffin BT, Cryan JF (2012). Interactions between antidepressants and P-glycoprotein at the blood-brain barrier: clinical significance of in vitro and in vivo findings. *Br J Pharmacol*, 165(2), 289–312. doi:10.1111/j.1476-5381.2011.01557.x.

Oesch F, Raphael D, Schwind H, Glatt HR (1977). Species differences in activating and inactivating enzymes related to the control of mutagenic metabolites. *Arch Toxicol*, 39(1–2), 97–108.

Ohmori O, Suzuki T, Kojima H, et al. (1998). Tardive dyskinesia and debrisoquine 4-hydroxylase (CYP2D6) genotype in Japanese schizophrenics. *Schizophr Res*, 32(2), 107–113.

Ohtsuki S, Schaefer O, Kawakami H, et al. (2012). Simultaneous absolute protein quantification of transporters, cytochromes P450, and UDP-glucuronosyltransferases as a novel approach for the characterization of individual human liver: comparison with mRNA levels and activities. *Drug Metab Dispos*, 40(1), 83–92. doi:10.1124/dmd.111.042259.

Okubo M, Murayama N, Shimizu M, et al. (2013). CYP3A4 intron 6 C>T polymorphism (CYP3A4*22) is associated with reduced CYP3A4 protein level and function in human liver microsomes. *J Toxicol Sci*, 38(3), 349–354.

Olesen OV, Linnet K (2000). Identification of the human cytochrome P450 isoforms mediating in vitro N-dealkylation of perphenazine. *Br J Clin Pharmacol*, 50(6), 563–571.

Oscarson M, Hidestrand M, Johansson I, Ingelman-Sundberg M (1997). A combination of mutations in the CYP2D6*17 (CYP2D6Z) allele causes alterations in enzyme function. *Mol Pharmacol*, 52(6), 1034–1040.

Oscarson M, Gullsten H, Rautio A, et al. (1998). Genotyping of human cytochrome P450 2A6 (CYP2A6), a nicotine C-oxidase. *FEBS Lett*, 438(3), 201–205.

Ouzzine M, Magdalou J, Burchell B, Fournel-Gigleux S (1999). An internal signal sequence mediates the targeting and retention of the human UDP-glucuronosyltransferase 1A6 to the endoplasmic reticulum. *J Biol Chem*, 274(44), 31401–31409.

Ouzzine M, Gulberti S, Ramalanjaona N, Magdalou J, Fournel-Gigleux S (2014). The UDP-glucuronosyltransferases of the blood-brain barrier: their role in drug metabolism and detoxication. *Front Cell Neurosci*, 8, 349. doi:10.3389/fncel.2014.00349.

Owens MJ (1996). Molecular and cellular mechanisms of antidepressant drugs. *Depress Anxiety*, 4(4), 153–159. doi:10.1002/(SICI)1520-6394(1996)4:4<53::aid-da1>3.0.CO;2-G.

Owens MJ, Morgan WN, Plott SJ, Nemeroff CB (1997). Neurotransmitter receptor and transporter binding profile of antidepressants and their metabolites. *J Pharmacol Exp Ther*, 283(3), 1305–1322.

Owens MJ, Knight DL, Nemeroff CB (2001). Second-generation SSRIs: human monoamine transporter binding profile of escitalopram and R-fluoxetine. *Biol Psychiatry*, 50(5), 345–350.

Ozdemir V, Naranjo CA, Herrmann N, et al. (1997). Paroxetine potentiates the central nervous system side effects of perphenazine: contribution of cytochrome P4502D6 inhibition in vivo. *Clin Pharmacol Ther*, 62(3), 334–347. doi:10.1016/S0009-9236(97)90037-0.

Ozdemir V, Bertilsson L, Miura J, et al. (2007). CYP2D6 genotype in relation to perphenazine concentration and pituitary pharmacodynamic tissue sensitivity in Asians: CYP2D6-serotonin-dopamine crosstalk revisited. *Pharmacogenet Genomics*, 17(5), 339–347. doi:10.1097/FPC.0b013e32801a3c10.

Pacifici GM, Bencini C, Rane A (1986). Acetyltransferase in humans: development and tissue distribution. *Pharmacology*, 32(5), 283–291. doi:10.1159/000138181.

Palleria C, Di Paolo A, Giofrè C, et al. (2013). Pharmacokinetic drug-drug interaction and their implication in clinical management. *J Res Med Sci*, 18(7), 601–610.

Pan YZ, Gao W, Yu AM (2009). MicroRNAs regulate CYP3A4 expression via direct and indirect targeting. *Drug Metab Dispos*, 37(10), 2112–2117. doi:10.1124/dmd.109.027680.

Pariente-Khayat A, Pons G, Rey E, et al. (1991). Caffeine acetylator phenotyping during maturation in infants. *Pediatr Res*, 29(5), 492–495. doi:10.1203/00006450-199105010-00015.

Parker AC, Pritchard P, Preston T, Choonara I (1998). Induction of CYP1A2 activity by carbamazepine in children using the caffeine breath test. *Br J Clin Pharmacol*, 45(2), 176–178.

Pelkonen O, Rautio A, Raunio H, Pasanen M (2000). CYP2A6: a human coumarin 7-hydroxylase. *Toxicology*, 144(1), 139–147.

Pelkonen O, Turpeinen M, Hakkola J, et al. (2008). Inhibition and induction of human cytochrome P450 enzymes: current status. *Arch Toxicol*, 82(10), 667–715. doi:10.1007/s00204-008-0332-8.

Perry PJ, Pfohl BM, Holstad SG (1987). The relationship between antidepressant response and tricyclic antidepressant plasma concentrations. A retrospective analysis of the literature using logistic regression analysis. *Clin Pharmacokinet*, 13(6), 381–392. doi:10.2165/00003088-198713060-00003.

Persson I, Aklillu E, Rodrigues F, Bertilsson L, Ingelman-Sundberg M (1996). S-mephenytoin hydroxylation phenotype and CYP2C19 genotype among Ethiopians. *Pharmacogenetics*, 6(6), 521–526.

Phillips EJ, Sukasem C, Whirl-Carrillo M, et al. (2018). Clinical Pharmacogenetics Implementation Consortium Guideline for HLA Genotype and Use of Carbamazepine and Oxcarbazepine: 2017 Update. *Clin Pharmacol Ther*, 103(4), 574–581. doi:10.1002/cpt.1004.

Phillips IR, Shephard EA (2017). Drug metabolism by flavin-containing monooxygenases of human and mouse. *Expert Opin Drug Metab Toxicol*, 13(2), 167–181. doi:10.1080/17425255.2017.1239718.

Piatkov I, Caetano D, Assur Y, et al. (2017). ABCB1 and ABCC1 single-nucleotide polymorphisms in patients treated with clozapine. *Pharmgenomics Pers Med*, 10, 235–242. doi:10.2147/PGPM.S142314.

Pinto N, Dolan ME (2011). Clinically relevant genetic variations in drug metabolizing enzymes. *Curr Drug Metab*, 12(5), 487–497.

Pisanu C, Melis C, Squassina A (2016). Lithium pharmacogenetics: where do we stand? *Drug Dev Res*, 77(7), 368–373. doi:10.1002/ddr.21341.

Pollock BG, Mulsant BH, Sweet RA, et al. (1995). Prospective cytochrome P450 phenotyping for neuroleptic treatment in dementia. *Psychopharmacol Bull*, 31(2), 327–331.

Preskorn SH (2003). Reproducibility of the in vivo effect of the selective serotonin reuptake inhibitors on the in vivo function of cytochrome P450 2D6: an update (part I). *J Psychiatr Pract*, 9(2), 150–158.

Preskorn SH (2012). Changes in the product label for pimozide illustrate both the promises and the challenges of personalized medicine. *J Clin Psychiatry*, 73(9), 1191–1193. doi:10.4088/JCP.12com07963.

Preskorn SH (2013). Complexities of personalized medicine: how genes, drug-drug interactions, dosing schedules, and other factors can combine to produce clinically meaningful differences in a drug's effect. *J Psychiatr Pract*, 19(5), 397–405. doi:10.1097/01.pra.0000435038.91049.cb.

Preskorn SH, Jerkovich GS (1990). Central nervous system toxicity of tricyclic antidepressants: phenomenology, course, risk factors, and role of therapeutic drug monitoring. *J Clin Psychopharmacol*, 10(2), 88–95.

Pringsheim T, Marras C (2009). Pimozide for tics in Tourette's syndrome. *Cochrane Database Syst Rev*, (2), CD006996. doi:10.1002/14651858.CD006996.pub2.

Puangpetch A, Vanwong N, Nuntamool N, et al. (2016). CYP2D6 polymorphisms and their influence on risperidone treatment. *Pharmgenomics Pers Med*, 9, 131–147. doi:10.2147/PGPM.S107772.

Puranik YG, Birnbaum AK, Marino SE, et al. (2013). Association of carbamazepine major metabolism and transport pathway gene polymorphisms and pharmacokinetics in patients with epilepsy. *Pharmacogenomics*, 14(1), 35–45. doi:10.2217/pgs.12.180.

Qin XP, Xie HG, Wang W, et al. (1999). Effect of the gene dosage of CgammaP2C19 on diazepam metabolism in Chinese subjects. *Clin Pharmacol Ther*, 66(6), 642–646. doi:10.1016/S0009-9236(99)90075-9.

Raimundo S, Fischer J, Eichelbaum M, et al. (2000). Elucidation of the genetic basis of the common 'intermediate metabolizer' phenotype for drug oxidation by CYP2D6. *Pharmacogenetics*, 10(7), 577–581.

Raimundo S, Toscano C, Klein K, et al. (2004). A novel intronic mutation, 2988G>A, with high predictivity for impaired function of cytochrome P450 2D6 in white subjects. *Clin Pharmacol Ther*, 76(2), 128–138. doi:10.1016/j.clpt.2004.04.009.

Raskin A, Crook TH (1975). Antidepressants in black and white inpatients. Differential response to a controlled trial of chlorpromazine and imipramine. *Arch Gen Psychiatry*, 32(5), 643–649.

Rau T, Diepenbruck S, Diepenbruck I, Eschenhagen T (2006). The 2988G>A polymorphism affects splicing of a CYP2D6 minigene. *Clin Pharmacol Ther*, 80(5), 555–558; author reply 558–560. doi:10.1016/j.clpt.2006.08.008.

Raunio H, Rahnasto-Rilla M (2012). CYP2A6: genetics, structure, regulation, and function. *Drug Metabol Drug Interact*, 27(2), 73–88. doi:10.1515/dmdi-2012-0001.

Reale M, Costantini E, Di Nicola M, et al. (2018). Butyrylcholinesterase and acetylcholinesterase polymorphisms in Multiple sclerosis patients: implication in peripheral inflammation. *Sci Rep*, 8(1), 1319. doi:10.1038/s41598-018-19701-7.

Relling MV, Klein TE (2011). CPIC: Clinical Pharmacogenetics Implementation Consortium of the Pharmacogenomics Research Network. *Clin Pharmacol Ther*, 89(3), 464–467. doi:10.1038/clpt.2010.279.

Relling MV, Gardner EE, Sandborn WJ, et al.; Clinical Pharmacogenetics Implementation, Consortium (2011). Clinical Pharmacogenetics Implementation Consortium guidelines for thiopurine methyltransferase genotype and thiopurine dosing. *Clin Pharmacol Ther*, 89(3), 387–391. doi:10.1038/clpt.2010.320.

Rettie AE, Jones JP (2005). Clinical and toxicological relevance of CYP2C9: drug-drug interactions and pharmacogenetics. *Annu Rev Pharmacol Toxicol*, 45, 477–494. doi:10.1146/annurev.pharmtox.45.120403.095821.

Ribaudo HJ, Haas DW, Tierney C, et al.; Adult AIDS Clinical Trials Group Study (2006). Pharmacogenetics of plasma efavirenz exposure after treatment discontinuation: an Adult AIDS Clinical Trials Group Study. *Clin Infect Dis*, 42(3), 401–407. doi:10.1086/499364.

Riches Z, Stanley EL, Bloomer JC, Coughtrie MW (2009). Quantitative evaluation of the expression and activity of five major sulfotransferases (SULTs) in human tissues: the SULT 'pie'. *Drug Metab Dispos*, 37(11), 2255–2261. doi:10.1124/dmd.109.028399.

Rietveld EC, Broekman MM, Houben JJ, Eskes TK, van Rossum JM (1984). Rapid onset of an increase in caffeine residence time in young women due to oral contraceptive steroids. *Eur J Clin Pharmacol*, 26(3), 371–373.

Riordan JR, Deuchars K, Kartner N, et al. (1985). Amplification of P-glycoprotein genes in multidrug-resistant mammalian cell lines. *Nature*, 316(6031), 817–819.

Rizzo N, Hispard E, Dolbeault S, et al. (1997). Impact of long-term ethanol consumption on CYP1A2 activity. *Clin Pharmacol Ther*, 62(5), 505–509. doi:10.1016/S0009-9236(97)90045-X.

Robbins MG, Andersen G, Somoza V, et al. (2011). Heat treatment of Brussels sprouts retains their ability to induce detoxification enzyme expression in vitro and in vivo. *J Food Sci*, 76(3), C454–C461. doi:10.1111/j.1750-3841.2011.02105.x.

Roberts RL, Mulder RT, Joyce PR, Luty SE, Kennedy MA (2004). No evidence of increased adverse drug reactions in cytochrome P450 CYP2D6 poor metabolizers treated with fluoxetine or nortriptyline. *Hum Psychopharmacol*, 19(1), 17–23. doi:10.1002/hup.539.

Rochat B, Amey M, Gillet M, Meyer UA, Baumann P (1997). Identification of three cytochrome P450 isozymes involved in N-demethylation of citalopram enantiomers in human liver microsomes. *Pharmacogenetics*, 7(1), 1–10.

Rogers HL, Bhattaram A, Zineh I, et al. (2012). CYP2D6 genotype information to guide pimozide treatment in adult and pediatric patients: basis for the U.S. Food and Drug Administration's new dosing recommendations. *J Clin Psychiatry*, 73(9), 1187–1190. doi:10.4088/JCP.11m07572.

Roh HK, Dahl ML, Tybring G, et al. (1996). CYP2C19 genotype and phenotype determined by omeprazole in a Korean population. *Pharmacogenetics*, 6(6), 547–551.

Roninson IB, Chin JE, Choi KG, et al. (1986). Isolation of human mdr DNA sequences amplified in multidrug-resistant KB carcinoma cells. *Proc Natl Acad Sci U S A*, 83(12), 4538–4542.

Rost KL, Brosicke H, Heinemeyer G, Roots I (1994). Specific and dose-dependent enzyme induction by omeprazole in human beings. *Hepatology*, 20(5), 1204–1212.

Rotger M, Tegude H, Colombo S, et al. (2007). Predictive value of known and novel alleles of CYP2B6 for efavirenz plasma concentrations in HIV-infected individuals. *Clin Pharmacol Ther*, 81(4), 557–566. doi:10.1038/sj.clpt.6100072.

Rothman RB, Baumann MH, Dersch CM, et al. (2001). Amphetamine-type central nervous system stimulants release norepinephrine more potently than they release dopamine and serotonin. *Synapse*, 39(1), 32–41. doi:10.1002/1098-2396(20010101)39:1<32::aid-syn5>3.0.CO;2-3.

Rudberg I, Mohebi B, Hermann M, Refsum H, Molden E (2007). Impact of the ultrarapid CYP2C19*17 allele on serum concentration of escitalopram in psychiatric patients. *Clin Pharmacol Ther*, 83(2), 322–327.

Rudorfer MV, Robins E (1982). Amitriptyline overdose: clinical effects on tricyclic antidepressant plasma levels. *J Clin Psychiatry*, 43(11), 457–460.

Saeed LH, Mayet AY (2013). Genotype-phenotype analysis of CYP2C19 in healthy Saudi individuals and its potential clinical implication in drug therapy. *Int J Med Sci*, 10(11), 1497–1502. doi:10.7150/ijms.6795.

Saez-Valero J, Sberna G, McLean CA, Small DH (1999). Molecular isoform distribution and glycosylation of acetylcholinesterase are altered in brain and cerebrospinal fluid of patients with Alzheimer's disease. *J Neurochem*, 72(4), 1600–1608.

Sakuyama K, Sasaki T, Ujiie S, et al. (2008). Functional characterization of 17 CYP2D6 allelic variants (CYP2D6.2, 10, 14A-B, 18, 27, 36, 39, 47–51, 53–55, and 57). *Drug Metab Dispos*, 36(12), 2460–2467. doi:10.1124/dmd.108.023242.

Sanchez C, Hyttel J (1999). Comparison of the effects of antidepressants and their metabolites on reuptake of biogenic amines and on receptor binding. *Cell Mol Neurobiol*, 19(4), 467–489.

Saruwatari J, Ishitsu T, Nakagawa K (2010). Update on the genetic polymorphisms of drug-metabolizing enzymes in antiepileptic drug therapy. *Pharmaceuticals (Basel)*, 3(8), 2709–2732. doi:10.3390/ph3082709.

Schrag ML, Wienkers LC (2001). Covalent alteration of the CYP3A4 active site: evidence for multiple substrate binding domains. *Arch Biochem Biophys*, 391(1), 49–55. doi:10.1006/abbi.2001.2401.

Sezutsu H, Le Goff G, Feyereisen R (2013). Origins of P450 diversity. *Philos Trans R Soc Lond B Biol Sci*, 368(1612), 20120428.

Shimada T, Yamazaki H, Mimura M, Inui Y, Guengerich FP (1994). Interindividual variations in human liver cytochrome P-450 enzymes involved in the oxidation of drugs, carcinogens and toxic chemicals: studies with liver microsomes of 30 Japanese and 30 Caucasians. *J Pharmacol Exp Ther*, 270(1), 414–423.

Shin JG, Park JY, Kim MJ, et al. (2002). Inhibitory effects of tricyclic antidepressants (TCAs) on human cytochrome P450 enzymes in vitro: mechanism of drug interaction between TCAs and phenytoin. *Drug Metab Dispos*, 30(10), 1102–1107.

Siegle I, Fritz P, Eckhardt K, Zanger UM, Eichelbaum M (2001). Cellular localization and regional distribution of CYP2D6 mRNA and protein expression in human brain. *Pharmacogenetics*, 11(3), 237–245.

Sim E, Westwood I, Fullam E (2007). Arylamine N-acetyltransferases. *Expert Opin Drug Metab Toxicol*, 3(2), 169–184. doi:10.1517/17425255.3.2.169.

Sim E, Abuhammad A, Ryan A (2014). Arylamine N-acetyltransferases: from drug metabolism and pharmacogenetics to drug discovery. *Br J Pharmacol*, 171(11), 2705–2725. doi:10.1111/bph.12598.

Sim SC, Risinger C, Dahl ML, et al. (2006). A common novel CYP2C19 gene variant causes ultrarapid drug metabolism relevant for the drug response to proton pump inhibitors and antidepressants. *Clin Pharmacol Ther*, 79(1), 103–113. doi:10.1016/j.clpt.2005.10.002.

Sindrup SH, Gram LF, Brøsen K, Eshoj O, Mogensen EF (1990). The selective serotonin reuptake inhibitor paroxetine is effective in the treatment of diabetic neuropathy symptoms. *Pain*, 42(2), 135–144.

Sindrup SH, Grodum E, Gram LF, Beck-Nielsen H (1991). Concentration-response relationship in paroxetine treatment of diabetic neuropathy symptoms: a patient-blinded dose-escalation study. *Ther Drug Monit*, 13(5), 408–414.

Sindrup SH, Brøsen K, Hansen MG, et al. (1993). Pharmacokinetics of citalopram in relation to the sparteine and the mephenytoin oxidation polymorphisms. *Ther Drug Monit*, 15(1), 11–17.

Singh D, Cho WC, Upadhyay G (2015). Drug-induced liver toxicity and prevention by herbal antioxidants: an overview. *Front Physiol*, 6, 363. doi:10.3389/fphys.2015.00363.

Sjöqvist F, Bertilsson L (1984). Clinical pharmacology of antidepressant drugs: pharmacogenetics. *Adv Biochem Psychopharmacol*, 39, 359–372.

Sjöqvist F, Bertilsson L, Asberg M (1980). Monitoring tricyclic antidepressants. *Ther Drug Monit*, 2(1), 85–93.

Skoda RC, Demierre A, McBride OW, Gonzalez FJ, Meyer UA (1988). Human microsomal xenobiotic epoxide hydrolase. Complementary DNA sequence, complementary DNA-directed expression in COS-1 cells, and chromosomal localization. *J Biol Chem*, 263(3), 1549–1554.

Smith RL (1986). Special Issue – Human Genetic Variations in Oxidative Drug-Metabolism – Introduction. *Xenobiotica*, 16(5), 361–365. doi:10.3109/00498258609050244.

Sobanski T, Bagli M, Laux G, Rao ML (1997). Serotonin syndrome after lithium add-on medication to paroxetine. *Pharmacopsychiatry*, 30(3), 106–107. doi:10.1055/s-2007-979491.

Spina E, Gitto C, Avenoso A, et al. (1997). Relationship between plasma desipramine levels, CYP2D6 phenotype and clinical response to desipramine: a prospective study. *Eur J Clin Pharmacol*, 51(5), 395–398.

Sproule BA, Naranjo CA, Brenmer KE, Hassan PC (1997). Selective serotonin reuptake inhibitors and CNS drug interactions. A critical review of the evidence. *Clin Pharmacokinet*, 33(6), 454–471.

Staudinger JL, Xu C, Cui YJ, Klaassen CD (2010). Nuclear receptor-mediated regulation of carboxylesterase expression and activity. *Expert Opin Drug Metab Toxicol*, 6(3), 261–271. doi:10.1517/17425250903483215.

Steimer W, Zöpf K, von Amelunxen S, et al. (2004). Allele-specific change of concentration and functional gene dose for the prediction of steady-state serum concentrations of amitriptyline and nortriptyline in CYP2C19 and CYP2D6 extensive and intermediate metabolizers. *Clin Chem*, 50(9), 1623–1633. doi:10.1373/clinchem.2003.030825.

Steimer W, Zopf K, von Amelunxen S, et al. (2005). Amitriptyline or not, that is the question: pharmacogenetic testing of CYP2D6 and CYP2C19 identifies patients with low or high risk for side effects in amitriptyline therapy. *Clin Chem*, 51(2), 376–385. doi:10.1373/clinchem.2004.041327.

Stern RS, Divito SJ (2017). Stevens-Johnson syndrome and toxic epidermal necrolysis: associations, outcomes, and pathobiology – thirty years of progress but still much to be done. *J Invest Dermatol*, 137(5), 1004–1008. doi:10.1016/j.jid.2017.01.003.

Sukasem C, Chaichan C, Nakkrut T, et al. (2018). Association between HLA-B alleles and carbamazepine-induced maculopapular exanthema and severe cutaneous reactions in Thai patients. *J Immunol Res*, 2018, 2780272. doi:10.1155/2018/2780272.

Sweet RA, Pollock BG, Mulsant BH, et al. (2000). Pharmacologic profile of perphenazine's metabolites. *J Clin Psychopharmacol*, 20(2), 181–197.

Takagi S, Nakajima M, Mohri T, Yokoi T (2008). Post-transcriptional regulation of human pregnane X receptor by micro-RNA affects the expression of cytochrome P450 3A4. *J Biol Chem*, 283(15), 9674–9680. doi:10.1074/jbc.M709382200.

Takeuchi F, McGinnis R, Bourgeois S, et al. (2009). A genome-wide association study confirms VKORC1, CYP2C9, and CYP4F2 as principal genetic determinants of warfarin dose. *PLoS Genet*, 5(3), e1000433. doi:10.1371/journal.pgen.1000433.

Tang MH, Pinsky EG (2015). Mood and affect disorders. *Pediatr Rev*, 36(2), 52–60; quiz 61. doi:10.1542/pir.36-2-52.

Tanner JA, Prasad B, Claw KG, et al. (2017). Predictors of variation in CYP2A6 mRNA, protein, and enzyme activity in a human liver bank: influence of genetic and nongenetic factors. *J Pharmacol Exp Ther*, 360(1), 129–139. doi:10.1124/jpet.116.237594.

Taskinen J, Ethell BT, Pihlavisto P, et al. (2003). Conjugation of catechols by recombinant human sulfotransferases, UDP-glucuronosyltransferases, and soluble catechol O-methyltransferase: structure-conjugation relationships and predictive models. *Drug Metab Dispos*, 31(9), 1187–1197. doi:10.1124/dmd.31.9.1187.

Teitelbaum AM, Murphy SE, Akk G, et al. (2018). Nicotine dependence is associated with functional variation in FMO3, an enzyme that metabolizes nicotine in the brain. *Pharmacogenomics J*, 18(1), 136–143. doi:10.1038/tpj.2016.92.

Thomas DR, Nelson DR, Johnson AM (1987). Biochemical effects of the antidepressant paroxetine, a specific 5-hydroxytryptamine uptake inhibitor. *Psychopharmacology (Berl)*, 93(2), 193–200.

Tirona RG, Lee W, Leake BF, et al. (2003). The orphan nuclear receptor HNF4alpha determines PXR- and CAR-mediated xenobiotic induction of CYP3A4. *Nat Med*, 9(2), 220–224. doi:10.1038/nm815.

Tolson AH, Wang H (2010). Regulation of drug-metabolizing enzymes by xenobiotic receptors: PXR and CAR. *Adv Drug Deliv Rev*, 62(13), 1238–1249. doi:10.1016/j.addr.2010.08.006.

Toscano C, Klein K, Blievernicht J, et al. (2006). Impaired expression of CYP2D6 in intermediate metabolizers carrying the *41 allele caused by the intronic SNP 2988G>A: evidence for modulation of splicing events. *Pharmacogenet Genomics*, 16(10), 755–766. doi:10.1097/01.fpc.0000230112.96086.e0.

Tsuchiya K, Gatanaga H, Tachikawa N, et al. (2004). Homozygous CYP2B6 *6 (Q172H and K262R) correlates with high plasma efavirenz concentrations in HIV-1 patients treated with standard efavirenz-containing regimens. *Biochem Biophys Res Commun*, 319(4), 1322–1326. doi:10.1016/j.bbrc.2004.05.116.

Tucker GT, Houston JB, Huang SM (2001). Optimizing drug development: strategies to assess drug metabolism/transporter interaction potential – towards a consensus. *Br J Clin Pharmacol*, 52(1), 107–117.

Tunbridge EM, Harrison PJ, Weinberger DR (2006). Catechol-O-methyltransferase, cognition, and psychosis: Val158Met and beyond. *Biol Psychiatry*, 60(2), 141–151. doi:10.1016/j.biopsych.2005.10.024.

Turpeinen M, Tolonen A, Chesne C, et al. (2009). Functional expression, inhibition and induction of CYP enzymes in HepaRG cells. *Toxicol In Vitro*, 23(4), 748–753. doi:10.1016/j.tiv.2009.03.008.

Ueda K, Clark DP, Chen CJ, et al. (1987). The human multidrug resistance (mdr1) gene. cDNA cloning and transcription initiation. *J Biol Chem*, 262(2), 505–508.

Ufer M, Dilger K, Leschhorn L, et al. (2008). Influence of CYP3A4, CYP3A5, and ABCB1 genotype and expression on budesonide pharmacokinetics: a possible role of intestinal CYP3A4 expression. *Clin Pharmacol Ther*, 84(1), 43–46. doi:10.1038/sj.clpt.6100505.

Uhr M, Tontsch A, Namendorf C, et al. (2008). Polymorphisms in the drug transporter gene ABCB1 predict antidepressant treatment response in depression. *Neuron*, 57(2), 203–209. doi:10.1016/j.neuron.2007.11.017.

US National Library of Medicine (2016). Abilify – aripiprazole tablet. Available at: https://dailymed.nlm.nih.gov/dailymed/drugInfo.cfm?setid=c040bd1d-45b7-49f2-93ea-aed7220b30ac (last accessed 5.12.18).

Václavíková R, Hughes DJ, Souček P (2015). Microsomal epoxide hydrolase 1 (EPHX1): gene, structure, function, and role in human disease. *Gene*, 571(1), 1–8. doi:10.1016/j.gene.2015.07.071.

Vaishnavi SN, Nemeroff CB, Plott SJ, et al. (2004). Milnacipran: a comparative analysis of human monoamine uptake and transporter binding affinity. *Biol Psychiatry*, 55(3), 320–322.

van der Weide J, Steijns LSW (1999). Cytochrome P450 enzyme system: genetic polymorphisms and impact on clinical pharmacology. *Ann Clin Biochem*, 36(6), 722–729.

van der Weide K, van der Weide J (2015). The influence of the CYP3A4*22 polymorphism and CYP2D6 polymorphisms on serum concentrations of aripiprazole, haloperidol, pimozide, and risperidone in psychiatric patients. *J Clin Psychopharmacol*, 35(3), 228–236. doi:10.1097/JCP.0000000000000319.

van Kempen GMJ (1971). Urinary excretion of perphenazine and its sulfoxide during administration in oral and long-acting injectable form. *Psychopharmacology (Berl)*, 21(3), 283–286.

Veeramah KR, Thomas MG, Weale ME, et al. (2008). The potentially deleterious functional variant flavin-containing monooxygenase 2*1 is at high frequency throughout sub-Saharan Africa. *Pharmacogenet Genomics*, 18(10), 877–886. doi:10.1097/FPC.0b013e3283097311.

Vistisen K, Poulsen HE, Loft S (1992). Foreign compound metabolism capacity in man measured from metabolites of dietary caffeine. *Carcinogenesis*, 13(9), 1561–1568.

von Moltke LL, Greenblatt DJ, Giancarlo GM, et al. (2001). Escitalopram (S-citalopram) and its metabolites in vitro: cytochromes mediating biotransformation, inhibitory effects, and comparison to R-citalopram. *Drug Metab Dispos*, 29(8), 1102–1109.

von Richter O, Burk O, Fromm MF, et al. (2004). Cytochrome P450 3A4 and P-glycoprotein expression in human small intestinal enterocytes and hepatocytes: a comparative analysis in paired tissue specimens. *Clin Pharmacol Ther*, 75(3), 172–183. doi:10.1016/j.clpt.2003.10.008.

Wacher VJ, Salphati L, Benet LZ (2001). Active secretion and enterocytic drug metabolism barriers to drug absorption. *Adv Drug Deliv Rev*, 46(1–3), 89–102.

Wang D, Poi MJ, Sun X, et al. (2014). Common CYP2D6 polymorphisms affecting alternative splicing and transcription: long-range haplotypes with two regulatory variants modulate CYP2D6 activity. *Hum Mol Genet*, 23(1), 268–278. doi:10.1093/hmg/ddt417.

Wang D, Papp AC, Sun X (2015). Functional characterization of CYP2D6 enhancer polymorphisms. *Hum Mol Genet*, 24(6), 1556–1562. doi:10.1093/hmg/ddu566.

Wang H, Tompkins LM (2008). CYP2B6: new insights into a historically overlooked cytochrome P450 isozyme. *Curr Drug Metab*, 9(7), 598–610.

Ward BA, Gorski JC, Jones DR, et al. (2003). The cytochrome P450 2B6 (CYP2B6) is the main catalyst of efavirenz primary and secondary metabolism: implication for HIV/AIDS therapy and utility of efavirenz as a substrate marker of CYP2B6 catalytic activity. *J Pharmacol Exp Ther*, 306(1), 287–300. doi:10.1124/jpet.103.049601.

Watson CP (2000). The treatment of neuropathic pain: antidepressants and opioids. *Clin J Pain*, 16(2 Suppl), S49–S55.

Weinshilboum RM, Otterness DM, Szumlanski CL (1999). Methylation pharmacogenetics: catechol O-methyltransferase, thiopurine methyltransferase, and histamine N-methyltransferase. *Annu Rev Pharmacol Toxicol*, 39, 19–52. doi:10.1146/annurev.pharmtox.39.1.19.

Werk AN, Lefeldt S, Bruckmueller H, et al. (2014). Identification and characterization of a defective CYP3A4 genotype in a kidney transplant patient with severely diminished tacrolimus clearance. *Clin Pharmacol Ther*, 95(4), 416–422. doi:10.1038/clpt.2013.210.

Whetstine JR, Yueh MF, McCarver DG, et al. (2000). Ethnic differences in human flavin-containing monooxygenase 2 (FMO2) polymorphisms: detection of expressed protein in African-Americans. *Toxicol Appl Pharmacol*, 168(3), 216–224. doi:10.1006/taap.2000.9050.

Windmill KF, Gaedigk A, Hall PM, et al. (2000). Localization of N-acetyltransferases NAT1 and NAT2 in human tissues. *Toxicol Sci*, 54(1), 19–29.

Wong DT, Horng JS, Bymaster FP, Hauser KL, Molloy BB (1974). A selective inhibitor of serotonin uptake: Lilly 110140, 3-(p-trifluoromethylphenoxy)-N-methyl-3-phenylpropylamine. *Life Sci*, 15(3), 471–479.

Wong DT, Bymaster FP, Horng JS, Molloy, BB (1975). A new selective inhibitor for uptake of serotonin into synaptosomes of rat brain: 3-(p-trifluoromethylphenoxy). N-methyl-3-

phenylpropylamine. *J Pharmacol Exp Ther*, 193(3), 804–811.

Woosley RL, Chen Y, Freiman JP, Gillis RA (1993). Mechanism of the cardiotoxic actions of terfenadine. *JAMA*, 269(12), 1532–1536.

Wu B, Kulkarni K, Basu S, Zhang S, Hu M (2011). First-pass metabolism via UDP-glucuronosyltransferase: a barrier to oral bioavailability of phenolics. *J Pharm Sci*, 100(9), 3655–3681. doi:10.1002/jps.22568.

Wu FS, Gibbs TT, Farb DH (1991). Pregnenolone sulfate: a positive allosteric modulator at the N-methyl-D-aspartate receptor. *Mol Pharmacol*, 40(3), 333–336.

Xie Y, Ke S, Ouyang N, et al. (2009). Epigenetic regulation of transcriptional activity of pregnane X receptor by protein arginine methyltransferase 1. *J Biol Chem*, 284(14), 9199–9205. doi:10.1074/jbc.M806193200.

Xu C, Li CY, Kong AN (2005). Induction of phase I, II and III drug metabolism/transport by xenobiotics. *Arch Pharm Res*, 28(3), 249–268.

Yamazaki H, Inui Y, Yun C-H, Guengerich FP, Shimada T (1992). Cytochrome P450 2E1 and 2A6 enzymes as major catalysts for metabolic activation of N-nitrosodialkylamines and tobacco-related nitrosamines in human liver microsomes. *Carcinogenesis*, 13(10), 1789–1794.

Yasukochi Y, Satta Y (2011). Evolution of the CYP2D gene cluster in humans and four non-human primates. *Genes Genet Syst*, 86(2), 109–116.

Yeung CK, Lang DH, Thummel KE, Rettie AE (2000). Immunoquantitation of FMO1 in human liver, kidney, and intestine. *Drug Metab Dispos*, 28(9), 1107–1111.

Yimer G, Amogne W, Habtewold A, et al. (2012). High plasma efavirenz level and CYP2B6*6 are associated with efavirenz-based HAART-induced liver injury in the treatment of naive HIV patients from Ethiopia: a prospective cohort study. *Pharmacogenomics J*, 12(6), 499–506. doi:10.1038/tpj.2011.34.

Yokota H, Tamura S, Furuya H, et al. (1993). Evidence for a new variant CYP2D6 allele CYP2D6J in a Japanese population associated with lower in vivo rates of sparteine metabolism. *Pharmacogenetics*, 3(5), 256–263.

Yoshinari K, Ueda R, Kusano K, et al. (2008). Omeprazole transactivates human CYP1A1 and CYP1A2 expression through the common regulatory region containing multiple xenobiotic-responsive elements. *Biochem Pharmacol*, 76(1), 139–145. doi:10.1016/j.bcp.2008.04.005.

Yu AM, Idle JR, Herraiz T, Kupfer A, Gonzalez FJ (2003). Screening for endogenous substrates reveals that CYP2D6 is a 5-methoxyindolethylamine O-demethylase. *Pharmacogenetics*, 13(6), 307–319. doi:10.1097/01.fpc.0000054094.48725.b7.

Yue Q-Y, Zhong Z-H, Tybring G, et al. (1998). Pharmacokinetics of nortriptyline and its 10-hydroxy metabolite in Chinese subjects of different CYP2D6 genotypes. *Clin Pharmacol Ther*, 64(4), 384–390.

Zanger UM, Klein K (2013). Pharmacogenetics of cytochrome P450 2B6 (CYP2B6): advances on polymorphisms, mechanisms, and clinical relevance. *Front Genet*, 4, 24.

Zanger UM, Schwab M (2013). Cytochrome P450 enzymes in drug metabolism: regulation of gene expression, enzyme activities, and impact of genetic variation. *Pharmacol Ther*, 138(1), 103–141. doi:10.1016/j.pharmthera.2012.12.007.

Zanger UM, Klein K, Saussele T, et al. (2007). Polymorphic CYP2B6: molecular mechanisms and emerging clinical significance. *Pharmacogenomics*, 8(7), 743–759. doi:10.2217/14622416.8.7.743.

Zhou H, Josephy PD, Kim D, Guengerich FP (2004). Functional characterization of four allelic variants of human cytochrome P450 1A2. *Arch Biochem Biophys*, 422(1), 23–30.

Ziegler VE, Biggs JT (1977). Tricyclic plasma levels. Effect of age, race, sex, and smoking. *JAMA*, 238(20), 2167–2169.

Ziegler VE, Clayton PJ, Biggs JT (1977). A comparison study of amitriptyline and nortriptyline with plasma levels. *Arch Gen Psychiatry*, 34(5), 607–612.

Zukunft J, Lang T, Richter T, et al. (2005). A natural CYP2B6 TATA box polymorphism (-82T-> C) leading to enhanced transcription and relocation of the transcriptional start site. *Mol Pharmacol*, 67(5), 1772–1782. doi:10.1124/mol.104.008086.

Good Clinical Practice in Psychopharmacology

Peter M. Haddad and Thomas R. E. Barnes

6.1 Introduction

This chapter discusses a range of issues related to good clinical practice in psychopharmacology. It has been written to address the wide readership of care professionals who are involved in prescribing, monitoring and/or advising patients about psychiatric medication, which includes psychiatrists, pharmacists, psychiatric nurses, primary care physicians and hospital doctors.

Most people who are treated for a psychiatric disorder are managed in primary care by their primary care physician and never consult a psychiatrist. Those who do come under the care of a psychiatrist are also likely to see other mental healthcare professionals, including psychiatric nurses, clinical psychologists, social workers and occupational therapists. Often, they will have more frequent contact with these professionals than with their psychiatrist or primary care physician and so will tend to raise queries about medication with them. Within secondary care mental health services in the UK, care coordinators often have a formal role in monitoring the effectiveness of psychiatric medication and screening for potential adverse effects. Psychiatric nurses usually administer long-acting injectable (LAI/depot) antipsychotic preparations. Nurse-led clozapine and lithium clinics have been shown to be effective; the monitoring of the patients who attend includes relevant blood tests and assessment of side effects (Clark et al., 2014; Gage et al., 2015; Shaw, 2004). Further, a significant proportion of patients under the care of secondary care physicians are likely to be prescribed psychotropic medication, partly because of the increased prevalence of depressive and anxiety disorders in patients with chronic medical conditions (Wells et al., 1988) and the increased prevalence of diabetes and cardiovascular disease in people with schizophrenia and bipolar disorder (Hoang et al., 2011).

Non-medical prescribing is another reason why psychopharmacology is not just the province and interest of doctors. It was introduced in the UK in 1992, allowing healthcare professionals other than doctors or dentists to prescribe medicines after obtaining a prescribing qualification. In the UK, the largest group of non-medical prescribers are nurses, followed by pharmacists, with a third and much smaller group made up of miscellaneous health professionals (Cope et al., 2016). Currently, nurses can be granted prescribing authority in many other countries, including Australia, Canada, New Zealand, various European countries and several states in the United States.

When medication is used to treat a psychiatric disorder, it is usually only one part of a wider treatment plan, which should be tailored to the individual and devised and agreed by the patient and prescriber working in collaboration. As such, pharmacotherapy is commonly accompanied by appropriate social and psychological treatments, the complexity of which can vary greatly. Such interventions may include simple lifestyle advice such as avoiding stress, reducing excess alcohol consumption and engaging in regular physical activity and exercise. Social treatment may encompass regular voluntary work, a support worker to provide assistance with practical activities, assessment by an occupational therapist regarding adaptations to the home or a social worker to help with the management of complex social issues. Psychological treatment can include interventions such as guided self-help, family therapy, cognitive behavioural treatment (CBT) and mindfulness.

6.2 Ensuring a Favourable Benefit-to-Risk Balance

Every time a prescriber starts a medication or initiates a pharmacological strategy such as a high-dose or augmentation regimen, it should be as an individual patient trial (Barnes et al., 2014; Maxwell, 2009), the outcome of which is uncertain. There should be agreement between the prescriber and the patient on the goals of therapy, such as relief of acute symptoms or long-term prevention, and the rationale for the particular medication prescribed, including its expected risks and likely gains. It should be clear what will be required in terms of the frequency and nature of review appointments and monitoring in order to assess the effects of the treatment over an appropriate timescale. At review, the extent to which the treatment aims have been achieved and the extent to which these are offset by any harms should be assessed. On this evidence, a decision can be made to continue the medication, change the dose, or withdraw it, or possibly introduce some other treatment strategy, such as augmentation with another medication.

A core principle behind the choice of a drug treatment is that its likely benefits, in terms of clinical improvement, should outweigh the risk of adverse effects. Furthermore, this balance should be more favourable than for alternative treatments, whether these be other medications or psychological interventions, or, in the case of a mild disorder, monitoring progress without active treatment. For example, antidepressants are a first-line treatment for moderate and severe major depressive disorder (MDD) in adults but are not recommended for the treatment of short duration, subthreshold depression (i.e. depressive symptoms that do not meet the criteria for DSM-5 major depression) where low-intensity psychosocial and psychological interventions are preferable (Cleare et al., 2015). This is because the diagnostic threshold for DSM-5 major depression is an approximate marker for benefit from antidepressant medication over placebo, with the strongest evidence for antidepressant efficacy being when major depression is of at least moderate severity (Cleare et al., 2015). However, the adverse effects of antidepressants remain the same irrespective of the severity of the depression. Psychological treatments are less likely to cause adverse effects than antidepressants and have been shown to be effective in subthreshold depression (Cuijpers et al., 2007). In summary, the risk–benefit ratio for antidepressant treatment is more favourable for major depression of moderate or greater severity than for short duration, subthreshold depression. The duration of depression, as well as its severity, should be considered when making treatment recommendations. The British Association for Psychopharmacology Guidelines recommend that antidepressant medication should be considered for subthreshold depression that has persisted for more than two to three months and for depression of any severity that has persisted for two years or more (Cleare et al., 2015).

Another example, that illustrates the importance of balancing benefit against risk, is the treatment of a moderate depressive episode in a person with epilepsy. In many cases, CBT will be preferred to an antidepressant because of concerns about an increased risk of seizures with such medication (Hill et al., 2015) and possible pharmacokinetic interactions with anticonvulsant medication, whereas CBT carries no such risks but is equally effective for moderate depression (Cleare et al., 2015). If the depression were to fail to respond to CBT and/or worsen then the risk–benefit ratio might shift to favouring the prescription of an antidepressant. In such a case, a clinician would be likely to recommend starting treatment with a selective serotonin reuptake inhibitor (SSRI) antidepressant rather than a tricyclic antidepressant (TCA), as SSRIs have a lower liability for causing seizures (Maguire et al., 2014).

Assessing the risk–benefit balance of pharmacological treatment involves the prescriber having a good knowledge of the evidence base for different treatments and also being able to judge the risks of not offering treatment. Box 6.1 summarizes relevant factors that should be considered in making safe prescribing decisions. Ensuring that a medication has a favourable risk–benefit balance for an individual patient also dictates that medication should be withdrawn if it proves to be ineffective after an adequate trial in terms of dose, duration and adherence; it is not good practice to continue an ineffective medication. However, in clinical practice, ineffective medication is sometimes continued, and new medication added, thereby contributing to unnecessary and persistent polypharmacy.

6.3 Shared Decision Making and Prescribing

Shared decision making (SDM) has been defined as '*an approach where clinicians and patients share the best available evidence when faced with the task of making decisions, and where patients are supported to consider options, to achieve informed preferences*' (Elwyn et al., 2010). SDM is encouraged and supported in the UK and many other countries, both in mental health and health care in general (National Institute for Health and Care Excellence, NICE, 2011). The justification is partly ethical and partly clinical. SDM respects patient autonomy, a fundamental principle of medical ethics, and this alone warrants its promotion.

While SDM is widely considered to be associated with better clinical outcomes, for example in terms of patient understanding of the disease area, patient satisfaction, symptom reduction and medication adherence, there is only limited evidence to support such positive outcomes. The reality is that SDM is under-researched in both mental

Box 6.1 Factors to consider in making safe prescribing decisions

Patient age

- elderly and children/adolescents are more vulnerable to many side effects
- in these groups use lower doses and slower titrations.

Is the patient pregnant or likely to become pregnant? If yes:

- obtain expert advice
- avoid known teratogens (e.g. lithium, valproate, carbamazepine)
- choose a drug where there is evidence of safety in pregnancy
- consider adverse effects on fetus and newborn other than teratogenesis (e.g. impairment of IQ with valproate)
- consider risk to newborn if breastfeeding while maternal prescribing continues
- consider risks to mother and unborn child if psychiatric illness is not treated pharmacologically.

Are there coexisting medical disorders? In particular consider:*

- cardiovascular disease
- epilepsy
- renal impairment
- hepatic impairment
- respiratory disease
- gastrointestinal disorders
- dementia and cerebrovascular disease.

Is there a potential for drug interactions?*[+]

- with other prescribed medication
- with over-the-counter medication
- with alcohol
- with illicit drugs
- with smoking.

Is the patient at risk of overdose?

- consider prescribing a less toxic drug
- consider dispensing in limited quantities
- consider asking a relative to give out medication (if the patient agrees).

Is there a history of drug allergies or serious drug side effects?

- if so, avoid the drug or similar drugs.

* Co-morbidity and pharmacodynamic interactions with co-prescribed drugs may increase susceptibility to adverse effects and require dose reduction or avoidance of certain drugs. [+] Pharmacokinetic interactions with co-prescribed medication may necessitate either dose reduction or dose decrease.

Reproduced with permission from Haddad PM and Wieck A (2016). Prescribing in clinical practice. Chapter 10 in *Fundamentals of Clinical Psychopharmacology* (editors Ian M Anderson, RH McAllister-Williams), 4th ed. British Association for Psychopharmacology.

health and general medicine. A 2010 Cochrane review of SDM in mental health identified only two randomized controlled trials (RCTs), one conducted in people with schizophrenia and the other in depression (Duncan et al., 2010). SDM was associated with greater patient satisfaction in the depression study but no difference was seen in the schizophrenia study. There was no evidence that SDM was associated with harm and the authors highlighted the need for further research. A subsequent study, conducted among patients in community mental health teams, showed that SDM (in this case, involving the use of an electronic decision aid) was associated with greater patient satisfaction with care planning (Woltmann et al., 2011). A systematic review of RCTs that compared SDM with care as usual in people with mood disorders concluded that SDM was associated with significant improvement in depression outcomes or medication adherence (Samalin et al., 2018).

Where possible, decisions about medication should be made through SDM. The clinician will need to provide the patient with information about their illness and different treatments, answer any questions that the patient may have and address any concerns and misconceptions. Depending on the psychiatric disorder and its severity, the treatment plan may include psychological treatment as an alternative, or adjunct, to drug treatment or the option of no active treatment with a period of 'watchful waiting'. In practice, the resources available to deliver an evidence-based psychological intervention may be insufficient and waiting lists can be long, which may limit this as a viable treatment choice. The prescriber should try to offer choice from a range of alternative medications. While some patients will wish to follow the prescriber's recommendation, others will be keen to take a more active role in deciding which medication to take (Paton & Esop, 2005).

As a general rule, individual antidepressants used in the treatment of MDD show little difference in efficacy (Cleare et al., 2015). Similarly, in the management of acute schizophrenia, antipsychotics show only minor differences in efficacy (Leucht et al., 2013). The only exception is clozapine, which has superior efficacy to other antipsychotics in treatment-resistant schizophrenia and is therefore the treatment of choice for this condition (Siskind et al., 2016). Both antidepressant and antipsychotic medications are heterogeneous in their adverse effect profiles (Cleare et al., 2015; Leucht et al., 2013). For this reason, the relative liability of medications for particular adverse effects and patients' tolerability of side effects are often major determinants of choice of an antidepressant or antipsychotic medication (Zimmerman et al., 2004). However, individuals vary greatly in their susceptibility to and tolerance of side effects and clinical data on the relative risk of particular side effects across the medications being considered may be incomplete (Pope et al., 2010). In some cases, adverse effects may be turned to therapeutic advantage, e.g. when using a sedating antidepressant such as mirtazapine in people whose depression is associated with significant insomnia.

6.4 Acute and Long-Term Drug Treatment

The pharmacological treatment of many psychiatric disorders can be divided into two phases, acute treatment and long-term treatment. However, in clinical practice the distinction between the two phases is often less than clear. Acute treatment refers to the use of medication to treat symptoms of an illness, for example an episode of depression, mania or psychosis. There is no fixed duration for acute treatment and in theory it continues until all acute symptoms have resolved; this is termed remission. If one medication is ineffective in eradicating symptoms it will often be switched to an alternative or combined with a new medication. Despite this, in practice incomplete remission is common and so acute treatment often merges into long-term treatment.

Long-term treatment refers to continuing a drug beyond the point at which acute symptoms have resolved in order to reduce the likelihood of a relapse or recurrence of the underlying psychiatric disorder. The effectiveness of long-term or maintenance treatment in reducing relapse, following successful use of the same drug for acute treatment of an illness, has been demonstrated by meta-analyses of RCTs in various disorders. These include antipsychotic medication in schizophrenia (Leucht et al., 2012), antidepressants in MDD (Geddes et al., 2003) and lithium and several other drugs in bipolar disorder (Miura et al., 2014). Figure 6.1 shows the efficacy of maintenance antipsychotic medication versus placebo in schizophrenia, from the meta-analysis by Leucht et al. (2012). The data are from 65 trials (n = 6493) and show that the number needed to benefit in terms of preventing relapse is 3 and to prevent hospitalization is 5. These data also show that there is a 'cost' for this benefit. Compared with those study participants assigned to placebo, those treated with antipsychotic medication have a higher risk of adverse effects including movement disorder, weight gain and sedation, as well as being more likely to be prescribed an anticholinergic drug (a proxy for extrapyramidal symptoms).

We have highlighted the distinction between acute and long-term treatment as many patients, their relatives and healthcare professionals who are new to psychiatry may question why a person, who is apparently well, continues to be prescribed medication. Many patients find it difficult to accept the need for long-term medication, especially if they have made a full recovery from an acute episode of illness.

The duration of long-term treatment will be influenced by various factors that include the nature of the underlying psychiatric disorder, the number and severity of previous episodes of illness, whether the person has totally recovered from the last episode or has residual symptoms, the presence of adverse drug effects and the potential impact of a recurrence. Individuals with MDD who have responded to antidepressant treatment are generally recommended to continue antidepressant medication for six to nine months after full remission (Cleare et al., 2015). Most schizophrenia treatment guidelines recommend continuing antipsychotic treatment for at least one to two years after the resolution of a first episode of psychosis (Barnes et al., 2011). In both depression and schizophrenia, a longer period of treatment is recommended if there is judged to be a higher risk of relapse, with the duration being tailored to the individual relapse risk.

Decisions on the duration of long-term treatment should be made jointly by the prescriber and the patient. Essentially, the benefits of continuing medication in terms of reducing the risk of relapse need to be weighed against the downsides, which include the inconvenience of taking medication and adverse effects. Given the potentially harmful consequences of relapse, a careful assessment and joint discussion is essential before a decision to withdraw maintenance medication in any disorder is made. As a general rule, medication that has been prescribed long term is best withdrawn gradually and followed by a period of monitoring to facilitate the early detection of relapse. Patients should be aware of the particular signs and symptoms that have characteristically heralded past episodes of relapse and know how to access help urgently if these early signs emerge, their health deteriorates or a crisis develops.

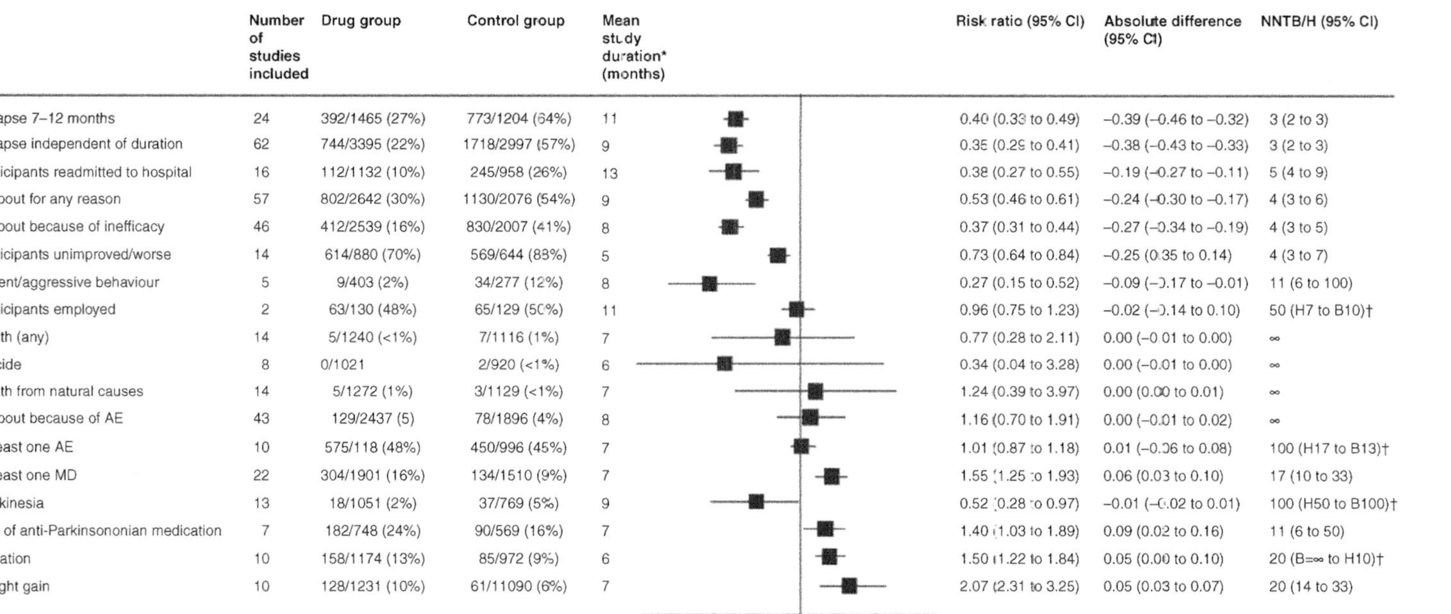

Figure 6.1 Efficacy of maintenance antipsychotic medication versus placebo in schizophrenia (65 trials, n = 6493). Reprinted from Leucht S et al. (2012). Antipsychotic drugs versus placebo for relapse prevention in schizophrenia: a systematic review and meta-analysis. *Lancet*, 379(9831), 2063–2071, Copyright 2012, with permission from Elsevier.

6.5 Off-Label Prescribing

Patients should be treated, whenever possible, with medicines that have an appropriate marketing authorization rather than with off-label or unlicensed medicines. However, off-label medicines and, less commonly, unlicensed medicines may sometimes be necessary to provide the best treatment for patients, although they should only be used if there is a clear clinical justification and relevant evidence of safety and efficacy.

A drug is within licence, or label, when it is prescribed in accordance with the marketing authorization (previously termed a product licence) in the country concerned. The marketing authorization is intended to guarantee the quality, safety and efficacy of the drug and states the clinical indication, dose and route of administration as well as the age group of the patients for whom the drug may be used. It also includes other relevant information, including a list of the known adverse effects. Licensing is the remit of the Medicines and Healthcare products Regulatory Agency (MHRA) in the UK and the Food and Drug Administration (FDA) in the USA. Marketing authorization, or approval, is only granted when a rigorous review of all the relevant data (animal studies and clinical trials) concludes that the benefits of using the drug for a particular indication outweigh the potential risks.

'Off-label' prescribing refers to using a drug outside of the terms of its marketing authorization, in relation to the indication, age group, dosage or duration. It also includes unapproved forms of administration, for example crushing a tablet before it is taken. It follows that using a drug outside the terms of its marketing authorization may involve some uncertainty, in that the licensing authority will either not have examined any data on the benefits and risks of using the drug in that way or, if they have, the evidence provided did not meet the requirement for approval. Prescribers can legally prescribe medicines outside the licensing terms with certain caveats but when they do so they take on a greater professional responsibility and liability. In the UK, general guidance on off-label prescribing is provided by the General Medical Council (General Medical Council, 2013). The term 'near label' prescribing is sometimes encountered in the literature to refer to a drug being used off-label but in a way that is close to the terms of the licence.

Off-label prescribing needs to be distinguished from the use of an unlicensed drug, i.e. a drug that has no licence for use in the country concerned. This includes the use of drugs that have a licence in another country or have no licence in any country. An example of the latter would be a drug that is in development and still undergoing clinical trials.

Prescribing drugs within label does not guarantee their safety or efficacy. The fact that drugs are occasionally withdrawn from the market due to the identification of serious adverse effects after licensing is the clearest demonstration of this. An example in psychiatry is nomifensine which was first marketed in the UK in 1977 for the treatment of depression. A series of reports of haemolytic anaemia and hepatotoxicity led to its worldwide withdrawal in 1986 (Committee on Safety of Medicines, 1986). Conversely, using a drug off-label does not necessarily imply that treatment is ineffective or unsafe. Off-label prescribing can be appropriate or inappropriate depending on the supporting evidence and clinical circumstances. Where a patient's condition has failed to respond to all approved treatments (or approved treatment options are contraindicated), then prescribing a drug off-label on the basis of supportive clinical trial evidence may be appropriate. Rigidly adhering to the licence may limit patient choice, reduce the chance of recovery and deny a patient a treatment which is supported by a reasonable evidence base. In contrast, poorly thought out off-label prescribing can be ineffective and dangerous.

Why do marketing authorizations sometimes exclude evidence-based indications for a drug? A drug's marketing authorization will normally only be extended if the relevant pharmaceutical company makes an application. The application process is expensive and time-consuming, partly because comprehensive data relating to the new indication will be required by the regulator. If existing trials that supported the new indication did not meet the specific requirements of the regulatory authority, new and costly clinical trials would need to be conducted. Further, if a drug were near the end of its patent life, or already available as a generic, financial considerations would mean that a company would be highly unlikely to apply for a revised marketing authorization, even if convincing data for its effectiveness and safety were available.

A recent study examined off-label prescribing of antidepressants in primary care in Canada in adults (Wong et al., 2017). Overall, 29% of all antidepressant prescriptions were for an off-label indication. TCAs were the antidepressant class with the highest prevalence of off-label indications (81%). The authors highlighted that these findings largely reflected amitriptyline being prescribed for pain, insomnia and migraine (note: in the UK, some formulations of amitriptyline are licensed to treat neuropathic pain in adults and for migraine prophylaxis in adults). The most frequent use of an off-label antidepressant was trazodone, being prescribed for insomnia and accounting for 26% of all off-label prescriptions. Examining the scientific rationale for this off-label prescribing of antidepressant medications, the researchers concluded that only 16% of all such prescriptions were supported by strong evidence. In 40% of off-label prescriptions, the prescribed drug lacked strong supportive evidence for the indication for which it was prescribed but another antidepressant in the same class had strong evidence for that indication (irrespective of whether on-label or off-label). In the remaining 45% of off-label prescriptions, neither the prescribed antidepressant nor any other antidepressant in its class had robust evidence for efficacy for the clinical indication. An accompanying editorial highlighted that, when it comes to making prescribing decisions, the '*strength of evidence matters more than presence or absence of a specific licence*' (Morales & Guthrie, 2017).

As a general rule, off-label prescribing of psychotropic drugs should only be commenced or recommended by a psychiatrist with appropriate experience. The corollary is that a non-specialist prescriber should ensure that psychiatric drugs are prescribed within the terms of their licence unless there is clear advice to the contrary from an appropriate senior colleague. There should always be an evidence-based rationale to support off-label prescribing and it should be fully discussed with the patient (Baldwin & Kosky, 2007; Royal College of Psychiatrists, 2017). The report by the Royal College of Psychiatrists (2017) on the *Use of licensed medicines for unlicensed applications in psychiatric practice* recommends that the agreement of the patient to the proposed intervention is recorded and if the patient is 'unable to provide consent to a necessary treatment, document that it has not been possible to obtain formal consent'. If a medication is used for an off-label indication and subsequently proves ineffective then it should be withdrawn. Similarly, if the off-label use relates to an increase in dosage above the maximum recommended for that disorder in the marketing authorization, and the higher dose confers no additional benefit, then the dose should be reduced so that it is again within the licensed dose range. Marketing authorizations often differ between countries and a drug may have different approved dose ranges for different indications. Licences can change over time. The best source of information on drug indications and doses in the UK is the SPC (Summary of Product Characteristics) for the particular medication. The *British National Formulary* (BNF) is a useful source of abbreviated information, the data for each drug reflecting that in the SPC.

6.6 Polypharmacy

Polypharmacy refers to prescribing multiple medications for a person at the same time, though beyond this there is no uniformly accepted or more specific definition. A helpful distinction is between polypharmacy that may be considered clinically appropriate and that which may be problematic (Duerden et al., 2013). Appropriate polypharmacy occurs when the potential benefits of the co-prescribed medications outweigh their potential harms. It can result from co-morbid conditions, each of which requires medication to be prescribed, or from a single medical disorder that requires several drugs for optimal management. Problematic polypharmacy occurs when the drug combination is inappropriate, for one or more of the following reasons:

- There is a lack of robust evidence for the potential risks and benefits of the combination.
- The benefits of the combination are outweighed by the risk of harm, including drug interactions.
- A drug is being used to treat the side effects of another medication but other solutions exist that would reduce the number of prescribed medications.
- The demands of the medication regimen make it unacceptable to the patient.

Prescribed drugs account for most polypharmacy but over-the-counter products, including herbal remedies, can also contribute. Before considering polypharmacy in psychiatry it is helpful to briefly consider polypharmacy in medicine generally. Polypharmacy is common worldwide, is becoming more prevalent and occurs in both primary and secondary care. The greater use of polypharmacy may be partly explained by an ageing population with increasing co-morbidity and the introduction of new medications for conditions that were previously untreatable. While appropriate polypharmacy may improve quality of life and life expectancy, inappropriate polypharmacy can be associated with poor medication adherence, a greater risk of drug interactions and an increased burden of adverse effects, which at their most serious can be fatal (Bourgeois et al., 2010; Maher et al., 2014). Inappropriate polypharmacy can lead to greater financial costs, partly due to the prescription of unnecessary medication but also due to the costs of treating the resultant medical complications. A final problem with polypharmacy is that it can be difficult for the prescriber to know which of several medications a patient is taking is responsible for any perceived benefit or emergent side effects.

Various attempts have been made to categorize psychiatric polypharmacy, including the following system from the National Association of State Mental Health Program Directors (NASMHPD) (2001):

1. Same-class polypharmacy: this refers to using two or more medications with the same basic pharmacology, e.g. using two benzodiazepine receptor hypnotic drugs to treat insomnia or two SSRIs to treat depression.
2. Multi-class polypharmacy: this refers to using medications from two different pharmacological classes to manage the same symptom cluster, e.g. combining valproate and an antipsychotic to treat mania.

3. Adjunctive polypharmacy: this refers to a medication being used to treat the side effects of a medication from a different class, e.g. an antimuscarinic agent (e.g. procyclidine) is used to treat parkinsonism caused by an antipsychotic drug.
4. Augmentation polypharmacy: this refers to adding a medication from one pharmacological class, sometimes at a lower dose than would be used in monotherapy, to a full therapeutic dose of a drug in another class that has proved only partially effective. The combination aims to treat a single symptom cluster. An example would be adding a serotonin-dopamine antagonist (i.e. second-generation) antipsychotic to an SSRI for the treatment of MDD.
5. Total polypharmacy: this refers to the total number of medications taken by an individual.

This categorization illustrates that psychiatric polypharmacy can arise in different ways. However, the subdivisions proposed above may not always be clear in clinical practice. The authors (NASMHPD, 2001) highlighted that 'class' refers to mechanism of action but the categorization of polypharmacy will be very different if this is ignored and drugs are classified by indication. For example, reboxetine and fluoxetine are both traditionally classified as 'antidepressants' but have different mechanisms of action, reboxetine is an inhibitor of noradrenaline reuptake and fluoxetine is an inhibitor of serotonin reuptake. The newly proposed Neuroscience-based Nomenclature (NbN) aims to overcome some of the problems inherent in the traditional classification of psychiatric drugs (see Editor's Note on Nomenclature). Although NbN has much to commend it, the reality is that clinicians are likely to continue to use traditional terminology in some of their work. In practice, the division of polypharmacy into appropriate and inappropriate may have most clinical utility.

Polypharmacy is common in psychiatry. A study of office-based psychiatric practice in the United States showed that in 2005–6 approximately a third of patients were taking three or more medications, a percentage that had nearly doubled over the preceding 10 years (Mojtabai & Olfson, 2010). Data from the Clinical Antipsychotic Trials of Intervention Effectiveness (CATIE) study, the largest randomized trial of antipsychotic treatment in schizophrenia (and also conducted in the United States), showed that for those patients at baseline who were prescribed at least one psychotropic medication, the mean number of psychotropic medications prescribed for each was 2.03 (SD ±1.1): 38% were prescribed antidepressant medications, 22% anxiolytics, 4% lithium and 15% other mood stabilizers, while 6% were prescribed two antipsychotics (Chakos et al., 2006). Psychiatric polypharmacy has been found to be more commonly prescribed for men than women and for those with a diagnosis of schizophrenia (De las Cuevas & Sanz, 2004).

Several practical steps can help reduce inappropriate polypharmacy (see Box 6.2). Medicine management, also termed medicines optimization, centres on improving medication use, one aspect of which is reducing inappropriate polypharmacy.

6.7 Managing Adverse Effects and Drug Interactions

The adverse effects of medication are clinically important as they can cause suffering, impair quality of life, stigmatize patients and lead to poor adherence to medication, which may result in a relapse of the underlying psychiatric disorder (Haddad & Sharma, 2007). In some cases, they may also confound the clinical assessment of the psychiatric illness. Minimizing adverse effects involves several steps: (i) discussing potential adverse

Box 6.2 Some practical strategies to help reduce inappropriate polypharmacy

- Consider whether non-pharmacological treatments (e.g. cognitive behavioural treatment) may be more appropriate than adding a new drug.
- Explore adherence to current medication before increasing dosages or adding new drugs.
- Be clear on the goals of treatment before medication is started
  - record the treatment targets clearly to assist future reviews especially if these will be by other healthcare professionals
  - review treatment targets periodically and stop medication if it proves to be ineffective.
- Consider drug interactions when adding a new medication.
- Keep medication regimens simple, ideally medication to be taken once or twice daily.
- Try to substitute rather than add medicines.
- Ask patients about over-the-counter products they may be taking including herbal remedies.
- Review medication regimens regularly especially in patients with long-term co-morbid conditions.
- Involve patients in prescribing decisions and medication reviews.

effects with the patient prior to commencing medication; (ii) avoiding excessive doses; (iii) considering the potential for drug interactions; (iv) systematically screening for adverse effects during treatment; and (v) appropriately managing adverse effects when they occur.

Discussing potential adverse effects with patients prior to starting treatment is important for several reasons. Talking about the relative liability for adverse effects of the possible medications is an important part of SDM and medication choice. If a person is prone to develop a certain adverse effect then a drug with a lower risk of causing that problem can be selected. Furthermore, patients who have been warned about potential adverse effects are less likely to unilaterally stop a medication if they subsequently develop an adverse effect they have been informed about. Their trust and confidence in the prescriber are likely to be increased.

While most psychiatric drugs have a therapeutic dose range, the dose within this range at which an individual will respond may be difficult if not impossible to predict. Many adverse effects become more frequent and severe as the dosage is increased. Tolerance for some adverse effects can develop over a period of days or weeks and in some cases a slow increase in dose initially can reduce their severity and frequency. As a general rule, doses should be increased gradually, especially in the elderly who are more prone to adverse effects for a variety of pharmacological and physiological reasons (see Chapter 18). Most antidepressants, other than TCAs, and most antipsychotics can be started at a therapeutic dose, though there are exceptions. For example, the SPC recommends that quetiapine immediate release is started at a subtherapeutic dose in the treatment of schizophrenia before being titrated to a therapeutic dose. Similarly, clozapine needs to be gradually titrated to a therapeutic dose. Although a licence may permit a drug to be commenced at a therapeutic dose, it is sometimes advisable to start at a subtherapeutic dose when treating patients who are judged to be more prone to adverse effects. Examples include patients with a history of poor tolerance to the class of drug that is to be used, the elderly, children, and those with hepatic or renal impairment or who are taking other drugs with which there is a potential interaction. However, it is important that this principle does not inadvertently result in a patient being left permanently on a subtherapeutic dose of medication.

To avoid potentially serious drug interactions, history taking should include documenting all currently prescribed and over-the-counter medications (including herbal remedies). Drug interactions may be due to pharmacokinetic or pharmacodynamic interactions. Examples of drugs used in psychiatry where there are well-documented and potentially serious drug interactions include the following (please note that this list is not extensive and merely describes a few examples):

- **Lithium:** Lithium has a narrow therapeutic index. Consequently, drugs that interact pharmacokinetically to elevate the serum level of lithium, even to a minor degree, can lead to lithium toxicity. Examples of such drugs are non-steroidal anti-inflammatory drugs (NSAIDs), thiazide diuretics, loop diuretics, angiotensin-converting enzyme (ACE) inhibitors and angiotensin II receptor antagonists (Finley, 2016).
- **Serotonergic antidepressants:** If two drugs that increase serotonergic transmission in the central nervous system are co-prescribed, especially if they increase serotonin transmission through different mechanisms, there is a risk of serotonin toxicity. This occurs on a spectrum of severity and at its gravest can be life-threatening. Most serious cases of serotonin toxicity involving antidepressants have occurred when monoamine oxidase inhibitors (MOAIs) have been co-prescribed with another serotonergic medication.
- **Lamotrigine:** There are a range of potential drug interactions with lamotrigine. Focusing on the interaction between lamotrigine and valproate, if these two medications are co-prescribed, lamotrigine plasma levels may be elevated because of inhibition of its metabolism (glucuronidation) by valproate. Lamotrigine can cause skin reactions especially early in treatment. These vary in severity but at their most serious include Stevens–Johnson syndrome and toxic epidermal necrolysis which are potentially life-threatening. The risk of skin rashes is much higher when the dose of lamotrigine is escalated more rapidly than the drug licence dictates. When lamotrigine is started in a patient who is already prescribed valproate, it is recommended that the starting dose for lamotrigine is lower, the dose is increased more gradually and the final recommended target dose is lower than it would be for a patient not taking valproate.

After a new drug is initiated, the clinician should enquire about adverse effects rather than simply waiting for the patient to volunteer information. However, the answers to simple questions to a patient about how their medication is suiting them or if they have noticed any problems are likely to underestimate the extent of their side effects (Yusufi et al., 2007). Patients may not report adverse effects for a variety of reasons; for example, they may not have attributed them to medication or may be reluctant to discuss problems they find embarrassing. For a patient prescribed antipsychotic medication, the use of a comprehensive rating scale, such as the Antipsychotic Non-Neurological Side Effects Rating Scale (ANNSERS) (Ohlsen et al., 2008), administered with sensitive and systematic questioning is perhaps the only way to determine a patient's full side-effect burden. Several patient-completed checklists and/or rating scales are also available to aid detection of adverse effects, depending on the medication that is prescribed. An example is the Glasgow Antipsychotics Adverse-effect Scale (GASS) (Waddell & Taylor, 2008). A patient can complete this before a consultation and it can form the basis for a discussion with the clinician. The discussion is essential as what is recorded on a patient-completed checklist/rating scale as an apparent adverse effect may have another cause including being a symptom of psychiatric illness or a concurrent medical disorder. Even if it is an adverse effect, discussion will be necessary in those prescribed more than one medication to identify which drug is most likely to be responsible.

Assessment of potential adverse effects may require physical examination and appropriate blood tests in addition to taking a history. For example, monitoring of weight and fasting serum lipids and glucose is recommended during treatment with antipsychotic medication given the risk of associated weight gain and metabolic abnormalities. With lithium, serial assessment of renal and thyroid function is required (lithium can cause thyroid and renal impairment) as well as monitoring of the serum lithium level, given lithium's low therapeutic index.

If adverse effects are detected, their consequences for the patient should be explored and options for treatment should be discussed. These will depend on the nature and severity of the adverse effect, whether it is likely to be transient or persistent, its impact on the patient and the results of a careful assessment of both the benefits and drawbacks of the current medication versus alternatives. Some adverse effects may be managed by simple lifestyle changes (e.g. sipping water if an antidepressant causes a dry mouth) but some may require a dose reduction or switch of medication. Management may be aided by the time course of the adverse effect in relation to prescribing. Some adverse effects, for example nausea with SSRIs and serotonin and noradrenaline reuptake inhibitors (SNRIs), are usually transient and spontaneously resolve over the first few weeks of treatment (Demyttenaere et al., 2005; Greist et al., 2004). Some adverse effects, for example sexual dysfunction with antidepressants, tend to persist, while others tend to become more marked with time, for example weight gain with antipsychotic medication (Bushe et al., 2012).

6.8 Medication Adherence

Medication adherence can be defined as the extent to which a patient's medication taking matches that agreed with the prescriber. Poor medication adherence is a common problem in all chronic conditions, both psychiatric and physical. A comprehensive literature review reported that the mean amount of prescribed medication taken was 58% for antipsychotics, 65% for antidepressants and 76% for a range of medications prescribed for physical disorders (Cramer & Rosenheck, 1998). Adherence is influenced by multiple patient, clinician, illness, medication and service factors (Figure 6.2). Non-adherence is a particular challenge in schizophrenia due to the impact of positive and negative symptoms, lack of insight, depression and cognitive impairment, as well as the association between the illness and social isolation, stigma and co-morbid substance use (Haddad et al., 2014). A useful distinction is between intentional and unintentional non-adherence though both can occur simultaneously in the same person. Intentional non-adherence is when a patient decides not to take their medication as prescribed, usually because they perceive its disadvantages as outweighing its benefits. Unintentional non-adherence occurs when practical problems

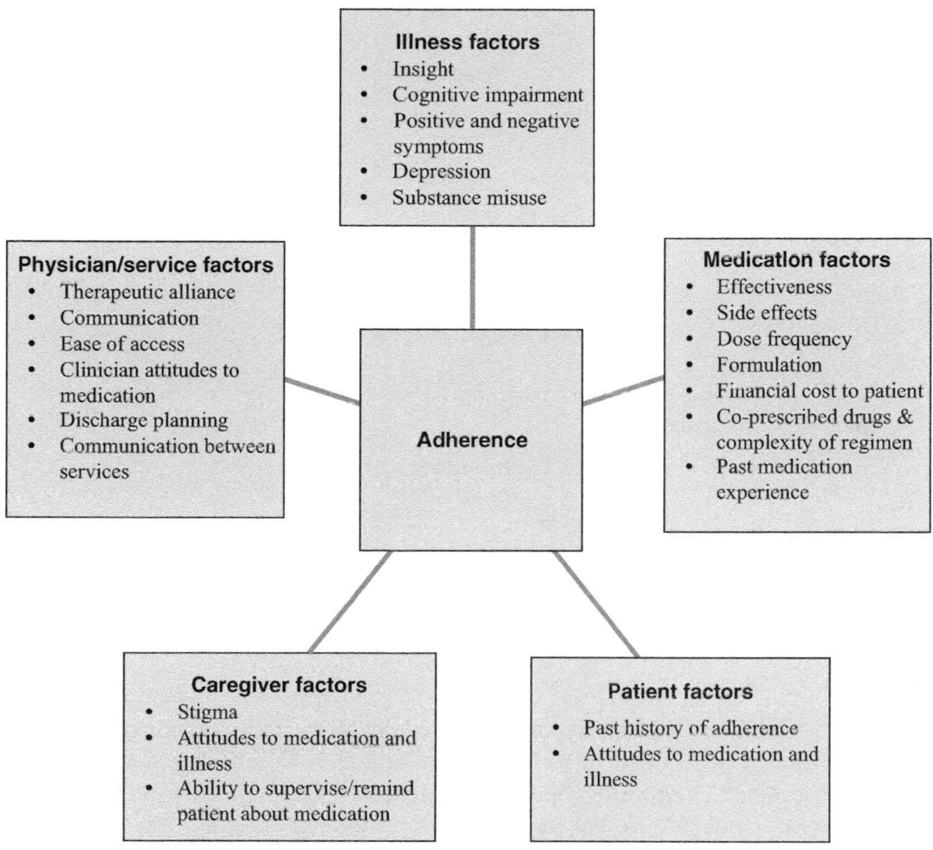

Figure 6.2 Factors associated with adherence. This figure has been adapted from Haddad PM et al. (2014), *Patient Related Outcome Measures*, 5, 43–62.

interfere with medication taking, for example a person does not understand the instructions that they were given about taking their medication or forgets to take it.

Non-adherence leads to poorer clinical outcomes. Observational studies demonstrate a strong association between poor medication adherence and relapse and rehospitalization in schizophrenia (Novick et al., 2010) and in bipolar disorder (Hong et al., 2011). As non-adherence is often covert (i.e. unrecognized by the prescriber) it is a common reason for an apparently poor response to medication. Thus, covert non-adherence may lead to inappropriate prescribing decisions such as a dose increase, switching or augmentation. Non-adherence has significant economic implications, especially in terms of increased inpatient costs, in both schizophrenia and bipolar disorder (Dilla et al., 2013; Hong et al., 2011; Knapp et al., 2004). Figure 6.3 summarizes the potential consequences of non-adherence to antipsychotic medication in schizophrenia.

Before a new medication is prescribed, the prescriber needs to try to understand the patient's beliefs and concerns about their illness and medication so that potential barriers to adherence can be identified and tackled (NICE, 2009). This will involve providing the patient with information about their illness and

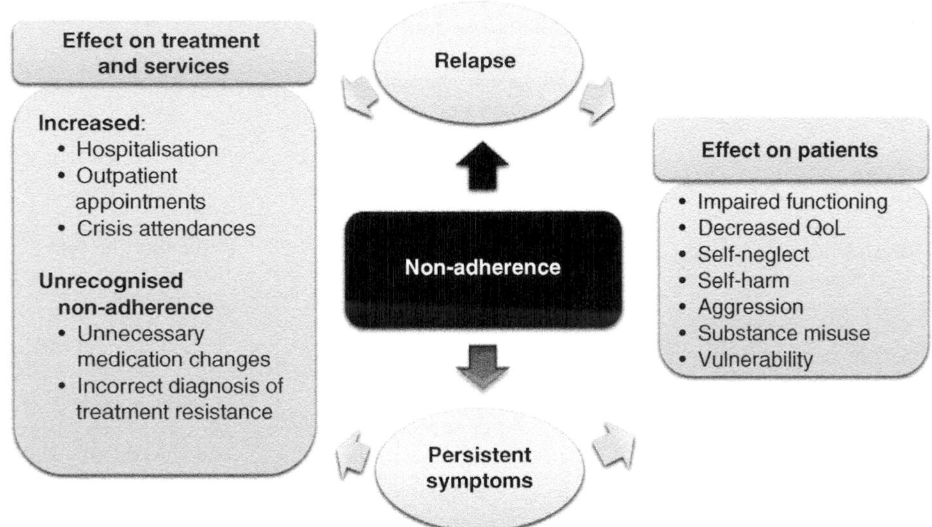

Figure 6.3 Consequences of non-adherence to antipsychotic medication in schizophrenia. Reproduced from Haddad P, Lambert T and Lauriello J (2016). The role of antipsychotic long-acting injections in clinical practice. Chapter 15 in *Antipsychotic Long-Acting Injections* (editors P Haddad, T Lambert and J Lauriello), 2nd ed. Oxford University Press.

treatment. Adherence is likely to be improved by some of the principles of good practice already discussed in this chapter, including SDM when choosing medication, adverse effect monitoring and the avoidance of unnecessary polypharmacy. Other generic strategies to enhance adherence include keeping the medication regimen simple and maintaining a positive therapeutic alliance between the prescriber and patient. Medication adherence should be enquired about, in a non-judgemental way, whenever the patient is seen.

When non-adherence is identified its causes should be explored and addressed, for example, managing adverse effects, enhancing efficacy and countering misperceptions associated with the medication and the underlying illness. More specific approaches to tackle non-adherence include psychosocial interventions, service interventions (e.g. intensive case management), electronic reminders, financial incentives and in the case of antipsychotics switching from an oral to a depot/LAI preparation. Sometimes several interventions will need to be combined. It is crucial that interventions are tailored to the individual patient and chosen in collaboration with them. In the rest of this section we review some strategies that have been used to improve antipsychotic adherence in schizophrenia.

Psychosocial interventions to improve medication adherence in schizophrenia include adherence therapy, behavioural interventions, cognitive adaptation training (CAT), motivational interviewing and psychoeducation. The distinction between these interventions is not absolute and studies have often combined elements of several models. Psychoeducation programmes are more effective in improving adherence when the focus is on adherence and environmental or behavioural interventions are included (Barkhof et al., 2012).

Adherence or compliance therapy utilizes motivational interviewing, psychoeducation and cognitive behavioural approaches to highlight the benefits of treatment to an individual, modify their illness and treatment beliefs, and resolve ambivalence towards medication. Many of the elements build on what would be regarded as good practice when discussing antipsychotic medication with a patient. However, a systematic review of four trials of adherence therapy failed to show an improvement in antipsychotic adherence compared with treatment as usual or a control intervention (Hegedüs & Kozel, 2014), leading to guideline recommendations that it should not be used (Barnes et al., 2011; NICE, 2014). In the studies reviewed by Hegedüs and Kozel (2014) baseline adherence was high, which may create a ceiling effect, i.e. it is difficult for such studies to demonstrate an improvement. The findings of a subsequent meta-analysis of six studies of adherence therapy in schizophrenia spectrum disorders suggested that although there was no significant effect on medication adherence, the intervention was associated with a significant reduction in psychiatric symptoms compared to treatment as usual (Gray et al., 2016).

One of the main advantages of LAI antipsychotic preparations is that they make antipsychotic adherence transparent. There is increasing evidence that LAIs can improve outcomes in schizophrenia compared with oral antipsychotic medication (OAPs) though this derives largely from observational studies rather than RCTs. In the most recent meta-analysis of RCTs, pooled LAIs did not reduce relapse compared with OAPs in people with schizophrenia (Kishimoto et al., 2014). This may partly reflect selective recruitment of adherent patients into RCTs plus the design of RCTs distorting the ecology of treatment as used in clinical practice. Since this meta-analysis was conducted, the results of three RCTs, with designs that better reflect real-world practice, have been published and each showed superiority of LAIs to OAPs (Alphs et al., 2014; Schreiner et al., 2015; Subotnik et al., 2015). It is notable that two of the three trials recruited people early in the course of schizophrenia (Alphs et al., 2014; Subotnik et al., 2015).

Observational studies have the advantage of studying patients that are representative of clinical practice and include mirror-image studies and parallel group cohort studies. A meta-analysis of mirror-image studies showed reduced hospitalization with LAIs compared with prior use of oral antipsychotics (Kishimoto et al., 2013). Cohort studies are methodologically stronger than mirror-image studies. A database study of all adult patients in Sweden with a schizophrenia diagnosis assessed the risk of rehospitalization and treatment failure (i.e. psychiatric rehospitalization, suicide attempt, stopping or switching medication, or death) for various antipsychotic medications (Tiihonen et al., 2017). The highest rates of relapse prevention were seen with LAI antipsychotics and clozapine. Compared with equivalent oral formulations, LAIs were associated with a 20% to 30% lower risk of rehospitalization.

A meta-analysis of retrospective and prospective cohort studies showed that LAIs were superior to OAPs for hospitalization rate, i.e. number of hospitalizations per person-year (Kishimoto et al., 2018). There was no significant difference between treatment with LAIs and OAPs for hospitalization risk (i.e. proportion of patients experiencing ≥1 hospitalizations) and total hospital days. Interpreting these findings should take account of the naturalistic treatment selection (indication bias) and that illness severity/chronicity was greater for those treated with LAIs compared with OAPs. Furthermore, the impact of LAIs on the hospitalization rate may not be due to better adherence; patients prescribed a LAI antipsychotic will usually have more clinical contact (from the healthcare professional administering the injections) than those on oral medication, and therefore potentially greater support, more regular review of mental state and side effects and enhanced adherence monitoring. Nevertheless, the authors' overall conclusion was that LAIs were superior to OAPs (Kishimoto et al., 2018).

The NICE schizophrenia guideline (NICE, 2014) recommends considering a LAI antipsychotic for people with schizophrenia who would prefer such a treatment after an acute episode or where avoiding covert non-adherence (either intentional or unintentional) to antipsychotic medication is a clinical priority.

Electronic reminders have been used to improve medication adherence in several illness areas. A systematic review of electronic reminders to improve patients' adherence with long-term medication in physical health disorders identified 13 controlled studies that used short message service (SMS) reminders, audio-visual reminders or pager messages (Vervolet et al., 2012). It found evidence for the short-term effectiveness of all three electronic reminders, especially SMS reminders, but the authors highlighted that their long-term effectiveness was unknown. In a study by Montes et al. (2012), SMS reminders improved patient-rated adherence to antipsychotic medication compared with a control group, over a three-month period. Although not widely used at present, electronic medication dispensers can be wirelessly linked to a central server to allow real-time electronic medication monitoring for individual patients. The dispensers register when a daily medication compartment is opened and convey this information wirelessly to a server. This can be programmed to allow various interventions, e.g. sending a 'medication reminder' text message to the patient if the dispenser is not opened within a specified time frame or alerting staff (Velligan et al., 2013).

In 2017 the FDA approved aripiprazole tablets with an embedded Ingestible Event Marker or 'sensor' ('Abilify MyCite') (Otsuka America Pharmaceutical, 2018). Following ingestion of the tablet, the sensor is activated by gastric acid and transmits a signal to a skin patch monitor worn by the patient. The skin patch monitor records the date and time of ingestion and the patient's rest and activity level and transfers the data wirelessly to an application (app) on the patient's smartphone which in turn relays it to a secure web-based portal (the 'dashboard'). This 'dashboard' allows healthcare professionals, with the patient's consent, to monitor the data including that on medication ingestion. The patient can view their data on their smartphone app and scroll through information for past months. The final design of this digital medicine system (DMS) incorporated feedback from patients and healthcare professionals (Peters-Strickland et al., 2018). The acceptability and effectiveness of the system, and whether it improves adherence and clinical outcomes, in real-world practice remains to be determined. The ingestible sensor can be embedded within most tablets. Outside of psychiatry, small feasibility studies have assessed this technology in patients with various disorders including hypertension, heart failure and tuberculosis (Au-Yeung et al., 2011; Belknap et al., 2013).

One RCT has investigated financial incentives to improve adherence with LAI antipsychotic medication (Priebe et al., 2013). The study was conducted in the UK and recruited patients prescribed LAIs who had shown poor adherence in the preceding year. Over the one-year trial period, the intervention group, who received £15 (€17; $22) per LAI administered, had significantly better adherence to the LAI and better patient-rated quality of life than the control group who received treatment as usual. However, the two groups did not differ in terms of clinician ratings of clinical improvement. When the trial ended, and the incentive stopped being paid, adherence returned to approximately baseline level (Priebe et al., 2016). The finding that a modest financial incentive can improve adherence to LAI antipsychotics is consistent with studies that show that financial incentives can improve medication adherence in general medicine as well as improve health behaviours in a range of areas, for example reducing the use of alcohol and illicit drugs, decreasing smoking and assisting weight loss (Petry et al., 2012). However, despite a growing evidence base, the use of financial incentives in health care is controversial and raises ethical and logistical issues (Petry et al., 2012).

6.9 Role of Audit as a Tool to Enhance Good Practice

Clinical audit can be an effective tool to improve the quality of prescribing in psychiatric services (Paton & Barnes, 2014) and has been defined as a '*quality improvement process that seeks to improve patient care and outcomes through systematic review of care against explicit criteria and the implementation of change*' (NICE, 2002). The collection and feedback of data relevant to the performance of clinicians and clinical teams against evidence-based practice standards can stimulate and support reflection on actual clinical practice. In an organization with a supportive, quality-improvement culture, this can then spur the implementation of change interventions and subsequent monitoring for continuing improvement. A range of change interventions may be considered; these may be implemented at an organizational level, targeted at clinicians (provision of educational material, reminders and knowledge support tools) or targeted at patients (educational materials). Barriers to such behavioural change may best be overcome with multifaceted interventions (Robertson & Jochelson, 2006).

A standard in this context may be considered as a '*definable measure against which existing structures, processes or outcomes can be compared*' (National Clinical Effectiveness Committee, 2015). The practice standards derived for clinical audit should be recognized by the clinicians taking part as defining optimal prescribing practice, being universally applicable, and realistic to achieve in routine care. They commonly relate to the quality of pretreatment screening and monitoring and review of continuing treatment.

The audit data collected will focus on measures of compliance with the practice standards. But other contextual data should be collected to provide some indication of the organizational, administrative and clinical factors that may be associated with variation in clinical performance and thus inform the change interventions. Clinicians' interpretation of the audit findings relating to their own clinical service may be enhanced by providing benchmarked performance data, allowing comparison with other, similar services. For local clinical audit, this may involve benchmarked data across clinical teams. For national, audit-based quality improvement programmes like those run by the Prescribing Observatory for Mental Health (POMH-UK; Barnes & Paton, 2012), use of a standard data collection tool by all the participating clinical services allows for local performance to be compared with equivalent data on performance from other services nationally. Topics addressed by POMH-UK quality improvement programmes tend to focus on discrete, defined aspects of prescribing practice, and have included high-dose and combined antipsychotic medication (Paton et al., 2008), screening for the metabolic side effects of antipsychotic medication (Barnes et al., 2015), monitoring of lithium treatment

(Paton et al., 2013), prescribing valproate for bipolar disorder (Paton et al., 2018) and the pharmacological management of acute behavioural disturbance, including rapid tranquillisation (Paton et al., 2019).

References

Alphs L, Mao L, Rodriguez SC, Hulihan J, Starr HL (2014). Design and rationale of the Paliperidone Palmitate Research in Demonstrating Effectiveness (PRIDE) study: a novel comparative trial of once-monthly paliperidone palmitate versus daily oral antipsychotic treatment for delaying time to treatment failure in persons with schizophrenia. *J Clin Psychiatry*, 75(12), 1388–1393.

Au-Yeung KY, Moon GD, Robertson TL, et al. (2011). Early clinical experience with networked system for promoting patient self-management. *Am J Manag Care*, 17, e277–e287.

Baldwin DS, Kosky N (2007). Off-label prescribing in psychiatric practice. *Adv Psychiatr Treat*, 13, 414–422.

Barkhof E, Meijer CJ, de Sonneville LM, Linszen DH, de Haan L (2012). Interventions to improve adherence to antipsychotic medication in patients with schizophrenia – a review of the past decade. *Eur Psychiatry*, 27, 9–18.

Barnes TR, Paton C (2012). Role of the Prescribing Observatory for Mental Health. *Br J Psychiatry*, 201, 428–429.

Barnes TR; Schizophrenia Consensus Group of British Association for Psychopharmacology (2011). Evidence-based guidelines for the pharmacological treatment of schizophrenia: recommendations from the British Association for Psychopharmacology. *J Psychopharmacol*, 25(5), 567–620.

Barnes TRE, Dye S, Ferrier N, et al. (2014). *Consensus Statement on High-Dose Antipsychotic medication*. College Report CR190. London: Royal College of Psychiatrists.

Barnes TRE, Bhatti SF, Adroer R, Paton C (2015). Screening for the metabolic side effects of antipsychotic medication: findings of a 6-year quality improvement programme in the UK. *BMJ Open*, 5, e007633.

Belknap R, Weis S, Brookens A, et al. (2013). Feasibility of an ingestible sensor-based system for monitoring adherence to tuberculosis therapy. *PLoS One*, 8(1), e53373.

Bourgeois FT, Shannon MW, Valim C, et al. (2010). Adverse drug events in the outpatient setting: an 11-year national analysis. *Pharmacoepidemiol Drug Saf*, 19, 901–910.

Bushe CJ, Slooff CJ, Haddad PM, Karagianis JL (2012). Weight change from 3-year observational data: findings from the worldwide schizophrenia outpatient health outcomes database. *J Clin Psychiatry*, 73(6), e749–e755.

Chakos MH, Glick ID, Miller AL, et al. (2006). Baseline use of concomitant psychotropic medications to treat schizophrenia in the CATIE trial. *Psychiatr Serv*, 57, 1094–1101.

Clark SR, Wilton L, Baune BT, et al. (2014). A state-wide quality improvement system utilising nurse-led clinics for clozapine management. *Australas Psychiatry*, 22(3), 254–259.

Cleare A, Pariante CM, Young AH, et al.; Members of the Consensus Meeting (2015). Evidence-based guidelines for treating depressive disorders with antidepressants: a revision of the 2008 British Association for Psychopharmacology guidelines. *J Psychopharmacol*, 29(5), 459–525.

Committee on Safety of Medicines (1986). CSM Update: withdrawal of nomifensine. *Br Med J (Clin Res Ed)*, 293(6538), 41.

Cope LC, Abuzour AS, Tully MP (2016). Nonmedical prescribing: where are we now? *Ther Adv Drug Saf*, 7(4), 165–172.

Cramer JA, Rosenheck R (1998). Compliance with medication regimens for mental and physical disorders. *Psychiatr Serv*, 49(2), 196–201.

Cuijpers P, Smit F, van Straten A (2007). Psychological treatments of subthreshold depression: a meta-analytic review. *Acta Psychiatr Scand*, 115(6), 434–441.

De las Cuevas C, Sanz EJ (2004). Polypharmacy in psychiatric practice in the Canary Islands. *BMC Psychiatry*, 4, 18.

Demyttenaere K, Albert A, Mesters P, et al. (2005). What happens with adverse events during 6 months of treatment with selective serotonin reuptake inhibitors? *J Clin Psychiatry*, 66, 859–863.

Dilla T, Ciudad A, Alvarez M. (2013). Systematic review of the economic aspects of nonadherence to antipsychotic medication in patients with schizophrenia. *Patient Prefer Adherence*, 7, 275–284.

Duerden M, Avery T, Payne R (2013). *Polypharmacy and medicines optimisation: Making it safe and sound*. London: The King's Fund. Available at: www.kingsfund.org.uk/publications/polypharmacy-and-medicines-optimisation (last accessed 1.10.14).

Duncan E, Best C, Hagen S (2010). Shared decision making interventions for people with mental health conditions. *Cochrane Database Syst Rev*, (1), CD007297.

Elwyn G, Coulter A, Laitner S, et al. (2010). Implementing shared decision making in the NHS. *BMJ*, 341, c5146.

Finley PR (2016). Drug interactions with lithium: an update. *Clin Pharmacokinet*, 55(8), 925–941.

Gage H, Family H, Murphy F, et al. (2015). Comparison of sole nurse and team-delivered community clozapine services for people with treatment-resistant schizophrenia. *J Adv Nurs*, 71(3), 547–558.

Geddes JR, Carney SM, Davies C, et al. (2003). Relapse prevention with antidepressant drug treatment in depressive disorders: a systematic review. *Lancet*, 361, 653–661.

General Medical Council (2013). *Good practice in prescribing and managing medicines and devices*. Available at: www.gmc-uk.org/ethical-guidance/ethical-guidance-for-doctors/prescribing-and-managing-medicines-and-devices (last accessed 2.8.19).

Gray R, Bressington D, Ivanecka A, et al. (2016). Is adherence therapy an effective adjunct treatment for patients with schizophrenia spectrum disorders? A systematic review and meta-analysis. *BMC Psychiatry*, 16, 90.

Greist J, McNamara RK, Mallinckrodt CH, Rayamajhi JN, Raskin J (2004). Incidence and duration of antidepressant induced nausea: duloxetine compared with paroxetine and fluoxetine. *Clin Ther*, 26, 1446–1455.

Haddad PM, Sharma SG (2007). Adverse effects of atypical antipsychotics: differential risk and clinical implications. *CNS Drugs*, 21(11), 911–936.

Haddad PM, Brain C, Scott J (2014). Nonadherence with antipsychotic medication in schizophrenia: challenges and management strategies. *Patient Relat Outcome Meas*, 5, 43–62.

Haddad P, Lambert T, Lauriello J (2016). The role of antipsychotic long-acting injections in clinical practice. In P Haddad, T Lambert, J Lauriell, eds., *Antipsychotic Long-Acting Injections*, 2nd ed. Oxford: Oxford University Press, pp. 337–360.

Hegedüs A, Kozel B (2014). Does adherence therapy improve medication adherence among patients with schizophrenia? A systematic review. *Int J Ment Health Nurs*, 23(6), 490–497.

Hill T, Coupland C, Morriss R, et al. (2015). Antidepressant use and risk of epilepsy and seizures in people aged 20 to 64 years: cohort study using a primary care database. *BMC Psychiatry*, 15, 315.

Hoang U, Stewart R, Goldacre MJ (2011). Mortality after hospital discharge for people with schizophrenia or bipolar disorder: retrospective study of linked English hospital episode statistics, 1999–2006. *BMJ*, 343, d5652.

Hong J, Reed C, Novick D, et al. (2011). Clinical and economic consequences of medication non-adherence in the treatment of patients with a manic/mixed episode of bipolar disorder: results from the European Mania in Bipolar Longitudinal Evaluation of Medication (EMBLEM) study. *Psychiatry Res*, 190(1), 110–114.

Kishimoto T, Nitta M, Borenstein M, Kane JM, Correll CU (2013). Long-acting injectable versus oral antipsychotics in schizophrenia: a systematic review and meta-analysis of mirror-image studies. *J Clin Psychiatry*, 74(10), 957–965.

Kishimoto T, Robenzadeh A, Leucht C, et al. (2014). Long-acting injectable vs oral antipsychotics for relapse prevention in schizophrenia: a meta-analysis of randomized trials. *Schizophr Bull*, 40(1), 192–213.

Kishimoto T, Hagi K, Nitta M, et al. (2018). Effectiveness of long-acting injectable vs oral antipsychotics in patients with schizophrenia: a meta-analysis of prospective and retrospective cohort studies. *Schizophr Bull*, 44(3), 603–619.

Knapp M, King D, Pugner K, Lapuerta P (2004). Non-adherence to antipsychotic medication regimens: associations with resource use and costs. *Br J Psychiatry*, 184, 509–516.

Leucht S, Tardy M, Komossa K, et al. (2012). Antipsychotic drugs versus placebo for relapse prevention in schizophrenia: a systematic review and meta-analysis. *Lancet*, 379(9831), 2063–2071.

Leucht S, Cipriani A, Spineli L, et al. (2013). Comparative efficacy and tolerability of 15 antipsychotic drugs in schizophrenia: a multiple-treatments meta-analysis. *Lancet*, 382(9896), 951–962.

Maguire MJ, Weston J, Singh J, Marson AG (2014). Antidepressants for people with epilepsy and depression. *Cochrane Database Syst Rev*, (12), CD010682.

Maher RL, Hanlon J, Hajjar ER (2014). Clinical consequences of polypharmacy in elderly. *Expert Opin Drug Saf*, 13(1), 57–65.

Maxwell S (2009). Rational prescribing: the principles of drug selection. *Clin Med (Lond)*, 9, 481–485.

Miura T, Noma H, Furukawa TA, et al. (2014). Comparative efficacy and tolerability of pharmacological treatments in the maintenance treatment of bipolar disorder: a systematic review and network meta-analysis. *Lancet Psychiatry*, 1(5), 351–359.

Mojtabai R, Olfson M (2010). National trends in psychotropic medication polypharmacy in office-based psychiatry. *Arch Gen Psychiatry*, 67, 26–36.

Montes JM, Medina E, Gomez-Beneyto M, Maurino J (2012). A short message service (SMS)-based strategy for enhancing adherence to antipsychotic medication in schizophrenia. *Psychiatry Res*, 200, 89–95.

Morales DR, Guthrie B (2017). Off-label prescribing of antidepressants. *BMJ*, 356, j849.

National Association of State Mental Health Program Directors (NASMHPD) (2001). *NASMHPD Medical Directors' Technical Report on Psychiatric Polypharmacy*. Available at: www.nasmhpd.org/sites/default/files/Polypharmacy.pdf (last accessed 2.8.19).

National Clinical Effectiveness Committee (2015). *Standards for Clinical Practice Guidance*. Department of Health, Ireland.

National Institute for Clinical Excellence (NICE) (2002). *Principles for Best Practice in Clinical Audit*. Oxford: Radcliffe Medical Press.

National Institute for Health and Care Excellence (NICE) (2009). *Medicines adherence: involving patients in decisions about prescribed medicines and supporting adherence*. Clinical guideline [CG76]. London: National Institute for Health and Clinical Excellence.

National Institute for Health and Care Excellence (NICE) (2011). *Service user experience in adult mental health: improving the experience of care for people using adult NHS mental health services*. Clinical guideline [CG136]. London: National Institute for Health and Care Excellence.

National Institute for Health and Care Excellence (NICE) (2014). *Psychosis and schizophrenia in adults: prevention and management*. Clinical guideline [CG178]. London: National Institute for Health and Care Excellence.

Novick D, Haro JM, Suarez D, et al. (2010). Predictors and clinical consequences of non-adherence with antipsychotic medication in the outpatient treatment of schizophrenia. *Psychiatry Res*, 176, 109–113.

Ohlsen RI, Williamson RJ, Yusufi B, et al. (2008). Interrater reliability of the Antipsychotic Non-Neurological Side-Effects Rating Scale (ANNSERS). *J Psychopharmacol*, 22, 323–329.

Otsuka America Pharmaceutical (2018). www.abilifymycite.com (last accessed 21.12.18).

Paton C, Barnes TRE (2014). Undertaking clinical audit, with reference to a Prescribing Observatory for Mental Health audit of lithium monitoring. *Psychiatr Bull*, 38, 128–131.

Paton C, Esop R (2005). Patients' perceptions of their involvement in decision making about antipsychotic drug choice as outlined in the NICE guidance on the use of atypical antipsychotics in schizophrenia. *J Mental Health*, 14, 305–310.

Paton C, Barnes TRE, Cavanagh M-R, Taylor D; POMH-UK project team (2008). High-dose and combination antipsychotic prescribing in acute adult wards in the UK; the challenges posed by PRN. *Br J Psychiatry*, 192, 435–439.

Paton C, Adroer R, Barnes TR (2013). Monitoring lithium therapy: the impact of a quality improvement programme in the UK. *Bipolar Disord*, 15, 865–875.

Paton C, Cookson J, Ferrier IN, et al. (2018). UK clinical audit addressing the quality of prescribing of sodium valproate for bipolar disorder in women of childbearing age. *BMJ Open*, 8, e020450.

Paton C, Adams CE, Dye S, et al. (2019). The pharmacological management of acute behavioural disturbance: data from a clinical audit conducted in UK mental health services. *J Psychopharmacol*, 33, 472–481.

Peters-Strickland T, Hatch A, Adenwala A, Atkinson K, Bartfeld B (2018). Human factors evaluation of a novel digital medicine system in psychiatry. *Neuropsychiatr Dis Treat*, 14, 553–565.

Petry NM, Rash CJ, Byrne S, Ashraf S, White WB (2012). Financial reinforcers for improving medication adherence: findings from a meta-analysis. *Am J Med*, 125(9), 888–896.

Pope A, Adams C, Paton C, Weaver T, Barnes TRE (2010). Assessment of adverse effects in clinical studies of antipsychotic medication: survey of methods used. *Br J Psychiatry*, 197, 67–72.

Priebe S, Yeeles K, Bremner S, et al. (2013). Effectiveness of financial incentives to improve adherence to maintenance treatment with antipsychotics: cluster randomised controlled trial. *BMJ*, 347, f5847.

Priebe S, Bremner SA, Pavlickova H, (2016). Discontinuing financial incentives for adherence to antipsychotic depot medication: Long-term outcomes of a cluster randomised controlled trial. *BMJ Open*, 6(9), e011673.

Royal College of Psychiatrists (2017). *Use of Licensed Medicines for Unlicensed Applications in Psychiatric Practice*, 2nd ed. College Report CR210. London: Royal College of Psychiatrists.

Samalin L, Genty JB, Boyer L, et al. (2018). Shared decision-making: a systematic review focusing on mood disorders. *Curr Psychiatry Rep*, 20, 23.

Shaw M (2004). The role of lithium clinics in the treatment of bipolar disorder. *Nurs Times*, 100(27), 42–46.

Siskind D, McCartney L, Goldschlager R, Kisely S (2016). Clozapine v. first- and second-generation antipsychotics in treatment-refractory schizophrenia: systematic review and meta-analysis. *Br J Psychiatry*, 209(5), 385–392.

Subotnik KL, Casaus LR, Ventura J, et al. (2015). Long-acting injectable risperidone for relapse prevention and control of breakthrough symptoms after a recent first episode of schizophrenia. A randomized clinical trial. *JAMA Psychiatry*, 72(8), 822–829.

Tiihonen J, Mittendorfer-Rutz E, Majak M, et al. (2017). Real-world effectiveness of antipsychotic treatments in a nationwide cohort of 29 823 patients with schizophrenia. *JAMA Psychiatry*, 74(7), 686–693.

Velligan D, Mintz J, Maples N, et al. (2013). A randomized trial comparing in person and electronic interventions for improving adherence to oral medications in schizophrenia. *Schizophr Bull*, 39, 999–1007.

Vervloet M, Linn AJ, van Weert JC, et al. (2012). The effectiveness of interventions using electronic reminders to improve adherence to chronic medication: a systematic review of the literature. *J Am Med Inform Assoc*, 19, 696–704.

Waddell L, Taylor M (2008). A new self-rating scale for detecting atypical or second-generation antipsychotic adverse effects. *J Psychopharmacol*, 22, 238–243.

Wells KB, Golding JM, Burnam MA (1988). Psychiatric disorder in a sample of the general population with and without chronic medical conditions. *Am J Psychiatry*, 145(8), 976–981.

Woltmann EM, Wilkniss SM, Teachout A, McHugo GJ, Drake RE (2011). Trial of an electronic decision support system to facilitate shared decision making in community mental health. *Psychiatr Serv*, 62 (1), 54–60.

Wong J, Motulsky A, Abrahamowicz M, et al. (2017). Off-label indications for antidepressants in primary care: descriptive study of prescriptions from an indication based electronic prescribing system. *BMJ*, 356, j603.

Yusufi BZ, Mukherjee S, Flanagan RJ, et al. (2007). Prevalence and nature of side effects during clozapine maintenance treatment and the relationship with clozapine dose and plasma concentration. *Int Clin Psychopharmacol*, 22(4), 238–243.

Zimmerman M, Posternak M, Friedman M, et al. (2004). Which factors influence psychiatrists' selection of antidepressants? *Am J Psychiatry*, 161(7), 1285–1289.

Drugs to Treat Depression

Patrick McLaughlin and Anthony Cleare

7.1 Introduction

This chapter reviews the main drugs used in the treatment of unipolar depressive disorders. At the outset it should be noted that the term 'antidepressant' is problematic given that drugs traditionally regarded as 'antidepressants' are effective in treating psychiatric syndromes other than depression, most notably various anxiety disorders. Furthermore, some drugs not traditionally classified as 'antidepressants' are effective in treating depression either in monotherapy or as adjunctive agents to antidepressants. Examples of the former include lamotrigine and quetiapine, which have efficacy in treating bipolar depression, and lithium and some antipsychotics, which are effective in augmenting the efficacy of reuptake inhibiting antidepressants in major depressive disorder. Despite these issues, the term 'antidepressant' is widely used and is likely to remain so. This chapter uses the traditional classification of antidepressants but the weaknesses are acknowledged and Section 7.2.7 reviews the categorization of these drugs as recommended by the Neuroscience-based Nomenclature (NbN) group (see Editor's Note on Nomenclature for further details of NbN).

This chapter addresses the pharmacological treatment of unipolar depressive syndromes. Randomized controlled trials (RCTs) have failed to show that antidepressants are effective in either the acute or maintenance treatment of bipolar depression (Sachs et al., 2007). The main drug options that are supported by RCT evidence in the acute treatment of bipolar depression are lamotrigine, quetiapine, lurasidone, olanzapine and the combination of olanzapine and fluoxetine (Goodwin et al., 2016). Despite the lack of evidence antidepressants are widely used in clinical practice to treat bipolar depression and it is possible that some individual patients do benefit. If antidepressants are used in bipolar I disorder, then it should always be under the cover of an appropriate antimanic agent to prevent switching to mania and cycle acceleration.

The first effective antidepressants were discovered serendipitously. In the early 1950s tuberculosis patients treated with iproniazid, a monoamine oxidase inhibitor (MAOI) which was thought to be effective in the treatment of tuberculosis, showed substantial elevations in mood. This led to the earliest studies demonstrating the efficacy of MAOIs in treating depression and it was from the action of these drugs that the monoamine theory of depression was developed; drugs that promoted monoamine activity appeared to relieve symptoms of depression while monoamine-depleting drugs, such as reserpine, led to the emergence of depressive symptoms. The monoamine theory has developed over later decades to incorporate additional mechanisms including receptor regulation and second messenger signalling. In more recent times and in acknowledgement of the limitations of the monoamine hypothesis, additional neurobiological hypotheses have also been proposed including hypothalamic–pituitary–adrenal axis abnormalities, glutamate up-regulation, reduced neuroplasticity and inflammatory processes. Such mechanisms may lead to development of novel treatment targets. Despite the emergence of these additional hypothesized pathophysiological mechanisms, it remains the case however that all available antidepressants prescribed in clinical practice have prominent effects on monoamine neurotransmission.

Antidepressants have proven to be eective in the acute treatment of major depression of moderate and greater severity in adults. The effect sizes of antidepressants are similar to those seen for treatments used in medicine as a whole (Leucht et al., 2012). Response to antidepressant treatment is typically defined as a 50% reduction in Hamilton Depression Rating Scale (HDRS) or Montgomery–Asberg Depression Rating Scale (MADRS) scores. Antidepressants compare favourably with treatment with placebo with response rates of about 48–50% compared with 30–32% on placebo (number needed to treat (NNT) 9–10) (Melander et al., 2008; Walsh et al., 2002). This benefit for antidepressants over placebo appears to increase with duration of the depressive episode. It appears that the clinical presentation of the depressive episode, and whether or not there was a preceding life event, affects response to antidepressants relatively little (Angst et al., 1993; Brown, 2007; Ezquiaga et al., 1998; Fava et al., 1997; Tomaszewska et al., 1996; Vallejo et al., 1991). Greater severity and melancholia may be associated with a greater benefit to antidepressant treatment. Acknowledging that antidepressant responders may experience significant residual symptoms, and that residual symptoms increase risk of future relapse, increasing emphasis is being placed on remission as a goal of treatment and maximizing antidepressant efficacy from the outset.

7.2 Classification of Antidepressants

7.2.1 Traditional Classification of Antidepressants

Antidepressants are a heterogeneous group of compounds all having effects on monoamine neurotransmission and sharing the property of being effective in the treatment of pathological depression. Methods of grouping antidepressants can be confusing; at times drugs have been defined on the basis of their pharmacology (e.g. selective serotonin reuptake inhibitors, SSRIs) and at times on the basis of their chemical structure (e.g. tricyclic antidepressants, TCAs). Recognizing these confusions, efforts have been to standardize antidepressant nomenclature based specifically on a drug's pharmacology and its mode of action. In this chapter, for the purposes of outlining the mechanism of action, pharmacokinetics, drug interactions, contraindications and common side effects of prescribed antidepressants, the traditional antidepressant classifications will be used as these will be familiar to prescribing clinicians. While commonality exists between the drugs classified within these groups with regards to side effects and drug interactions, the move towards a more standardized system of nomenclature, based on pharmacology and mode of action, should be acknowledged; this is discussed in the relevant sections that follow.

7.2.2 Selective Serotonin Reuptake Inhibitors (SSRIs)

Compounds: citalopram, escitalopram, fluoxetine, fluvoxamine, paroxetine, sertraline.

Neurochemistry and mechanism of action: SSRIs all share the property of selective inhibition of serotonin (5-hydroxytryptamine (5-HT)) uptake with consequent potentiation of postsynaptic 5-HT effect. As a group SSRIs are structurally quite heterogeneous and most SSRIs have some minor degree of action on other neurotransmitter systems.

Pharmacokinetics: All SSRIs are hepatically metabolized and have long elimination half-lives ranging from 15 hours with fluvoxamine to 72 hours with fluoxetine. The active metabolite of fluoxetine (norfluoxetine) has a half-life of 146 hours necessitating a five-week washout period before the effects of the medication fully dissipate. Low concentrations of SSRIs are found in breast milk (highest with fluoxetine and citalopram, lowest with sertraline and paroxetine). Discontinuation symptoms are noted particularly with shorter half-life drugs (paroxetine and fluvoxamine).

Interactions: Serotonin toxicity (including the clinical triad of locomotor, autonomic and cognitive abnormalities) is possible if SSRIs are co-prescribed with MAOIs, L-tryptophan and St John's wort. SSRIs can inhibit CYP2D6 and CYP3A3/4 enzymes and increase levels of antipsychotics, TCAs and opiates, amongst other drugs. Lithium may enhance serotonergic effects of SSRIs, thereby increasing the risk of serotonergic side-effects, although in some cases this effect may also be therapeutically advantageous. Fluvoxamine can inhibit CYP1A2 and so increase levels of clozapine, theophylline and caffeine.

Contraindications: An absolute contraindication exists with co-prescription of MAOIs due to the high risk of serotonin toxicity. At least one week is required between discontinuation of SSRI and the initiation of MAOI (five weeks for fluoxetine given the long half-life described above). SSRIs are contraindicated in mania due to a potentiating effect on the manic state and in general should be used with caution in bipolar disorder and not without antimanic cover, particularly in bipolar I disorder, because of the risk of precipitating mania, cycle acceleration and the relative lack of efficacy in studies specifically in bipolar depression.

Side effects: Gastrointestinal effects are common with SSRIs; nausea, vomiting and diarrhoea have been reported in up to 20% in clinical trials (Edwards & Anderson, 1999). Sexual dysfunction with anorgasmia is common in both sexes; delayed ejaculation is also seen in men. Hyponatraemia is a particular risk in the elderly due to syndrome of inappropriate antidiuretic hormone (SIADH) secretion and citalopram and to a lesser extent escitalopram are associated with a dose-dependent QTc increase. There is an increased risk of bleeding due to blockade of platelet 5-HT reuptake; gastroprotective agents are therefore recommended in those considered at high risk (see relevant section below).

7.2.3 Serotonin and Noradrenaline Reuptake Inhibitors (SNRIs)

Compounds: venlafaxine, duloxetine.

Neurochemistry and mechanism of action: SNRIs, often known as 'dual action' uptake inhibitors in the form of venlafaxine and duloxetine, combine the 5-HT reuptake inhibition of SSRIs with various degrees of inhibition of noradrenaline (NA) reuptake. Whether this additional effect of NA reuptake inhibition confers additional benefit over SSRIs remains debated although SNRIs remain valuable treatment options in those who have failed to respond to SSRI treatment.

Venlafaxine: The action of 5-HT and NA reuptake inhibition with venlafaxine is dose dependent. At lower doses venlafaxine functions as an SSRI with NA reuptake inhibition occurring at doses above 150 mg/day. Venlafaxine is also associated with a dose-dependent increase in blood pressure and regular blood pressure monitoring is recommended, particularly at doses higher than 300 mg/day. In line with its mechanism of action, the side-effect profile of venlafaxine is similar to SSRIs with noradrenergic effects, including sweating, becoming evident at higher doses.

Duloxetine: Duloxetine's relative affinity for 5-HT and NA reuptake inhibition is similar throughout its dose range; this contrasts to venlafaxine, which shows preferential 5-HT action at lower doses. The side-effect profile of duloxetine is similar to that of venlafaxine although it is less likely to cause a dose-related increased in blood pressure. As is the case with venlafaxine and SSRIs, duloxetine should not be co-prescribed with an MAOI due to high risk of serotonin toxicity. Duloxetine also has additional use in pain syndromes (neuropathic pain and fibromyalgia) and is sometimes prescribed for this purpose frequently in the absence of depression.

7.2.4 Tricyclic Antidepressants (TCAs)

Compounds: desipramine, protriptyline, lofepramine, amoxapine, imipramine, dosulepin, clomipramine, amitriptyline, doxepin, nortriptyline, trimipramine.

Neurochemistry and mechanism of action: TCAs are a structurally similar group of drugs, each sharing a three-ringed structure; they may be subdivided structurally as either secondary amines (desipramine, nortriptyline and amoxapine) or tertiary amines (imipramine, amitriptyline, trimipramine, lofepramine, dosulepin, doxepin). While structurally similar, TCAs are a pharmacologically heterogeneous group with varying degrees of NA and 5-HT reuptake inhibition. They may therefore act similarly to an SSRI (clomipramine), an SNRI (amitriptyline) or a noradrenaline reuptake inhibitor (NARI; lofepramine). Most possess some antimuscarinic activity contributing to additional side-effects; amitriptyline has potent antimuscarinic activity in contrast to desipramine which has relatively weak antimuscarinic activity.

Pharmacokinetics: The half-life of TCAs varies from 8 hours with lofepramine to 36 hours with nortriptyline. They are extensively metabolized in the liver. Tertiary amines are metabolized to active secondary amines; for example, amitriptyline is metabolized to nortriptyline and lofepramine is metabolized to desipramine. The rate of metabolism is reduced in the elderly leading to higher plasma levels and increased risk of toxicity.

Interactions: Co-prescription of a TCA and a MAOI carries a high risk of serotonin toxicity, especially in agents with strong serotonergic reuptake inhibition such as clomipramine. Co-prescription of TCAs with SSRIs may lead to high TCA levels due to SSRI inhibition of the CYP2D6 isoenzyme (paroxetine and fluoxetine are potent inhibitors whereas citalopram and escitalopram have minimal effect). Alcohol may potentiate the sedative effects seen with some TCAs. Cimetidine, a commonly prescribed histamine receptor antagonist that inhibits gastric acid production, also increases TCA levels.

Contraindications: Due to their effects on myocardial contractibility TCAs are contraindicated in those with a recent myocardial infarction, arrhythmias or a bundle branch block. They can lower seizure threshold; therefore, cautious use is advised in epilepsy. TCAs are contraindicated in mania due to a potentiating effect on the manic state and in general should be used with caution in bipolar disorder and not without antimanic cover, particularly in bipolar I disorder where the risk of precipitating mania appears even higher than with SSRIs (Gijsman et al., 2004).

Side effects: The side-effect profile of TCAs relates to their broad pharmacological action. Anticholinergic effects include blurred vision, dry mouth, constipation and urinary retention. Antihistaminergic effects can lead to sedation and weight gain. α_1-adrenoceptor blockade can lead to postural hypotension, dizziness and sedation. Sodium and calcium channel blockade underlie cardiotoxic effects and arrhythmic potential.

7.2.5 Monoamine Oxidase Inhibitors (MAOIs)

Compounds: isocarboxazid, phenelzine, moclobemide, tranylcypromine, selegiline.

Neurochemistry and mechanism of action: Monoamine oxidase (MAO) exists in two forms, MAO-A and MAO-B. MAO-A metabolizes NA, 5-HT, dopamine (DA) and tyramine. MAO-B metabolizes DA, tyramine and phenylethylamine. Consequently, MAOIs have the effect of increasing concentrations of NA, DA and 5-HT within synapses. The traditional MAOIs (phenelzine, tranylcypromine and isocarboxazid) irreversibly inhibit both MAO-A and MAO-B, which means that new enzyme has to be synthesized in order to relieve the blockade. Moclobemide functions as a reversible inhibitor of MAO-A and therefore has reduced propensity for tyramine interactions. Tranylcypromine has an additional effect in that it releases catecholamines from nerve terminals, which contributes to its alerting potential.

Pharmacokinetics: MAOIs are extensively metabolized in the liver. Substantial time is needed to restore MAO enzyme function after irreversible blockade; at least two weeks are therefore needed before switching from an irreversible MAOI to an antidepressant with a potential interaction. Moclobemide, with its reversible mode of action, requires no washout period. About half of the White population are 'fast acetylators' so clear these drugs more quickly. A higher proportion of the Oriental population are 'slow acetylators', which can be associated with higher plasma levels and a greater potential for side effects. Selegiline can be given transdermally as a patch, avoiding first-pass metabolism.

Interaction: An important dietary interaction is with tyramine which can result in a hypertensive crisis. Tyramine functions as a 'pressor amine' and has the propensity to increase blood pressure. Dietary tyramine is normally inactivated in the gut by MAO-A. Traditional MAOIs prevent degradation of tyramine in the gut and therefore tyramine-containing foods (including mature cheese, broad bean pods, improperly stored meat, poultry and fish; patients are given a full list with the prescription) need to be avoided. Moclobemide has very limited potential for a tyramine interaction due to its reversible mode of action although it still carries the dietary restriction warnings of the irreversible agents. Sympathomimetic medications (including over-the-counter 'cold cures') also need to be avoided with MAOIs as the combination can also lead to a hypertensive crisis. The combination of an MAOI with a serotonergic agent (SSRIs, SNRIs or TCAs with strong serotonergic activity such as clomipramine) can result in serotonin toxicity which at its most severe can be fatal.

Contraindications: Risk of hypertensive crisis renders MAOIs hazardous in those with cardiovascular and cerebrovascular disease. Caution is also advised in those with pheochromocytoma, as the secretion of catecholamines can potentiate the effect of a hypertensive crisis.

Side effects: Side effects are more common with traditional MAOIs and include nausea, dizziness, restless, tremor, insomnia and sexual dysfunction. Postural hypotension, particularly in the elderly, is common. Peripheral oedema is noted to occur, especially with phenelzine. The risk of hypertensive reactions with foodstuffs and sympathomimetic medications, and the corresponding list of contraindicated foods, drinks and medications mean that MAOIs are more complex to use than other antidepressants. As such, they are generally used when a range of other antidepressants have proved ineffective. Currently, their use is largely restricted to clinicians with experience in their use, particularly those working in tertiary affective disorder centres. Clinical experience suggests that some patients respond to MAOIs when other antidepressants have proved ineffective. Therefore, it is recommended that a higher proportion of psychiatrists who treat depression become familiar with prescribing MAOIs.

7.2.6 Other Antidepressants

Compounds: mirtazapine, vortioxetine, agomelatine, bupropion, reboxetine.

Mirtazapine: Mirtazapine is an α_2-adrenergic, 5-HT$_2$, 5-HT$_3$ and H$_1$ antagonist. Blockade of 5-HT$_2$ is thought to minimize sexual side effects and blockade of 5-HT$_3$ is thought to minimize nausea, although H$_1$ antagonism can result in excessive sedation and (together with the 5-HT receptor antagonism) weight gain potential. The net effect of mirtazapine is increased activity in both NA and 5-HT systems. Mirtazapine has the advantage of being able to be safely combined with SSRIs and SNRIs and the combination is widely used in clinical practice to treat antidepressant-refractory patients though its efficacy was not supported by a large recent RCT (Kessler et al., 2018; for further details see Section 7.5.3.4).

Vortioxetine: Vortioxetine is a 5-HT transporter blocker with a strong affinity for several serotonergic receptors (Alvarez et al., 2014). It is an antagonist of the 5-HT$_3$ and 5-HT$_7$ receptors, a partial agonist of 5-HT$_{1B}$ and an agonist of the 5-HT$_{1A}$ receptor. Overall, its combined action on the 5-HT transporter and four subtypes of serotonergic receptors increases the extracellular concentration of 5-HT, DA and NA. Vortioxetine may have a comparative advantage over SSRIs in having reduced sexual side effects and improving cognition compared with SSRIs.

Agomelatine: Agomelatine is an agonist at melatonin MT$_1$ and MT$_2$ receptors and an antagonist of 5-HT$_{2C}$ receptors. It is reported to increase DA and NA concentrations and appears to have equal efficacy in comparison with other antidepressants. It has a generally favourable side-effect profile but can cause liver function test (LFT) elevation and is contraindicated in patients with hepatic impairment. It is recommended that LFTs are checked when initiating agomelatine and at three weeks, six weeks, three months and six months after starting treatment, as well as whenever clinically indicated (see below).

Bupropion (amfebutamone): Bupropion is the only licensed example of a NA and DA uptake inhibitor and is unrelated in structure to other antidepressants. It does not appear to cause sexual side effects, is generally activating or stimulating and may be useful for those who cannot tolerate serotonergic effects of SSRIs. It can be safely combined with SSRIs and can therefore be considered in treatment-refractory patients (see below).

Reboxetine: Reboxetine functions as a NA reuptake inhibitor. Uncertainty exists regarding the efficacy of reboxetine and this combined with its relatively poor tolerability means that routine use of reboxetine is not recommended. It may however be considered in patients unresponsive to primarily serotonergic antidepressants.

7.2.7 Towards a New Classification System

Recognizing the confusion that might arise when drugs are named according to descriptors based on indication (e.g. antidepressants, antipsychotics, mood stabilizer etc.) or chemical structure (e.g. TCAs) efforts have been made to standardize the nomenclature based specifically on a drug's pharmacology and its mode of action. While the traditional antidepressant groupings have been used in this chapter and will be familiar to prescribing clinicians, the inconsistencies in using this approach should be acknowledged. The moves towards a standardized nomenclature based on pharmacology and mode of action, such as that proposed by the NbN group (see Table 7.1), should be welcomed. Further details of NbN are provided in the Editor's Note on Nomenclature.

7.3 General Issues in Antidepressant Prescribing

7.3.1 When to Prescribe an Antidepressant

Even in the absence of antidepressant use high natural recovery rates in the first three months may be observed in those suffering from a depressive relapse (Posternak et al., 2006). There is however evidence suggesting that magnitude of the response to antidepressants decreases if the duration of untreated illness is left longer than three to six months (Bukh et al., 2013; Okuda et al., 2010). Taking these two factors into consideration there is a balance to be made between unnecessarily over-treating self-limiting depressive episodes with antidepressants and undertreating a depression that is going to persist. Naturally, it would be helpful if it were possible to distinguish between those depressive states that are relatively transient and likely to improve spontaneously or with low-intensity support and those which are precursors of a more severe or chronic condition where antidepressants may be necessary (Kessing, 2007), although making such distinctions in clinical practice is incredibly challenging with few predictive factors. It is important, therefore, to consider the current episode in the context of the overall history of depression, and the nature of previous episodes, when considering treatment options. It is also important not to consider solely duration of symptoms in treatment decisions. Thus, the British Association of Psychopharmacology (BAP) Guidelines (Cleare et al., 2015) recommend antidepressants as first-line treatment for a moderate to severe major depressive disorder (MDD) of any duration, or a depression of any severity persisting for more than two years. They should also be considered for an MDD of mild severity persisting for more than two to three months, or earlier if there is a prior history of a moderate to severe MDD.

Table 7.1 Neuroscience-based Nomenclature for antidepressants

Indication-based name	Pharmacological-based name		
Former terminology	Pharmacology	Mode of action	Drugs
Antidepressants (TCA)	Drugs for depression		
	Noradrenaline	Reuptake inhibitor (NET)	Desipramine
	Noradrenaline, serotonin	Reuptake inhibitor (NET and SERT)	Protriptyline, lofepramine, amoxapine
	Serotonin, noradrenaline	Reuptake inhibitor (SERT and NET)	Imipramine, dosulepin
	Serotonin	Reuptake inhibitor (SERT)	Clomipramine
	Serotonin, noradrenaline	(MM) reuptake inhibitor (SERT and NET), 5-HT_2 receptor antagonist	Amitriptyline
	Noradrenaline, serotonin	(MM) reuptake inhibitor (NET and SERT), 5-HT_2 receptor antagonist	Doxepin, nortriptyline
	Serotonin, dopamine	Receptor antagonist (5-HT_2 and D_2)	Trimipramine
MAOI	Serotonin, noradrenaline, dopamine	Enzyme inhibitor (MAO-A and -B)	Isocarboxazid, phenelzine
		Reversible enzyme inhibitor (MAO-A)	Moclobemide
		(MM) enzyme inhibitor (MAO-A and -B), releaser (dopamine and noradrenaline)	Tranylcypromine
	Dopamine, noradrenaline, serotonin	Enzyme inhibitor (MAO-B and -A)	Selegiline
SSRI	Serotonin	Reuptake inhibitor (SERT)	Citalopram, escitalopram, fluoxetine, fluvoxamine, paroxetine, sertraline
SNRI, NARI	Serotonin, noradrenaline	Reuptake inhibitor (SERT and NET)	Venlafaxine, duloxetine
	Noradrenaline, serotonin	Reuptake inhibitor (NET and SERT)	Milnacipran
	Noradrenaline	Reuptake inhibitor (NET)	Reboxetine

MM, multimodal; NET, noradrenaline transporter; SERT, serotonin transporter.

7.3.2 Efficacy Considerations

Although many systematic reviews and meta-analyses suggest that there is no one antidepressants class with superior efficacy over the others there is ongoing debate about whether some individual antidepressants may be marginally more effective. There is a paucity of head-to-head comparisons of antidepressants to allow conclusions and so network meta-analyses are important. After reviewing existing evidence, the BAP concluded that there are small advantages for escitalopram, sertraline, venlafaxine, mirtazapine, amitriptyline and clomipramine (Cleare et al., 2015). In individual patients where maximal efficacy is required, such as severely ill or treatment-resistant patients, these differences may become more relevant. More recently, in the largest network meta-analysis of its kind, 21 antidepressants were compared for efficacy and tolerability (Cipriani et al., 2018). All antidepressants were demonstrated to be more effective than placebo although differences between individual antidepressants were modest. Greater differences were seen with regards to tolerability however and indeed this may be the predominant issue when deciding which antidepressant to prescribe for an individual patient. Whether subtypes of depression (e.g. atypical, seasonal, melancholic, psychotic) or characterizations based on symptom profile (e.g. cognitive dimensions or neurovegetative symptoms) should guide choice of antidepressants remains largely unresolved. These are discussed in further detail below, as well as antidepressant considerations based on the presence of co-morbid disorders and pain syndromes.

7.3.2.1 Depression Subtype

'Atypical' depression is currently defined by mood reactivity (i.e. mood which can improve in response to environmental stimulation) and at least one of the following four associated symptoms: increased appetite/weight gain, increased sleep, severe fatigue/leaden heaviness of limbs and sensitivity to rejection as a personality trait (American Psychiatric Association, 2013). Limited evidence exists to suggest a marginal advantage with the use of MAOIs (Henkel et al., 2006; Thase et al., 1995). It should be noted that atypical depression has historically been subjected to varying definitions over time distinguishing it from 'typical' or 'endogenous' depression. In those with melancholic depression, it has been suggested that TCAs may be more effective than SSRIs; the evidence however is patchy with studies mostly retrospective, open or using secondary analysis with insufficient information to guide first-line choice of antidepressant. Again, there are also difficulties in the definition of 'melancholic' depression with psychomotor disturbance being proposed as a key criterion (Parker, 2000). With regards to psychotic depression, the evidence is now sufficient to recommend what most clinicians do in current practice, namely the co-prescription of an antidepressant and antipsychotic combination. A meta-analysis of two small comparative studies found imipramine more efficacious than mirtazapine or fluvoxamine in psychotic depression (Wijkstra et al., 2006). The evidence for antidepressant efficacy in seasonal depression is very limited with the strongest being for SSRIs; a positive placebo-controlled study exists for sertraline (Moscovitch et al., 2004) as well as a suggestive study with fluoxetine (Lam et al., 1995). Comparative (non-placebo-controlled) data and relapse prevention data also suggest efficacy for moclobemide (Partonen & Lonnqvist, 1996) and bupropion (Modell et al., 2005).

One RCT assessed the efficacy of lurasidone, a DA receptor antagonist, for the treatment of MDD with mixed features (i.e. two or three protocol-defined manic symptoms) but no past history of mania or hypomania (Suppes et al., 2016). This is the only study we are aware of that has investigated pharmacological treatment of MDD with mixed features. Furthermore, the status of this category, in particular whether it is best seen as part of the bipolar spectrum, is uncertain. After six weeks of treatment lurasidone was significantly superior to placebo in treating depressive and anxiety symptoms. Lurasidone is not approved for the treatment of MDD; it is approved in the USA for the acute treatment of bipolar depression and in both Europe and the USA for the treatment of schizophrenia. The dose of lurasidone used in this study was relatively low compared with the dose range approved for use in schizophrenia. Further research is required to confirm the findings of this study and to ascertain the effects of other antipsychotics and also antidepressants in the treatment of MDD with mixed features.

7.3.2.2 Symptom Profile

In considering symptom profile rather than depression subtype, it has been suggested that neurovegetative symptoms (sleep disturbance, appetite loss, fatigue) may be preferentially linked to response to noradrenergic drugs and improving emotional reactivity (including anxiety and impulsivity) may preferentially respond to serotonergic drugs (Healy & McMonagle, 1997). While preliminary data were suggestive of a possible link (Dubini et al., 1997; Katz et al., 2004), subsequent analysis of two RCTs of reboxetine against fluoxetine found no reproducible difference in degree of improvement of different symptoms or in residual symptom profile as measured on the HDRS (Nelson et al., 2005a, 2005b); this suggested a lack of clinically important differential effects. In contrast, the large GENDEP study, which randomized 800 individuals to a noradrenergic antidepressant (nortriptyline) or a serotonergic one (escitalopram), found differences when using symptom dimensions as opposed to total depression scale scores (Uher et al., 2009). Escitalopram was more effective on observed mood and cognitive dimensions and nortriptyline on neurovegetative symptoms (see Figure 7.1). The two antidepressants did not differ on total scores on the clinician-rated Montgomery–Asberg Depression Rating Scale (MADRS) and 17-item Hamilton Rating Scale for Depression (HDRS–17) and the self-report Beck Depression Inventory (BDI) which combine all three symptoms dimensions. This was taken to suggest that drugs acting on both 5-HT and NA reuptake were more likely to be of benefit in those with more neurovegetative symptoms as part of their depressive syndrome. Despite these findings, however, evidence remains limited when choosing between antidepressants on the basis of symptom profile or depression subtype.

7.3.2.3 Co-morbidity and Pain Symptoms

Psychiatric co-morbidity predicts a generally poorer response to all antidepressant treatments (e.g. Trivedi et al., 2006b). However, the response to different types of antidepressants in those with co-morbid diagnoses has been little examined. Co-morbid anxiety disorders are especially common with depression. Antidepressants are generally effective in their treatment although there is most evidence for SSRIs (Baldwin et al., 2005). For co-morbid obsessive-compulsive disorder (OCD), the evidence that noradrenergic antidepressants are ineffective against OCD suggests that serotonergic drugs be prescribed in preference (Cleare et al., 2015). Pain symptoms are common in depression

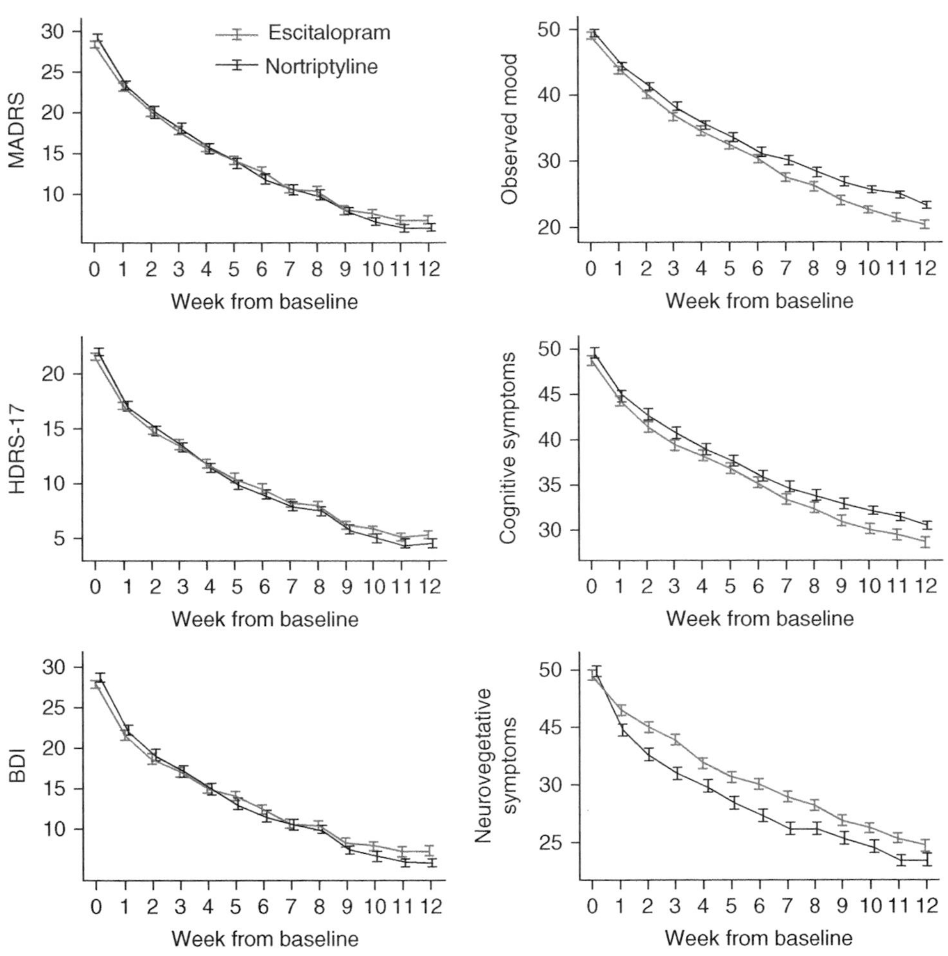

Figure 7.1 Mean symptom scores by study week, drug and outcome measure. Symptom dimensions are represented as T-scores with a mean of 50 and standard deviation of 10 at baseline. Error bars represent 1 standard error of the mean. MADRS, Montgomery–Asberg Depression Rating Scale; HDRS–17, Hamilton Rating Scale for Depression (17 items); BDI, Beck Depression Inventory. Reproduced with permission from Uher et al. (2009).

(Ohayon & Schatzberg, 2003) and have been associated with poorer response to treatment and an increase in suicide rate in some studies (Bair et al., 2004; DeVeaugh-Geiss et al., 2010; Karp et al., 2005), although this suicidal effect may be nullified by controlling for baseline depression severity, socio-economic status and demographic factors, therefore suggesting that pain in itself is not a causal factor in suicide (Leuchter et al., 2010). It has been proposed that SNRIs may be more effective than SSRIs in treating pain symptoms occurring co-morbidly with depression (Delgado, 2004), and indeed duloxetine has a licence for treating some pain syndromes such as painful diabetic neuropathy; however, there is little evidence for a large or consistent advantage on pain symptoms in RCTs of SNRIs versus SSRIs (Detke et al., 2004; Goldstein et al., 2004; Lee et al., 2007; Perahia et al., 2006).

Insomnia is very common in depression and often the major complaint. Though most antidepressants improve this over time, as the depression lifts, some practitioners prefer to use sedating antidepressants, e.g. mirtazapine, for patients with severe insomnia to gain more immediate symptom relief.

7.3.3 Tolerability Considerations

7.3.3.1 Introductory Comments

As discussed above, while modest differences in efficacy may be observed in different antidepressants, greater differences may be seen in their tolerability and their potential to interact with other drugs. A recent network meta-analysis examining all-cause discontinuation across 21 antidepressants found that all drugs were associated with higher discontinuation rates than placebo with the exception of agomelatine and fluoxetine (Cipriani et al., 2018). In comparing different classes, SSRIs are more associated with nausea, diarrhoea, anorexia and stimulatory side effects, including agitation, insomnia and anxiety, while TCAs are more associated with antimuscarinic side effects including dry mouth, constipation, blurred vision and urinary disturbance; the newer TCA lofepramine is known to cause fewer antimuscarinic side effects however. Data on sexual side effects, a significant problem across many classes of psychotropics, show a consistent picture of greater sexual side effects on SSRIs and SNRIs with relatively fewer side effects with agomelatine, bupropion, reboxetine, mirtazapine, moclobemide and vortioxetine. Where long-term maintenance treatment is used, these differences may be especially important, as the sexual side effects do seem to persist as long as medication is taken.

Paroxetine is associated with more sedation, sexual dysfunction, weight gain and discontinuation reactions compared with other SSRIs. In short-term studies mirtazapine caused fewer dropouts due to side effects, but not due to all causes, than SSRIs; it is however associated with sedation and weight gain (Anderson, 2001; Leinonen et al., 1999; Masand & Gupta, 2002; National Institute for Clinical Excellence, 2004 appendix 18c). With regards to SNRIs, studies with duloxetine have reported both equal and poorer tolerability compared with SSRIs, with the largest and most recent meta-analysis reporting a higher discontinuation rate for duloxetine due to adverse events (Schueler et al., 2011). Duloxetine has been reported however to cause fewer sexual side effects than paroxetine (Delgado et al., 2005). In pooled data from two studies against venlafaxine more patients on duloxetine discontinued due to side effects (Perahia et al., 2008). Overall, the evidence suggests slightly poorer tolerability with SNRIs compared with SSRIs, particularly where higher SNRI doses are used.

Despite its favourable side-effect profile agomelatine is known to cause LFT elevation and is consequently contraindicated in patients with hepatic impairment. The frequency of transaminase elevation, defined as three times the upper limit of the normal range, is 1.4% with 25 mg daily and 2.5% with 50 mg daily (Servier Laboratories Limited, 2012). LFTs should be checked at initiation, three weeks, six weeks, three months, six months after starting treatment and whenever clinically indicated; treatment should be discontinued if transaminase levels exceed three times the upper limit of normal range and enzyme levels usually return to normal after the drug is stopped. Tolerability studies of vortioxetine, a novel 5-HT transporter blocker with a strong affinity for several serotonergic receptors, indicate that the drug does not appear to cause any clinically significant effects on blood biochemistry, vital signs or electrocardiography. A lack of weight gain is also noted as well as the lack of a significant effect on QTc. At lower doses of 5–10 mg/day, the incidence of sexual dysfunction is low and similar to placebo, although increases with dose (Jacobsen et al., 2016).

7.3.3.2 Suicidality

There has been considerable concern as to whether antidepressants, particularly SSRIs, are associated with an increase in suicidal ideation or acts. Evidence suggests a lack of a specific link between antidepressant/SSRI use and suicide or suicidal behaviour in adults (Fergusson et al., 2005; Gunnell et al., 2005) with some evidence for a small increase in non-fatal suicidal ideation or self-harm behaviour in adolescents treated with SSRIs but not for completed suicide (Bridge et al., 2007). In ecological data however the association is generally for increased SSRI use to be linked to lower suicide rates; this has now been demonstrated using data across 29 European countries (Gusmao et al., 2013). Furthermore, data from the Netherlands and United States show an inverse relationship between decreases in SSRI use and increase in suicide in adolescents since warnings about SSRI use have been issued (Gibbons et al., 2007). Therefore, the risk–benefit analysis needs to take into account the reality that suicidal behaviour is relatively high in depressed adolescents before treatment and that the increased chance of successful treatment following an SSRI outweighs the increased risk of non-fatal self-harm.

7.3.3.3 Toxicity in Overdose

Antidepressant drugs are involved in 10–20% of drug poisoning deaths in England and Wales (Cheeta et al., 2004; Morgan et al., 2004). A number of studies have examined the fatal toxicity index (ratio of rates of deaths to prescriptions) in England and Wales between 1993 and 2002 (Buckley & McManus, 2002; Cheeta et al., 2004; Hawton et al., 2010; Morgan et al., 2004). In cases where only antidepressants were mentioned, TCAs and MAOIs had the highest toxicity with about a 10- to 27-fold increase over SSRIs. TCAs are noted to be cardiotoxic, mainly due to cardiac sodium channel blockade leading to conduction defects (Thanacoody & Thomas, 2005). It should be noted however that within the TCA class a wide range of toxicity is observed; dosulepin (dothiepin) has particularly high toxicity, lofepramine a relatively low toxicity while clomipramine is intermediate. MAOIs are dangerous in overdose and have interactions with tyramine-containing foodstuffs and a variety of medications; toxic effects include hypertensive crises, 5-HT and NA toxicity and central nervous system excitation and depression (Bateman, 2003). Within the SSRI group citalopram is associated with a greater cardiac toxicity than other SSRIs in overdose (Isbister et al., 2004). In the study by Hawton et al. (2010) the relative fatal toxicity of citalopram was approximately twice that seen with SSRIs as a group, though it was still less than half of that seen with mirtazapine and venlafaxine and approximately a tenth of that seen with TCAs as a group. Venlafaxine and mirtazapine have toxicities substantially less than TCAs as a group but higher than that of SSRIs as a group (Hawton et al., 2010). In summary, there are wide differences in toxicity between and within classes of antidepressants. This is relevant to prescribing especially in those at risk of overdose.

7.3.3.4 QTc Prolongation

The QTc interval is the heart rate-corrected QT interval measured on ECG representing the time between the onset of electrical depolarization of the ventricles and the end of repolarization. The degree of QTc prolongation caused by a drug is a surrogate marker for its ability to cause torsade de pointes, a polymorphic ventricular arrhythmia that can progress to ventricular fibrillation and sudden death (Haddad & Anderson, 2002). A recent pharmacovigilance study that used records from a US healthcare system to investigate the effect of various antidepressants on the QTc interval (Castro et al., 2013) showed that escitalopram, citalopram and amitriptyline had a dose-dependent effect on QTc prolongation. In contrast, bupropion was associated with QTc shortening while seven other antidepressants (fluoxetine, paroxetine, sertraline, nortriptyline, duloxetine, venlafaxine and mirtazapine) had no significant effect (Castro et al., 2013). In 2011 the Medicines and Healthcare products Regulatory Agency (MHRA) issued a warning about the QTc prolonging effect of citalopram and escitalopram and set new maximum daily dose restrictions and contraindications (MHRA, 2011). The guidance specified that citalopram and escitalopram should not be prescribed to patients with congenital long QT syndrome, known pre-existing QT interval prolongation, or in combination with other medicines that prolong the QT interval. The last point is particularly relevant given the frequent co-prescription of SSRIs with antipsychotics; antipsychotics vary in their ability to prolong the QTc interval but most have the potential to cause some degree of QTc prolongation (Haddad & Anderson, 2002).

The situation in clinical practice however may be more complicated. Zivin et al. (2013) reviewed outcomes in a cohort of US veterans who received a prescription for citalopram (n = 618 450) or sertraline (n = 365 898). Citalopram prescribed at higher doses (greater than 20 mg/day) was associated with *lower* risks of ventricular arrhythmia and all-cause mortality compared with lower doses. Higher doses of sertraline were similarly associated with a lower risk of ventricular arrhythmia. These finding suggest the possibility that depression itself is a risk factor for adverse cardiac events and that its successful treatment is associated with improved mortality rates. Thase et al. (2013) reviewed cardiovascular effects of escitalopram (5–20 mg/day) versus placebo in over 3000 patients and found that the mean difference from placebo in the QTc was considered clinically insignificant (3.5 ms for all escitalopram doses, 1.3 ms for 10 mg and 1.7 ms for escitalopram 20 mg). Only one out of 2407 escitalopram patients had a QTc interval >500 ms and a change from baseline >60 ms (both are regarded as clinically significant degrees of QTc prolongation). Rates of cardiac adverse events were similar between patients treated with escitalopram and those treated with placebo up to 24 weeks. Based on these findings concerns about QTc alone should not prevent effective use of citalopram and escitalopram in patients for whom these drugs are indicated. It is also worth remembering that other antidepressants (e.g. TCAs) may increase the QTc interval and that this issue is not unique to citalopram and escitalopram. If using such drugs in high doses, or in combination with other drugs that may have an effect on QTc such as antipsychotics, it is recommended that a baseline ECG is obtained before a change in dose or starting the combination, soon after it is started and subsequently after any significant dose increase.

7.3.3.5 Drug Interactions

Most modern antidepressants have selective receptor profiles and so less potential for pharmacodynamic interactions compared with the older TCAs and MAOIs with their broad receptor profiles. MAOIs can interact with a wide range of medications and foodstuffs (see earlier). The risk of a hypertensive reaction is lower with moclobemide than other MAOIs by virtue of it being a reversible inhibitor of MAO. Serotonin toxicity can occur when any two or more drugs that increase serotonergic transmission, particularly by different mechanisms, are co-prescribed. Symptoms occur on a spectrum of severity ranging from mild to fatal and this is predictable from the pharmacology of the drugs involved. Most severe cases of serotonin toxicity involve MAOIs.

Antidepressants differ in their effects on the cytochrome system. Among modern agents, citalopram, escitalopram, venlafaxine, mirtazapine and reboxetine cause minimal inhibition of cytochrome isoenzymes and have a low risk of pharmacokinetic interactions. Fluvoxamine strongly inhibits CYP1A2 and CYP2C19 and fluoxetine and paroxetine strongly inhibit CYP2D6. Duloxetine and bupropion are moderate inhibitors of CYP2D6 as is sertraline (Spina et al., 2008).

7.4 Optimizing Antidepressant Treatment

7.4.1 Accuracy of Diagnostic Assessment

Taking an accurate longitudinal history in order to distinguish accurately between unipolar and bipolar depression is of the utmost importance due to the different evidence base for treatment interventions in both disorders. The BRIDGE study reported that amongst those presenting with an ongoing episode of MDD 16% met formal DSM-IV criteria for bipolar disorder and many more had some sub-syndromal features of bipolar disorder, up to 47% on some definitions (Angst et al., 2012). There are few studies to guide the management of patients with sub-syndromal bipolar symptoms. Despite the evidence that patients with bipolar depression benefit poorly from antidepressants (Pacchiarotti et al., 2013), the consensus view of clinicians working in the area is that individual bipolar patients may derive some benefit from antidepressant treatment. In choosing an antidepressant in the presence of bipolarity, SSRIs and bupropion are generally recommended over TCAs and SNRIs due to their association with lower rates of manic switch. In bipolar I disorder, antidepressants should be prescribed only as an adjunct to mood-stabilizing medications due to the increased frequency and severity of antidepressant-associated mood elevations compared with bipolar II disorder, and the risks of cycle acceleration and rapid cycling precipitation. In addition to failure to recognize bipolarity, additional diagnostic factors associated with a poor response to antidepressant treatment include a failure to accurately characterize the presence of psychotic or atypical features, or co-morbid anxiety disorders.

7.4.2 Frequency of Monitoring and Adherence to Treatment

Direct evidence for the optimum frequency of monitoring of patients with depression is lacking but systematic follow-up has been shown to improve treatment adherence and outcome. A meta-analysis of 41 studies that reported weekly HDRS scores found that the response to placebo was enhanced if there were a greater number of follow-up visits (Posternak & Zimmerman, 2007). The risk of suicide attempts during treatment is highest in the first few weeks (Jick et al., 2004; Simon & Savarino, 2007; Simon et al., 2006) and the need to monitor this risk together with side effects and adherence to treatment indicate that early follow-up and more frequent monitoring are advisable in the first phase of treatment. Although patients report that educational materials are somewhat helpful, simply providing information about antidepressants or reminders about the need for adherence appears largely ineffective in improving adherence (Hoffman et al., 2003; Robinson et al., 1997; Vergouwen et al., 2003).

Although by no means unanimous, many studies suggest that the use of standardized symptom ratings to monitor outcomes systematically (sometimes called 'measurement-based care') can improve outcomes compared to relying solely on a clinical global impression. For example, Guo et al. (2015) conducted an RCT that compared measurement-based care with standard treatment in outpatients with major depression. In both groups, antidepressant treatment was limited to paroxetine or mirtazapine with clinicians being able to alter the dose and switch between the two drugs. Psychiatrists treating patients in the standard treatment group based their treatment decisions on clinical judgement. Treatment decisions for those in the measurement-based care group were based on an algorithm informed by two patient-completed rating scales, one for depressive symptoms and one for medication side effects. The algorithm specified starting dosages and when to adjust the dose and switch to the alternative antidepressant. Time to response and remission were significantly shorter with measurement-based care and response and remission rates were significantly higher compared with the standard treatment group.

Generally, standardized symptoms ratings are recommended to form the basis of guidance about when to implement treatment changes at 'critical decision points'. A self-rating measure for this purpose suitable for both primary and secondary care is the Quick Inventory of Depressive Symptoms (QIDS-SR) as utilized by Guo et al. (2015), although if feasible clinician-rated measures such as the QIDS-C or the HDRS may be preferable.

Adherence counselling involving special educational sessions does improve adherence to antidepressants although most studies have included it as part of collaborative care (Vergouwen et al., 2003). With regards to frequency of dosing, a database study of over 3000 patients found considerably better treatment adherence with once-daily versus twice-daily bupropion (McLaughlin et al., 2007). A meta-analysis of 22 studies found that even in antidepressants with a short half-life (<12 hours) no difference in either efficacy or the number of dropouts was observed when the antidepressant was administered once a day or on multiple occasions. (Yildiz et al., 2004; Yyldyz & Sachs, 2001). Taken together these data support once-daily administration of antidepressants. Older people may if anything adhere more closely to antidepressant treatment than their younger counterparts, though cognitive impairment, absence of a carer and lack of information about drug treatment and possible side effects may decrease treatment adherence in some people (Maidment et al., 2002). Further information on medication adherence is provided in Chapter 6.

7.4.3 Dosing, Onset of Action and Plasma Drug Monitoring

The improved tolerability of more recent antidepressants means that they can be initiated at doses known to be therapeutic. There has long been a debate about effective doses of TCAs however. Recommended doses are equivalent to >125 mg of imipramine/amitriptyline, although there is some conflicting evidence, including a meta-analysis of TCA studies that found low-dose TCAs (<100 mg) were more effective than placebo and higher doses were no more effective than lower doses but caused more dropouts

(Furukawa et al., 2002). To improve tolerability, TCAs should be started at a low dose and titrated upwards but data are lacking about the optimal rate of dose titration. If a patient appears to respond to a 'low' dose of an antidepressant there is no controlled evidence about whether or not to continue dose titration; limited evidence from continuation studies suggests that it is best to achieve a dose of proven efficacy if possible, particularly in more severely depressed patients. The elderly generally have higher plasma concentrations for a given dose (Hammerlein et al., 1998) and they have a higher rate of side-effect-related dropouts in RCTs (Anderson, 2000); lower doses are therefore usually recommended in this population.

The existence of a delay in the onset of antidepressant action has become an accepted belief. This does not accord with trial data and is likely to reflect time to appreciable improvement rather than onset of antidepressant action per se. Significant antidepressant-placebo differences are apparent in the first week (Posternak & Zimmerman, 2005; Stassen et al., 1996; Taylor et al., 2006); indeed, a meta-analysis of 47 studies found that 35% of the eventual rating scale improvement occurred during this period (Posternak & Zimmerman, 2005). A substantial improvement in the first two weeks (typically >25–30% reduction) strongly predicts final response (Aberg-Wistedt et al., 2000; Nierenberg et al., 2000; Stassen et al., 1996; Szegedi et al., 2003) and most but not all studies find that only a minority of those with lack of improvement in the first two weeks go on to demonstrate therapeutic response (Nierenberg et al., 1995; Quitkin et al., 2003; Szegedi et al., 2003).

Therapeutic drug monitoring is an established procedure for lithium and some anticonvulsants but is rarely used for antidepressants. It potentially has a use where there is relatively low therapeutic index and/or a therapeutic window; in practice this applies to TCAs, either when there is a high risk of toxicity or when there is lack of efficacy and side effects despite adequate doses (Baumann et al., 2005). Pragmatically, in patients who have not responded to treatment, plasma levels may help with detecting non-adherence or identifying fast metabolizers, and plasma levels may also help when using especially high doses or complex combinations of drugs with potential pharmacokinetic interactions. Although the correlation between dose and plasma level is often poor, there are now data detailing the expected plasma level ranges for many antidepressants based on large patient samples (Reis et al., 2009).

7.4.4 Managing Side Effects

Antidepressants differ in their pattern of adverse effects and managing side effects is a common clinical necessity. Managing side effects is complicated by the overlap in presentation between side effects caused by the drug and symptoms related to the depression; indeed, the relative contribution of drug and condition can be difficult to determine. Many side effects are most troublesome at the start of treatment and subside over time (Demyttenaere et al., 2005). Nausea associated with SSRIs and SNRIs starts almost immediately and lasts on average for a week before reducing to near placebo levels (Greist et al., 2004). In contrast, anticholinergic side effects seen with TCAs have been reported not to diminish with long-term treatment (Bryant et al., 1987). Sexual side effects can also be persistent and may be especially relevant for those needing to take medication for the longer term. Using a drug with a lower propensity for sexual side effects, for example agomelatine, vortioxetine or bupropion, or using the interventions described below may be helpful.

There is relatively little good evidence relating to the management of side effects. Common clinical strategies include dose reduction, slower titration, switching antidepressant to a drug with less tendency to cause that side-effect and symptomatic treatment with another drug. Sleep disturbance and anxiety/agitation early in treatment can be treated with adjunctive benzodiazepines although potential benefit should be balanced against the risk that benzodiazepine use may continue into the long term. Both sildenafil and tadalafil are reported to improve sexual functioning in men with antidepressant-related erectile dysfunction (Taylor et al., 2013); there is less evidence for use of sildenafil for the treatment of sexual dysfunction in women although one RCT did find positive benefits (Nurnberg et al., 2008). A study combining data from two RCTs of modafinil augmentation in patients with partial response to SSRIs with persisting fatigue and sleepiness found an improvement of depression and sleepiness over placebo with separation from week one, but early benefit for fatigue did not separate from placebo at endpoint (Fava et al., 2007).

SSRIs are known to decrease platelet aggregability and activity and prolong bleeding time; fluoxetine, paroxetine and sertraline are the most frequently implicated (Halperin & Reber, 2007). Fewer studies have investigated the risk with SNRIs or other antidepressant classes, but some studies suggest the risk also applies to venlafaxine (de Abajo et al., 2008) whereas others suggest SNRIs as a group (venlafaxine, duloxetine and milnacipran) are not associated with higher risk (Cheng et al., 2015). As a result, available data suggest that non-SSRI antidepressants should be favoured in patients with bleeding disorders. A recent meta-analysis which included 15 case-control studies and four cohort studies looking at upper gastrointestinal bleeding with SSRI use found an increased risk of bleeding with an odds ratio of 1.66 in the case-control and 1.68 in the cohort studies (Anglin et al., 2014). A substantially heightened risk was found where an SSRI and non-steroidal anti-inflammatory drugs (NSAIDs) were co-prescribed (odds ratio 4.25). Studies suggest that proton pump inhibitors (PPIs) decrease the risk of gastrointestinal bleeds with SSRIs alone or in combination with NSAIDs. Targownik et al. (2009) found that PPI co-prescription reduced the risk of SSRI-associated upper gastrointestinal bleeding by 60% (odds ratio 0.39). The National Institute for Health and Clinical Excellence (NICE, 2009) recommends that SSRIs should not be offered as first line to those taking NSAIDs or anticoagulant medication, and if SSRIs are ultimately required, they should be given with a PPI.

7.5 Next-Step Treatments

Treatment response in drug trials is typically defined as 50% reduction in HDRS scores. A failure to show improvement at the four- to six-week stage, often defined as a 20–30% reduction in HDRS scores, has been associated with very low subsequent response rates at eight weeks of the order of 10–20% (Nierenberg et al., 1995, 2000). Based on this, and related data, NICE recommends that in patients showing *no response* to optimized treatment after four weeks, consideration should be given to moving to next-step treatments (NICE, 2009). If *some improvement* is observed at the four-week stage, however, treatment should continue for another two to four weeks before reassessing. *Minimal improvement* at the six- to eight-week stage of treatment should trigger consideration for next-step treatment (Cleare et al., 2015). In those patients who have failed to respond to antidepressant treatment, it is important to review the diagnosis, to check that the initial treatment has been adequately given and to reassess for presence of concurrent medical or psychiatric conditions. With this in mind, the next-stage pharmacological treatment options that can be considered after initial poor response include:

- dose increase
- switching antidepressant
- antidepressant combination/augmentation.

The largest prospective study investigating sequential treatment outcomes is the Sequenced Treatment Alternatives for the Relief of Depression (STAR*D). This study found that response rates dropped from 49% to 16% and remission from 37% to 13% over four steps of treatment; early discontinuation for side effects increased from 16% to 30% over the four stages (Rush et al., 2006a). Nevertheless, cumulatively about half of those completing two trials and two-thirds completing four did enter remission (Warden et al., 2007). Studies of next-step treatments are mostly small, many are non-replicated and the stage of treatment resistance, methodology and patient populations differ, thereby making conclusions difficult to reach.

Medication non-adherence can be an additional significant factor to be considered; a mean non-adherence rate with antidepressants of about 40–50% has been found with different reviews (Cramer & Rosenheck, 1998; Sansone & Sansone, 2012). Identification of potentially remedial factors that are associated with poorer response such as chronic social difficulties and continuing life events (Mazure et al., 2000; Ronalds et al., 1997) may indicate therapeutic targets for intervention in addition to antidepressants. In clinical practice patients are encountered at different stages in their illness and treatment history. In addition to severity and duration of illness, the amount of previous treatment is another important factor in predicting outcome. Definitions of treatment resistance vary although most describe it as a failure to respond to two or more adequate antidepressant treatment trials (Anderson, 2003). In reality, treatment resistance is a continuum; older staging models relied entirely on number and type of prior treatments, whereas newer models such as the Maudsley Staging Model (Fekadu et al., 2009) incorporate duration and severity of depression in a multidimensional assessment. Problems can arise however in defining what comprises an adequate treatment trial, which drugs are to be included, and in taking account of psychological treatments; standardized assessment tools such as the Maudsley Treatment Inventory may help in this regard (Fekadu et al., 2018). The severe end of the continuum has been formulated as multi-therapy-resistant-major depressive disorder (MTR-MDD) and indicates when tertiary care and non-standard treatments need to be actively considered (McAllister-Williams et al., 2018).

7.5.1 Dose Increase

There is a lack of direct evidence for the efficacy of increasing the dose after initial treatment non-response for many antidepressants. A systematic review found no consistent evidence for increased efficacy after dose escalation in non-responders compared with continuing lower doses for SSRIs in seven RCTs (Adli et al., 2005). Three large randomized double-blind studies also found that raising the dose of sertraline and fluoxetine had no benefit over staying on the original dose (Dornseif et al., 1989; Licht & Qvitzau, 2002; Schweizer et al., 2001). Indeed, Licht and Qvitzau (2002) reported that raising the dose of sertraline in non-responders at six weeks from 100 mg to 200 mg per day under randomized double-blind conditions led to a significantly poorer outcome than staying on the lower dose. Higher doses of antidepressants are associated with a greater risk of adverse events and discontinuation effects and so raising the dose may increase these side effects without the benefit of better efficacy. It is important to note however that indirect evidence from differential dose studies in non-resistant patients suggests a possible slightly greater efficacy for higher doses for *some* antidepressants including TCAs (200–300 mg imipramine-dose equivalent versus standard doses) (Adli et al., 2005), venlafaxine (225–375 mg vs. 75 mg) (Rudolph et al., 1998), escitalopram (20 mg vs. 10 mg) (Burke et al., 2002) and vortioxetine (20 mg vs. 5–10 mg) (Thase et al., 2016). In view of this, increasing the dose (provided side effects and safety allow), particularly with the aforementioned drugs, may be a reasonable step. The case for increasing doses may also be made in view of wide interindividual variability in plasma concentration of antidepressants and associated uncertainty about what is an effective dose for an individual patient. A Swedish laboratory has prepared a reference guide to expected plasma levels and dose of common antidepressants (Reis et al., 2009).

7.5.2 Switching Antidepressants

Switching antidepressant should be considered when there has been no treatment response after an adequate trial or if troublesome or dose-limiting side effects emerge. Response rates to an antidepressant switch, including to a drug in the same class, have varied widely in different studies (12–70%). Switching to a second SSRI in open studies and SSRI arms of RCTs shows response rates of between 25% and 70% (Ruhe et al., 2006). Switching from a reuptake inhibitor to an MAOI and from an SSRI to venlafaxine is associated with short-term response rates >50% in some studies with switches between other antidepressants showing <50% response rates (Anderson, 2003; Ruhe et al., 2006) without a clear benefit between classes. In pooling the data from three studies with different methodologies, a significant but modest advantage was observed in switching from an SSRI to venlafaxine rather than a second SSRI (Ruhe et al., 2006) and this was confirmed in a subsequent meta-analysis (Papakostas et al., 2008). This meta-analysis included five studies and found a small advantage of switching from an SSRI to venlafaxine, bupropion or mirtazapine versus switching to another SSRI (Papakostas et al., 2008). A comparison of switching to high dose (mean 309 mg/day) versus standard dose (mean 148 mg/day) venlafaxine after SSRI failure or intolerance found a tendency to faster and greater response, but poorer tolerability, at the higher dose (Thase et al., 2006).

When switching antidepressants, an abrupt switch or cross-titration is generally preferable unless a potential drug interaction is identified, in which case the recommended taper/washout period should be followed. Potentially toxic interactions need to be considered especially when the initial drug has long-lasting effects (e.g. fluoxetine to TCA, MAOIs to serotonergic drugs) and it is recommended that appropriate reference books are consulted such as the *British National Formulary* (BNF; Joint Formulary Committee, 2018) or the *Maudsley Prescribing Guidelines* (Taylor et al., 2015). Direct switching (without washout) from an initial SSRI to another SSRI, nortriptyline, mirtazapine, bupropion, reboxetine, venlafaxine and duloxetine appears well tolerated and may reduce discontinuation symptoms (Ruhe et al., 2006; Wohlreich et al., 2005). Direct switching from citalopram to sertraline, venlafaxine and bupropion was used in the STAR*D study without apparent problems (Rush et al., 2006b). A small randomized open study found no difference in the severity of discontinuation symptoms between a 3-day and 14-day taper when switching from SSRIs to other antidepressants, with significant discontinuation symptoms with shorter-acting SSRIs but not fluoxetine (Tint et al., 2007).

7.5.3 Augmentation and Combination Treatment

Adding a second agent tends to be called 'augmentation' when the drug is not primarily an antidepressant and 'combination' when two antidepressants are used. Augmenting and add-on medications for depression are discussed in other chapters so only a brief summary is provided here. Reviewing available evidence, the BAP Guidelines concluded that the best evidence of efficacy in augmentation of antidepressants is for quetiapine, aripiprazole and lithium with less robust evidence for risperidone, olanzapine, tri-iodothyronine, bupropion, mirtazapine and buspirone (Cleare et al., 2015). The potential for increased side-effect burden with the addition of augmenting agents should also be noted. Unfortunately, few direct comparisons of augmentation strategies have been undertaken. A network meta-analysis attempted to use indirect comparison to gain some indication of relative efficacy of augmentation agents (Zhou et al., 2015). Notwithstanding limitations of the methodology and the variable quality of the underlying studies, quetiapine, aripiprazole, lithium and tri-iodothyronine emerged as most effective in terms of treatment response; unfortunately, the first three of these were also amongst the least well tolerated, although tri-iodothyronine was amongst the best tolerated.

7.5.3.1 Antipsychotics (i.e. Dopamine Receptor Antagonists)

The efficacy of certain 'atypical' or newer antipsychotics as augmenting agents has now been firmly established by the developing evidence base, though most studies to date have only looked at short-term efficacy. A recent meta-analysis identified 14 studies where atypical antipsychotic augmentation was compared with placebo (Spielmans et al., 2013); higher remission rates and responses were observed for quetiapine, aripiprazole and risperidone. An earlier meta-analysis of 16 RCTs of atypical antipsychotic augmentation in patients failing to respond to an antidepressant including olanzapine, quetiapine, aripiprazole and risperidone, mostly added to fluoxetine or venlafaxine, showed a benefit for augmentation over placebo (Nelson & Papakostas, 2009). Discontinuation rates due to adverse effects however were fourfold higher in the augmented versus placebo groups. In patients with a prospectively determined inadequate antidepressant response at eight weeks, and who continued on the same treatment, aripiprazole was more effective than placebo augmentation (response 34% vs. 24%) and had good tolerability (Berman et al., 2007).

Although there are few comparisons over the full dose ranges, effective doses of atypical antipsychotics when used for augmentation are generally lower than when used to treat psychosis. For quetiapine, one study found that 300 mg did not show greater rates of sustained remission than 150 mg (Vieta et al., 2013), but in another 300 mg was more effective than placebo whereas 150 mg was not (El-Khalili et al., 2010). Recommended dose ranges for aripiprazole are 2.5–10 mg/day, for olanzapine 2.5–10 mg/day and risperidone 0.5–2 mg/day (Taylor et al., 2014). There are no direct comparisons between the atypical antipsychotics. Differences in side effects and other actions may be helpful in choosing the most appropriate augmenting agent for an individual patient. For example, aripiprazole has more activating effects whereas quetiapine has more sedating and anxiolytic effects, and these profiles may better suit individual patients. Furthermore, clinical experience suggests that one 'atypical' antipsychotic may prove effective where another has failed; the degree to which modes of action are shared or different between the individual drugs is unclear.

7.5.3.2 Lithium

While modest, there is also reasonably sound evidence supporting lithium augmentation of monoamine reuptake inhibitors; a meta-analysis of 10 small studies in treatment-resistant depression found a response rate of 41% versus 14 % (Crossley & Bauer, 2007) with most studies using lithium in the dose range 600 mg to 1200 mg. Lithium augmentation as the second stage in a four-step treatment programme in inpatients resulted in a 59% response rate (Birkenhager et al., 2006) but the results were disappointing in the STAR*D study when lithium was added as a third-stage treatment with only 16% remitting and a 23% rate of discontinuation due to side effects (Nierenberg et al., 2006). Patient characteristics with high co-morbidity and greater degree of treatment resistance together with unknown adequacy of lithium treatment (only ascertained in 57% of patients, with a median concentration of 0.6 mmol/L) could have contributed to these differences. A recent systematic review (Bauer et al., 2014) identified more than 30 open-label studies and 10 placebo-controlled trials of lithium augmentation. The main limitations of these studies have been the relatively small numbers of study participants and the fact that most studies included augmentation of TCAs, rather than newer drugs. Increasing evidence is now available however to support the efficacy of lithium augmentation of newer antidepressants, with lithium augmentation of SSRIs or venlafaxine being more effective when plasma levels above 0.6 mmol/L are achieved (Bauer et al., 2013). Evidence from continuation-phase studies is sparse but suggests that lithium augmentation should be maintained in the lithium-antidepressant combination for at least one year to prevent early relapses. There is emerging evidence that the long-term prophylactic anti-suicide effects of lithium in bipolar disorder may also extend to unipolar depression (Cipriani et al., 2013). Chapter 11 provides further information on the use of lithium to augment antidepressants.

7.5.3.3 Thyroid Hormone

A meta-analysis of augmentation of TCAs with tri-iodothyronine (T3), 25 μg to 37.5 μg, in four small RCTs of treatment-resistant depression found significant benefit with regard to improvement in HDRS score (effect size 0.6) but a non-significant improvement in response rate (NNT = 13) (Aronson et al., 1996). The STAR*D study found a non-significantly higher remission rate on T3 (25–50 μg) than lithium (23% vs. 16%, NNT = 14) but with significantly fewer patients discontinuing due to side effects (10% vs. 23%, number needed to harm (NNH) = 8); it should be noted that lithium levels were not consistently monitored in this study (Nierenberg et al., 2006).

7.5.3.4 Antidepressant Combinations

The rationale behind combining antidepressants is to broaden pharmacological action in the hope that multiple actions will be of benefit. The most common antidepressant combinations reported are:

- an SSRI with mirtazapine, reboxetine, bupropion or a TCA

- mirtazapine with a TCA or venlafaxine
- mianserin with a TCA or SSRI (Rojo et al., 2005).

Clinical experience and open studies indicate that tolerability and safety are usually good but there is limited controlled data examining the efficacy of most combinations (Rojo et al., 2005).

SSRI/SNRI augmentation with mirtazapine has been explored in two settings, i.e. as an add-on treatment option when there has been an inadequate response to an initial antidepressant and as an initial starting treatment compared with monotherapy. The evidence for these two scenarios will be examined in turn. However, in both cases initial positive results in small trials were not supported by subsequent larger and more rigorous studies.

In the case of add-on treatment, a small placebo-controlled study conducted by Carpenter et al. (2002) found that mirtazapine augmentation of predominantly SSRI non-responders was significantly more effective than placebo augmentation at four weeks post-randomization. However, the recently reported MIR trial did not show any advantage for combining mirtazapine with a SSRI or SNRI compared with continuing SNRI or SSRI monotherapy in treatment-resistant depression (Kessler et al., 2018). This study recruited UK primary care patients who had taken an SSRI or an SNRI antidepressant for at least six weeks at an adequate dose but remained depressed according to standardized criteria. The starting dose of mirtazapine was 15 mg daily for 2 weeks and increasing to 30 mg daily for up to 12 months. Mean depression scores at 12 weeks showed no significant difference, clinically or statically, between the two groups and differences became smaller at subsequent assessment points. More participants in the mirtazapine augmentation group withdrew from the trial medication due to side effects. Despite the negative results, it should be noted that the MIR study was undertaken in more mildly ill primary care patients with early stage treatment resistance (failure to respond to just one antidepressant) and may not apply to more severely ill or treatment-resistant populations.

With regard to initial treatment, two separate studies reported that initiating treatment with mirtazapine plus another antidepressant was more effective than using the antidepressant in question alone (Blier et al., 2009, 2010). In contrast, the far larger CO-MED study (Rush et al., 2011) found no advantage of either venlafaxine-mirtazapine or an escitalopram-bupropion combination versus escitalopram-placebo at 12 weeks or 7 months.

Three small RCTs of mianserin added to a TCA or SSRI in patients not responding to antidepressant treatment were positive (Ferreri et al., 2001; Maes et al., 1999; Medhus et al., 1994) but the fourth and largest with sertraline was not (Licht & Qvitzau, 2002). A pooled analysis of mianserin augmentation of SSRIs shows a non-significant advantage to the combination (three studies, response 66% vs. 57%, NNT = 13) with significant heterogeneity.

Interpreting the results from STAR*D is limited by the study's methodological shortcoming. Nevertheless, the results shed further light on the relative efficacy of antidepressant combinations. Bupropion augmentation of citalopram as a second stage treatment was better tolerated and marginally more effective than buspirone (Trivedi et al., 2006a). Combined mirtazapine and venlafaxine as a fourth stage treatment was non-significantly better than the MAOI tranylcypromine in terms of response (24% vs. 12%) but led to significantly greater symptom reduction and fewer side-effect-related dropouts (McGrath et al., 2006a).

The combination of a TCA with an MAOI, used historically for treatment-resistant depression, has the potential for dangerous interaction with a lack of controlled evidence for its benefit (Lader, 1983).

In summary, the evidence to support the use of antidepressant combinations when there has been limited response to a first antidepressant remains very thin or negative depending on the combination in question. However, this is based on mean results seen in groups and it does not rule out the possibility that some individual patients may benefit from a certain combination. If a combination is adopted it should be seen as a therapeutic trial for that individual and if there has not been a benefit after a suitable period, for example, 6 weeks, then the combination should be withdrawn.

7.5.3.5 Antiepileptics

There are few data using antiepileptics as augmenting agents in unipolar depression. A small RCT of lamotrigine plus fluoxetine compared with fluoxetine in patients non-responsive to at least one previous treatment found significant benefit on secondary but not primary outcome measures (response 77% vs. 40%, NNT = 3) (Barbosa et al., 2003) and a randomized open comparison with lithium found a non-significantly better response to lamotrigine (53% vs. 41%, NNT = 9) (Schindler & Anghelescu, 2007). A more recent RCT of lamotrigine added to paroxetine however found no advantage for lamotrigine over placebo (Barbee et al., 2011). No evidence exists for antidepressant augmentation with sodium valproate or carbamazepine in unipolar depression.

7.5.3.6 Buspirone

Buspirone augmentation of SSRIs was not effective in two studies (Appelberg et al., 2001; Landen et al., 1998) although a secondary analysis of more severely depressed patients did report a benefit in one study (Appelberg et al., 2001). The STAR*D trial reported poorer tolerability and possibly slightly poorer efficacy compared with bupropion augmentation (see above, Trivedi et al., 2006a).

7.5.3.7 Ketamine

In recent years there has been increasing research interest in the ability of a non-anaesthetic dose of the NMDA receptor antagonist, ketamine, to produce a rapid resolution of symptoms in patients with treatment-resistant depression (both bipolar and unipolar) in about 50% of participants. Short-term efficacy of the intravenous formulation has been demonstrated against placebo and against an active comparator, midazolam (NNT of 3 versus midazolam, Murrough et al., 2013a). Two meta-analyses have been published. The first identified nine non-ECT studies including 192 patients with MDD (Fond et al., 2014), with an effect size for short-term reduction in depressive symptoms of −0.91. Four ECT trials were identified, including 118 patients predominantly with MDD; receiving ketamine as part of ECT anaesthesia reduced depressive symptoms after ECT more than ECT alone (effect size −0.56). The interest sparked by these findings stimulated several subsequent RCTs of adding ketamine to ECT protocols; evidence remains mixed, with the most recent meta-analysis (17 RCTs, 1035 patients) suggesting that speed of antidepressant onset may be increased but not final post-ECT response rates (Zheng et al., 2019).

Ketamine alone was used in seven RCTs (McGirr et al., 2015), six employing an intravenous infusion and one RCT employing intranasal ketamine (149 with MDD, 34 with bipolar disorder). Remission rates were higher with ketamine relative to comparator (saline or midazolam) at 24 hours, 3 days and 7 days, as were response rates. However, where studies have performed sequential follow-up the antidepressant effect usually subsides over the following several days and thus far there is no established means of maintaining the response with oral glutamatergic medications (Aan Het Rot et al., 2012). Repeated intravenous administration of ketamine may be possible (Murrough et al., 2013b) but there are concerns regarding toxicity in chronic use, particularly bladder inflammation. Other more serious adverse effects include transient blood pressure elevation that may require treatment and transient psychotomimetic effects, but no persistent psychosis or affective switches. A more readily deliverable intranasal formulation (esketamine) is under clinical development, with ongoing trials for treatment-resistant depression and for rapid reduction in suicidality (Canuso et al., 2018). As of February 2019, on the basis of both short-term and long-term Phase III trials, the US Food and Drug Administration (FDA) Psychopharmacologic Drug Advisory Committee and Drug Safety and Risk Management Advisory Committee has recommended esketamine, in combination with a newly administered antidepressant, for use in treatment-resistant depression, suggesting it is likely to be available in the near future. In this regard, it is of interest that a recent meta-analysis that compared augmention therapies in those with more stringently defined treatment-resistant depression (failure to respond to two adequate antidepressant trials) found that treatments targeting the NMDA receptor as a group had the largest effect size in terms of reduction in severity of symptoms (see Figure 7.2) (Strawbridge et al., 2019).

7.5.3.8 Other Treatments

Other strategies with preliminary evidence for efficacy in treatment-resistant patients are tryptophan addition (although tryptophan is not easily obtainable in many countries), especially to MAOIs (Anderson, 2003), and oestrogen in perimenopausal women (Morgan et al., 2005). In men with depression not responding to antidepressants and

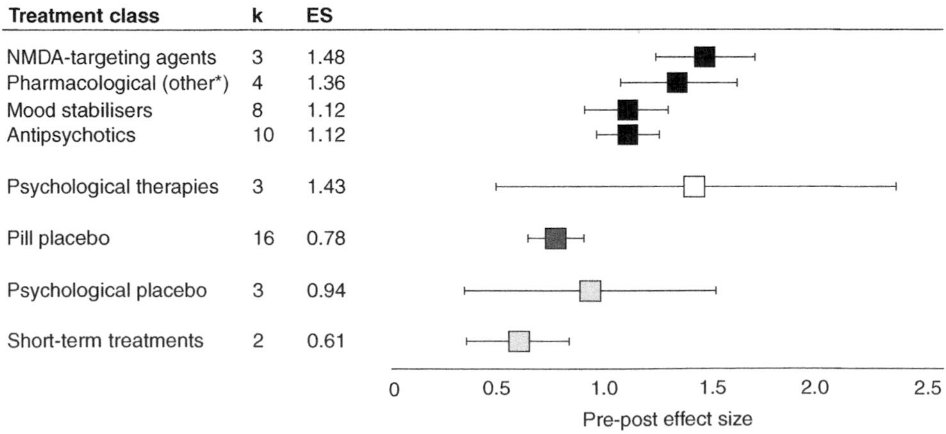

Treatment class	k	ES
NMDA-targeting agents	3	1.48
Pharmacological (other*)	4	1.36
Mood stabilisers	8	1.12
Antipsychotics	10	1.12
Psychological therapies	3	1.43
Pill placebo	16	0.78
Psychological placebo	3	0.94
Short-term treatments	2	0.61

Figure 7.2 Treatment effects by class. Augmentation treatments for treatment-resistant depression, pre-post effect size (Hedges' *g*) and 95% confidence intervals are shown. *Pharmacological treatments categorized with mechanisms not akin to *N*-methyl-D-aspartate (NMDA) agents, mood stabilizers or antipsychotics: this comprised trazodone (serotonin antagonist and reuptake inhibitor), buspirone (anxiolytic), dexmecamylamine (nicotinic channel modulator) or thyroid hormone. k, number of studies; ES, effect size. Reproduced with permission from Strawbridge et al. (2019).

who had borderline or low testosterone, a small RCT (n = 22) of testosterone gel replacement found an active-placebo difference of six points on the HDRS after eight weeks of treatment (Pope et al., 2003), although a subsequent larger study did not replicate this finding (Pope et al., 2010). A meta-analysis of the use of testosterone to treat depression identified seven studies with a heterogeneous study population, but concluded that testosterone replacement is more effective than placebo (response rates 54% vs. 33%), with benefits most apparent in those with low testosterone levels (Zarrouf et al., 2009). More recently, a systematic review and meta-analysis of 27 RCTs involving a total of 1890 men found that testosterone treatment was associated with a significant reduction of depressive symptoms, particularly in participants who received higher-dosage regimens, although with significant heterogeneity between trials (Walther et al, 2019).

There are many other interventions that may be used in specialist centres, and which are regularly revised in publications such as the annual *Maudsley Prescribing Guidelines* (Taylor et al., 2018). Of particular note is the increasing interest in anti-inflammatory strategies as adjuvant to antidepressants. A recent meta-analysis of a variety of anti-inflammatory agents found benefits for add-on treatment with NSAIDs (predominantly celecoxib), cytokine inhibitors, statins, corticosteroids and minocycline (39 RCTs, overall effect size −0.64), although most studies were short-term and potential side effects poorly ascertained (Köhler-Forsberg et al., 2019). There is also as yet unreplicated evidence from a small trial benefit of anti-inflammatory treatment with the tumour necrosis factor antagonist infliximab is specific to those with raised pro-inflammatory markers (Raison et al., 2013). A novel and still experimental approach is the use of psilocybin in treatment-resistant depression, with governmental approval for studies and medicinal grade formulations now available. Treatment efficacy and durability has not yet been demonstrated and may relate more to psychotherapeutic input and insights during the psychedelic experience rather than to a direct pharmacological effect.

ECT has an important place in treatment-resistant depression. The evidence base for other neuromodulation treatments in resistant depression (including rTMS, vagal nerve stimulation and deep brain stimulation) is less clear. ECT and other neuromodulation treatments are not considered further in this chapter as they are dealt with in Chapter 16.

7.6 Prevention and Treatment of Relapse

7.6.1 Relapse Prevention

Relapse rates are high in the months after remission and decline with time. Age of onset does not appear to be a consistent factor in increasing rate of relapse but a number of other factors have been implicated including:

- increased number of previous episodes (Kessing & Andersen, 2005; Solomon et al., 2000)
- presence of residual depressive symptoms (Dombrovski et al., 2007; Kanai et al., 2003; Paykel et al., 1995)
- depression severity (Ramana et al., 1995)
- longer episode duration (Dotoli et al., 2006; McGrath et al., 2006b)
- presence of psychosis (Flint & Rifat, 1998; Kessing, 2003)
- degree of treatment resistance (Rush et al., 2006a)

- female sex (Kessing, 1998; McGrath et al., 2006b; Mueller et al., 1999)
- social stress/poor social adjustment (Kanai et al., 2003; Reimherr et al., 2001)
- life events (Ghaziuddin et al., 1990; Paykel & Tanner, 1976)
- co-morbid medical illness (Iosifescu et al., 2004; Reynolds et al., 2006).

Antidepressants have shown consistent efficacy over placebo in reducing relapse rates and increased duration of remission is associated with a decreased rate of further relapse (Franchini et al., 2000a; Solomon et al., 2000). A recent meta-analysis of second-generation antidepressants found a pooled relapse rate of patients kept on antidepressants of 22% compared with 42% on placebo up to 12 months (Hansen et al., 2008). Consistent with the RCT data, naturalistic studies have found that medication adherent patients have better outcomes in terms of relapse or time to relapse than those stopping antidepressants (Akerblad et al., 2006; Dawson et al., 1998). No differences have been observed in relapse rates when individual antidepressants are compared (Bump et al., 2001; Franchini et al., 2000a; Lonnqvist et al., 1995; Montgomery et al., 1998; Walters et al., 1999).

After antidepressant discontinuation the greatest risk of relapse occurs in the first six months (Thase, 2006) but can continue to over two years (Frank et al., 1990). Published studies are consistent in supporting continuing antidepressant use for a minimum of six to nine months after any episode of depression, with persisting benefit from continuing further in those with more recurrent depression (Dawson et al., 1998; Geddes et al., 2003; Reimherr et al., 1998). A number of studies with TCAs and related drugs have favoured ongoing treatment with the dose required to achieve remission compared to a reduced 'maintenance dose' (Dawson et al., 1998; Frank et al., 1993; Reynolds et al., 1999; Rouillon et al., 1991); while the evidence with SSRIs in this regard is less clear there are data suggesting greater protection at higher doses (Franchini et al., 2000b). Taken together these data would support ongoing prescription of antidepressant at the dose taken to achieve remission. Despite the proven efficacy of antidepressants over placebo in reducing relapse rates published trials have shown that a cohort of patients will suffer a relapse while purportedly continuing to take medication. It is not clear if this is a true loss of effect to the drug, a loss of placebo effect, non-adherence or due to illness factors (Byrne & Rothschild, 1998; Thase, 2006). In this context the long-term use of antidepressants may be better conceived of as modifying risk or severity of depressive relapse rather than 'curing' depression.

7.6.2 Treatment of Relapse

The treatment of patients relapsing while continuing on prophylactic treatment is a major clinical problem. The first question that arises is whether to change treatment or persist with the current antidepressants. Existing data with regards to 'next-step treatments' (switching or combining drug treatments after relapse) is limited. Open studies of increasing the dose of the current antidepressant (SSRIs/SNRIs) report 57–90% response rates (Fava et al., 2002; Fava et al., 1995, 2006; Franchini et al., 2000b; Schmidt et al., 2002). Taken together this evidence suggests that increasing the dose of the current antidepressant may be effective in the majority of patients while there is presently a lack of evidence for other strategies. It should also be remembered that a significant proportion of depressive relapses appear self-limiting over a three-month period; in a group of patients followed for up to 15 years of those who suffered a relapse 52% of patients (including those receiving and not receiving antidepressants) recovered in the first three months (Posternak et al., 2006).

7.6.3 Stopping Antidepressants

The reasons for stopping antidepressants are complex and depend on the stage of treatment. Common reasons are patient choice, including feeling better, perceptions regarding continued prophylaxis and dissatisfaction with efficacy or tolerability. Pregnancy is another important reason for discontinuation (Petersen et al., 2011). Discontinuation or withdrawal symptoms have been described with all of the main classes including TCAs, MAOIs, SSRIs, SNRIs and mirtazapine (Howland, 2010) although symptoms are variable and differ between classes. The mean time to onset of symptoms is about two days with resolution usually after five to eight days.

The range of symptoms induced by antidepressant discontinuation include sleep disturbance, gastrointestinal symptoms, affective symptoms and general somatic symptoms such as lethargy and headache. In addition, drugs inhibiting 5-HT reuptake are associated with sensory symptoms such as electric shock feelings and paraesthesia, disequilibrium symptoms and tinnitus. MAOIs may cause more severe symptoms including worsening depression and anxiety, confusion and psychotic symptoms. In most patients, discontinuation symptoms are self-limiting and of short duration; however, in a minority of cases they can be severe and last several weeks and there is potential for misdiagnosis as depressive relapse. Reintroduction of the same class of antidepressant appears to suppress symptoms rapidly (Ruhe et al., 2006) and with SSRIs (or SNRIs) an option is to switch to fluoxetine which can then be stopped abruptly due to its long half-life.

It is presumed that tapering is an effective strategy to minimize discontinuation symptoms but there is a lack of evidence for the optimal rate of taper, with opinions varying from a few weeks to a year (Greden, 1993). A study randomizing patients on SSRIs/venlafaxine to a 3-day or 14-day taper found a discontinuation syndrome in 46% of patients with no difference according to rate of taper (Tint et al., 2007). However, a case note review of nearly 400 patients followed up for an average of nearly three years suggested that the risk of relapse into a new episode of illness is higher following rapid (one to seven days) versus gradual (14 days or more) discontinuation of antidepressants (Baldessarini et al., 2010).

An additional factor that should be considered when stopping antidepressants is the consequence of relapse given that the highest risk of relapse is in the six months after stopping. If antidepressants are stopped at a critical time in a person's life (e.g. examinations, starting a new job or going to university etc.) then the impact of a relapse is likely to be more serious than if discontinuation is attempted when the person is not at a critical point in their life.

The BAP guidelines for treating depressive disorders with antidepressants recommend taking into account the clinical situation to determine the rate of taper when antidepressants are to be stopped (Cleare et al., 2015). Serious adverse events may warrant rapid withdrawal of treatment. Outside of this scenario, a minimum four-week taper is recommended after longer-term treatment. However, tapering over several months may be appropriate for planned withdrawal after long-term prophylaxis.

References

Aan Het Rot M, Zarate CA Jr, Charney DS, Mathew SJ (2012). Ketamine for depression: where do we go from here? *Biol Psychiatry*, 72(7), 537–547. doi:10.1016/j.biopsych.2012.05.003.

Aberg-Wistedt A, Agren H, Ekselius L, Bengtsson F, Akerblad AC (2000). Sertraline versus paroxetine in major depression:

clinical outcome after six months of continuous therapy. *J Clin Psychopharmacol*, 20, 645–652.

Adli M, Baethge C, Heinz A, Langlitz N, Bauer M (2005). Is dose escalation of antidepressants a rational strategy after a medium-dose treatment has failed? A systematic review. *Eur Arch Psychiatry Clin Neurosci*, 255, 387–400.

Akerblad AC, Bengtsson F, von Knorring L, Ekselius L (2006). Response, remission and relapse in relation to adherence in primary care treatment of depression: a 2-year outcome study. *Int Clin Psychopharmacol*, 21, 117–124.

Alvarez E, Perez V, Artigas F (2014). Pharmacology and clinical potential of vortioxetine in the treatment of major depressive disorder. *Neuropsychiatr Dis Treat*, 10, 1297–1307.

American Psychiatric Association (2013). *Diagnostic and Statistical Manual of Mental Disorders*, 5th ed. Arlington, VA: American Psychiatric Association.

Anderson IM (2000). Selective serotonin reuptake inhibitors versus tricyclic antidepressants: a meta-analysis of efficacy and tolerability. *J Affect Disord*, 58, 19–36.

Anderson IM (2001). Meta-analytical studies on new antidepressants. *Br Med Bull*, 57, 161–178.

Anderson IM (2003). Drug treatment of depression: reflections on the evidence. *Adv Psychiatr Treat*, 9, 11–20.

Anglin R, Yuan Y, Moayyedi P, et al. (2014). Risk of upper gastrointestinal bleeding with selective serotonin reuptake inhibitors with or without concurrent nonsteroidal anti-inflammatory use: a systematic review and meta-analysis. *Am J Gastroenterol*, 109(6), 811–819. doi:10.1038/ajg.2014.82.

Angst J, Scheidegger P, Stabl M (1993). Efficacy of moclobemide in different patient groups. Results of new subscales of the Hamilton Depression Rating Scale. *Clin Neuropharmacol*, 16(Suppl 2), S55–S62.

Angst J, Gamma A, Bowden CL, et al. (2012). Diagnostic criteria for bipolarity based on an international sample of 5,635 patients with DSM-IV major depressive episodes. *Eur Arch Psychiatry Clin Neurosci*, 262(1), 3–11. doi:10.1007/s00406-011-0228-0.

Appelberg BG, Syvalahti EK, Koskinen TE, et al. (2001). Patients with severe depression may benefit from buspirone augmentation of selective serotonin reuptake inhibitors: results from a placebo-controlled, randomized, double-blind, placebo wash-in study. *J Clin Psychiatry*, 62, 448–452.

Aronson R, Offman HJ, Joffe RT, Naylor CD (1996). Triiodothyronine augmentation in the treatment of refractory depression. A meta-analysis. *Arch Gen Psychiatry*, 53, 842–848.

Bair MJ, Robinson RL, Eckert GJ, et al. (2004). Impact of pain on depression treatment response in primary care. *Psychosom Med*, 66, 17–22.

Baldessarini RJ, Tondo L, Ghiana C, Lepri B (2010). Illness risk following rapid versus gradual discontinuation of antidepressants. *Am J Psychiatry*, 167, 934–994.

Baldwin DS, Anderson IM, Nutt DJ, et al. (2005). Evidence-based guidelines for the pharmacological treatment of anxiety disorders: recommendations from the British Association for Psychopharmacology. *J Psychopharmacol*, 19, 567–596.

Barbee JG, Thompson TR, Jamhour NJ, et al. (2011). A double-blind placebo-controlled trial of lamotrigine as an antidepressant augmentation agent in treatment-refractory unipolar depression. *J Clin Psychiatry*, 72(10), 1405–1412. doi:10.4088/JCP.09m05355gre.

Barbosa L, Berk M, Vorster M (2003). A double-blind, randomized, placebo-controlled trial of augmentation with lamotrigine or placebo in patients concomitantly treated with fluoxetine for resistant major depressive episodes. *J Clin Psychiatry*, 64, 403–407.

Bateman DN (2003). Poisonous substances: antidepressants. *Medicine*, 31, 32–34.

Bauer M, Dell'osso L, Kasper S, et al. (2013). Extended-release quetiapine fumarate (quetiapine XR) monotherapy and quetiapine XR or lithium as add-on to antidepressants in patients with treatment-resistant major depressive disorder. *J Affect Disord*, 151(1), 209–219. doi:10.1016/j.jad.2013.05.079.

Bauer M, Adli M, Ricken R, Severus E, Pilhatsch M (2014). Role of lithium augmentation in the management of major depressive disorder. *CNS Drugs*, 28(4), 331–342. doi:10.1007/s40263-014-0152-8.

Baumann P, Ulrich S, Eckermann G, et al. (2005). The AGNP-TDM Expert Group Consensus Guidelines: focus on therapeutic monitoring of antidepressants. *Dialogues Clin Neurosci*, 7, 231–247.

Berman RM, Marcus RN, Swanink R, et al. (2007). The efficacy and safety of aripiprazole as adjunctive therapy in major depressive disorder: a multicenter, randomized, double-blind, placebo-controlled study. *J Clin Psychiatry*, 68, 843–853.

Birkenhager TK, van den Broek WW, Moleman P, Bruijn JA (2006). Outcome of a 4-step treatment algorithm for depressed inpatients. *J Clin Psychiatry*, 67, 1266–1271.

Blier P, Gobbi G, Turcotte JE, et al. (2009). Mirtazapine and paroxetine in major depression: a comparison of monotherapy versus their combination from treatment initiation. *Eur Neuropsychopharmacol*, 19(7), 457–465.

Blier P, Ward HE, Tremblay P, et al. (2010). Combination of antidepressant medications from treatment initiation for major depressive disorder: a double-blind randomized study. *Am J Psychiatry*, 167(3), 281–288.

Bridge JA, Iyengar S, Salary CB, et al. (2007). Clinical response and risk for reported suicidal ideation and suicide attempts in pediatric antidepressant treatment: a meta-analysis of randomized controlled trials. *JAMA*, 297, 1683–1696.

Brown WA (2007). Treatment response in melancholia. *Acta Psychiatr Scand*, 115(Suppl 433), 125–129.

Bryant SG, Fisher S, Kluge RM (1987). Long-term versus short-term amitriptyline side effects as measured by a postmarketing surveillance system. *J Clin Psychopharmacol*, 7, 78–82.

Buckley NA, McManus PR (2002). Fatal toxicity of serotoninergic and other antidepressant drugs: analysis of United Kingdom mortality data. *BMJ*, 325, 1332–1333.

Bukh JD, Bock C, Vinberg M, Kessing LV (2013). The effect of prolonged duration of untreated depression on antidepressant treatment outcome. *J Affect Disord*, 145(1), 42–48. doi:10.1016/j.jad.2012.07.008.

Bump GM, Mulsant BH, Pollock BG, et al. (2001). Paroxetine versus nortriptyline in the continuation and maintenance treatment of depression in the elderly. *Depress Anxiety*, 13, 38–44.

Burke WJ, Gergel I, Bose A (2002). Fixed-dose trial of the single isomer SSRI escitalopram in depressed outpatients. *J Clin Psychiatry*, 63, 331–336.

Byrne SE, Rothschild AJ (1998). Loss of antidepressant efficacy during maintenance therapy: possible mechanisms and treatments. *J Clin Psychiatry*, 59, 279–288.

Canuso CM, Singh JB, Fedgchin M, et al. (2018). Efficacy and safety of intranasal esketamine for the rapid reduction of symptoms of depression and suicidality in patients at imminent risk for suicide: results of a double-blind, randomized, placebo-controlled study. *Am J Psychiatry*, 175, 620–630. doi:10.1176/appi.ajp.2018.17060720.

Carpenter LL, Yasmin S, Price LH (2002). A double-blind, placebo-controlled study of antidepressant augmentation with mirtazapine. *Biol Psychiatry*, 51, 183–188.

Castro VM, Clements CC, Murphy SN, et al. (2013). QT interval and antidepressant use: a cross sectional study of electronic health records. *BMJ*, 346, f288. doi:10.1136/bmj.f288.

Cheeta S, Schifano F, Oyefeso A, Webb L, Ghodse AH (2004). Antidepressant-related deaths and antidepressant prescriptions in England and Wales, 1998–2000. *Br J Psychiatry*, 184, 41–47.

Cheng YL, Hu HY, Lin XH, et al. (2015). Use of SSRI, but not SNRI, increased upper and lower gastrointestinal bleeding: a nationwide population-based cohort study in Taiwan. *Medicine (Baltimore)*, 94(46), e2022. doi:10.1097/MD.0000000000002022.

Cipriani A, Hawton K, Stockton S, Geddes JR (2013). Lithium in the prevention of suicide in mood disorders: updated systematic review and meta-analysis. *BMJ*, 346, f3646. https://doi.org/10.1136/bmj.f3646.

Cipriani A, Furukawa TA, Salanti G, et al. (2018). Comparative efficacy and acceptability of 21 antidepressant drugs for the acute treatment of adults with major depressive disorder: a systematic review and network meta-analysis. *Lancet*, 391(10128), 1357–1366.

Cleare A, Pariante CM, Young AH, et al. (2015). Evidence-based guidelines for treating depressive disorders with antidepressants: a revision of the 2008 British Association for Psychopharmacology guidelines. *J Psychopharmacology*, 29(5), 459–525.

Cramer JA, Rosenheck R (1998). Compliance with medication regimens for mental and physical disorders. *Psychiatr Serv*, 49, 196–201.

Crossley NA, Bauer M (2007). Acceleration and augmentation of antidepressants with lithium for depressive disorders: two meta-analyses of randomized, placebo-controlled trials. *J Clin Psychiatry*, 68, 935–940.

Dawson R, Lavori PW, Coryell WH, Endicott J, Keller MB (1998). Maintenance strategies for unipolar depression: an observational study of levels of treatment and recurrence. *J Affect Disord*, 49, 31–44.

de Abajo FJ, Garcia-Rodriguez LA (2008). Risk of upper gastrointestinal tract bleeding associated with selective serotonin reuptake inhibitors and venlafaxine therapy: interaction with nonsteroidal anti-inflammatory drugs and effect of acid-suppressing agents. *Arch Gen Psychiatry*, 65, 795–803.

Delgado PL (2004). Common pathways of depression and pain. *J Clin Psychiatry*, 65(Suppl 12), 16–19.

Delgado PL, Brannan SK, Mallinckrodt CH, et al. (2005). Sexual functioning assessed in 4 double-blind placebo- and paroxetine-controlled trials of duloxetine for major depressive disorder. *J Clin Psychiatry*, 66, 686–692.

Demyttenaere K, Albert A, Mesters P, et al. (2005). What happens with adverse events during 6 months of treatment with selective serotonin reuptake inhibitors? *J Clin Psychiatry*, 66, 859–863.

Detke MJ, Wiltse CG, Mallinckrodt CH, et al. (2004). Duloxetine in the acute and long-term treatment of major depressive disorder: a placebo- and paroxetine-controlled trial. *Eur Neuropsychopharmacol*, 14, 457–470.

DeVeaugh-Geiss AM, West SL, Miller WC, et al. (2010). The adverse effects of comorbid pain on depression outcomes in primary care patients: results from the ARTIST trial. *Pain Med*, 11(5), 732–741. doi:10.1111/j.1526-4637.2010.00830.x.

Dombrovski AY, Mulsant BH, Houck PR, et al. (2007). Residual symptoms and recurrence during maintenance treatment of late-life depression. *J Affect Disord*, 103, 77–82.

Dornseif BE, Dunlop SR, Potvin JH, Wernicke JF (1989). Effect of dose escalation after low-dose fluoxetine therapy. *Psychopharmacol Bull*, 25, 71–79.

Dotoli D, Spagnolo C, Bongiorno F, et al. (2006). Relapse during a 6-month continuation treatment with fluvoxamine in an Italian population: the role of clinical, psychosocial and genetic variables. *Prog Neuropsychopharmacol Biol Psychiatry*, 30, 442–448.

Dubini A, Bosc M, Polin V (1997). Noradrenaline-selective versus serotonin-selective antidepressant therapy: differential effects on social functioning. *J Psychopharmacol*, 11, S17–S23.

Edwards JG, Anderson I (1999). Systematic review and guide to selection of selective serotonin reuptake inhibitors. *Drugs*, 57(4), 507–533.

El-Khalili N, Joyce M, Atkinson S, et al. (2010). Extended-release quetiapine fumerate (quetiapine XR) as adjunctive therapy in major depressive disorder (MDD) in patients with an inadequate response to ongoing antidepressant treatment: a multicentre, randomized, double-blind, placebo-controlled study. *Int J Neuropsychopharmacol*, 13, 917–932.

Ezquiaga E, Garcia A, Bravo F, Pallares T (1998). Factors associated with outcome in major depression: a 6-month prospective study. *Soc Psychiatry Psychiatr Epidemiol*, 33, 552–557.

Fava GA, Ruini C, Rafanelli C, Grandi S (2002). Cognitive behavior approach to loss of clinical effect during long-term antidepressant treatment: a pilot study. *Am J Psychiatry*, 159, 2094–2095.

Fava M, Rappe SM, Pava JA, et al. (1995). Relapse in patients on long-term fluoxetine treatment: response to increased fluoxetine dose. *J Clin Psychiatry*, 56, 52–55.

Fava M, Uebelacker LA, Alpert JE, et al. (1997). Major depressive subtypes and treatment response. *Biol Psychiatry*, 42, 568–576.

Fava M, Detke MJ, Balestrieri M, et al. (2006). Management of depression relapse: re-initiation of duloxetine treatment or dose increase. *J Psychiatr Res*, 40, 328–336.

Fava M, Thase ME, DeBattista C, et al. (2007). Modafinil augmentation of selective serotonin reuptake inhibitor therapy in MDD partial responders with persistent fatigue and sleepiness. *Ann Clin Psychiatry*, 19, 153–159.

Fekadu A, Wooderson S, Donaldson C, et al. (2009). A multidimensional tool to quantify treatment resistance in depression: the Maudsley staging method. *J Clin Psychiatry*, 70, 177–184.

Fekadu A, Donocik J, Cleare AJ (2018). Standardisation framework for the Maudsley staging method for treatment resistance in depression. *BMC Psychiatry*, 18, 100. Available at: https://bmcpsychiatry.biomedcentral.com/articles/10.1186/s12888-018-1679-x.

Fergusson D, Doucette S, Glass KC, et al. (2005). Association between suicide attempts and selective serotonin reuptake inhibitors: systematic review of randomised controlled trials. *BMJ*, 330, 396.

Ferreri M, Lavergne F, Berlin I, Payan C, Puech AJ (2001). Benefits from mianserin augmentation of fluoxetine in patients with major depression non-responders to fluoxetine alone. *Acta Psychiatr Scand*, 103, 66–72.

Flint AJ, Rifat SL (1998). Two-year outcome of psychotic depression in late life. *Am J Psychiatry*, 155, 178–183.

Fond G, Loundou A, Rabu C, et al. (2014). Ketamine administration in depressive disorders: a systematic review and meta-analysis. *Psychopharmacology (Berl)*, 231(18), 3663–3676. doi:10.1007/s00213-014-3664-5.

Franchini L, Gasperini M, Zanardi R, Smeraldi E (2000a). Four-year follow-up study of sertraline and fluvoxamine in long-term treatment of unipolar subjects with high recurrence rate. *J Affect Disord*, 58, 233–236.

Franchini L, Rossini D, Bongiorno F, et al. (2000b). Will a second prophylactic treatment with a higher dosage of the same antidepressant either prevent or delay new depressive episodes? *Psychiatry Res*, 96, 81–85.

Frank E, Kupfer DJ, Perel JM, et al. (1990). Three-year outcomes for maintenance therapies in recurrent depression. *Arch Gen Psychiatry*, 47, 1093–1099.

Frank E, Kupfer DJ, Perel JM, et al. (1993). Comparison of full-dose versus half-dose pharmacotherapy in the maintenance treatment of recurrent depression. *J Affect Disord*, 27, 139–145.

Furukawa TA, McGuire H, Barbui C (2002). Meta-analysis of effects and side effects of low dosage tricyclic antidepressants in depression: systematic review. *BMJ*, 325, 991.

Geddes JR, Carney SM, Davies C, et al. (2003). Relapse prevention with antidepressant drug treatment in depressive disorders: a systematic review. *Lancet*, 361, 653–661.

Ghaziuddin M, Ghaziuddin N, Stein GS (1990). Life events and the recurrence of depression. *Can J Psychiatry*, 35, 239–242.

Gibbons RD, Brown CH, Hur K, et al. (2007). Early evidence on the effects of regulators' suicidality warnings on SSRI prescriptions and suicide in children and adolescents. *Am J Psychiatry*, 164, 1356–1363.

Gijsman HJ, Geddes JR, Rendell JM, et al. (2004). Antidepressants for bipolar depression: a systematic review of randomized, controlled trials. *Am J Psychiatry*, 161 1537–1547.

Goldstein DJ, Lu Y, Detke MJ, et al. (2004). Duloxetine in the treatment of depression: a double-blind placebo-controlled comparison with paroxetine. *J Clin Psychopharmacol*, 24, 389–399.

Goodwin GM, Haddad PM, Ferrier IN, et al. (2016). Evidence-based guidelines for treating bipolar disorder: revised third edition recommendations from the British Association for Psychopharmacology. *J Psychopharmacol*, 30(6), 495–553.

Greden JF (1993). Antidepressant maintenance medications: when to discontinue and how to stop. *J Clin Psychiatry*, 54 Suppl, 39–45.

Greist J, McNamara RK, Mallinckrodt CH, Rayamajhi JN, Raskin J (2004). Incidence and duration of antidepressant-induced nausea: duloxetine compared with paroxetine and fluoxetine. *Clin Ther*, 26, 1446–1455.

Gunnell D, Saperia J, Ashby D (2005). Selective serotonin reuptake inhibitors (SSRIs) and suicide in adults: meta-analysis of drug company data from placebo controlled, randomised controlled trials submitted to the MHRA's safety review. *BMJ*, 330, 385.

Guo T, Xiang YT, Xiao L, et al. (2015). Measurement-based care versus standard care for major depression: a randomized controlled trial with blind raters. *Am J Psychiatry*, 172(10), 1004–1013.

Gusmao R, Quintao S, McDaid D, et al. (2013). Antidepressant utilization and suicide in Europe: an ecological multi-national study. *PLoS One*, 8, e66455.

Haddad PM, Anderson IM (2002). Antipsychotic-related QTc prolongation, torsade de pointes and sudden death. *Drugs*, 62, 1649–1671.

Halperin D, Reber G (2007). Influence of antidepressants on hemostasis. *Dialogues Clin Neurosci*, 9, 47–59.

Hammerlein A, Derendorf H, Lowenthal DT (1998). Pharmacokinetic and pharmacodynamic changes in the elderly. Clinical implications. *Clin Pharmacokinet*, 35, 49–64.

Hansen R, Gaynes B, Thieda P, et al. (2008). Meta-analysis of major depressive disorder relapse and recurrence with second-generation antidepressants. *Psychiatr Serv*, 59 (10), 1121–1130. doi:10.1176/appi.ps.59.10.1121.

Hawton K, Bergen H, Simkin S, et al. (2010). Toxicity of antidepressants: rates of suicide relative to prescribing and non-fatal overdose. *Br J Psychiatry*, 196(5), 354–358. doi:10.1192/bjp.bp.109.070219.

Healy D, McMonagle T (1997). The enhancement of social functioning as a therapeutic principle in the management of depression. *J Psychopharmacol*, 11, S25–S31.

Henkel V, Mergl R, Allgaier AK, et al. (2006). Treatment of depression with atypical features: a meta-analytic approach. *Psychiatry Res*, 141, 89–101.

Hoffman L, Enders J, Luo J, et al. (2003). Impact of an antidepressant management program on medication adherence. *Am J Manag Care*, 9, 70–80.

Howland RH (2010). Potential adverse effects of discontinuing psychotropic drugs: part 2: antidepressant drugs. *J Psychosoc Nurs Ment Health Serv*, 48, 9–12. doi:10.3928/02793695-20100527-98.

Iosifescu DV, Nierenberg AA, Alpert JE, et al. (2004). Comorbid medical illness and relapse of major depressive disorder in the continuation phase of treatment. *Psychosomatics*, 45, 419–425.

Isbister GK, Bowe SJ, Dawson A, Whyte IM (2004). Relative toxicity of selective serotonin reuptake inhibitors (SSRIs) in overdose. *J Toxicol Clin Toxicol*, 42, 277–285.

Jacobsen PL, Mahableshwarkar AR, Palo WA, et al. (2016). Treatment-emergent sexual dysfunction in randomized trials of vortioxetine for major depressive disorder or generalized anxiety disorder: a pooled analysis. *CNS Spectr*, 21, 367–378.

Jick H, Kaye JA, Jick SS (2004). Antidepressants and the risk of suicidal behaviors. *JAMA*, 292, 338–343.

Joint Formulary Committee (2018). *British National Formulary*, 75th ed. London: BMJ Group and Pharmaceutical Press.

Kanai T, Takeuchi H, Furukawa TA, et al. (2003). Time to recurrence after recovery from major depressive episodes and its predictors. *Psychol Med*, 33, 839–845.

Karp JF, Scott J, Houck P, et al. (2005). Pain predicts longer time to remission during treatment of recurrent depression. *J Clin Psychiatry*, 66, 591–597.

Katz MM, Tekell JL, Bowden CL, et al. (2004). Onset and early behavioral effects of pharmacologically different antidepressants and placebo in depression. *Neuropsychopharmacology*, 29, 566–579.

Kessing LV (1998). Recurrence in affective disorder. II. Effect of age and gender. *Br J Psychiatry*, 172, 29–34.

Kessing LV (2003). Subtypes of depressive episodes according to ICD-10: prediction of risk of relapse and suicide. *Psychopathology*, 36, 285–291.

Kessing LV (2007). Epidemiology of subtypes of depression. *Acta Psychiatr Scand*, 433 Suppl, 85–89.

Kessing LV, Andersen PK (2005). Predictive effects of previous episodes on the risk of recurrence in depressive and bipolar disorders. *Curr Psychiatry Rep*, 7, 413–420.

Kessler D, Burns A, Tallon D, et al. (2018). Combining mirtazapine with SSRIs or SNRIs for treatment-resistant depression: the MIR RCT. *Health Technol Assess*, 22(63), 1–136.

Köhler-Forsberg O, Lydholm N, Hjorthøj C, et al. (2019). Efficacy of anti-inflammatory treatment on major depressive disorder or depressive symptoms: meta-analysis of clinical trials. *Acta Psychiatr Scand*, 139, 404–419.

Lader M (1983). Combined use of tricyclic antidepressants and monoamine oxidase inhibitors. *J Clin Psychiatry*, 44, 20–24.

Lam RW, Gorman CP, Michalon M, et al. (1995). Multicenter, placebo-controlled study of fluoxetine in seasonal affective disorder. *Am J Psychiatry*, 152, 1765–1770.

Landen M, Bjorling G, Agren H, Fahlen T (1998). A randomized, double-blind, placebo-controlled trial of buspirone in combination with an SSRI in patients with treatment-refractory depression. *J Clin Psychiatry*, 59, 664–668.

Lee P, Shu L, Xu X, et al. (2007). Once-daily duloxetine 60 mg in the treatment of major depressive disorder: multicenter, double-blind, randomized, paroxetine-controlled, non-inferiority trial in China, Korea, Taiwan and Brazil. *Psychiatry Clin Neurosci*, 61, 295–307.

Leinonen E, Skarstein J, Behnke K, Agren H, Helsdingen JT (1999). Efficacy and tolerability of mirtazapine versus citalopram: a double-blind, randomized study in patients with major depressive disorder. Nordic Antidepressant Study Group. *Int Clin Psychopharmacol*, 14, 329–337.

Leucht S, Hierl S, Kissling W, Dold M, Davis JM (2012). Putting the efficacy of psychiatric and general medicine medication into perspective: review of meta-analyses. *Br J Psychiatry*, 200(2), 97–106. doi:10.1192/bjp.bp.111.096594.

Leuchter AF, Husain MM, Cook IA, et al. (2010). Painful physical symptoms and treatment outcome in major depressive disorder: a STAR*D (Sequenced Treatment Alternatives to Relieve Depression) report. *Psychol Med*, 40(2), 239–251. doi:10.1017/S0033291709006035.

Licht RW, Qvitzau S (2002). Treatment strategies in patients with major depression not responding to first-line sertraline treatment. A randomised study of extended duration of treatment, dose increase or mianserin augmentation. *Psychopharmacology (Berl)*, 161, 143–151.

Lonnqvist J, Sihvo S, Syvalahti E, et al. (1995). Moclobemide and fluoxetine in the prevention of relapses following acute treatment of depression. *Acta Psychiatr Scand*, 91, 189–194.

Maes M, Libbrecht I, van Hunsel F, Campens D, Meltzer HY (1999). Pindolol and mianserin augment the antidepressant activity of fluoxetine in hospitalized major depressed patients, including those with treatment resistance. *J Clin Psychopharmacol*, 19, 177–182.

Maidment R, Livingston G, Katona C (2002). Just keep taking the tablets: adherence to antidepressant treatment in older people in primary care. *Int J Geriatr Psychiatry*, 17(8), 752–757.

Masand PS, Gupta S (2002). Long-term side effects of newer-generation antidepressants: SSRIs, venlafaxine, nefazodone, bupropion, and mirtazapine. *Ann Clin Psychiatry*, 14, 175–182.

Mazure CM, Bruce ML, Maciejewski PK, Jacobs SC (2000). Adverse life events and cognitive-personality characteristics in the prediction of major depression and antidepressant response. *Am J Psychiatry*, 157, 896–903.

McAllister-Williams RH, Christmas D, Cleare AJ, et al. (2018). Multiple-therapy-resistant-major depressive disorder: a clinically important concept. *Br J Psychiatry*, 212(5), 274–278. doi:10.1192/bjp.2017.33.

McGirr A, Berlim MT, Bond DJ, et al. (2015). A systematic review and meta-analysis of randomized, double-blind, placebo-controlled trials of ketamine in the rapid treatment of major depressive episodes. *Psychol Med*, 45(4), 693–704. doi:10.1017/S0033291714001603.

McGrath PJ, Stewart JW, Fava M, et al. (2006a). Tranylcypromine versus venlafaxine plus mirtazapine following three failed antidepressant medication trials for depression: a STAR*D report. *Am J Psychiatry*, 163, 1531–1541.

McGrath PJ, Stewart JW, Quitkin FM, et al. (2006b). Predictors of relapse in a prospective study of fluoxetine treatment of major depression. *Am J Psychiatry*, 163, 1542–1548.

McLaughlin T, Hogue SL, Stang PE (2007). Once-daily bupropion associated with improved patient adherence compared with twice-daily bupropion in treatment of depression. *Am J Ther*, 14, 221–225.

Medhus A, Heskestad S, Tjemsland L (1994). Mianserin added to tricyclic antidepressant in depressed patients not responding to a tricyclic antidepressant alone. A randomised, placebo-controlled, double-blind trial. *Nord J Psychiatry*, 48, 355–358.

Medicines and Healthcare products Regulatory Agency (2011). Citalopram and escitalopram: QT interval prolongation (online). Available at: www.gov.uk/drug-safety-update/citalopram-and-escitalopram-qt-interval-prolongation (last accessed 16.10.19).

Melander H, Salmonson T, Abadie E, et al. (2008). A regulatory Apologia – a review of placebo-controlled studies in regulatory submissions of new-generation antidepressants. *Eur Neuropsychopharmacol*, 18(9), 623–627.

Modell JG, Rosenthal NE, Harriett AE, et al. (2005). Seasonal affective disorder and its prevention by anticipatory treatment with bupropion XL. *Biol Psychiatry*, 58, 658–667.

Montgomery SA, Reimitz PE, Zivkov M (1998). Mirtazapine versus amitriptyline in the long-term treatment of depression: a double-blind placebo-controlled study. *Int Clin Psychopharmacol*, 13, 63–67.

Morgan ML, Cook IA, Rapkin AJ, Leuchter AF (2005). Estrogen augmentation of antidepressants in perimenopausal depression: a pilot study. *J Clin Psychiatry*, 66, 774–780.

Morgan O, Griffiths C, Baker A, Majeed A (2004). Fatal toxicity of antidepressants in England and Wales, 1993–2002. *Health Stat Q*, 23, 18–24.

Moscovitch A, Blashko CA, Eagles JM, et al. (2004). A placebo-controlled study of sertraline in the treatment of outpatients with seasonal affective disorder. *Psychopharmacology (Berl)*, 171, 390–397.

Mueller TI, Leon AC, Keller MB, et al. (1999). Recurrence after recovery from major depressive disorder during 15 years of observational follow-up. *Am J Psychiatry*, 156, 1000–1006.

Murrough JW, Iosifescu DV, Chang LC, et al. (2013a). Antidepressant efficacy of ketamine in treatment-resistant major depression: a two-site randomized controlled trial. *Am J Psychiatry*, 170(10), 1134–1142. doi:10.1176/appi.ajp.2013.13030392.

Murrough JW, Perez AM, Pillemer S, et al. (2013b). Rapid and longer-term antidepressant effects of repeated ketamine infusions in treatment-resistant major depression. *Biol Psychiatry*, 74(4), 250–256. doi:10.1016/j.biopsych.2012.06.022.

National Institute for Clinical Excellence (2004). *Depression: the management of depression in primary and secondary care.* Clinical guideline [CG23]. Available at: www.nice.org.uk/guidance/cg23 (last accessed 20.10.19).

National Institute for Health and Clinical Excellence (NICE) (2009). *Depression in adults: the treatment and management of depression in adults (update).* Clinical guideline [CG90]. London: National Institute for Health and Care Excellence. Available at: www.nice.org.uk/guidance/cg90/chapter/1-guidance (last accessed 16.10.19).

Nelson JC, Papakostas GI (2009). Atypical antipsychotic augmentation in major depressive disorder: a meta-analysis of placebo-controlled randomized trials. *Am J Psychiatry*, 166(9), 980–991. doi:10.1176/appi.ajp.2009.09030312.

Nelson JC, Portera L, Leon AC (2005a). Are there differences in the symptoms that respond to a selective serotonin or norepinephrine reuptake inhibitor? *Biol Psychiatry*, 57, 1535–1542.

Nelson JC, Portera L, Leon AC (2005b). Residual symptoms in depressed patients after treatment with fluoxetine or reboxetine. *J Clin Psychiatry*, 66, 1409–1414.

Nierenberg AA, McLean NE, Alpert JE, et al. (1995). Early nonresponse to fluoxetine as a predictor of poor 8-week outcome. *Am J Psychiatry*, 152, 1500–1503.

Nierenberg AA, Farabaugh AH, Alpert JE, et al. (2000). Timing of onset of antidepressant response with fluoxetine treatment. *Am J Psychiatry*, 157, 1423–1428.

Nierenberg AA, Fava M, Trivedi MH, et al. (2006). A comparison of lithium and T(3) augmentation following two failed medication treatments for depression: a STAR*D report. *Am J Psychiatry*, 163, 1519–1530.

Nurnberg H, Hensley PL, Heiman JR, et al. (2008). Sildenafil treatment of women with antidepressant-associated sexual dysfunction: a randomized controlled trial. *JAMA*, 300, 395–404.

Ohayon MM, Schatzberg AF (2003). Using chronic pain to predict depressive morbidity in the general population. *Arch Gen Psychiatry*, 60, 39–47.

Okuda A, Suzuki T, Kishi T, et al. (2010). Duration of untreated illness and antidepressant fluvoxamine response in major depressive disorder. *Psychiatry Clin Neurosci*, 64(3), 268–273. doi:10.1111/j.1440-1819.2010.02091.x.

Pacchiarotti I, Bond DJ, Baldessarini RJ, et al. (2013). The International Society for Bipolar Disorders (ISBD) task force report on antidepressant use in bipolar disorders. *Am J Psychiatry*, 170(11), 1249–1262. doi:10.1176/appi.ajp.2013.13020185.

Papakostas GI, Fava M, Thase ME (2008). Treatment of SSRI-resistant depression: a meta-analysis comparing within- versus across-class switches. *Biol Psychiatry*, 63(7), 699–704.

Parker G (2000). Classifying depression: should paradigms lost be regained? *Am J Psychiatry*, 157, 1195–1203.

Partonen T, Lonnqvist J (1996). Moclobemide and fluoxetine in treatment of seasonal affective disorder. *J Affect Disord*, 41, 93–99.

Paykel ES, Tanner J (1976). Life events, depressive relapse and maintenance treatment. *Psychol Med*, 6, 481–485.

Paykel ES, Ramana R, Cooper Z, et al. (1995). Residual symptoms after partial remission: an important outcome in depression. *Psychol Med*, 25, 1171–1180.

Perahia DG, Wang F, Mallinckrodt CH, Walker DJ, Detke MJ (2006). Duloxetine in the treatment of major depressive disorder: a placebo- and paroxetine-controlled trial. *Eur Psychiatry*, 21, 367–378.

Perahia DG, Pritchett YL, Kajdasz DK, et al. (2008). A randomized, double-blind comparison of duloxetine and venlafaxine in the treatment of patients with major depressive disorder. *J Psychiatr Res*, 42, 22–34.

Petersen I, Gilbert RE, Evans SJ, Man SL, Nazareth I (2011). Pregnancy as a major determinant for discontinuation of antidepressants: an analysis of data from The Health Improvement Network. *J Clin Psychiatry*, 72(7), 979–985. doi:10.4088/JCP.10m06090blu.

Pope HG Jr, Cohane GH, Kanayama G, Siegel AJ, Hudson JI (2003). Testosterone gel supplementation for men with refractory depression: a randomized, placebo-controlled trial. *Am J Psychiatry*, 160(1), 105–111.

Pope HG, Amiaz R, Brennan BP, et al. (2010). Parallel-group placebo-controlled trial of testosterone gel in men with major depressive disorder displaying an incomplete response to standard antidepressant treatment. *J Clin Psychopharmacol*, 30(2), 126–134. doi:10.1097/JCP.0b013e3181d207ca.

Posternak MA, Zimmerman M (2005). Is there a delay in the antidepressant effect? A meta-analysis. *J Clin Psychiatry*, 66, 148–158.

Posternak MA, Zimmerman M (2007). Therapeutic effect of follow-up assessments on antidepressant and placebo response rates in antidepressant efficacy trials: meta-analysis. *Br J Psychiatry*, 190, 287–292.

Posternak MA, Solomon DA, Leon AC, et al. (2006). The naturalistic course of unipolar major depression in the absence of somatic therapy. *J Nerv Ment Dis*, 194, 324–329.

Quitkin FM, Petkova E, McGrath PJ, et al. (2003). When should a trial of fluoxetine for major depression be declared failed? *Am J Psychiatry*, 160, 734–740.

Raison CL, Rutherford RE, Woolwine BJ, et al. (2013). A randomized controlled trial of the tumor necrosis factor antagonist infliximab for treatment-resistant depression: the role of baseline inflammatory biomarkers. *JAMA Psychiatry*, 70(1), 31–41. doi:10.1001/2013.jamapsychiatry.4.

Ramana R, Paykel ES, Cooper Z, et al. (1995). Remission and relapse in major depression: a two-year prospective follow-up study. *Psychol Med*, 25, 1161–1170.

Reimherr FW, Amsterdam JD, Quitkin FM, et al. (1998). Optimal length of continuation therapy in depression: a prospective assessment during long-term fluoxetine treatment. *Am J Psychiatry*, 155, 1247–1253.

Reimherr FW, Strong RE, Marchant BK, Hedges DW, Wender PH (2001). Factors affecting return of symptoms 1 year after treatment in a 62-week controlled study of fluoxetine in major depression. *J Clin Psychiatry*, 62(Suppl 22), 16–23.

Reis M, Aamo T, Spigset O, Ahlner J (2009). Serum concentrations of antidepressant drugs in a naturalistic setting: compilation based on a large therapeutic drug monitoring database. *Ther Drug Monit*, 31(1), 42–56. doi:10.1097/FTD.0b013e31819114ea.

Reynolds CF, III, Perel JM, Frank E, et al. (1999). Three-year outcomes of maintenance nortriptyline treatment in late-life depression: a study of two fixed plasma levels. *Am J Psychiatry*, 156, 1177–1181.

Reynolds CF, III, Dew MA, Pollock BG, et al. (2006). Maintenance treatment of major depression in old age. *N Engl J Med*, 354, 1130–1138.

Robinson P, Katon W, Von Korff M, et al. (1997). The education of depressed primary care patients: what do patients think of interactive booklets and a video?*J Fam Pract*, 44, 562–571.

Rojo JE, Ros S, Aguera L, de la Gandara J, de Pedro JM (2005). Combined antidepressants: clinical experience. *Acta Psychiatr Scand Suppl*, 428, 25–31.

Ronalds C, Creed F, Stone K, Webb S, Tomenson B (1997). The outcome of anxiety and depressive disorders in general practice. *Br J Psychiatry*, 171, 427–433.

Rouillon F, Serrurier D, Miller HD, Gerard MJ (1991). Prophylactic efficacy of maprotiline on unipolar depression relapse. *J Clin Psychiatry*, 52, 423–431.

Rudolph RL, Fabre LF, Feighner JP, et al. (1998). A randomized, placebo-controlled, dose-response trial of venlafaxine hydrochloride in the treatment of major depression. *J Clin Psychiatry*, 59, 116–122.

Ruhe HG, Huyser J, Swinkels JA, Schene AH (2006). Switching antidepressants after a first selective serotonin reuptake inhibitor in major depressive disorder: a systematic review. *J Clin Psychiatry*, 67, 1836–1855.

Rush AJ, Trivedi MH, Wisniewski SR, et al. (2006a). Acute and longer-term outcomes in depressed outpatients requiring one or several treatment steps: a STAR*D report. *Am J Psychiatry*, 163, 1905–1917.

Rush AJ, Trivedi MH, Wisniewski SR, et al. (2006b). Bupropion-SR, sertraline or venlafaxine-XR after failure of SSRIs for depression. *N Engl J Med*, 354, 1231–1242.

Rush AJ, Trivedi MH, Stewart JW, et al. (2011). Combining medications to enhance depression outcomes (CO-MED): acute and long-term outcomes of a single-blind randomized study. *Am J Psychiatry*, 168, 689–701.

Sachs GS, Nierenberg AA, Calabrese JR, et al. (2007). Effectiveness of adjunctive antidepressant treatment for bipolar depression. *N Engl J Med*, 356(17), 1711–1722.

Sansone RA, Sansone, LA (2012). Antidepressant adherence: are patients taking their medications? *Innov Clin Neurosci*, 9(5–6), 41–46.

Schindler F, Anghelescu IG (2007). Lithium versus lamotrigine augmentation in treatment resistant unipolar depression: a randomized, open-label study. *Int Clin Psychopharmacol*, 22, 179–182.

Schmidt ME, Fava M, Zhang S, et al. (2002). Treatment approaches to major depressive disorder relapse. Part 1: dose increase. *Psychother Psychosom*, 71, 90–94.

Schueler Y-B, Koesters M, Wieseler B, et al. (2011). A systematic review of duloxetine and venlafaxine in major depression, including unpublished data. *Acta Psychiatr Scand*, 123, 247–265.

Schweizer E, Rynn M, Mandos LA, et al. (2001). The antidepressant effect of sertraline is not enhanced by dose titration: results from an outpatient clinical trial. *Int Clin Psychopharmacol*, 16, 137–143.

Servier Laboratories Limited (2012). SPC for Valdoxan.

Simon GE, Savarino J (2007). Suicide attempts among patients starting depression treatment with medications or psychotherapy. *Am J Psychiatry*, 164, 1029–1034.

Simon GE, Savarino J, Operskalski B, Wang PS (2006). Suicide risk during antidepressant treatment. *Am J Psychiatry*, 163, 41–47.

Solomon DA, Keller MB, Leon AC, et al. (2000). Multiple recurrences of major depressive disorder. *Am J Psychiatry*, 157, 229–233.

Solomon DA, Leon AC, Mueller TI, et al. (2005). Tachyphylaxis in unipolar major depressive disorder. *J Clin Psychiatry*, 66, 283–290.

Spielmans GI, Berman MI, Linardatos E, et al. (2013). Adjunctive atypical antipsychotic treatment for major depressive disorder: a meta-analysis of depression, quality of life, and safety outcomes. *PLoS Med*, 10(3), e1001403.

Spina E, Santoro V, D'Arrigo C (2008). Clinically relevant pharmacokinetic drug interactions with second-generation antidepressants: an update. *Clin Ther*, 30(7), 1206–1227.

Stassen HH, Angst J, Delini-Stula A (1996). Delayed onset of action of antidepressant drugs? Survey of results of Zurich meta-analyses. *Pharmacopsychiatry*, 29, 87–96.

Strawbridge R, Carter B, Marwood L, et al. (2019). Augmentation therapies for treatment-resistant depression: systematic review and meta-analysis. *Br J Psychiatry*, 214(1), 42–51. doi:10.1192/bjp.2018.233.

Suppes T, Silva R, Cucchiaro J, et al. (2016). Lurasidone for the treatment of major depressive disorder with mixed features: a randomized, double-blind, placebo-controlled study. *Am J Psychiatry*, 173, 400–407.

Szegedi A, Muller MJ, Anghelescu I, et al. (2003). Early improvement under mirtazapine and paroxetine predicts later stable response and remission with high sensitivity in patients with major depression. *J Clin Psychiatry*, 64, 413–420.

Targownik LE, Bolton JM, Metge CJ, Leung S, Sareen J (2009). Selective serotonin reuptake inhibitors are associated with a modest increase in the risk of upper gastrointestinal bleeding. *Am J Gastroenterol*, 104(6), 1475–1482. doi:10.1038/ajg.2009.128.

Taylor D, Cornelius V, Smith L, Young AH (2014). Comparative efficacy and acceptability of drug treatments for bipolar depression: a multiple-treatments meta-analysis. *Acta Psychiatr Scand*, 130(6), 452–469. doi:10.1111/acps.12343.

Taylor D, Barnes TRE, Young A (2018). *The Maudsley Prescribing Guidelines in Psychiatry*, 13th ed. Wiley-Blackwell.

Taylor MJ, Freemantle N, Geddes JR, Bhagwagar Z (2006). Early onset of selective serotonin reuptake inhibitor antidepressant action: systematic review and meta-analysis. *Arch Gen Psychiatry*, 63, 1217–1223.

Taylor MJ, Rudkin L, Bullemor-Day P, et al. (2013). Strategies for managing sexual dysfunction induced by antidepressant medication. *Cochrane Database Syst Rev*, (5), CD003382. doi:10.1002/14651858.CD003382.pub3.

Thanacoody HK, Thomas SH (2005). Tricyclic antidepressant poisoning: cardiovascular toxicity. *Toxicol Rev*, 24, 205–214.

Thase ME (2006). Preventing relapse and recurrence of depression: a brief review of therapeutic options. *CNS Spectr*, 11, 12–21.

Thase ME, Trivedi MH, Rush AJ (1995). MAOIs in the contemporary treatment of depression. *Neuropsychopharmacology*, 12, 185–219.

Thase ME, Shelton RC, Khan A (2006). Treatment with venlafaxine extended release after SSRI nonresponse or intolerance: a randomized comparison of standard- and higher-dosing strategies. *J Clin Psychopharmacol*, 26, 250–258.

Thase ME, Larsen KG, Reines E, Kennedy SH (2013). The cardiovascular safety profile of escitalopram. *Eur Neuropsychopharmacol*, 23(11), 1391–1400. doi:10.1016/j.euroneuro.2013.05.011.

Thase ME, Mahableshwarkar AR, Dragheim M, Loft H, Vieta, E (2016). A meta-analysis of randomized, placebo-controlled trials of vortioxetine for the treatment of major depressive disorder in adults. *Eur Neuropsychopharmacol*, 26, 979–993.

Tint A, Haddad PM, Anderson IM (2008). The effect of rate of antidepressant tapering on the incidence of discontinuation symptoms: a randomised study. *J Psychopharmacol*, 22(3), 330–332.

Tomaszewska W, Peselow ED, Barouche F, Fieve RR (1996). Antecedent life events, social supports and response to antidepressants in depressed patients. *Acta Psychiatr Scand*, 94, 352–357.

Trivedi MH, Fava M, Wisniewski SR, et al. (2006a). Medication augmentation after the failure of SSRIs for depression. *N Engl J Med*, 354, 1243–1252.

Trivedi MH, Rush AJ, Wisniewski SR, et al. (2006b). Evaluation of outcomes with citalopram for depression using measurement-based care in STAR*D: implications for clinical practice. *Am J Psychiatry*, 163, 28–40.

Uher R, Maier W, Hauser J, et al. (2009). Differential efficacy of escitalopram and nortriptyline on dimensional measures of depression. *Br J Psychiatry*, 194, 252–259. doi:10.1192/bjp.bp.108.057554.

Vallejo J, Gasto C, Catalan R, Bulbena A, Menchon JM (1991). Predictors of antidepressant treatment outcome in melancholia: psychosocial, clinical and biological indicators. *J Affect Disord*, 21, 151–162.

Vergouwen AC, Bakker A, Katon WJ, Verheij TJ, Koerselman F (2003). Improving adherence to antidepressants: a systematic review of interventions. *J Clin Psychiatry*, 64, 1415–1420.

Vieta E, Bauer M, Montgomery S, et al. (2013). Pooled analysis of sustained response rates for extended release quetiapine fumarate as monotherapy or adjunct to antidepressant therapy in patients with major depressive disorder. *J Affect Disord*, 150(2), 639–643. doi:10.1016/j.jad.2013.01.052.

Walsh BT, Seidman SN, Sysko R, Gould M (2002). Placebo response in studies of major depression: variable, substantial, and growing. *JAMA*, 287, 1840–1847.

Walters G, Reynolds CF, III, Mulsant BH, Pollock BG (1999). Continuation and maintenance pharmacotherapy in geriatric depression: an open-trial comparison of paroxetine and nortriptyline in patients older than 70 years. *J Clin Psychiatry*, 60(Suppl 20), 21–25.

Walther A, Breidenstein J, Miller R (2019). Association of testosterone treatment with alleviation of depressive symptoms in men: a systematic review and meta-analysis. *JAMA Psychiatry*, 76(1), 31–40. doi:10.1001/jamapsychiatry.2018.2734.

Warden D, Rush AJ, Trivedi MH, Fava M, Wisniewski SR (2007). The STAR*D Project results: a comprehensive review of findings. *Curr Psychiatry Rep*, 9(6), 449–459.

Wijkstra J, Lijmer J, Balk JF, Geddes JR., Nolen WA (2006). Pharmacological treatment for unipolar psychotic depression: systematic review and meta-analysis. *Br J Psychiatry*, 188(5), 410–415.

Wohlreich MM, Mallinckrodt CH, Watkin JG, et al. (2005). Immediate switching of antidepressant therapy: results from a clinical trial of duloxetine. *Ann Clin Psychiatry*, 17, 259–268.

Yildiz A, Pauler DK, Sachs GS (2004). Rates of study completion with single versus split daily dosing of antidepressants: a meta-analysis. *J Affect Disord*, 78, 157–162.

Yyldyz A, Sachs GS (2001). Administration of antidepressants. Single versus split dosing: a meta-analysis. *J Affect Disord*, 66, 199–206.

Zarrouf FA, Artz S, Griffith J, Sirbu C, Kommor M (2009). Testosterone and depression: systematic review and meta-analysis. *J Psychiatr Pract*, 15(4), 289–305. doi:10.1097/01.pra.0000358315.88931.fc.

Zheng W, Li X-H, Zhu X-M, et al. (2019). Adjunctive ketamine and electroconvulsive therapy for major depressive disorder: a meta-analysis of randomized controlled trials. *J Affective Disord*, 250, 123–131.

Zhou X, Ravindran AV, Qin B, et al. (2015). Comparative efficacy, acceptability, and tolerability of augmentation agents in treatment-resistant depression: systematic review and network meta-analysis. *Clin Psychiatry*, 76(4), e487–e498. doi:10.4088/JCP.14r09204.

Zivin K, Pfeiffer PN, Bohnert AS, et al. (2013). Evaluation of the FDA warning against prescribing citalopram at doses exceeding 40 mg. *Am J Psychiatry*, 170(6), 642–650. doi:10.1176/appi.ajp.2013.12030408.

Chapter

8 Drugs to Treat Anxiety and Insomnia

David S. Baldwin and Nathan T. M. Huneke

8.1 Introduction

Anxiety is an understandable response to perceived threat or experienced stress, and is usually fleeting and feels controllable: it represents an 'alarm', facilitating physical and psychological responses to perceived danger. *Anxiety symptoms* are mostly mild and transient, but many people experience severe and persistent symptoms that cause distress and impair everyday function. An *anxiety disorder* can be diagnosed when distressing and impairing anxiety exceeds specified severity thresholds and persists beyond minimum duration requirements, providing symptoms are not explicable by another condition. Insomnia is a common disorder in which sleep is reduced in amount or quality so that daytime well-being and functioning is impaired. It is more common in women than in men and is often a long-term disorder. About half of all diagnosed insomnia is related to an underlying psychiatric disorder. In such cases it is essential to treat the underlying disorder, though some additional intervention may be needed especially in the short term. This chapter reviews pharmacological treatments for anxiety disorders and insomnia. It should be highlighted that in anxiety and insomnia of mild to moderate severity, the first-line treatment is usually a psychological intervention. Medication is generally reserved for severe anxiety disorders or moderate cases where first-line psychological interventions have proved ineffective.

8.2 Overview of the Presumed Neuropsychobiology of Anxiety Disorders

The anxiety disorders share some psychological and physical symptoms but differ in the characteristic features that aid their specific diagnosis. These varying characteristics may reflect differences between disorders in their presumed underlying neuropsychobiological features, but disturbances in monoaminergic (serotonin, dopamine, noradrenaline) systems are probably common to all conditions. Other major neurotransmitters (glutamate, gamma-aminobutyric acid) are also important in influencing mechanisms underlying anxiety, and awareness of the potential role of neuroendocrine and immunological factors is also increasing (Bandelow et al., 2017).

Serotonin (5-hydroxytryptamine, 5-HT) both exerts an inhibitory effect on fight/flight responses to threat mediated by the periaqueductal grey matter (PGM) and facilitates anxiety responses to threat mediated by the amygdala (Deakin, 2013). Reactions to threat mediated by the PGM are characterized by the emotion of fearfulness, physical symptoms and the desire to escape (seen in panic attacks and phobic disorders); whereas responses to threat mediated by the amygdala are more characterized by apprehensiveness, psychological symptoms and endured distress (seen in generalized anxiety disorder (GAD) and obsessive-compulsive disorder (OCD)). This difference in 5-HT function between fear-related and anxiety-related disorders is supported by the findings of acute tryptophan depletion studies, through which brain 5-HT is lowered briefly but substantially: depletion leads to the transient reappearance of physical and psychological symptoms in previously remitted patients with panic disorder and social anxiety disorder, but not in patients with GAD or OCD (Corchs et al., 2015).

Dopamine is involved in reward-motivated behaviour and motor control and has a probable role in the pathophysiology of anergia and anhedonia in depressive states, but dopaminergic disturbances in anxiety disorders in the absence of accompanying depression have not been investigated extensively and may be only slight. By contrast, potential disturbances in *noradrenaline* (*norepinephrine*) pathways have been examined widely and may be important in panic disorder, although findings have been inconsistent (Bandelow et al., 2017).

Glutamate is the primary excitatory neurotransmitter, involved in physiological processes associated with emotion and cognition, acting through ionotropic (NMDA, AMPA and kainate) and G-protein-coupled metabotropic ($mGlu_{1\text{-}8}$) receptors. The principal inhibitory neurotransmitter *gamma-aminobutyric acid* (GABA) is synthesized from glutamate and exerts its effects through three differing receptors: $GABA_A$ and $GABA_c$ receptors are ligand-gated ion channels, whereas the $GABA_B$ receptor is a transmembrane receptor linked to G-proteins and second messenger systems. Fast inhibitory effects of GABA are mediated through $GABA_A$ receptors. Anxiety disorders may be associated with altered balance of GABA- and glutamate-mediated neurotransmission. Psychotropic drugs which enhance the actions of GABA (most notably, benzodiazepines, barbiturates and alcohol) exert anxiolytic effects, whereas 'negative modulators' at $GABA_A$ receptors elicit anxiety-like responses (Kalueff & Nutt, 2007). Some metabotropic glutamate receptors are targets for novel anxiolytics – including agonists at $mGlu_2$ and $mGlu_3$ receptors and antagonists at the $mGlu_5$ receptor (Peterlik et al., 2016; Pitsikas, 2014).

8.3 General Considerations in Pharmacological Treatment of Anxiety Disorders

The persistence and associated disability of anxiety disorders means that most patients exceeding threshold criteria for diagnosis are likely to benefit from pharmacological or psychological interventions. Need for treatment should be judged by ascertaining the severity and persistence of symptoms, their impact on everyday life, the level of coexisting depressive symptoms, and other features such as a previous good response to medication or psychotherapy. Choice of treatment is influenced

Table 8.1 Properties of the 'ideal' anxiolytic drug

Effectiveness considerations	Acceptability considerations
Effective across full range of anxiety disorders	Once-daily dosage
Effective across the spectrum of symptom severity	Minimal adverse effects
Effective across age range	Minimal interference with everyday life
Effective in achieving remission in acute treatment	No development of tolerance
Effective in preventing relapse of symptoms	No withdrawal symptoms
Rapid onset of action	Suitable in physically ill patients
Effective in treating coexisting depression	Free from interactions
Cost-effective	Safe in overdose

by clinical characteristics, patient preferences and availability of potential interventions. However, the 'ideal' anxiolytic drug does not exist (Table 8.1). Response rates to initial treatment can be disappointing, many patients experience unwanted side-effects (such as drowsiness with benzodiazepines or pregabalin, sexual dysfunction with selective serotonin reuptake inhibitors (SSRIs)), others relapse despite continuing treatment and some will be affected by troublesome discontinuation symptoms.

The overall efficacy of psychological and pharmacological approaches in acute treatment of anxiety disorders has been regarded as broadly similar, although this assumption has been questioned (Bandelow et al., 2015). There is much overlap between the anxiety disorders for evidence-based effective therapies – such as prescription of an SSRI or a course of individual cognitive behavioural therapy (CBT) – though there are some differences in evidence-based treatments between disorders, such as the lack of evidence of efficacy for benzodiazepines in OCD (Table 8.2). Depressive symptoms often accompany anxiety disorders: around one-third of people with anxiety disorders meet diagnostic criteria for a depressive episode. Treatment of depression will usually reduce anxiety symptoms when depression is the primary diagnosis, but if depression is co-morbid with an anxiety disorder, each condition requires separate consideration and treatment (Baldwin et al., 2014).

Strongest evidence for acute treatment is for judicious prescription of an SSRI or undertaking manualized CBT delivered by trained and supervised staff: it is uncertain whether combining these approaches is associated with greater improvement than with either treatment given alone, at least in some disorders. Continuation treatment, following a satisfactory response to acute treatment (ideally resulting in remission of symptoms) is needed in all patients with anxiety disorders, to consolidate the response and reduce the risk of relapse. It has been argued that psychological treatments may be more effective than pharmacological treatments in keeping patients well: but there is clear evidence that 'antidepressants' are highly effective in preventing relapse of symptoms in long-term treatment of patients with anxiety disorders (Batelaan et al., 2017).

Table 8.2 Summary of possible treatment options in anxiety disorders

	GAD	Panic disorder[a]	Specific phobia	Social anxiety disorder	OCD	PTSD
First line						
Psychological	CBT	CBT	Exposure-based therapy	CBT	Behaviour therapy or CBT	Trauma-focused CBT
Pharmacological	SSRI	SSRI	SSRI	SSRI	SSRI	SSRI
Second line						
Psychological	Applied relaxation	Supportive psychotherapy	CBT	Combination (CBT + SSRI)	Combination (CBT + SSRI)	EMDR
Pharmacological	SSRI, SNRI, pregabalin	SSRI, SNRI	SSRI	SSRI, SNRI, SSRI plus benzodiazepine	SSRI, clomipramine	Venlafaxine
Third line						
Psychological	Uncertain	Combination (CBT + SSRI) Psychodynamic psychotherapy	Uncertain	Uncertain	Combination (CBT + SSRI)	Trauma-focused CBT plus SSRI
Pharmacological	Agomelatine, buspirone, quetiapine, TCA, benzodiazepine	TCA, MAOI, benzodiazepine	Uncertain	MAOI, pregabalin, benzodiazepine	SSRI plus antipsychotic SSRI plus 5-HT_3 antagonist	SSRI plus anti-psychotic SSRI plus prazosin

EMDR, eye movement desensitization and reprocessing; MAOI, monoamine oxidase inhibitor; PTSD, post-traumatic stress disorder; SNRI, serotonin and noradrenaline reuptake inhibitor; TCA, tricyclic antidepressant.

[a] With or without agoraphobia.

8.4 Benzodiazepine Hypnotics and Anxiolytics

Benzodiazepines can be grouped according to chemical structure and pharmacokinetic properties, but all share a common mechanism of action and produce a range of similar clinical effects. Beneficial effects include reduction of anxiety; induction and maintenance of sleep; muscle relaxation; and treatment and prevention of epileptic seizures. These properties are shared by most benzodiazepines to varying degrees, depending on their potency and pharmacokinetic profile. They have a range of untoward adverse effects that may outweigh benefits in certain patients, so limiting their use in clinical practice. The balance of risk and benefit remains disputed but is undergoing a reconsideration (Baldwin et al., 2013).

8.4.1 Pharmacodynamic Properties

Benzodiazepines are 'positive allosteric modulators' at the $GABA_A$ receptor, which comprises five transmembrane glycoprotein subunits arranged around a central chloride channel. Each $GABA_A$ receptor contains two α subunits, two β subunits and either a γ or δ subunit: differing subunits are combined to produce a variety of receptor subtypes, which have distinct distributions and specific pharmacological properties (Sieghart & Sperk, 2002) (Figure 8.1). Anxiolytic effects of benzodiazepines are thought to be mediated through the α_2 and α_3 subunit, sedative effects through the α_1 subunit and amnestic effects through the α_5 subunit: suggesting that α_2/α_3 subtype selective ligands might have beneficial anxiolytic effects while avoiding the problems of non-selective agents (Chagraoui et al., 2016). Flumazenil is a drug that competitively blocks the binding of benzodiazepine anxiolytics at their active site on the $GABA_A$ receptor complex. It has little intrinsic activity so only exerts its alerting effects when administered concurrently with a benzodiazepine and therefore can be used to reverse the effects of benzodiazepine overdose (for example, respiratory depression).

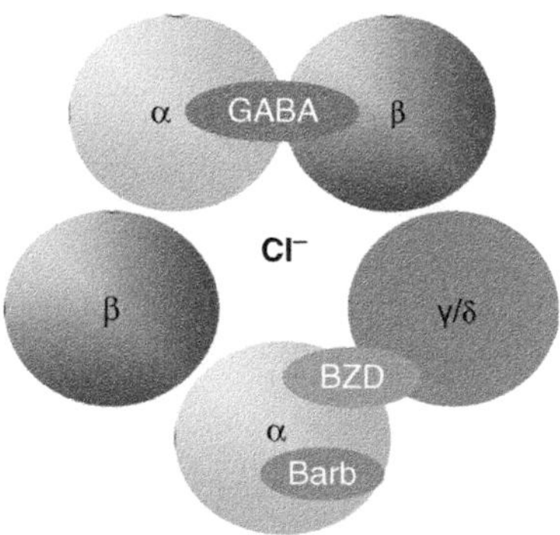

Figure 8.1 The $GABA_A$ receptor and important binding sites. Each $GABA_A$ receptor comprises five transmembrane glycoprotein subunits: two α subunits, two β subunits and either a γ or δ subunit. These glycoprotein subunits are arranged around a central chloride ion channel. Benzodiazepines are 'positive allosteric modulators' at the $GABA_A$ receptor: they increase the affinity of the receptor for GABA, which increases the likelihood of the receptor 'opening' to allow the passage of chloride ions through the membrane. Benzodiazepines bind to a specific site on the receptor membrane complex, distinct from the GABA binding site. $GABA_A$ receptors have additional binding sites for barbiturates and neurosteroids. Abbreviations: GABA, gamma-aminobutyric acid; BZD, benzodiazepine; Barb, barbiturate.

Benzodiazepines bind to a specific site on the receptor membrane complex, distinct from the GABA binding site. $GABA_A$ receptors have additional binding sites, including those for barbiturates and neurosteroids (Sigel & Steinmann, 2012). Rather than acting as a GABA receptor agonist, binding of a benzodiazepine to its site increases the affinity of the receptor for GABA, so increasing the likelihood of the receptor 'opening' to allow the passage of chloride ions through the membrane. This influx normally results in neuronal hyperpolarization and thus reduced 'excitability' of the target cell. Unlike barbiturates at high doses, benzodiazepines do not activate chloride channels directly, which makes them safer in overdose.

8.4.2 Pharmacokinetic Properties

Benzodiazepines differ in potency, time to effect and duration of action: some need repeated daily dosing but others are suitable for once-daily dosing to achieve the desired clinical effects (Table 8.3). Many benzodiazepines (for example, diazepam) have long-lasting active metabolites, which can accumulate with repeated dosing, especially in elderly patients and those with physical health problems, or in those with genetic variants leading to low or absent activity of relevant cytochrome P450 enzymes. Due to drug accumulation, drugs with longer half-lives may be more hazardous than drugs with a shorter half-life.

Table 8.3 Pharmacokinetic parameters and prescribing correlates in some benzodiazepines

Compound	Bioavailability (%)	Time to peak level (h)	Biological half-life (h)	Dosage and use(s)	Onset of effect
Midazolam	96 (IM route)	1.5–2.5	1.5–2.5	Single dose, sedation	Very fast
Temazepam	96	2–3	8–20	Night-time, sleep induction	Fast
Flunitrazepam	64–77	1–2	18–26	Night-time, sleep induction	Fast
Lorazepam	85	2	10–20	As required, panic attack	Fast
Oxazepam	95	1.5–3.0	4–15	3–4 times daily, anxiolysis	Fast
Chlordiazepoxide	~100	~4	5–30	3 times daily, anxiolysis	Intermediate
Alprazolam	80–90	1–2	4–6 (IR) 10–16 (XR)	3 times daily, anxiolysis	Intermediate
Diazepam	76	0.5–1.5	20–100	Twice daily, anxiolysis	Intermediate
Clonazepam	90	1–8	19–60	Once daily, anticonvulsant	Intermediate

IR, immediate release; XR, extended release.

With the exception of lorazepam (which is conjugated with glucuronic acid), all benzodiazepines undergo extensive hepatic metabolism, so medications which act as either inducers or inhibitors of hepatic enzymes can cause changes in plasma levels which may be clinically significant. As examples, the SSRIs fluoxetine and fluvoxamine can impair the elimination of alprazolam and diazepam, presumably through inhibition of metabolism via CYP2C19 (diazepam) and CYP3A4 (both drugs) (Muscatello et al., 2012).

8.4.3 Treatment of Anxiety Disorders

Randomized controlled trials demonstrate efficacy of some benzodiazepines in some anxiety disorders, usually in acute treatment for reducing anxiety symptom severity and sometimes in long-term treatment for preventing relapse. There is good evidence for efficacy in acute treatment of generalized anxiety disorder, social anxiety disorder and panic disorder, but limited evidence for efficacy in OCD and post traumatic stress disorder (Baldwin et al., 2014). Benzodiazepines differ in potency and this may be reflected in clinical efficacy with only highly potent ones such as alprazolam and clonazepam being effective in the treatment of more severe anxiety such as panic disorder.

There have been few direct comparisons of benzodiazepines with other medications such as the SSRIs, but alternative compounds are somewhat better tolerated. For this reason, most guidance suggests that alternatives should be preferred over benzodiazepines, which are generally reserved for patients who do not respond to a series of other treatments. Benzodiazepines have limited antidepressant effects, which is troublesome in anxious patients who are also markedly depressed. Benzodiazepine anxiolytics should be prescribed either for short-term relief of severe symptoms, or where anxiety disorders are disabling, severe and causing significant distress and substantial impairment of activities (Baldwin et al., 2013).

8.4.4 Treatment of Insomnia

Benzodiazepine hypnotics can be effective in short-term treatment of insomnia that is severe, impairing and causing distress: they can reduce the time to fall asleep (sleep latency), increase the overall duration and efficiency of sleep, and reduce periods of wakefulness after onset of sleep. Drugs with a short half-life have a lower risk of residual daytime drowsiness ('hangover') than drugs with long half-lives. The Z-drugs (zolpidem, zopiclone and zaleplon) were developed for these reasons.

Prescriptions should generally be limited to a maximum of four weeks, preferably at the lowest effective dosage with medication taken intermittently. In chronic insomnia, benzodiazepines should be prescribed only briefly, while longer-term treatments (such as CBT for insomnia) are started.

8.4.5 Cognitive and Psychomotor Effects

Benzodiazepine administration can result in dose-dependent sedation and drowsiness, mental slowing and anterograde amnesia (difficulty in forming new memories): somnolence typically becomes less prominent with continued use, though memory problems tend to persist. Withdrawal from benzodiazepines is often associated with an improvement in cognitive performance (Barker et al., 2004).

Longitudinal studies indicate a possible link between benzodiazepine use and development of dementia (Billioti de Gage et al., 2015) but 'confounding by indication' may be important in some studies. Benzodiazepine administration can also cause a dose-dependent impairment of driving performance, which potentiates the impairment due to alcohol consumption. Epidemiological studies suggest benzodiazepine use is associated with an increased risk of road traffic accidents, above that seen with untreated mental disorders. Elderly patients are more vulnerable to adverse cognitive and psychomotor effects and eliminate drugs more slowly than younger patients, so an increased risk of falls should be considered before benzodiazepines are prescribed to older individuals.

8.4.6 Tolerance and Dependence

Tolerance to the effects of benzodiazepines can occur and is most pronounced for the anticonvulsant and sedative effects. Tolerance to hypnotic and anxiolytic effects can develop, though probably less often and more slowly. It is unusual for patients to steadily increase the dosage, but this can occur particularly in those with a history of substance use disorders. Dependence on benzodiazepines is usually recognized following the emergence of withdrawal symptoms on either abruptly stopping or rapidly reducing long-term treatment. A broad range of physical and psychological symptoms is described (Table 8.4): these can be hard to distinguish from symptoms of underlying anxiety disorders, but perceptual disturbances are infrequent in untreated patients with anxiety disorders. Withdrawal phenomena are usually short-lived (lasting less than four weeks), although their duration is influenced by individual pharmacokinetic factors.

8.4.7 Management of Dependence

To reduce the risk of dependence, benzodiazepines should generally not be prescribed as a regularly administered medication for longer than four weeks. Ideally, they should be taken intermittently and only 'as required'. Compounds with higher potency and a short half-life are associated with a greater likelihood of developing dependence. After short-term use, a downwards tapering regime (over at least two weeks) may reduce the risk of

Table 8.4 Clinical features reported or observed after benzodiazepine withdrawal

Psychological symptoms	Physical symptoms	Complications
Increased anxiety	Trembling	Increased risk of seizures
Nervousness	Sweating	Poor motor coordination
Sleep disorders	Nausea and vomiting	Cognitive impairment
Inner restlessness	Motor agitation	Impairment of memory
Depressive symptoms	Dyspnoea	Perceptual impairments
Irritability	Increased heart rate	Hyperacusis
Psychosis-like conditions	Elevated blood pressure	Photophobia
Depersonalization-derealization	Headaches	Hypersomnia
Confusion	Muscle tension	Dysaesthesia and dyskinesia

'rebound' phenomena. Established dependence is preferably treated by gradual dosage down-titration and psychological support, evidence being less robust for pharmacological optimization or substitution (Soyka, 2017). Some patients cannot stop taking benzodiazepines: identified risk factors include other substance misuse, co-morbid depression, personality disorder and physical ill-health.

8.4.8 Benzodiazepine Abuse

Some benzodiazepines are abused as part of a wider pattern of drug and alcohol misuse, often being taken as an alternative when supplies of other drugs are scarce. The complications of overdose are greater when benzodiazepines are mixed with other respiratory depressants, including alcohol. 'Repeat prescriptions' should be reviewed regularly, as prescribed medication may be diverted to the 'black market'. Prescription of benzodiazepines in conjunction with methadone should be avoided. Altering the formulation of certain benzodiazepines has made them less easy to inject and restricting the availability of temazepam has probably limited its abuse by that route.

8.4.9 Long-Term Treatment with Benzodiazepines

Long-term prescriptions may be desirable when the alternatives are probably worse than continued use of benzodiazepines: this may be the case in patients with previously chronic and treatment-resistant anxiety disorders who have responded to but developed dependence on benzodiazepine anxiolytics (Baldwin et al., 2013). Longer-term but regularly reviewed prescriptions may represent a form of 'harm reduction' in patients who would otherwise consume illicit benzodiazepines or intoxicate themselves with alcohol to 'cope' with anxiety: but further efforts should be made to reduce the dosage over time.

8.5 'Z-Drugs' in the Treatment of Insomnia

The 'Z-drugs' (zaleplon, zolpidem, zopiclone (and eszopiclone)) were developed as potentially preferable alternatives to benzodiazepine hypnotics: as with benzodiazepines, most also have some anxiolytic, myorelaxant and anticonvulsant properties. They differ subtly from benzodiazepines in pharmacodynamic properties, and their pharmacokinetic profiles result in sleep induction but reduced risk of 'hangover'.

8.5.1 Pharmacodynamic Properties

Current Z-drugs are $GABA_A$ receptor positive allosteric modulators, and all share the property of acting as full agonists at the $GABA_A$ α_1 subunit. Zopiclone (a cyclopyrrolone) may have relative selectivity for α_1 and α_5 subunits, although it also binds to α_2 and α_3 subunits: its metabolite desmethylzopiclone has partial agonist properties. Eszopiclone is the dextrorotatory stereoisomer of zopiclone and the two do not differ notably in pharmacodynamic effects. Zolpidem (an imidazopyridine) and zaleplon (a pyrazolopyrimidine) both have lower affinity for α_2 and α_3 than for α_1 subunits, and zolpidem has no appreciable affinity for α_5 subunits.

8.5.2 Pharmacokinetic Properties

Z-drugs differ markedly in pharmacokinetic parameters (Drover, 2004). For zopiclone, plasma levels usually peak within 2 hours and the terminal elimination half-life is around 5 hours: up to 10% is excreted unchanged in urine but hepatic metabolism is through cytochromes CYP3A4 and CYP2E1, plasma levels being increased by erythromycin but decreased by rifampicin. Zolpidem levels peak within 3 hours, and its terminal elimination half-life is approximately 3 hours: metabolism is through cytochromes CYP3A4, CYP1A2 and CYP2D6, plasma levels being altered by chlorpromazine, imipramine, fluconazole, itraconazole, ketoconazole, rifampicin and ritonavir. Zaleplon is absorbed rapidly, plasma levels typically peaking within 60 minutes: it has an elimination half-life of approximately 90 minutes and is primarily metabolized by aldehyde oxidase to 5-oxozaleplon and 5-oxodesethylzaleplon, less than 1% of the parent compound being excreted intact in urine.

8.5.3 Clinical Uses

Z-drugs have a role in the short-term (two to four weeks) treatment of insomnia: long-term treatment with Z-drugs is not recommended because of risks of tolerance and dependence. They can reduce the time taken to fall asleep (sleep latency) but have less effects on sleep maintenance (Wilson et al., 2010). A controlled-release version of zolpidem enhances sleep continuity, but to a small degree. A meta-analysis which compared benzodiazepine and non-benzodiazepine hypnotics (primarily Z-drugs) found few differences in terms of sleep-onset latency, total sleep duration, number of awakenings, quality of sleep, adverse events, tolerance, rebound insomnia and daytime alertness (Dündar et al., 2004). A series of case reports indicate that zolpidem administration may be followed by a paradoxical arousing effect in patients with persistent vegetative states following stroke, anoxia or trauma (Sutton & Clauss, 2017). Newer variants of Z-drugs, especially eszopiclone (not available in the UK), have shown efficacy without the development of tolerance over six months (Walsh et al., 2007).

8.5.4 Adverse Effects

Approximately 50% of zopiclone-treated patients describe a persistent bitter or metallic taste (dysguesia), which is also reported frequently during eszopiclone treatment. Electroencephalographic studies indicate that zopiclone alters 'sleep architecture' with a reduction in rapid eye movement (REM) sleep, and abrupt discontinuation of zopiclone can be followed by vivid dreams and nightmares. Zopiclone and zolpidem can increase postural sway and psychomotor impairment (leading to increased risks of falls and driving accidents), and dependence, withdrawal symptoms and abuse have been reported for both drugs (Hajak et al., 2003): but the short half-life of zaleplon probably mitigates these risks. Z-drugs may have limited advantages over benzodiazepines in terms of dependence and withdrawal, so should be considered when there is a potential need for longer-term treatment or in patients at increased risk of dependence.

8.6 Other Medications Used in the Treatment of Insomnia

Sleep induction and maintenance involves a complex, phased and changing balance of pathways involved in arousal, wakefulness and drowsiness. Sleep-promoting pathways are centred on the ventrolateral preoptic nucleus of the hypothalamus and involve GABA, but wakefulness-promoting pathways are complex and involve multiple neurotransmitters (acetylcholine, dopamine, glutamate, histamine, noradrenaline and 5-HT) and the neuropeptide orexin: the balance of sleep and wakefulness also being influenced by adenosine, galanin and melatonin. Novel approaches to pharmacological management of patients with insomnia have included medications with effects on histamine and melatonin receptors, or with effects on orexin.

8.6.1 Agents Targeting Histaminergic Pathways

Sedative antihistamines (diphenhydramine, promethazine) have been taken widely as 'over-the-counter' preparations for short-term management of sleep disturbance, but randomized placebo-controlled evidence of efficacy is limited (Culpepper & Wingertzahn, 2015) and daytime drowsiness and increased appetite may become troublesome with prolonged use. Certain antidepressants with pharmacological properties which include antagonist effects at histamine H_1 receptors (for example, mianserin, mirtazapine and trazodone) have also been used in attempts to reduce insomnia, but again evidence is limited and inconsistent. Doxepin has long been used for treating depressed patients, typically at doses between 75 and 300 mg/day, when its pharmacological properties include serotonin and noradrenaline reuptake inhibitor (SNRI)-like and anticholinergic effects: at lower dosage (below 25 mg) it is a highly potent and selective H_1 antagonist, and even lower night-time doses (below 6 mg) promote sleep maintenance and increase sleep duration (Yeung et al., 2015).

8.6.2 Agents Targeting Melatonin Receptors

The pineal gland hormone melatonin has a role in synchronizing various circadian rhythms, including regulation of sleep and wakefulness. Melatonin release is affected by light–dark information from retinal photosensitive cells relayed through the suprachiasmatic nuclei, secretion being regulated by noradrenaline, its effects being mediated through M_1 and M_2 receptors, leading to drowsiness and facilitation of sleep. Immediate-release melatonin is included within some over-the-counter remedies for insomnia and has been used to manage sleep disturbance in children, but a prolonged-release formulation (Circadin – containing 2 mg of melatonin) is available for short-term use in older patients (aged 55 years and above) who are troubled by primary insomnia characterized by poor quality sleep. The M_1/M_2 receptor agonist ramelteon has efficacy in reducing subjective sleep latency (by approximately 13 minutes), but not in increasing total sleep duration, in randomized controlled trials lasting up to 24 weeks (Kuriyama et al., 2014).

8.6.3 Agents Influencing Orexin Secretion

Orexinergic neurons originate in lateral and posterior hypothalamic areas and project widely to brain nuclei involved in wakefulness: orexin-A and orexin-B integrate circadian, metabolic and sleep debt influences to determine the balance of wakefulness and sleepiness and are also involved in regulation of food intake and lipid metabolism. The hypnotic drug suvorexant exerts antagonist effects at orexin type 1 and type 2 receptors, thereby suppressing wakefulness: its hepatic metabolism is through cytochromes CYP3A4 and CYP2C19, the elimination half-life being approximately 12 hours. Meta-analysis indicates its rather limited efficacy in reducing subjective time-to-sleep-onset (by 6 minutes) and increasing subjective total-sleep-time (by 16 minutes) in patients with primary insomnia (Kishi et al., 2015). It does however reduce the duration of within-night wakenings.

8.7 Antidepressant Drugs to Treat Anxiety Disorders

8.7.1 Introduction

Antidepressant drugs are widely used in the treatment of patients with anxiety disorders. Chapter 7 reviews the major classes of antidepressant drugs, i.e. SSRIs, serotonin and noradrenaline reuptake inhibitors (SNRIs), tricyclic antidepressants (TCAs) and monoamine oxidase inhibitors (MAOIs), and also provides information on other antidepressants, namely agomelatine, bupropion, mirtazapine, reboxetine and vortioxetine. Chapter 7 considered each of the major antidepressant groups in terms of neurochemistry and mechanism of action, pharmacokinetics, interactions, contraindications and side effects. These issues remain the same irrespective of the disorder for which these drugs are given. Readers of this chapter should refer to Chapter 7 for this information: the following paragraphs are limited to reviewing the role of antidepressants in managing anxiety disorders. Chapter 7 also dealt with the classification of antidepressant drugs and the problem inherent in the term 'antidepressant'. Neuroscience-based Nomenclature (NbN) offers advantages over the traditional classification of psychiatric drugs by primary indication. However, these advantages are more apparent to researchers and academics. Realistically, older terms such as 'antidepressants' are likely to remain in use in many clinical consultations.

8.7.2 General Principles

Routinely combining drug and psychological treatments is not recommended for first-line treatment of anxiety disorders though the combination is often helpful when there has been a partial response to one treatment modality (Baldwin et al., 2014). As with depressive syndromes, antidepressants appear more effective in treating patients with more severe symptoms of anxiety disorders. A clinically meaningful response of anxiety symptoms to antidepressant treatment usually only appears several weeks after starting treatment. For the treatment of GAD, a treatment period of up to 12 weeks may be required to assess efficacy. However, if there has been no improvement after four weeks, the likelihood of a later response is low and consideration should be given to a change of medication (Baldwin et al., 2014). Some patients show a transient worsening of symptoms after an antidepressant is started, so for panic disorder in particular a low initial dose is usually used. If a patient with an anxiety disorder responds to drug treatment, this should be followed by a phase of maintenance treatment, in the same way as for depression.

The choice of antidepressant 'class' (and the specific drug to use within that 'class') depends primarily on the evidence base. One cannot assume that a drug that lacks a licensed indication does not have evidence of efficacy in that indication. Conversely, if one member of an antidepressant class has proven efficacy in a specific anxiety disorder, one cannot assume that all other drugs in the same class possess efficacy. This partly reflects the fact that the traditional drug classes (e.g. TCAs) can encompass drugs with significantly different pharmacodynamic properties. If an anxiety disorder coexists with a major depressive episode of moderate or greater severity this should guide treatment towards an antidepressant medication rather than another anxiolytic drug such as pregabalin.

8.7.3 Efficacy in Anxiety Disorders

SSRIs and SNRIs have been shown to be efficacious in the short-term and long-term treatment of anxiety disorders (Baldwin et al., 2014). These drugs are generally well tolerated, more so for SSRIs, though sexual dysfunction can be a significant long-term side effect for both SSRIs and SNRIs. Abrupt cessation of virtually all antidepressants can cause troublesome discontinuation symptoms (Haddad & Anderson, 2007). An exception to this is agomelatine, which seems to show placebo-level discontinuation symptoms following abrupt cessation (Goodwin et al., 2009). Fluoxetine has a lower propensity to cause discontinuation symptoms, probably due to the long half-life of the parent compound and its main active metabolite. Many guidelines for the treatment of anxiety disorders, including those from the British Association for Psychopharmacology (Baldwin et al., 2014), list SSRIs and SNRIs as the first-line pharmacological treatment for people with anxiety disorders or OCD. With regard to specific drugs, duloxetine and venlafaxine (both SNRIs) are efficacious in the acute treatment of GAD and in preventing relapse. Venlafaxine is also efficacious in the acute treatment of panic disorder and in preventing relapse. The doses of SSRIs that are needed to treat patients with OCD are often higher than those needed in the treatment of depression.

Specific TCAs are efficacious in some anxiety disorders. However, TCAs are generally less well tolerated than either SSRIs or SNRIs, so they should usually be used when SSRIs and SNRIs have either proved ineffective or not been tolerated. Phenelzine, an irreversible MAOI, has proven efficacy in social phobia and panic disorder. Its side effects and wide range of potential interactions with drugs and foodstuffs, leading to strict dietary precautions, mean it is generally reserved for patients who have not responded to or not tolerated other drugs. Chapter 7 reviews the interactions of MAOIs. Among miscellaneous antidepressants, agomelatine has proven efficacy in acute treatment and prevention of relapse of GAD (Stein et al., 2008, 2012). The drug is generally well tolerated but regular monitoring of liver function tests is required in the first year of treatment and after any dose increase due to the risk of hepatic dysfunction.

8.8 Antipsychotic Drugs to Treat Anxiety Disorders

8.8.1 Introduction

Pignon et al. (2017) reviewed the efficacy of antipsychotics in the treatment of several anxiety disorders based on published randomized controlled trials (RCTs) or, if these were lacking, open-label studies. The authors' main conclusions were as follows:

- Evidence supports the use of quetiapine monotherapy to treat GAD.
- Evidence supports the use of risperidone and aripiprazole to augment antidepressants in the treatment of refractory OCD.
- There is no strong evidence for the effectiveness of antipsychotics in refractory social anxiety disorder and refractory panic disorder.
- First-generation antipsychotics are not recommended to treat anxiety disorders.

- Open-label studies support the efficacy of aripiprazole in antidepressant-refractory GAD but this requires testing in RCTs.

The following sections examine the role of quetiapine in GAD and of specific antipsychotics to augment antidepressants in refractory OCD given that their use in both indications are supported by RCTs.

8.8.2 Quetiapine for the Treatment of GAD

Maneeton et al. (2016) systematically reviewed the evidence from RCTs for extended-release quetiapine in treating adult patients with GAD. Data from three RCTs were meta-analyzed and outcomes included mean-changed score on the Hamilton Anxiety rating Scale (HAM-A), improvement in sleep quality, the overall discontinuation rate (acceptability) and the discontinuation for adverse events (tolerability). Data were analyzed for all doses of quetiapine-XR pooled together and for three individual doses (50 mg, 150 mg and 300 mg per day). The authors concluded that quetiapine-XR (50–150 mg/day) is efficacious in the treatment of GAD in adult patients being superior to placebo and equivalent to SSRIs in reducing overall anxiety scores; and superior to SSRIs in improving sleep quality. However, the tolerability of quetiapine-XR was less good than that of SSRIs with the exception of the lowest dose (50 mg/day) where tolerability was equivalent to SSRIs. It should be noted that quetiapine is not licensed for the treatment of GAD in the UK.

The efficacy of quetiapine in treating GAD may reflect the action of its active metabolite, *N*-desalkylquetiapine (norquetiapine), which shows moderate to high affinity for 5-HT_{1A}, 5-HT_{2A} and 5-HT_{2C} and D_2 receptors, as well as being an inhibitor of noradrenaline reuptake. The last action differentiates it from other serotonin-dopamine antagonists. Its benefits in terms of sleep probably reflect its sedative effects which in turn reflect antagonism at the 5-HT_{2A} and histamine H_1 receptors.

8.8.3 Antipsychotics as Augmenting Agents in Refractory OCD

Dold et al. (2015) reported a meta-analysis that included double-blind, randomized, placebo-controlled trials of antipsychotic augmentation of SSRIs in patients with treatment-resistant OCD. Data from 13 trials were analyzed, testing quetiapine, risperidone, aripiprazole, olanzapine, paliperidone and haloperidol (drugs listed in terms of decreasing sample size within the meta-analysis). For all drugs combined, antipsychotic augmentation was significantly more efficacious than placebo in reducing the Yale-Brown Obsessive Compulsive Scale (the primary outcome measure) and also on a range of secondary outcome measures. Antipsychotic treatment was associated with significantly more adverse effects compared with placebo, although the discontinuation rate did not differ between groups. When single drugs were analyzed, aripiprazole, haloperidol and risperidone were superior to placebo on the primary outcome measure, whereas olanzapine, paliperidone and quetiapine were not. An earlier meta-regression analysis (Ducasse et al., 2014) suggested that the effectiveness of antipsychotic augmentation of SSRIs in OCD was related to their D_2 and D_3 dopamine receptor binding affinities.

8.9 Pregabalin and Other Gabapentinoids

Gabapentinoids are substituted derivatives of GABA, which share a common property of blocking $\alpha_2\delta$ subunit-containing voltage-dependent calcium channels: some (gabapentin and pregabalin) have entered widespread clinical use, but others (gabapentin enacarbil, for restless legs syndrome; phenibut, for anxiety and insomnia) are available in only a few countries. Gabapentin and pregabalin have analgesic, anticonvulsant and anxiolytic effects, but only pregabalin has a licence for treating patients with GAD.

8.9.1 Pharmacodynamic Properties

Pregabalin is a branched-chain amino acid, with structural similarities to L-leucine, L-isoleucine and GABA. It shows high-affinity binding to the Type 1 and Type 2 proteins of the $\alpha_2\delta$ subunit of the P/Q type of voltage-gated calcium channels: mainly to $\alpha_2\delta$-1 subunits in the cortex, olfactory bulb, hypothalamus, amygdala and hippocampus, and $\alpha_2\delta$-2 subunits in the cerebellum. It does not bind directly to $GABA_A$, $GABA_B$ or $GABA_C$ receptors or to binding sites allosterically linked to GABA, but increases the density of GABA transporter proteins and increases extracellular GABA in the brain through a dose-dependent increase in L-glutamic acid decarboxylase activity (Micó & Prieto, 2012). Through its effects on calcium channels, pregabalin administration reduces glutamate release: it may also reduce the synthesis of excitatory synapses and block the 'trafficking' of new voltage-gated calcium channels to the cell surface.

8.9.2 Pharmacokinetic Properties

Pregabalin is absorbed rapidly after oral administration, maximal plasma levels occurring within 60 minutes: absorption is dependent upon active transport and is linear, with proportional increases in plasma levels across the dose range. Pharmacokinetic interactions are unlikely as pregabalin undergoes negligible metabolism, approximately 98% being excreted unchanged in urine, the renal clearance being around 75 ml/min. Angiotensin-converting enzyme (ACE) inhibitors may worsen adverse effects of pregabalin, and it may enhance the fluid-retaining effect of thiazolidinedione (an antidiabetic agent).

8.9.3 Clinical Uses

Pregabalin is effective as monotherapy in short- and long-term treatment of GAD and social anxiety disorder. In GAD, it has similar effects in reducing psychological and physical symptoms of anxiety and reduces the severity both of sleep disturbance and of coexisting depressive symptoms; and augmentation with pregabalin is beneficial in reducing anxiety symptoms after initial partial response to SSRI or SNRI antidepressants (Baldwin et al., 2015). It can reduce withdrawal symptoms from benzodiazepines and zolpidem and facilitate abstinence in previously alcohol-dependent patients (Freynhagen et al., 2016).

8.9.4 Adverse Effects

The most commonly reported problems are dizziness and drowsiness (both occurring in approximately 30% of patients with GAD), less common side effects include visual disturbances, unsteadiness and clumsiness (Baldwin et al., 2015). Weight gain occurs in approximately 4% of patients. Peripheral oedema is reported (in less than 3% of treated patients), but does not appear to be associated with hypertension, congestive heart failure, or declining renal or hepatic function. Symptoms after abrupt discontinuation can occur, probably less frequently than with benzodiazepines. 'Euphoria' was described in clinical trials and abuse is reported, particularly in patients with a history of substance use disorders or after high dosage, and prescription dosage and duration should be monitored carefully (Schjerning et al., 2016). There are potential pharmacodynamic interactions with other central nervous system depressants and pregabalin overdose can be hazardous when combined with alcohol, benzodiazepines and opioids (Bonnet & Scherbaum, 2017). Pregabalin (and gabapentin) were reclassified as Class C controlled substances in April 2019, after fatalities associated with the drug.

8.10 Buspirone and Related Azapirone Medications

The azapirone group includes buspirone (an anxiolytic), gepirone (which may have efficacy in certain forms of sexual dysfunction), ipsapirone (an investigational drug), perospirone (an antipsychotic, used in Japan) and tandospirone (used in China and Japan for its anxiolytic and antidepressant effects). Of these, only buspirone has entered widespread use in clinical practice in multiple countries.

8.10.1 Pharmacodynamic Properties

The anxiolytic effects of buspirone probably derives from its 5-HT_{1A} agonist properties (Loane & Politis, 2012). It is a high-affinity full agonist at presynaptic 5-HT_{1A} inhibitory autoreceptors and a partial agonist at postsynaptic 5-HT_{1A} receptors: it has low affinity for 5-HT_{2A}, 5-HT_{2B}, 5-HT_{2C}, 5-HT_6 and 5-HT_7 receptors. At low dosage it blocks presynaptic D_2 autoreceptors and enhances dopaminergic neurotransmission in the nigrostriatal pathway, but at higher dosage it blocks postsynaptic D_2 receptors, causing hypoactivity though not catalepsy: it also has high affinity as an antagonist at D_3 and D_4 receptors. It does not interact with the $GABA_A$ receptor complex but some actions may be mediated by oxytocin release secondary to 5-HT_{1A} agonist effects. In addition, the metabolite 1-(2-pyrimidinyl) piperazine is a potent terminal α_2-adrenergic autoreceptor antagonist and may enhance noradrenergic activity.

8.10.2 Pharmacokinetic Properties

Buspirone has low oral bioavailability, due to extensive first-pass hepatic metabolism. Peak plasma levels occur within 90 minutes and the elimination half-life is probably less than 11 hours. It should not be prescribed with MAOIs or in patients with liver or kidney disease. As its metabolism (hydroxylation and methylation) is primarily through cytochrome CYP3A4, plasma levels are increased by concomitant haloperidol or nefazodone (now withdrawn from clinical use) or drinking grapefruit juice, all of which are CYP3A4 inhibitors, and decreased by the CYP3A4 inducer carbamazepine (Muscatello et al., 2012).

8.10.3 Clinical Uses

Buspirone is licensed for the short-term treatment of anxiety (United Kingdom) and short- and long-term treatment of anxiety disorders (United States). It is mainly used in the treatment of patients with GAD, and may be most helpful when patients have not previously been treated with a benzodiazepine (Chessick et al., 2006). It has only limited efficacy in augmenting the response to antidepressants in depressed patients (Kishi et al., 2013). It can augment the response to antidepressants in patients with social phobia and can reduce symptoms of sexual dysfunction associated with SSRI treatment. It has shown beneficial effects in attention deficit hyperactivity disorder, and in managing irritability and behavioural problems in some patients with dementia. The onset of effect is slower than with benzodiazepines, and buspirone is not helpful in reducing symptoms associated with withdrawal from alcohol, barbiturates or benzodiazepines.

8.10.4 Adverse Effects

Although generally well tolerated, common problems include dizziness, headache, nausea and nervousness but unlike benzodiazepines, buspirone does not cause sedation or psychomotor impairment (nor does it have myorelaxant or anticonvulsant effects). It appears to be safe in overdose, when taken alone. It does not cause euphoria and there is no evidence of the development of tolerance or dependence. Studies in healthy volunteers (Cowen et al., 1990) indicate that buspirone lowers body temperature (mediated through its actions at 5-HT_{1A} presynaptic receptors) and increases plasma prolactin and growth hormone levels (through uncertain mechanisms).

8.11 Beta Blockers (β-Blockers)

Although best known as 'cardiac drugs' for managing hypertension, correcting dysrhythmias and secondary prevention of myocardial function, certain β-blockers (atenolol, propranolol) have long been used to reduce the severity of physical symptoms of anxiety, following the early discovery of beneficial effects in reducing symptoms associated with hyperthyroidism (Turner et al., 1965).

8.11.1 Pharmacodynamic Properties

Beta blockers are competitive antagonists for adrenaline (epinephrine) and noradrenaline (norepinephrine) at three types of β-adrenergic receptors. β_1-adrenergic receptors are located mainly in heart and kidneys; β_2-adrenergic receptors mainly in lungs, gastrointestinal tract, liver, uterus, vascular smooth muscle and skeletal muscle; and β_3-adrenergic receptors in adipocytes. Some β-blockers block all types of receptor, whereas others are selective for certain receptors: blockade of β-adrenergic receptors within the sympathetic branch of the autonomic nervous system reduces physical symptoms associated with the 'fight-or-flight' response. Some β-blockers (for example, oxprenolol) have intrinsic sympathomimetic activity (acting as partial agonists) rendering them unhelpful for managing anxiety.

8.11.2 Pharmacokinetic Properties

There are marked differences between β-blockers in their pharmacokinetic parameters and risk of drug interactions. For example, propranolol (a non-selective β_1- and β_2-adrenergic receptor antagonist) is rapidly and completely absorbed, peak plasma levels occurring within 3 hours of ingestion, but taking it with food increases its bioavailability, which is also variable because of extensive first-pass hepatic metabolism. Being highly lipophilic, propranolol crosses the blood–brain barrier and high concentrations can be present in the brain. Propranolol biotransformation is mediated mainly by CYP1A2 and CYP2D6 (with contributions from CYP2C19 and CYP3A4), and co-administration of inhibitors of CYP2D6 (fluoxetine, paroxetine) has occasionally resulted in severe adverse events (severe bradycardia and atrioventricular block) (Muscatello et al., 2012). The main metabolite 4-hydroxypropranolol has a longer half-life (up to 7.5 hours) than the parent compound (3–4 hours), and is pharmacologically active. By contrast, atenolol (selective β_1-adrenergic receptor antagonist) is hydrophilic and so does not cross the blood–brain barrier; and pindolol (non-selective β_1- and β_2-antagonist, with intrinsic sympathomimetic activity) undergoes less first-pass metabolism, but elimination is reduced in patients with renal disease.

8.11.3 Clinical Uses

Despite the traditional use of propranolol in reducing physical symptoms of anxiety, there is only limited evidence of efficacy in reducing psychological symptoms in patients with anxiety disorders (Steenen et al., 2016). Other potential uses of β-blockers include augmentation of serotonin reuptake inhibitors in depressed patients with pindolol (which also possesses 5-HT_{1A} partial agonist effects) (Whale et al., 2010), quelling agitation after acquired brain injury (propranolol) (Fleminger et al., 2006), reducing akathisia associated with antipsychotic and antidepressant drugs (principally propranolol) (Miller & Fleischhacker, 2000) and attenuating physiological responses to traumatic events (Argolo et al., 2015).

8.11.4 Adverse Effects

Well-known side effects of β-blockers, understandable from their psychopharmacological properties, include bronchospasm, dyspnoea, cold extremities, bradycardia, hypotension, heart failure, heart block and sexual dysfunction. Lipophilic compounds are more likely than hydrophilic compounds to cause insomnia, vivid dreams and nightmares. Adverse effects associated with β_2-adrenergic receptor antagonist activity (bronchospasm, peripheral vasoconstriction, altered glucose and lipid metabolism) are less common with β_1-selective agents. Hypoglycaemia can occur because β_2-adrenoceptors normally stimulate hepatic glycogen breakdown and pancreatic release of glucagon.

8.12 Pathways to Improving Treatments for Anxiety Disorders

Current recommendations for pharmacological treatment of anxiety disorders are derived mainly from the findings of randomized double-blind placebo-controlled trials, which demonstrate robust efficacy and reasonable tolerability for many interventions, both in acute treatment and in preventing relapse. However, the patients who participate in RCTs may have a better prognosis than patients treated in 'real-world' clinical settings, where the effects of treatment can often be disappointing. It is not currently possible to predict the likelihood of response in a given patient with great accuracy, and there are uncertainties about next steps in further management after non-response to first-line treatment approaches.

Attempts to optimize clinical outcomes rest on making best use of available treatments, and there is much scope for improving the treatments available and how they are used. Improved outcomes could result from additional medications with novel mechanisms of action, leading to greater efficacy and improved acceptability in all patient groups. Alternatively, the use of reliable biomarkers might lead to identification of specific patient subgroups in which novel or current treatments might have enhanced effectiveness and acceptability.

References

Argolo FC, Cavalcanti-Ribeiro P, Netto LR, Quarantini LC (2015). Prevention of posttraumatic stress disorder with propranolol: a meta-analytic review. *J Psychosom Res*, 79, 89–93.

Baldwin DS, Aitchison KBA, Curran HV, et al. (2013). Benzodiazepines: risks and benefits. A reconsideration. *J Psychopharmacol*, 27, 967–971.

Baldwin DS, Anderson IM, Nutt DJ, et al. (2014). Evidence-based pharmacological treatment of anxiety disorders, post-traumatic stress disorder and obsessive-compulsive disorder: a revision of the 2005 guidelines from the British Association for Psychopharmacology. *J Psychopharmacol*, 28, 403–439.

Baldwin DS, den Boer JA, Lyndon G, et al. (2015). Efficacy and safety of pregabalin in generalised anxiety disorder: a critical review of the literature. *J Psychopharmacol*, 29, 1047–1060.

Bandelow B, Reitt M, Röver C, et al. (2015). Efficacy of treatments for anxiety disorders: a meta-analysis. *Int Clin Psychopharmacol*, 30, 183–192.

Bandelow B, Baldwin D, Abelli M, et al. (2017). Biological markers for anxiety disorders, OCD and PTSD: a consensus statement. Part II: Neurochemistry, neurophysiology and neurocognition. *World J Biol Psychiatry*, 18, 162–214.

Barker MJ, Greenwood KM, Jackson M, Crowe SF (2004). Persistence of cognitive effects after withdrawal from long-term benzodiazepine use: a meta-analysis. *Arch Clin Neuropsychol*, 19, 437–454.

Batelaan NM, Bosman RC, Muntingh A, et al. (2017). Risk of relapse after antidepressant discontinuation in anxiety disorders, obsessive-compulsive disorder, and post-traumatic stress disorder: systematic review and meta-analysis of relapse prevention trials. *BMJ*, 358, j3927.

Billioti de Gage S, Pariente A, Bégaud B (2015). Is there really a link between benzodiazepine use and the risk of dementia? *Expert Opin Drug Saf*, 14, 733–747.

Bonnet U, Scherbaum N (2017). How addictive are gabapentin and pregabalin? A systematic review. *Eur Neuropsychopharmacol*, 27, 1185–1215.

Chagraoui A, Skiba M, Thuillez C, Thibaut F (2016). To what extent is it possible to dissociate the anxiolytic and sedative/hypnotic properties of GABAA receptors modulators? *Prog Neuropsychopharmacol Biol Psychiatry*, 71, 189–202.

Chessick CA, Allen MH, Thase ME, et al. (2006). Azapirones for generalized anxiety disorder. *Cochrane Database Syst Rev*, (3), CD006115.

Corchs F, Nutt DJ, Hince DA, et al. (2015). Evidence for serotonin function as a neurochemical difference between fear and anxiety disorders in humans? *J Psychopharmacol*, 29, 1061–1069.

Cowen PJ, Anderson IM, Grahame-Smith DG (1990). Neuroendocrine effects of azapirones. *J Clin Psychopharmacol*, 10, 21S–25S.

Culpepper L, Wingertzahn MA (2015). Over-the-counter agents for the treatment of occasional disturbed sleep or transient insomnia: a systematic review of efficacy and safety. *Prim Care Companion CNS Disord*, 17, 10.4088/PCC.15r01798.

Deakin JFW (2013). The origins of '5-HT and mechanisms of defence' by Deakin and Graeff: a personal perspective. *J Psychopharmacol*, 27, 1084–1089.

Dold M, Aigner M, Lanzenberger R, Kasper S (2015). Antipsychotic augmentation of serotonin reuptake inhibitors in treatment-resistant obsessive-compulsive disorder: an update meta-analysis of double-blind, randomized, placebo-controlled trials. *Int J Neuropsychopharmacol*, 18, pii: pyv047. doi:10.1093/ijnp/pyv047.

Drover DR (2004). Comparative pharmacokinetics and pharmacodynamics of short-acting hypnosedatives. *Clin Pharmacokinet*, 43, 227–238.

Ducasse D, Boyer L, Michel P, et al. (2014). D2 and D3 dopamine receptor affinity predicts effectiveness of antipsychotic drugs in obsessive-compulsive disorders: a metaregression analysis. *Psychopharmacology (Berl)*, 231, 3765–3770.

Dündar Y, Dodd S, Strobl J, et al. (2004). Comparative efficacy of newer hypnotic drugs for the short-term management of insomnia: a systematic review and meta-analysis. *Hum Psychopharmacol*, 19, 305–322.

Fleminger S, Greenwood RRJ, Oliver DL (2006). Pharmacological management for agitation and aggression in people with acquired brain injury. *Cochrane Database Syst Rev*, (4), CD003299.

Freynhagen R, Backonja M, Schug S, et al. (2016). Pregabalin for the treatment of drug and alcohol withdrawal symptoms: a comprehensive review. *CNS Drugs*, 30, 1191–1200.

Goodwin GM, Emsley R, Rembry S, et al. (2009). Agomelatine prevents relapse in patients with major depressive disorder without evidence of a discontinuation syndrome: a 24-week randomized, double-blind, placebo-controlled trial. *J Clin Psychiatry*, 70, 1128–1137.

Haddad PM, Anderson IM (2007). Recognising and managing antidepressant discontinuation symptoms. *Adv Psychiatr Treat*, 13, 447–457.

Hajak G, Müller WE, Wittchen HU, Pittrow D, Kirch W (2003). Abuse and dependence potential for the non-benzodiazepine hypnotics zolpidem and zopiclone: a review of case reports and epidemiological data. *Addiction*, 98, 1371–1378.

Kalueff AV, Nutt DJ (2007). Role of GABA in anxiety and depression. *Depress Anxiety*, 24, 495–517.

Kishi T, Meltzer HY, Matsuda Y, Iwata N (2013). Azapirone 5-HT1A receptor partial agonist treatment for major depressive disorder: systematic review and meta-analysis. *Psychol Med*, 44, 2255–2269.

Kishi T, Matsunaga S, Iwata N (2015). Suvorexant for primary insomnia: a systematic review and meta-analysis of randomized placebo-controlled trials. *PLoS One*, 10, e0136910.

Kuriyama A, Honda M, Hayashino Y (2014). Ramelteon for the treatment of insomnia in adults: a systematic review and meta-analysis. *Sleep Med*, 15, 385–392.

Loane C, Politis M (2012). Buspirone: what is it all about? *Brain Res*, 1461, 111–118.

Maneeton N, Maneeton B, Woottiluk P, et al. (2016). Quetiapine monotherapy in acute treatment of generalized anxiety disorder: a systematic review and meta-analysis of randomized controlled trials. *Drug Des Devel Ther*, 10, 259–276.

Micó J-A, Prieto R (2012). Elucidating the mechanism of action of pregabalin. *CNS Drugs*, 26, 637–648.

Miller CH, Fleischhacker WW (2000). Managing antipsychotic-induced acute and chronic akathisia. *Drug Saf*, 22, 73–81.

Muscatello MR, Spina E, Bandelow B, Baldwin DS (2012). Clinically relevant drug interactions in anxiety disorders. *Hum Psychopharmacol*, 27, 239–253.

Peterlik D, Flor PJ, Uschold-Schmidt N (2016). The emerging role of metabotropic glutamate receptors in the pathophysiology of chronic stress-related disorders. *Curr Neuropharmacol*, 14, 514–539.

Pignon B, Tezenas du Montcel C, Carton L, Pelissolo A (2017). The place of antipsychotics in the therapy of anxiety disorders and obsessive-compulsive disorders. *Curr Psychiatry Rep*, 19, 103.

Pitsikas N (2014). The metabotropic glutamate receptors: potential drug targets for the treatment of anxiety disorders? *Eur J Pharmacol*, 723, 181–184.

Schjerning O, Rosenzweig M, Pottegård A, Damkier P, Nielsen J (2016). Abuse potential of pregabalin. *CNS Drugs*, 30, 9–25.

Sieghart W, Sperk G (2002). Subunit composition, distribution and function of GABA-A receptor subtypes. *Curr Top Med Chem*, 2, 795–816.

Sigel E, Steinmann ME (2012). Structure, function and modulation of GABAA receptor. *J Biol Chem*, 287, 40224–40231.

Soyka M (2017). Treatment of benzodiazepine dependence. *N Engl J Med*, 376, 1147–1157.

Steenen SA, van Wijk AJ, van der Heijden GJ, et al. (2016). Propranolol for the treatment of anxiety disorders: systematic review and meta-analysis. *J Psychopharmacol*, 30, 128–139.

Stein DJ, Ahokas AA, de Bodinat C (2008). Efficacy of agomelatine in generalized anxiety disorder: a randomized, double-blind, placebo-controlled study. *J Clin Psychopharmacol*, 28, 561–566.

Stein DJ, Ahokas A, Albarran C, et al. (2012). Agomelatine prevents relapse in generalized anxiety disorder: a 6-month randomized, double-blind, placebo-controlled discontinuation study. *J Clin Psychiatry*, 73, 1002–1008.

Sutton JA, Clauss RP (2017). A review of the evidence of zolpidem efficacy in neurological disability after brain damage due to stroke, trauma and hypoxia: a justification of further clinical trials. *Brain Inj*, 31, 1019–1027.

Turner P, Granville-Grossman KL, Smart JV (1965). Effect of adrenergic receptor blockade on the tachycardia of thyrotoxicosis and anxiety state. *Lancet*, 286, 1316–1318.

Walsh JK, Krystal AD, Amato DA, et al. (2007). Nightly treatment of primary insomnia with eszopiclone for six months: effect on sleep, quality of life, and work limitations. *Sleep*, 30, 959–968.

Whale R, Terao T, Cowen P, Freemantle C, Geddes G (2010). Pindolol augmentation of serotonin reuptake inhibitors for the treatment of depressive disorder: a systematic review. *J Psychopharmacol*, 24, 513–520.

Wilson SJ, Nutt DJ, Alford C, et al. (2010). British Association for Psychopharmacology consensus statement on evidence-based treatment of insomnia, parasomnias and circadian rhythm disorders. *J Psychopharmacol*, 24, 1577–1601.

Yeung W-F, Chung K-F, Yung K-P, Ng TH-Y (2015). Doxepin for insomnia: a systematic review of randomized placebo-controlled trials. *Sleep Med Rev*, 19, 75–83.

Drugs to Treat Schizophrenia and Psychosis (Dopamine Antagonists and Partial Agonists Other Than Clozapine)

Robert McCutcheon, Stephen J. Kaar and Oliver D. Howes

9.1 Introduction

This chapter provides a wide-ranging review of the clinical pharmacology of drugs for the treatment of schizophrenia and psychosis other than clozapine. These are dopamine receptor antagonists and dopamine partial agonists (as per the new Neuroscience-based Nomenclature (NbN) classification). This chapter covers their pharmacodynamics, pharmacokinetics, adverse effects, the latest evidence regarding their 'antipsychotic' mechanism of action, their use in the acute and maintenance treatment of schizophrenia, other therapeutic indications and some controversies that surround their use.

Dopamine receptor antagonists and dopamine partial agonists are commonly referred to as antipsychotics. As a clinical shorthand the term 'antipsychotic' is likely to remain in use. However, it has its problems, principally that these drugs have proven efficacy in treating a range of disorders other than psychotic disorders (by proven we refer to evidence from randomized placebo-controlled trials). For example, most antipsychotics are effective in treating mania even when this is not associated with psychotic symptoms. In addition, individual antipsychotic drugs have shown efficacy in the maintenance treatment of bipolar disorder and as augmenting agents in the treatment of major depressive disorder and obsessive-compulsive disorder. A further example is that quetiapine monotherapy is efficacious in the treatment of bipolar depression. The issue of nomenclature is considered in a later section of this chapter. Clozapine is considered separately in Chapter 10.

9.2 The Discovery of Drugs to Treat Psychosis

Rauwolfia serpentina has been used in Ayurvedic medicine for centuries to treat insanity. In 1952 the active component, reserpine, was isolated. Reserpine was later found to block the uptake and storage of noradrenaline and dopamine into synaptic vesicles, markedly reducing monoamine-mediated neuronal signalling. In 1955 its clinical properties were formally investigated in the first randomized controlled trial (RCT) of an anti-dopaminergic agent for schizophrenia (Davies & Shepherd, 1955). However, its side effects, in particular lowering of mood likely linked to the depletion of noradrenaline, limited its use. Thus, while reserpine might be considered the first dopamine-modulating treatment for psychosis, the modern era of pharmacology for psychosis really took off with the discovery of another drug: chlorpromazine.

During the Second World War the production of phenothiazines was pursued for their potential as antimalarials though they ultimately failed to show any success. However, Paul Charpentier's team at the Rhône-Poulenc laboratories continued to study the clinical uses of phenothiazines and in 1949 when the surgeon Henri-Marie Laborit was investigating the management of surgical shock, the Rhône-Poulenc laboratories began to focus on this problem. One of the phenothiazines, the antihistamine promethazine, appeared a promising compound in this regard and several of its derivatives were synthesized, including, in December 1950, the compound 'RP-4560' or chlorpromazine as it was later named. Laborit noted that this new compound induced a sense of calm without any clouding of consciousness and, as a result, he encouraged his psychiatric colleagues to test the drug in psychotic patients. The initial reports were extremely encouraging, and news of this remarkable new drug reached Jean Delay and Pierre Denniker at Hôpital Sainte-Anne in Paris. Delay and Denniker were the first to administer the drug alone to treat psychosis and mania without any adjunctive treatments and over the course of 1952 they published six reports documenting their experiences and developed the initial treatment regimens. As a result, chlorpromazine became widely used in Europe and North America during the 1950s, but it was not until the early 1960s that the first large-scale double-blind placebo-controlled trials demonstrating its efficacy in schizophrenia were published (for a further discussion see Haddad & Correll, 2018).

Inspired by the success of chlorpromazine, there was considerable effort over the next decade to produce drugs that worked in a similar way, resulting in numerous agents coming to market. This extraordinary pace was accompanied by a clinical optimism that this rate of progress would continue, and lead to treatments of ever greater efficacy and tolerability. Over the ensuing 60 years, however, while the choice of drugs has expanded significantly, the clinical effectiveness of pharmacological treatments for psychosis has arguably not improved markedly since chlorpromazine's discovery. There have been only two further major developments in terms of the pharmacological mechanisms underlying the clinical efficacy of drugs. First was the discovery of clozapine, a medication that was shown to possess antipsychotic properties without accompanying motor side effects and showing relatively low $D_{2/3}$ occupancy at clinical doses (Shen, 1999), while the second was the development of drugs such as aripiprazole that demonstrated partial agonism, as opposed to full antagonism, at the D_2 receptor.

9.3 Dopamine and Schizophrenia

Following the discovery of antipsychotics, research into their mechanism of action did not take place in isolation but was a component of more general neuroscientific study that led to the discovery of dopamine, and the role that it plays in psychotic illnesses.

Dopamine was initially thought to be a biologically inactive molecule, existing solely as an intermediary in the metabolic pathway between tyramine and noradrenaline.

Towards the end of the 1950s, however, Arvid Carlsson showed that the movement inhibiting effects of reserpine could be reversed by administration of the dopamine precursor L-dopa, and that this was linked to the recovery of dopamine (not noradrenaline) in the brain. Furthermore, Carlsson's group identified dopamine in large concentrations in the brain, in areas of low noradrenaline concentration, supporting the theory that dopamine was a neurotransmitter in its own right.

Soon after these discoveries it was established that dopamine was distributed in the brain via four distinct pathways. The *mesolimbic* pathway projects from the ventral tegmental area (VTA) to the ventral striatum and limbic cortex, the *nigrostriatal* pathway projects from the substantia nigra to the dorsal striatum, the *mesocortical* pathway from the VTA to the prefrontal cortex, and the *tuberoinfundibular* pathway from the hypothalamus to the pituitary.

Preclinical experiments in 1963 had suggested that antipsychotics blocked monoamine receptors, but dopamine had not been specifically identified. Later work in the 1970s linked antipsychotic effects more specifically to their action on dopamine receptors (Creese et al., 1976; Seeman et al., 1975). Additional evidence implicating dopamine in psychosis came from studies demonstrating that substances such as methamphetamine, which increased dopaminergic neurotransmission, could induce psychosis in healthy individuals, and worsen psychotic symptoms in patients. The first direct evidence for dopaminergic abnormalities in schizophrenia came from post-mortem studies. These demonstrated dopaminergic abnormalities in the striata of individuals with schizophrenia; however, results were inconsistent. Furthermore, samples were mostly from individuals that had received extended periods of treatment with dopamine antagonists, and so it was not possible to establish that any abnormalities were a result of a disease process as opposed to a treatment confound (Howes et al., 2017b).

The findings discussed above implicated dopamine in the pathophysiology of schizophrenia only indirectly or after death. Neuroimaging studies of the dopamine system with positron emission tomography (PET) or single photon emission computed tomography (SPECT) involves the radiolabelling of compounds that either bind to receptors and other proteins or are involved in the synthesis of dopamine. The technique has enabled studies to be performed in vivo, in individuals with psychosis prior to treatment with dopamine antagonists. This has therefore avoided many of the drawbacks associated with post-mortem studies. The primary finding from these studies has been that psychosis is associated with increased striatal dopamine synthesis and release capacity, while the density of dopamine $D_{2/3}$ receptors appears to be relatively normal, at least prior to sustained antipsychotic treatment (Howes et al., 2012). Imaging of the mesocortical system has been more challenging, but recently evidence has emerged suggesting that cortical dopamine release may be reduced in schizophrenia (Slifstein et al., 2015).

The striatum receives topographically localized inputs from the cortex and can be divided into three *functional* subdivisions based on the topography of these cortical afferents. The limbic striatum (also known as ventral striatum) receives inputs from limbic areas of the brain such as the medial prefrontal cortex and amygdala, the associative striatum receives inputs from the dorsolateral prefrontal cortex, while the sensorimotor striatum receives inputs from the sensory and motor cortex. The mesolimbic hypothesis of schizophrenia originated with observations that epileptic seizures within limbic areas were associated with psychotic symptoms, and that electrodes implanted in individuals with schizophrenia showed increased activity during periods of psychosis. A link to dopamine specifically came from animal work linking dopamine excess within the limbic striatum to psychotic-like behaviours, and findings that dopamine antagonism extinguished these behaviours (McCutcheon et al., 2019).

Over the past 10 years the development of high-resolution PET cameras has allowed these subdivisions to be examined in detail, and the mesolimbic hypothesis to be tested directly in patients. These recent PET studies have demonstrated an unexpected finding – the major difference in dopaminergic functioning between patients and controls appears to be located dorsally in the associative and sensorimotor striatum as opposed to the limbic striatum (McCutcheon et al., 2018). This calls into question the theory that psychosis is related to mesolimbic dysfunction and has relevance for treatment given that a purported advantage of more recently developed dopamine antagonists was that these drugs might offer 'mesolimbic selectivity' – thereby maximizing efficacy while minimizing side effects.

9.4 Mechanisms Underlying Efficacy in Schizophrenia

9.4.1 Dopamine Receptors

The serendipitous nature of the discovery of chlorpromazine's antipsychotic effects meant that its mechanism of action was initially unknown. A decade passed following its introduction into psychiatric practice before the findings of Carlsson and Lindqvist demonstrated that antipsychotics increased monoamine turnover, and suggested that this might be a compensatory response following the blockade of monoamine receptors (Carlsson & Lindqvist, 1963).

It took a further 10 years before dopamine receptors were identified as intrinsic to the antipsychotic effects of drug treatments for psychosis. Seminal work by Philip Seeman and colleagues, and Solomon Snyder and colleagues in the 1970s (Creese et al., 1976; Seeman et al., 1975) demonstrated that chlorpromazine and other drugs used to treat psychosis bound to receptors in the brain, and that the clinical potency of these drugs was related to both the affinity of the drug for the receptor and the concentration of the drug required to block these receptors.

From early on, it became clear that dopamine bound to the same receptor these drugs bound to, but it was also evident that there existed other receptor sites in the brain that dopamine bound to that did not show a high affinity for antipsychotics. By the 1980s it was apparent that there were two main groups of dopamine receptors in the brain – D_1-like and D_2-like receptors. This was consistent with earlier preclinical work demonstrating that dopamine could have both excitatory and inhibitory effects. The receptor bound by the drugs used to treat psychosis was termed the D_2 receptor, and was shown to have inhibitory effects, while the D_1 receptor displayed excitatory effects (Kebabian & Calne, 1979). It has subsequently been discovered that there are in fact three inhibitory dopamine receptor subtypes (D_2, D_3, D_4) and two excitatory subtypes (D_1, D_5); however, it is primarily the D_2 receptor that is linked to the antipsychotic effect of dopamine antagonists (Seeman, 2001).

The D_2 receptor (like all G-protein-coupled receptors) exists in two states – a high-affinity state that is G-protein coupled and is responsible for the functional effects following agonist binding, and an inert uncoupled low-affinity state. D_2 antagonists bind equally to both states, while agonists such as dopamine preferentially bind to the high-affinity receptor. Animal and in vitro studies have suggested that schizophrenia could be associated with a selective increase in the density of high-affinity receptors (for reviews see Howes et al., 2015; Perreault et al., 2010; Seeman, 2011). The development of D_2 agonist radiotracers (e.g. 11C-PHNO), which preferentially bind to the high-affinity form of the D_2 receptors, provided the opportunity to test this in vivo. However, studies to date have found no evidence that there is a difference in the D_2 high-affinity state in schizophrenia (Graff-Guerrero et al., 2009, 2013), although subsequently it has been suggested that current tools are still unable to accurately distinguish between different affinity states (Howes et al., 2015; Seeman, 2012).

9.4.2 Determining the Mechanism of Action of Drugs In Vivo

As well as its utility in probing the pathophysiology of psychotic disorders, PET imaging has been a valuable tool for studying the action of dopamine antagonists in vivo. The first PET study of this kind demonstrated that at typical clinical doses dopamine receptor antagonists such as haloperidol and chlorpromazine displayed D_2 receptor occupancies of around 80%. Further research developed the idea that a 'therapeutic window' existed in terms of receptor occupancy, whereby D_2 occupancies above 60% were required for a high likelihood of clinical response, but occupancies above 80% were associated with an increased risk of side effects, in particular extrapyramidal motor side effects, without much greater likelihood of response (see Figure 9.1). In most first-episode patients, a dose of around 2 mg of haloperidol is sufficient to achieve $D_{2/3}$ receptor blockade in this window. Prior to this research being conducted in the 1990s, it was common to treat patients with doses well in excess of 20 mg of haloperidol per day, and some received doses of more than 100 mg per day. The PET findings contributed to a change in clinical practice to use lower doses of dopamine blockers (Kapur, 1998).

Roughly one third of individuals with schizophrenia do not respond to standard dopamine antagonists. PET studies have shown that this is not generally related to insufficient occupancy of D_2 receptors, although it may explain inadequate response in some patients (Kapur et al., 2000). More recent PET studies have suggested that in these treatment-resistant patients there is no increase in dopamine synthesis capacity, suggesting that a non-dopaminergic mechanism may underlie their symptoms (Howes & Kapur, 2014).

9.4.3 Non-Dopaminergic Mechanisms and the Concept of Atypicality

All drugs currently used to treat schizophrenia are dopamine $D_{2/3}$ receptor blockers to some degree, although they differ in their actions at other receptors. Shortly after the development of chlorpromazine and haloperidol it was found that these drugs could cause catalepsy in rodents and motor side effects in patients. It was originally thought that these effects were linked to the drugs' therapeutic effects. The development of clozapine in the 1960s challenged this hypothesis because it was an efficacious treatment with almost no movement side effects. However, clozapine was found to be associated with agranulocytosis in about 2% of patients, leading to it being removed from the market in many countries in 1975. Nevertheless, it continued to be used with careful monitoring of blood counts in some countries. Clinicians in these countries noted that it seemed effective in patients who did not respond to other drugs, and this clinical observation led to clinical trials in the late 1980s and early 1990s that showed it was

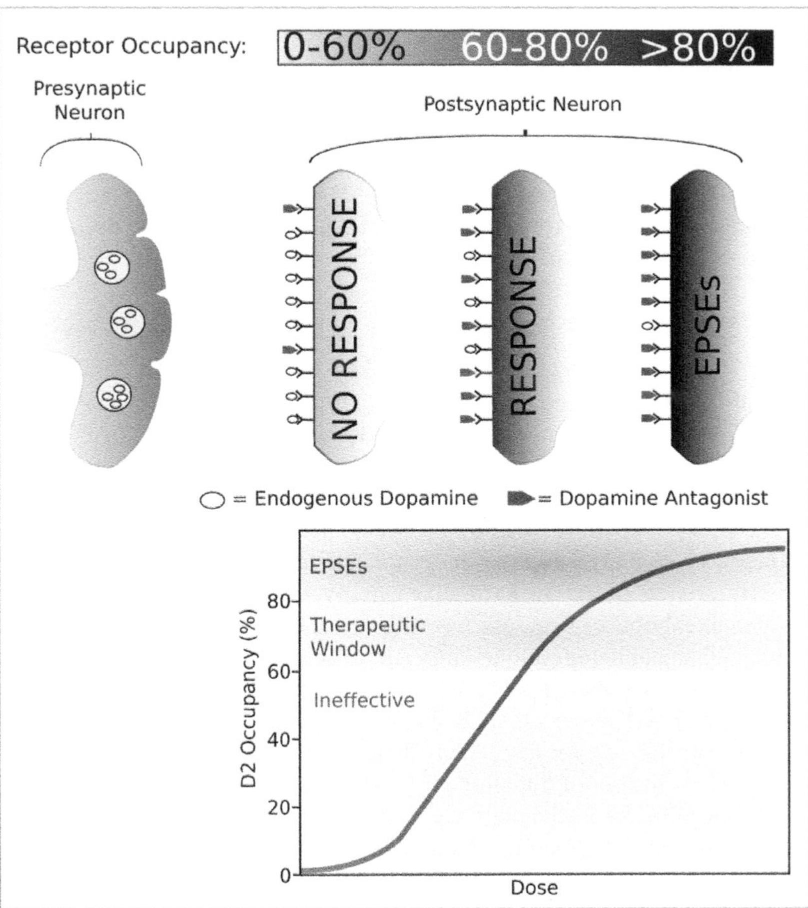

Figure 9.1 The 'therapeutic window' of response. Blocking of D_2 receptors by dopamine antagonists improves symptoms when this blockade is greater than 60%, but this leads to movement side effects when greater than 80%.

effective for patients who had not responded to standard $D_{2/3}$-blocking treatments such as chlorpromazine. Thus, clozapine was different to the other dopamine antagonists because it showed greater effectiveness in treatment-resistant patients but was much less likely to cause catalepsy in rodents and motor side effects in patients. Clozapine became the prototypical 'atypical antipsychotic' drug, and the other drugs were termed 'typical' because they showed catalepsy and motor side effects, and less efficacy in some patients. This, in turn, led to a search for other drug treatments that would display antipsychotic activity with greater efficacy and without movement side effects, similar to clozapine but without the risk of agranulocytosis.

The mechanism via which movement side effect could be avoided, yet antipsychotic effects retained and even enhanced, was not entirely clear and various hypotheses have been proposed. Rapid dissociation was proposed as one mechanism potentially contributing to a reduced extrapyramidal side-effect (EPSE) burden. The binding of a drug to a receptor is a dynamic process, in which molecules of the drug continuously bind, and then dissociate (are released) from the receptor. Differences in receptor affinity between dopamine antagonists are particularly driven by differences in the rate of dissociation, as association rates are generally uniform. Supporting this, clozapine and quetiapine show a higher dissociation rate constant than the 'typical' drugs, such as haloperidol, used to treat psychosis. Drugs that dissociate faster are more sensitive to changes in endogenous levels of dopamine, thereby potentially allowing more physiological dopaminergic transmission than drugs with slow dissociation rates. Thus, it was suggested that rapid dissociation could permit enough dopaminergic neurotransmission to avoid catalepsy and motor side effects. Preclinical work has also shown that drugs that display more sustained blockade of the D_2 receptor are more likely to lead to tolerance and up-regulation of receptors, potentially increasing the risk of tardive dyskinesia. This hypothesis was supported by PET studies of D_2 occupancy demonstrating that drugs noted for lower rates of EPSE such as quetiapine and clozapine displayed rapid reductions in dopamine receptor occupancy following dosing. Although the drugs show greater occupancy immediately after dosing, this fell to as low as 20% 12 hours after receiving the dose (Kapur & Seeman, 2001).

Clozapine was also noted to show a high ratio of binding to the serotonin 2A receptor (5-HT_{2A}) relative to binding to the dopamine $D_{2/3}$ receptor. Based on this, Meltzer and colleagues suggested that the preferential activity at the 5-HT_{2A} receptor could contribute to the special properties of clozapine (Meltzer et al., 1989). This contributed to the development of several drugs, including risperidone and olanzapine, which had high affinities for the 5-HT_{2A} receptor (see Figure 9.2).

'Atypicality' was also held to reflect an anatomical specificity. It had been proposed that psychotic symptoms were primarily driven by aberrant dopaminergic function of mesolimbic dopamine pathways. Animal studies suggested that atypical drugs had the ability to preferentially affect neuronal firing and gene expression in limbic, as opposed to motor, areas of the striatum. This was seen as potentially underlying both greater antipsychotic effects and lower movement side effects of atypical agents.

Multiple clinical and PET studies, however, have challenged the concept of 'atypicality'. There is no evidence for greater clinical effectiveness in schizophrenia of drugs other than clozapine that possess high levels of 5-HT_{2A} affinity, nor those that show rapid D_2 dissociation. Amisulpride, which displays almost no serotonergic activity, is no less effective than dopamine antagonists which possess a high affinity for the 5-HT_{2A} receptor (Leucht et al., 2013). Likewise, quetiapine rapidly dissociates from the D_2 receptor, yet shows no greater effectiveness than slow dissociators such as haloperidol (Leucht et al., 2013).

A lower burden of EPSE is another clinical characteristic associated with the concept of atypicality. Based on several PET studies, Kapur and colleagues proposed that a major contributing factor to this was not any difference in molecular mechanisms, but rather that this was primarily secondary to dosing. Drugs such as haloperidol were frequently given at doses that led to greater than 90% D_2 occupancy, whereas doses used for the drugs described as 'atypical' rarely exceed 80% D_2 occupancy, and generally when atypicals were given in higher doses, they too induced EPSE (Kapur et al., 2000). Quetiapine and clozapine are unusual because they rarely result in EPSE even at high doses. This also can be understood in terms of D_2 occupancy, because even high doses are unlikely to exceed 80% D_2 occupancy, and their fast dissociation from the D_2 receptor means occupancy drops rapidly after dosing (Kapur & Seeman, 2000) As a result, it appears that the concept of atypicality bears no established relationship to pharmacological mechanisms, or clinical outcomes, and is better understood as largely an artefact of

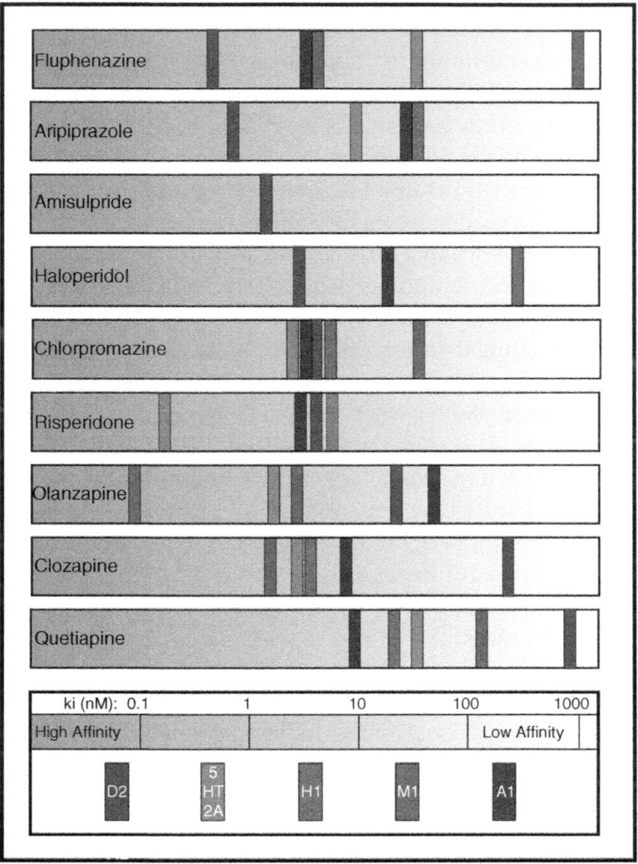

Figure 9.2 Affinities for the D_2 (dopamine D_2), 5-HT_{2A} (serotonin 2A), H_1 (histamine H_1), M_1 (muscarinic acetylcholine) and A1 (α_1-adrenergic) receptor for various antipsychotics. At lower doses the drugs primarily bind to receptors which they have a high affinity for (those to the left of the diagram); as dosage increases, they will start to bind to lower affinity receptors. This means that if a drug is dosed to achieve adequate D_2 occupancy for antipsychotic effects, any receptors to the left of, or close to the D_2 bar will also have relatively high levels of occupancy. Affinities taken from Correll (2010) and the PDSP Ki database (http://pdspdb.unc.edu/pdspWeb/).

dosing and pharmacodynamics at the dopamine D_2 receptor. It is therefore recommended that the term 'atypical antipsychotic' is abandoned as it does not provide accurate information regarding either the clinical or molecular profile of these drugs. However, in NbN the distinction is made between those drugs with a high 5-HT_{2A} receptor affinity (serotonin/dopamine antagonists) and those without this (dopamine antagonists) as there is some emerging evidence that drugs with pure 5-HT_{2A} antagonist activity, e.g. pimavanserin, do have antipsychotic activity in Parkinson's disease and maybe Alzheimer's disease (see below), and their actions at these receptors may contribute to therapeutic effects for mood and anxiety.

9.4.4 Targeting the Locus of Dysfunction in Schizophrenia

As discussed above, developments in PET imaging have suggested that dopaminergic overactivity in schizophrenia is unlikely to be restricted to the mesolimbic pathway. A consequence of this is that the proposed 'mesolimbic selectivity' of newer dopamine antagonists is unlikely to translate into meaningful benefits in terms of efficacy, a conclusion mirrored in the clinical trial literature. It has long been proposed that in addition to hyperdopaminergic functioning in the striatum, schizophrenia may be accompanied by a hypodopaminergic state in cortical areas (Slifstein et al., 2015; Weinberger, 1987). Dopamine antagonists therefore have the potential to block cortical dopamine receptors and so exacerbate some aspects of the disorder including negative symptoms and cognitive impairment. Treatments with the potential to augment dopaminergic transmission in cortical regions while blocking striatal dopamine (e.g. aripiprazole and low-dose amisulpride) have shown some evidence of effectiveness against negative symptoms (Murphy et al., 2006).

Current dopamine-modulating treatments for psychosis act on dopamine receptors (predominantly postsynaptically) despite the finding that dopaminergic abnormalities in schizophrenia appear to be predominantly presynaptic. Furthermore, the underlying cause of presynaptic dopaminergic dysfunction remains to be established. Therapeutic agents currently in development are investigating the possibility of intervening earlier in the causative chain, potentially at the site of primary pathology. There is interest both in directly modulating presynaptic dopamine function, for example by targeting dopamine D_2 autoreceptors to reduce excess dopamine synthesis (Jauhar et al., 2017), and in addressing targets further upstream that are proposed to lead to striatal dopamine dysfunction (Grace & Gomes, 2019; Howes & McCutcheon, 2017).

9.5 From Vegetative Stabilizers to Dopamine Antagonists; Classification and Nomenclature

9.5.1 Older Terminology

Chlorpromazine was initially described as a 'vegetative stabilizer' as it had been investigated with a view to its ability to dampen the activity of the autonomic nervous system during surgery (Laborit et al., 1952). In addition to descriptions of chemical structure such as 'phenothiazine' and 'dibenzodiazepine', this group of drugs has had a range of names that aims to capture their behavioural effects, including 'ataraxic', 'neuroleptic' and 'major tranquilliser' (King & Voruganti, 2002). In recent decades the term 'antipsychotic' has become most widely used, despite the fact that these agents are often used in the treatment of individuals with non-psychotic disorders. The terms 'second generation' and 'atypical' were used to distinguish the wave of compounds developed following the rediscovery of clozapine, from earlier antipsychotic agents. None of these terms reliably speak to the compounds' pharmacological properties.

This is an issue that is not unique to dopamine antagonists. There are significant drawbacks to the existing nomenclature used for psychopharmacological agents. Current terminology encourages the inappropriate grouping of drugs with significantly different pharmacological properties. It may also inappropriately shape clinical heuristics and discourage a neuroscientific approach to pharmacological research and clinical practice. For example, trials investigating the pharmacological treatment of psychotic depression have typically been framed as investigating the comparative efficacy of 'antidepressants' and 'antipsychotics' (Wijkstra et al., 2015). This is potentially misleading given the use of certain drugs typically classified as 'antipsychotic' in treating depressive symptoms (e.g. quetiapine, flupentixol). In addition, the development of drugs for the treatment of schizophrenia with no direct dopaminergic activity (Davidson et al., 2017) means pharmacologically informative descriptions are of increasing importance.

9.5.2 Neuroscience-Based Nomenclature

Neuroscience-based Nomenclature (NbN) (Zohar et al., 2015) aims to address a number of the deficiencies inherent to the drug classification systems discussed above. The method aims to primarily classify compounds by their receptor binding profiles (see below for further discussion). Drug affinities were determined from the published literature. Where there was more than one data source, the data were ranked as follows: in vivo > in vitro (primate brain imaging > cloned human receptors > rat tissue). The term serotonin-dopamine antagonist has been used to highlight the fact that some antipsychotic medications block very high numbers of serotonin receptors, principally 5-HT_{2A}, at clinical doses. For example olanzapine has near 100% 5-HT_{2A} occupancy at subtherapeutic doses (Kapur et al., 1998) and similarly, risperidone and clozapine also show high levels of 5-HT_{2A} occupancy (Kapur et al., 1999; Nyberg et al., 1993) relative to D_2 receptor occupancy. Pimavanserin, uniquely, is primarily serotonergic. It has shown efficacy in psychosis associated with Parkinson's disease, but has yet to be tested in schizophrenia. Further information on NbN is provided in the Editor's Note on Nomenclature.

9.6 Binding Affinities of Dopamine-Modulating Agents

The binding affinity (Ki) of a drug refers to the concentration of drug that would occupy 50% of the receptors if there was no competition for the receptor. A smaller value therefore represents a greater affinity (i.e. tighter binding) of the compound for the receptor. This is quite different to the concept of *potency*, as the affinity does not speak to the biological response engendered by the receptor binding.

Nevertheless, the binding affinity profile of a drug has clinical relevance for dosing as it influences the dose needed for adequate $D_{2/3}$ blockade and the likelihood of off-target effects at other receptors that increase the risk of side effects. For example, quetiapine has a Ki of 19 for the H_1 receptor, 31 for the 5-HT_{2A} receptor and 770 for the D_2 receptor. This means that at low doses quetiapine will have a large antihistaminergic action with relatively low anti-dopaminergic action. As dose is increased, H_1 receptors will rapidly become saturated so there will be little change in antihistaminergic properties, but anti-dopaminergic and anti-serotonergic properties will become evident. Moreover, as the relationship between dose and occupancy (and therefore clinical effect) is not linear, relatively small increases in dosing can have a marked clinical impact (see Figure 9.3). Relative receptor affinities for some of the more commonly used dopamine blockers are displayed in Figure 9.2.

9.7 Pharmacokinetics

The pharmacodynamic properties of a drug describe the effects of that drug on the organism, in particular drug–receptor interactions. Pharmacokinetic properties, meanwhile, describe how the organism processes the drug. Both have important clinical

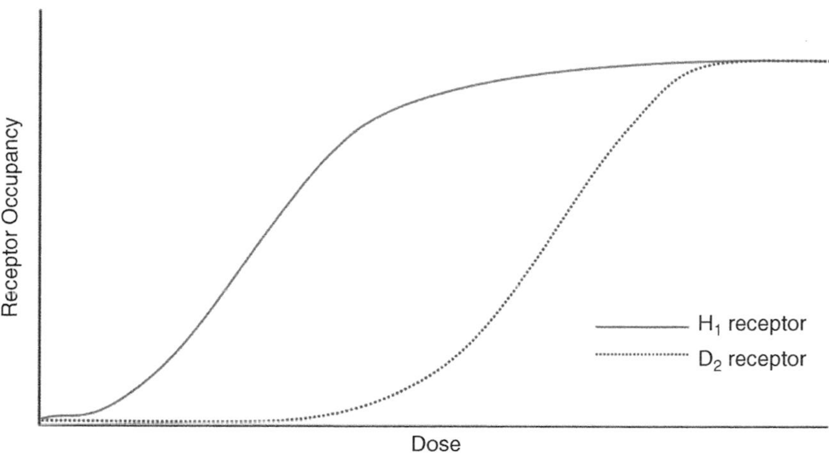

Figure 9.3 Example dose–occupancy curve. The hypothetical drug illustrated has a greater affinity for the H_1 receptor than the D_2 receptor and so at low doses predominantly antihistaminergic clinical effects will be observed. At higher doses some D_2 occupancy begins to occur and H_1 receptors become fully saturated.

implications. The rest of this section outlines important principles related to the pharmacokinetics of oral formulations of dopamine antagonists and partial agonists; a subsequent section discusses the pharmacokinetics of long-acting injectable (LAI) formulations while Chapter 4 provides a more detailed review of pharmacokinetics in general.

9.7.1 Half-Lives, Steady State and Washout

When a drug is orally administered its plasma concentration gradually rises, reaches a peak and then begins to fall. The half-life of a drug is the time required for the concentration of the drug to fall to half its initial concentration, after reaching the peak value. This typically refers to the plasma concentration, and so factors that increase the rate of removal of the drug from the plasma contribute to a shorter half-life.

The half-life of a drug will determine both the drug's time to steady state and the drug's washout time. The steady state of a drug refers to the situation in which the intake of the drug is in equilibrium with its elimination. The time to reach steady state is proportional to the half-life of a drug. In most situations, if the drug is dosed about every half-life, after one half-life the concentration of the drug will have reached 50% of steady state, after two 75%, after three 87.5% etc. It is a fair approximation to assume for clinical purposes that after five half-lives one has achieved close to steady state. The converse of *time to steady state* is *washout time*; this is the time for the drug to be effectively eliminated, generally after one half-life the drug will be 50% eliminated, and after five half-lives the concentration of the drug will have reduced to 3% of the steady-state value. Half-lives and washout times for a number of dopamine antagonists are displayed in Table 9.1.

Most dopamine antagonists are metabolized by the cytochrome P450 system (with some exceptions, e.g. amisulpride is renally excreted unchanged). Inhibition and

Table 9.1 Half-lives and washout times for a number of dopamine antagonists

Drug	Half-life (hours)	Time to steady state/ washout time (days)
Clozapine	12	2.5
Haloperidol	20	4.2
Olanzapine	30	6.3
Amisulpride	12	2.5
Risperidone	20[a]	4.2
Aripiprazole	60	13
Quetiapine	6/24[b]	1.3/5[b]

[a] Half-life of risperidone and its active metabolite 9-hydroxyrisperidone.
[b] Depending on whether instant or extended-release formulation.

induction of these enzymes by other drugs can have a significant impact on levels of dopamine antagonists and dosing may need to be adjusted (see the section on interactions below). The polycyclic aromatic hydrocarbons in tobacco smoke induce CYP1A2 enzymes and this can cause a significant reduction in clozapine and olanzapine levels. Discontinuation of smoking, including switching to e-cigarettes, can therefore lead to a marked increase in drug levels and plasma levels should be checked, particularly in the case of clozapine.

CYP450 genetic polymorphisms influence the plasma levels of many dopamine blockers (Ravyn et al., 2013). The CYP2D6 enzyme is involved in the metabolism of most dopamine antagonists, and individuals possessing inactive alleles will have higher plasma levels, compared with individuals with active alleles. Despite the impact of polymorphisms on drug metabolism, it is not clear whether routine pharmacogenetic testing improves patient outcomes, either in terms of efficacy or safety. It may be that potential benefits have not been identified due to the limitations of existing studies – which have predominantly been either small, or retrospective (Arranz et al., 2011; Grossman et al., 2008). Alternatively, given that in clinical practice dosing is titrated according to clinical benefit and side effects, it may be that to a large extent patients have plasma levels indirectly optimized. As such, the use of pharmacogenetics to more precisely adjust plasma levels may have little to offer. This applies to the issues accompanying plasma level testing of dopamine antagonists and is discussed further below.

Gender and ethnicity have pharmacokinetic relevance. Males typically require higher drug doses than females, this may be both due to larger volumes of distribution and more rapid clearance (Soldin & Mattison, 2009). Certain genetic variants involved in the metabolism of dopamine antagonists appear to be more common in certain ethnic groups. For example, in the Clinical Antipsychotic Trials of Intervention Effectiveness (CATIE) study olanzapine clearance was found to be significantly higher in African-American patients compared with other ethnic groups, and this was suggested to result from a CYP3A variant being more common in those of African origin

(Soderberg & Dahl, 2013). In general, however, ethnic differences in dopamine antagonist metabolism have not been well studied and should not routinely influence treatment decisions.

Where pharmacokinetic factors have clinical relevance is when switching dopamine antagonists. Abruptly switching from a dopamine antagonist with a short half-life to one with a longer half-life with no cross-over increases the likelihood of rebound phenomena, as the initial drug's concentration will have reduced markedly without the replacement medication having reached a sufficient concentration. The converse of abruptly switching from a long to short half-life drug does not carry the same risk.

9.7.2 Absorption and Modes of Administration

The bioavailability of a drug is the fraction of the administered dose that enters the systemic circulation. Following ingestion and prior to reaching the systemic circulation the drug will undergo absorption and potentially first-pass hepatic metabolism, each of which will potentially affect the drug's bioavailability. Most drugs used to treat psychosis have sufficient oral bioavailability that doses can be taken orally without the need to be too concerned about factors that may affect this. There are, however, several exceptions. Due to its high hepatic first-pass metabolism, asenapine must be taken sublingually rather than swallowed, and eating or drinking should be avoided for 10 minutes following administration. Lurasidone and ziprasidone meanwhile should be taken with food to optimize absorption from the gastrointestinal tract and hence maximize bioavailability.

Most dopamine antagonists are administered once daily. Due to a shorter half-life some drugs including amisulpride, asenapine, clozapine and immediate-release quetiapine are licensed for twice-daily administration. If unintentional non-adherence is a concern and treatment with one of these latter medications is indicated once-daily administration may be considered if it is felt this may improve adherence. This will however lead to greater variability in plasma levels so attention should be paid to potential worsening of side effects or changes in mental state.

Oral disintegrating forms of olanzapine and risperidone are available. Oral suspensions are also available for a range of dopamine antagonists. These modes of administration are used less commonly but may be useful if a patient has difficulty swallowing tablets or if covert non-adherence is a concern in an inpatient setting. Loxapine is available as an inhalation powder and its rapid onset of action means it can be used to manage acute agitation in schizophrenia and bipolar disorder (Kwentus et al., 2012; Lesem et al., 2011).

9.7.3 Plasma Level Monitoring

Assays are available to measure the plasma concentration of most commonly used dopamine antagonists and partial agonists. However, while plasma level monitoring is recommended for clozapine, for other dopamine antagonists there is little evidence that routine use offers any significant benefit (Horvitz-Lennon et al., 2017). This is partly due to the fact that for most dopamine antagonists a clearly defined therapeutic range has not been established (Mauri et al., 2007). Studies attempting to clarify therapeutic ranges are complicated by the fact that they require large sample sizes, randomization to different doses, repeated sampling and clinical measurements. As a result, evidence in this area is lacking. Furthermore, for most dopamine antagonists, dose–response relationships have been established to an extent that in routine clinical care the additional information provided by plasma level monitoring is not required.

While routine use is not advised, there are several clinical scenarios where the measurement of plasma levels is likely to have a favourable cost–benefit ratio. In cases of suspected toxicity plasma level monitoring should be undertaken urgently. There is also a role for the use of plasma levels in the assessment of treatment-resistant schizophrenia (Beck et al., 2014; McCutcheon et al., 2015, 2017). It is often not clear if inadequate response to treatment is due to inadequate dopamine antagonist exposure as opposed to true treatment resistance. It is important to distinguish between these two possibilities as management options are quite different – in the first case action will be taken to address underexposure, while in the second a trial of clozapine is likely indicated.

9.8 Therapeutic Uses of Dopamine Antagonists and Partial Agonists

9.8.1 Acute Treatment of Schizophrenia

Dopamine antagonists have demonstrated efficacy in the acute treatment of schizophrenia. These drugs increase the percentage of patients responding from 24% with placebo to 41%. Therefore, approximately twice as many patients improve with active treatment compared with placebo. Recent meta-analytic data suggest the standardized mean difference (SMD) between antipsychotics and placebo is 0.38, with a greater effect seen on positive symptoms (SMD 0.45) than negative symptoms (SMD 0.35), quality of life (SMD 0.35) or depression (SMD 0.27) (Leucht et al., 2017). Such effect sizes are comparable with or better than those found in treatments for physical health conditions including angiotensin-converting-enzyme inhibitors for reducing cardiac mortality and events due to hypertension (SMD 0.16) and statins for reducing risk of cardiac disease and stroke (SMD 0.15) (Leucht et al., 2012a).

Meta-analysis shows that the dopamine antagonist amisulpride and the dopamine-serotonin antagonists clozapine, olanzapine and risperidone had greater overall efficacy in the acute treatment of schizophrenia than the first-generation dopamine antagonists albeit with small to medium effect sizes for the additional benefit (Leucht et al., 2009). However, as differences are relatively modest, and many of the trials of the first-generation drugs used much higher doses than would be generally used today, there may be some bias in such findings against the first-generation drugs. Other second-generation drugs do not appear more efficacious than the first-generation drugs (Leucht et al., 2009). Thus, with the exception of clozapine for treatment resistance, efficacy differences between drugs are not a major factor in determining choice of drug. In contrast, there are large differences in side effects (Leucht et al., 2009), which has implications for drug choice.

In terms of efficacy and tolerability, network meta-analysis suggests that the dopamine-serotonin antagonists olanzapine and risperidone and the dopamine antagonist amisulpride rank highly for efficacy and tolerability in the acute phases of schizophrenia (Zhu et al., 2017). However, olanzapine can present significant metabolic side effects and risperidone and amisulpride have a higher propensity for hyperprolactinaemia and EPSE than other dopamine-serotonin antagonists.

The more potent dopamine antagonists such as haloperidol, flupentixol, zuclopenthixol, depixol and fluphenazine are effective in treating the positive symptoms of schizophrenia but the risk of inducing both acute and chronic EPSE, including tardive dyskinesia, is approximately double the risk of the dopamine-serotonin antagonists (Carbon et al., 2018). However, measures can be taken to reduce the impact of such long-term side effects by, for example, using the lowest effective maintenance dose possible. In all cases the most appropriate medication should be chosen following a considered review of the individual characteristics of the patient.

Most patients who fail to show any response after the first two to three weeks at an effective dose are unlikely to respond if given more, though some patients with a partial response may improve over time (Leucht et al., 2007). Plasma drug monitoring can be helpful in such cases (Horvitz-Lennon et al., 2017). If the first antipsychotic is unsuccessful then a different antipsychotic should be tried in a similar fashion. In most cases patients who do not respond to a therapeutic dose of an antipsychotic are unlikely to respond to doses above the licensed range, that is, high doses. However, there are some cases where patients may require high doses to be efficacious, for example due to the effect of smoking or genetic variants on the metabolism of some antipsychotics (Horvitz-Lennon et al., 2017).

If the patient has failed to respond to two different antipsychotics then guidelines indicate the patient's condition should be considered treatment resistant (Howes et al., 2017a) . In this case clozapine is recommended as the only antipsychotic drug licensed for treatment resistance and with established efficacy in treatment resistance (Siskind et al., 2016).

The administration of two or more antipsychotics to the same patient (other than with 'add-ons' to clozapine – see Chapter 10) is usually unnecessary and increases the risk of adverse effects without much evidence of increased benefit (Ortiz-Orendain et al., 2017). Combinations of more than one antipsychotic drug are also likely to lead to the inadvertent prescribing of net high doses, risking side effects. Only one antipsychotic drug should be given at a time, other than rare exceptions or for short periods during cross-titrations.

9.8.2 Maintenance Treatment of Schizophrenia

Results from RCTs clearly demonstrate the superiority of oral dopamine receptor antagonists compared with placebo in preventing relapse in schizophrenia at 7 to 12 months (Leucht et al., 2012b). However, randomized controlled evidence beyond one year is relatively limited because it is ethically and practically challenging to conduct such studies (Leucht et al., 2012b). This raises the question of how long to continue treatment given the potential risks associated with long-term treatment

(Murray et al., 2016). Naturalistic studies generally show lower rates of relapse and readmission in patients who continue treatment over the longer term (Tiihonen et al., 2017), although, as patients are not randomized in these studies, there is the risk that results are biased because more compliant patients who might be expected to do well anyway end up continuing treatment. LAI preparations of antipsychotics have an important role in maintenance treatment and are considered in a later section of this chapter.

9.8.3 Treatment of Mania

Several lines of evidence indicate that hyperdopaminergia contributes to acute mania (Ashok et al., 2017), and dopamine blockers have been used in its treatment for many years. Meta-analysis suggests that D_2 antagonists are slightly more effective than so-called 'mood stabilizers' (i.e. valproate and lithium) in acute mania (Cipriani et al., 2011) and that haloperidol, olanzapine, risperidone and quetiapine are particularly effective as short-term treatments, though haloperidol was associated with more drop-outs (Goodwin et al., 2016). Lithium and valproate, as monotherapy or in combination with an antipsychotic in more severe cases, are other potential treatments, and, while less effective for acute mania, they may be preferred if the clinical history indicates prophylaxis against depressive episodes is also warranted. The choice of drug to treat acute mania should be determined by the clinical presentation of the patient and patient preference. Other than in exceptional circumstances valproate should be avoided in women of childbearing potential due primarily to concerns about its teratogenic and neurodevelopmental effects on the fetus (for further details see Chapter 19).

9.8.4 Treatment of Acute Bipolar Depression

The dopamine-serotonin antagonists quetiapine, lurasidone or olanzapine are recommended as first-line treatment options in treating acute bipolar depression and have the advantage of having additional antimanic properties (Goodwin et al., 2016). However, it is something of a paradox that these are dopamine receptor blockers, which might be thought to worsen some depressive symptoms. It is presumed that it is their actions at serotonin receptors that contribute to their potential benefit for bipolar depression but this remains to be tested (Ashok et al., 2017).

There is very little evidence from RCTs for the efficacy of antidepressants in treating bipolar depression. Indeed, the largest placebo-controlled RCT of adjunctive antidepressants in bipolar depression showed that mood stabilizers plus antidepressant treatment was no more effective than mood stabilizer plus placebo (Sachs et al., 2007). Treatment of bipolar depression can be particularly challenging due to the risk of inducing a switch into mania or provoking mood instability. Antidepressant monotherapy increases the risk of switching and should be avoided.

9.8.5 Maintenance Treatment of Bipolar Disorder

Several dopamine antagonists and partial agonists have been approved in one or more countries to reduce the risk of relapse in bipolar disorder including aripiprazole, olanzapine, quetiapine, ziprasidone and LAI risperidone. These licences differ between countries, for example the only antipsychotics that are licensed for maintenance treatment of bipolar disorder in the UK are quetiapine, olanzapine and aripiprazole. Each of these drugs was shown in RCTs to reduce the risk of relapse in bipolar disorder compared with placebo. Most maintenance trials in bipolar disorder have randomized patients who had an acute episode of illness that responded to the drug in question, i.e. they have an enrichment design (selection bias) (Lindström et al., 2017). As such, maintenance licences usually specify that approval is for continued treatment when a manic or mixed episode responded to the drug in question. Quetiapine is unique in that its maintenance licence applies irrespective of whether an episode of depression or mania responded to treatment. This reflects the fact that quetiapine is the only dopamine receptor antagonist that has been shown to be effective in treating mania and bipolar depression and reduce the risk of relapse at both these poles. All the other dopamine receptor antagonists and partial agonists that are licensed as maintenance treatments in bipolar disorder are effective in reducing manic relapse but have not shown superiority to placebo in preventing relapse of bipolar depression.

In practice, the choice of a long-term maintenance agent in bipolar disorder is likely to be influenced by the drug that was successful in treating the last acute episode of illness. If adherence to oral medication is poor, then a LAI antipsychotic should be considered to reduce the risk of future manic episodes. At present LAI risperidone is the only LAI to be approved as a maintenance agent in bipolar disorder and this approval is in the USA and not the UK. The selection of a long-term agent will also be influenced by the relative risk of side effects of different medications.

Lamotrigine and lithium have also been shown to reduce the risk of relapse of bipolar disorder in RCTs and are approved as maintenance treatments in bipolar disorder in the UK. Lamotrigine reduces the risk of depressive relapses (see Chapter 13) while lithium (see Chapter 11) reduces the risk of both depressive and manic relapses. Most guidelines also regard valproate as an option for maintenance treatment of bipolar disorder though it is not approved for this indication (see Chapter 12). Valproate should not be prescribed to women of childbearing potential due to the risk of teratogenicity and neurodevelopmental impairment to the fetus and the risk of polycystic ovary syndrome (Chapter 19).

9.8.6 Treatment of Acute Agitation

Dopamine antagonists and partial agonists have an important role in the treatment of acute agitation. They may be administered orally but if a rapid onset of action is needed then certain drugs may be given intramuscularly and, in very rare cases, intravenously. In addition, loxapine is available as an orally inhaled preparation with absorption occurring in the lungs. It should be remembered that the underlying cause of the agitation should be treated in conjunction with the symptoms of agitation. Further details of using antipsychotics in control of agitation, and in rapid tranquillisation, are provided in Chapter 20.

9.8.7 Treatment of Anxiety Disorders

Dopamine and dopamine-serotonin antagonists have several potential uses in the treatment of anxiety disorders. This is only discussed briefly here as Chapter 8 provides a detailed review. Low-dose quetiapine (50–150 mg/day) is effective in monotherapy in treating generalized anxiety disorder in adults but does not have a UK licence for this indication (Maneeton et al., 2016). As it is less well tolerated than selective serotonin reuptake inhibitors (SSRIs) in generalized anxiety disorder it is usually reserved for those that fail to respond to or tolerate SSRIs or where sedation or a sleep-promoting effect is desired. Meta-analytic evidence supports the role of specific antipsychotics (aripiprazole, haloperidol, risperidone) in augmenting SSRIs in treatment-resistant obsessive-compulsive disorder (Dold et al., 2015). One open-label trial has suggested efficacy for augmenting SSRI treatment with olanzapine in treatment-resistant panic disorder (Sepede et al., 2006).

9.8.8 Treatment of Major Depressive Disorder

Spielmans et al. (2013) conducted a meta-analysis of randomized trials that compared adjunctive antipsychotic medication with placebo for treatment-resistant depression in adults. Fourteen trials of aripiprazole, olanzapine/fluoxetine combination (OFC), quetiapine and risperidone were identified. All four drugs improved remission to a statistically significant degree. The trials involved patients taking various antidepressants. The number needed to treat (NNT) was nine for each drug other than OFC where it was 19. However, there was little or no benefit on measures of functioning and quality of life with the exception of risperidone, which improved quality of life to a small to moderate degree. Adverse effects were more common with antipsychotic augmentation compared with placebo augmentation. The pattern of adverse effects differed somewhat depending on the agent used. For example, akathisia was more common with aripiprazole and weight gain with OFC. The authors concluded that specific antipsychotics were efficacious in augmenting antidepressants and reducing observer-rated depressive symptoms. However, they recommended that clinicians interpret the results with caution given the modest benefits, the very limited evidence for improvement in terms of quality of life or functioning and the adverse effect profile. Furthermore, there is a lack of long-term data in using antipsychotics in this indication. On the other hand, one needs to consider the severity and impact of the depressive syndrome that is being treated. Note the benefit of these specific drugs may relate to their serotonin antagonist properties as much as to their dopamine-blocking ones.

9.9 Long-Acting Injectable Dopamine Antagonists

9.9.1 Introduction

The development of LAI antipsychotics began in the late 1950s following experiments to prolong drug release into the circulation through esterification of antipsychotics with fatty acids. For a comprehensive history of depot antipsychotic medication see Johnson (2009). Fluphenazine enanthate and flupenazine decanoate were the first long-acting compounds. Both drugs proved efficacious in 'mirror studies' which compared duration and frequency of admission before and after treatment with the LAI (Hirsch et al., 1973). Subsequently, flupentixol decanoate (Depixol), zuclopenthixol decanoate (Clopixol) and haloperidol decanoate (Haldol) were produced and used in clinical practice.

These long-acting esterified dopamine antagonists are dissolved in an oil carrier, usually sesame oil (see Table 9.2), and injected intramuscularly deep into the gluteal muscle. As the esters are slowly released from the oil they are hydrolysed into the active drug over a number of days. This allows weekly to monthly dosing regimens and leads to such preparations being called depot antipsychotics.

The newer LAI dopamine-serotonin antagonists and dopamine partial agonists use an aqueous solution of microspheres/drug particles instead of an oil delivery system (see Table 9.2). An injection is usually given every one to six weeks with the exception of the three-monthly preparation of paliperidone palmitate.

Head-to-head comparisons between depot antipsychotics have generally not demonstrated greater efficacy for one preparation over another and frequency of injection (either two- or four-week intervals) does not appear to greatly affect clinical outcome (measured as Brief Psychiatric Rating Scale (BPRS), Positive and Negative Symptom Score (PANSS), Clinical Global Impression-Severity (CGI-S) or measures of EPSE) (Kisely et al., 2015). Given the similar efficacy between LAIs, the propensity to cause EPSE and other adverse effects is generally the determining factor in making a choice of drug. Dopamine-serotonin antagonist and dopamine partial agonist LAIs are significantly less likely to lead to EPSE so are likely to be the first choice, especially in first-episode populations (Leucht et al., 1999).

The slow pharmacokinetics mean the beneficial and adverse effects of the depot preparations may be evident for many months after the last injection. Thus, when these are discontinued many patients will continue to remain well and apparently 'drug free', so that both they and their carers begin to believe that maintenance medication is no longer necessary. However, relapse may occur 9–12 months later and such patients should, therefore, be closely followed up for at least this length of time before a decision is made that maintenance antipsychotic treatment is not required (Leucht et al., 2012b). By the same token, depot-induced EPSE can persist for an equally long time in spite of discontinuation of the injections. In such situations, patience is necessary, since too vigorous treatment with anticholinergic agents can be both ineffective and hazardous.

9.9.2 Pharmacokinetics

LAIs have the considerable advantage of assured drug delivery when administered regularly. However, there are a number of pharmacokinetic factors that need to be taken into account to minimize side effects and support adherence (see Table 9.2). One significant advantage is that the intramuscular route avoids first-pass effects as the hepatic circulation is avoided, leading to 100% bioavailability. The rate-limiting step with LAIs is absorption (whereas with oral it is metabolism). Some LAIs may have an absorption rate constant that is less than their elimination rate constant, which is an example of 'flip-flop' pharmacokinetics, i.e. that the elimination half-life is no longer determined by clearance and volume of distribution but by bioavailability and absorption. The older dopamine antagonist drugs such as haloperidol and fluphenazine decanoate have long half-lives, which means they reach steady state over many months. Some studies suggest patients may not reach steady state for up to six months (Marder et al., 1989). This means doses need to be increased slowly and patiently, and if a patient is switched to an alternative medication the long washout period of the previous LAI needs to be taken into account.

Table 9.2 Pharmacokinetics of commonly used long-acting injectable antipsychotic medication

Drug	Dopamine antagonist				Dopamine-serotonin antagonists			Dopamine partial agonist
	Flupentixol decanoate	**Fluphenazine decanoate**	**Haloperidol decanoate**	**Zuclopenthixol decanoate**	**Risperidone microspheres**	**Paliperidone palmitate**	**Olanzapine pamoate**	**Aripiprazole**
Brand name	Depixol/ Psytixol	Modecate	Haldol Decanoate	Clopixol	Risperdal Consta	Xeplion	Zypadhera	Abilify Maintena
Release mechanism	Prodrug: hydrolysis by esterases	Prodrug: hydrolysis by esterases	Prodrug: hydrolysis by esterases	Prodrug: hydrolysis by esterases	Microspheres: diffusion and erosion	Prodrug nanocrystals: hydrolysis by esterases	Salt: dissociation	Drug: slow absorption due to low solubility
Formulation	Fractionated coconut oil	Sesame oil solution	Sesame oil solution	Fractionated coconut oil	Aqueous suspension	Aqueous suspension	Aqueous suspension	Aqueous suspension
Administration frequency	Every 2–4 weeks	Every 2–5 weeks	Every 4 weeks	Every 1–4 weeks	Every 2 weeks	Every 4 weeks*	Every 2 weeks	Every 4 weeks
Storage	Room temperature (15–30 °C)	Room temperature (15–30 °C)	Room temperature (15–30 °C)	Room temperature (15–30 °C)	2–8 °C	Room temperature (15–30 °C)	Room temperature (15–30 °C)	Room temperature (15–30 °C)
Time to peak	3–7 days[a]	24 hours[b]	3–9 days[c]	7 days[a]	4–6 weeks[d]	13 days[d]	3–4 days[e]	5–7 days[d]
Half-life	17 days[a]	7–14 days**, [a]	3 weeks[c]	7–19 days[a]	4–6 days[a]	25–49 days (depending on dose)[d]	30 days[e]	28 days[d]
Time to steady state	2 months (with injections every 4 weeks)[a]	3 months (with injections every 4 weeks)[b]	3 months (with injections every 4 weeks)[b]	2 months[a]	2 months (with injections every 2 weeks)[a]	7–11 months (with injections every 4 weeks)[d]	3 months[f] (with injections every 2 or 4 weeks)	4–8 months[d] (400 mg injections every 4 weeks)

Adapted from Park et al. (2013) and Mallikaarjun et al. (2013).
[a] Taylor (2009), [b] Marder et al. (1989), [c] Beresford and Ward (1987), [d] Correll et al. (2016), [e] Frampton (2010), [f] Kane et al. (2010).
* 3-monthly paliperidone preparation uses the same technology but with larger nanoparticles.
** Fluphenazine decanoate can produce sharp transient post-injection peaks in blood levels from 2 to 24 hours which have been associated with dystonia (Stein & Wilkinson, 2007)

Unlike other LAIs, patients need to be observed for 3 hours after the first dose of olanzapine LAI because of the risk of a post-injection syndrome. Table 9.2 shows the drug characteristics and pharmacokinetics of some commonly prescribed LAIs.

A number of factors are thought to contribute to non-adherence that could be mitigated by the use of an LAI. These include a lack of social support which reduces the likelihood that the patient will be reminded to take oral medication, poor insight and cognitive deficits which lead to forgetfulness and complicated or inconvenient oral medication regimens which may be difficult to follow (Oehl et al., 2000). Depot administration thus has the significant advantage of removing the risk of covert non-adherence without resorting to plasma monitoring and offering the convenience of less frequent dosing. Young people, and males in particular, are thought to be at the highest risk of non-adherence, yet the use of antipsychotic depot/LAIs for first-episode schizophrenia patients remains controversial (Heres et al., 2006). Evidence on the efficacy, acceptability and tolerability of LAIs in first-episode patients is limited, but generally favourable (Emsley et al., 2008; Kim et al., 2008; Weiden et al., 2009).

9.9.3 Efficacy and Effectiveness Versus Oral Preparations

In terms of preventing relapse in schizophrenia, meta-analysis demonstrates that LAIs are more effective than placebo (Adams et al., 2001). The most recent meta-analysis of RCTs that compared the efficacy of oral antipsychotics and LAIs showed no difference in relapse rates (Kishimoto et al., 2014). However, such trials include patients who by virtue of being able to engage in an RCT are unlikely to be representative of the patient population who would most benefit from treatment with an LAI. Furthermore the level of monitoring required in the oral treatment arm of head-to-head trials is likely to be much greater than that in routine clinical practice (Kirson et al., 2013), which may lead to better outcomes in participants taking oral medication in trials than would be seen in standard practice (Buckley et al., 2016). In comparison with RCTs, large-scale naturalistic studies reveal benefits of LAIs versus oral antipsychotics, especially among first episode patients, with risk of rehospitalization reduced by 50–60% in those treated with LAIs compared with oral treatment (Kirson et al., 2013; Tiihonen et al., 2011).

9.9.4 Side Effects and Relative Contraindications

Patients may experience injection site pain and reactions with LAIs. Low volume preparations reduce the risk of injection site reactions and studies show two-weekly injections are less likely to lead to site pain (Kisely et al., 2015). If patients are sensitive to EPSE then lower doses should be used, and a cautious approach taken to allow the drug to reach steady state before additional dose changes are made. Older dopamine antagonist LAIs require the administration of a test dose to determine tolerability. It is likely that the negative experiences patients have with LAIs are in part a consequence of too rapid dose escalations, therefore clinicians need to be aware of the effect of a long half-life on time to steady state when dosing. In a patient with a history of neuroleptic malignant syndrome (NMS), use of LAIs is contraindicated due to their prolonged release pharmacokinetics. In patients who are dopamine blocker naive, a short trial of oral medication or a small test dose of the depot medication is judicious to ensure there are not significant acute tolerability concerns related to the drug or, in the case of oil-based depots, the oily vehicle. A trial of oral medication, often supervised in an inpatient setting, also allows one to determine that the antipsychotic is effective and then a decision can be made to switch to the comparable LAI formulation of that drug for maintenance treatment.

9.10 Contraindications to Dopamine Antagonists

Table 9.3 summarizes conditions in which dopamine blockers should be used with caution, if at all. Prescribers should refer to the individual drug's SPC for detailed information on contraindications.

9.11 Key Side Effects of Dopamine Antagonists

Antipsychotic medication can cause a wide variety of side effects some of which, such as EPSE, sedation and dry mouth, can be detected by careful history taking and examination. Other adverse effects, such as impaired glucose tolerance or prolonged QTc, require regular investigations and monitoring in order to prevent both acute and chronic health problems (e.g. diabetes, myocardial infarction or stroke). Polypharmacy in particular is associated with adverse events and should be minimized as much as possible (Young et al., 2015). Patients, when asked, rank sexual dysfunction and EPSE as the most distressing side effects (Lambert et al., 2004). Network meta-analysis has suggested that the dopamine antagonist amisulpride and the serotonin-dopamine antagonists olanzapine, clozapine, paliperidone and risperidone have significantly lower rates of all-cause discontinuation than other antipsychotics (Leucht et al., 2013, 2017; Samara et al., 2016).

Table 9.3 Cautions and contraindications to antipsychotics

Disorder	Concern with antipsychotic treatment
Blood dyscrasias	Dopamine antagonists may suppress bone marrow
Cardiovascular disease	Increased risk of arrhythmias and sudden cardiac death
Closed-angle glaucoma	Anticholinergic effects of antipsychotics can precipitate or exacerbate glaucoma
Conditions predisposing to seizures	Dopamine antagonists reduce the seizure threshold
Elderly patients with dementia	Elderly patients with dementia-related psychosis treated with antipsychotic drugs are at an increased risk of death
Jaundice	Most dopamine antagonists (except sulpiride/ amisulpride) are hepatically metabolized
Myasthenia gravis	Anticholinergic effects of antipsychotics may worsen myasthenia gravis
Parkinson's disease	Dopamine antagonist may worsen symptoms
Prostatic hypertrophy	Anticholingeric effects of antipsychotics may increase risk of urinary retention
Severe respiratory disease	Dose-dependent increase in pneumonia in patients with schizophrenia treated with serotonin-dopamine antagonists

9.11.1 Extrapyramidal Side Effects (EPSE)

EPSE are common side effects of antipsychotics and can be divided into four types:

1. Akathisia
2. Parkinsonism
3. Acute dystonias
4. Tardive dyskinesia.

Several meta-analyses of RCTs have shown that dopamine-serotonin antagonists and dopamine partial agonists are less likely to cause EPSE than dopamine antagonists. However, most trials used haloperidol at relatively high doses as the comparator drug and measured EPSE by the amount of anti-Parkinsonian medication used (Bagnall et al., 2003; Leucht et al., 2017).

The peak incidence of akathisia, Parkinsonism and dystonia occurs within the first three months of treatment and thereafter a tolerance develops in most cases and the incidence declines after six months. Tardive dyskinesia (TD) is a neurological side effects that usually develops after treatment with antipsychotic medication for many years, though there have been reports of TD developing after three to six months. Most cases of TD occur after two to three years of treatment and, unlike other EPSE, tolerance does not develop and it can persist, irreversibly in some cases. The elderly are at particular risk and TD needs to be carefully distinguished from senile chorea and other movement disorders unrelated to medication.

Akathisia is probably the most common psychomotor reaction to antipsychotics and has been reported to occur to some extent in up to 50% of patients. It is characterized by both motor restlessness and subjective agitation, dysphoria or intolerance of inactivity. In mild cases this can take the form of shifting of the legs or tapping of the feet but in more severe forms can lead to constant pacing and internal anxiety. It is important to consider dysphoria in the context of new or increased antipsychotic medication as an early prodrome of akathisia. Furthermore, patients might not attribute akathisia to their medication as there is often a delay of a few hours from last dose to onset.

Iatrogenic Parkinsonism induced by antipsychotic medication is manifest as bradykinesia (generalized slowing and loss of movements, in particular involuntary muscles of association and expression), muscle rigidity and tremor. These symptoms tend to develop in the first few weeks of treatment and are commoner in older people and in particular older women. It may also persist even when the offending drug has been withdrawn. Anticholinergic drugs may be used for up to the first six months of treatment but are usually unnecessary after that.

Acute dystonias occur after the first few doses of antipsychotic. They tend to be more common in men and younger people (Haddad & Dursun, 2008). The classical examples of acute dystonia are oculogyric crisis – fixed upward or lateral gaze, and torticollis – acute rigidity of neck muscles and jaw as well as spasms of the lips, tongue, face and throat. Acute dyskinesias (involuntary movements) with grimacing or exaggerated posturing and twisting of the head can also occur and can be distinguished from TD by the length of exposure to the antipsychotic drug and reversibility. Both these reactions occur rapidly and are reversed as quickly by the administration of anticholinergic medication.

9.11.2 Prolactin

Prolactin is a polypeptide hormone secreted by the anterior pituitary gland under the control of the hypothalamus via dopamine neurons. It regulates a number of biological functions including reproduction, pregnancy and lactation as well as bone growth and development. Dopamine, via D_2 receptors on the lactotroph cells in the anterior pituitary gland, inhibits prolactin release. Consequently, dopamine antagonists, in particular those with potent D_2 antagonism, can increase plasma prolactin. Dopamine partial agonists and some dopamine-serotonin antagonists show a lesser propensity to raise prolactin (Haddad & Wieck, 2004). A consequence of the pituitary being outside of the blood–brain barrier is that the levels of dopamine antagonists with relatively poor blood–brain barrier penetrance, such as amisulpride, paliperidone and risperidone, are higher at the pituitary than in the brain, because such drugs are dosed for sufficient brain D_2 occupancy. This is one explanation for the higher rates of hyperprolactinaemia with these drugs than other dopamine antagonists.

The point prevalence of hyperprolactinaemia among those treated with antipsychotics is influenced by a range of factors, most notably the antipsychotic prescribed, the dose and the sex distribution of the sample; for any given antipsychotic, the likelihood of raised prolactin occurring is higher in men than women (Haddad & Wieck, 2004). Bearing these risk factors in mind, raised prolactin is frequently encountered in clinical practice. Johnsen et al. (2008) found that it was present in nearly 40% of patients in a cross-sectional study. In many cases it can be asymptomatic so may require blood monitoring to detect and if hyperprolactinaemia is detected, then other causes of hyperprolactinaemia should be ruled out, e.g. stress (mild elevation), pituitary adenoma and primary hypothyroidism. Men may present with galactorrhoea, gynaecomastia and sexual dysfunction, while women may additionally develop dysmenorrhea, acne and hirsutism. This can progress to significant sexual and reproductive dysfunction as well as osteoporosis in the long term which can have serious effects on quality of life. Women of reproductive age, in particular parous women, appear to be at a higher risk of hyperprolactinaemia than post-menopausal women.

It is worth noting that a recent meta-analysis of antipsychotic-naive patients with schizophrenia found that such patients have elevated levels of prolactin prior to starting any dopamine antagonist treatment. This was particularly the case in males and did not appear related to age, body mass index, smoking or cortisol (González-Blanco et al., 2016).

9.11.3 Sedation

Sedation caused by dopamine antagonists is a dose-related effect that patients tend to build tolerance to. Drugs with actions at histamine and 5-HT_{2A} receptors, such as chlorpromazine, clozapine, olanzapine and quetiapine, tend to cause the most sedation. The dopamine partial agonist aripiprazole appears to be the most activating though, paradoxically, some patients do report sedation.

9.11.4 Cardiac Effects

Dopamine antagonists can cause postural hypotension, QTc prolongation and other, much rarer cardiac effects such as myocarditis, myopathy and pericarditis.

Postural hypotension is correlated with the degree to which the drug antagonizes α_1-adrenoceptors and the elderly and patients with underlying cardiovascular disease are more sensitive to such effects, as are those prescribed antihypertensive drugs. The best approach is to start with a low dose and increase slowly.

QTc prolongation is thought to be a marker of an increased risk of arrhythmias such as torsade de pointes and sudden cardiac death. Dopamine antagonists, and other drugs that can increase QTc, exert this effect by antagonism of potassium channels on cardiac myocytes leading to delayed repolarization (Haddad & Anderson, 2002). It is important to recognize that other factors, including dose, use of other medication, e.g. methadone, age, gender, ethnicity and drug and alcohol misuse, may also influence the QTc interval measurement, and the risks of discontinuing or switching treatment should also be considered before making changes. Amongst commonly used drugs, aripiprazole and lurasidone have relatively low risks of affecting the QTc interval.

Antipsychotics, in particular clozapine, can rarely be associated with myocarditis, cardiomyopathy, pericarditis and pericardial effusion. Estimates of the incidence of myocarditis incidence vary markedly, but it is probably less than 1 in 100, and the risk is highest in the first two months of treatment (Ronaldson, 2017). Clinicians should be mindful of any symptoms of myocarditis or myopathy developing, such as new-onset fatigue, dyspnoea, fever, chest pain, palpitations and any ECG changes, although it should be recognized that tachycardia is very common with clozapine and generally benign. It is helpful to measure ESR and CRP and cardiac markers in patients with these symptoms and have a low threshold for conducting an urgent echocardiogram.

9.11.5 Metabolic Effects

Weight gain and metabolic disturbance can be particularly problematic with drugs such as olanzapine and clozapine that have actions at histamine and 5-HT_2 receptors (Parsons et al., 2009), whereas purer dopamine antagonists and partial agonists tend to have lower risks of weight gain and metabolic side effects (Leucht et al., 2017; Rummel-Kluge et al., 2010). First-onset patients appear to be most susceptible to weight gain with increases of 7–8% of body weight on risperidone and 13% for olanzapine seen over the first three months of treatment in some studies (Zhang et al., 2004). Antipsychotic-induced weight gain may also be associated with elevation of liver enzymes.

Antipsychotic drugs can elevate blood glucose and lipid levels. Their relative liability to do so approximately mirrors their different liability to cause weight gain. Metabolic side effects can be mitigated by choosing a drug with a low propensity to cause dysregulation (such as lurasidone or aripiprazole), encouraging a healthy diet and lifestyle with regular exercise and augmentation strategies such as metformin. Chapter 21 provides a detailed review of weight gain and metabolic issues associated with antipsychotic drugs.

9.11.6 Neuroleptic Malignant Syndrome

Neuroleptic malignant syndrome (NMS) is an uncommon but severe and life-threatening reaction to dopamine antagonism. It is characterized by severe muscle rigidity, hyperpyrexia, fluctuating levels of consciousness and autonomic disturbance manifesting as diaphoresis (sweating), tachycardia, labile blood pressure and hypersalivation. Elevated levels of creatinine kinase (CK) are also found. For a detailed review of NMS see Pelonero et al. (1998).

All dopamine antagonists including those with serotonergic antagonist activity can cause NMS. Case reports of NMS in patients taking metoclopramide, lithium and antidepressants of various classes have also been reported (Haddad & Dursun, 2008). It is hypothesized that a sudden block of D_2 receptors in the hypothalamus affects thermoregulation, and in the striatum leads to rigidity, which causes peripheral heat production and further pyrexia.

The incidence of NMS is thought to be 0.2% and it is twice as common in men. It is important to differentiate NMS from catatonia, heat stroke (flaccid muscles and dry skin), serotonin syndrome (patient will usually present as restless and jerky as opposed to akinesia in NMS and show gastrointestinal signs such as diarrhoea, nausea and vomiting with onset over 24 hours compared with days from NMS) and anticholinergic delirium (no rigidity and dry hot skin).

NMS is a medical emergency and will require treatment in a general hospital. Management includes the cessation of all dopamine-blocking treatment and any other drugs that can cause the syndrome, rehydration and cooling of the patient, regular physical monitoring and daily CK monitoring. Rhabdomyolysis leading to myoglobinuria and renal failure may occur in severe cases. Benzodiazepines may help with muscle rigidity as may dantrolene.

9.11.7 Other Significant Side Effects

Many dopamine antagonists have the potential to cause anticholinergic effects, but agents such as chlorpromazine, clozapine and olanzapine, which have a high affinity for muscarinic receptors, carry the greatest risk (Bolden et al., 1992; Bymaster et al., 1996). Peripheral cholinergic blockade causes reduced salivation and dry mouth, reduced bronchial secretions and sweating, increased pupil size and the inhibition of the accommodation reflex, tachycardia, urinary retention and constipation (Lieberman, 2004). Cholinergic blockade within the central nervous system can cause cognitive impairment and delirium (Minzenberg et al., 2004). Paradoxically clozapine appears to have partial agonist properties at some muscarinic receptors so can induce sialorrhoea (Olianas et al., 1997; Zeng et al., 1997).

Most dopamine-blocking drugs, antidepressants and lithium lower the seizure threshold so should be used with caution in those with a history of seizures. Clozapine (Wu et al., 2016) and chlorpromazine (Hedges et al., 2003) are both associated with a relatively high risk of seizures. Observational data show an association between antipsychotics and pneumonia (Dzahini et al., 2018). The data are reviewed in Chapter 10 on clozapine as it appears most compelling for clozapine. Nevertheless, the association has been demonstrated for other individual drugs as well as in analyses that have considered the broad classes of first-generation and second-generation antipsychotics.

Meta-analyses have shown that elderly patients with dementia who are treated with dopamine blockers had a threefold risk of a cerebrovascular event (Douglas & Smeeth, 2008), and these drugs should be used cautiously, if at all, in this group. This effect has been demonstrated for individual antipsychotics as well as in analyses that have considered the broad classes of first-generation and second-generation antipsychotics.

9.12 Drug Interactions

Several drugs, when prescribed with dopamine blockers, can lead to a potentiation of side effects. There is an increased risk of QTc prolongation with medication such as methadone and escitalopram/citalopram. There can be a potentiation of the sedating effects of antipsychotics if they are co-administered with alcohol, antihistamines, benzodiazepines, sedating antidepressants and opioid analgesics. Patients are more likely to experience anticholinergic side effects if antipsychotics are given with anticholinergic drugs such as procyclidine, hyoscine and tricyclic antidepressants. Prescribing angiotensin-converting enzyme (ACE) inhibitors and other antihypertensives can increase the risk of hypotension and falls, as can alcohol consumption or tricyclic antidepressant use. Tricyclics and lithium can also reduce the seizure threshold as can sudden benzodiazepine withdrawal. Finally, the risk of metabolic side effects from antipsychotics are increased with co-administration of lithium, mirtazapine and other antipsychotics.

Most antipsychotics, along with a number of other substances, are metabolized by the hepatic cytochrome P450 enzymes (sulpiride, amisulpride and paliperidone are not extensively metabolized and are largely excreted unchanged). Therefore, other drugs that compete as substrates for the same enzyme can induce or inhibit activity. A list of the most common ones is found in Table 9.4.

9.13 Controversies Concerning Use in Schizophrenia/Psychosis

One prominent controversy concerning dopamine antagonists is whether they induce dopamine supersensitivity. The theory suggests dopamine blockade may induce changes in the dopamine system that increase a patient's biological vulnerability to relapse or breakthrough psychosis (Fallon et al., 2012). There are three main mechanisms that might underlie supersensitivity psychosis: increased receptor numbers, increased high-affinity dopamine receptor subtypes or increased postsynaptic transduction. PET studies suggest there is no change in high-affinity D_2 subtypes (Graff-Guerrero et al., 2009), but there may be an increase in D_2 receptor numbers in people who have antipsychotics long term (Howes et al., 2012), potentially supporting this as a mechanism, although it has yet to be linked to supersensitivity psychosis.

Another controversy is whether dopamine-blocking drugs cause structural brain changes during long-term treatment. Reduced brain volumes are seen in patients with

Table 9.4 The common CYP antipsychotic interactions

Substance	CYP enzyme	Antipsychotic concentration
Tobacco[a]	Induces 1A2	Reduces clozapine and to a lesser extent olanzapine and asenapine. Significantly reduces fluphenazine and haloperidol
Caffeine[b]	Inhibits 1A2	Increases clozapine and to a lesser extent olanzapine and asenapine
Fluvoxamine	Inhibits 1A2 and 2C9	Increases clozapine and to a lesser extent olanzapine and asenapine
Fluoxetine[c]	Inhibits 2D6	Increases perphenazine, risperidone, thioridazine
Paroxetine	Inhibits 2D6	Increases perphenazine, risperidone, thioridazine
Carbamazepine	Induces 1A2, 3A4 and UGT	Reduces clozapine, olanzapine, quetiapine, risperidone, zisprazidone
Valproic acid	Enzyme inhibition	Increases quetiapine, decreases aripiprazole
Grapefruit juice	Inhibits 3A4	May increase levels of clozapine
St John's wort	Induces 3A4	May reduce aripiprazole

[a] Smoking as few as 7–10 cigarettes can cause high levels of enzyme induction.
[b] Remember to ask about use of energy drinks which often contain caffeine when calculating daily caffeine intake.
[c] Due to its long half-life fluoxetine's 2D6 inhibition can last for several weeks.
Adapted from Bleakley (2012); Spina and de Leon (2007).

schizophrenia (Brugger & Howes, 2017). Whether this is due to the disorder, other factors or dopamine-blocking medication remains controversial. Reductions in both white and grey matter have been associated with antipsychotic exposure, but such associations could be explained by more severely ill patients receiving higher doses of treatment (Ho et al., 2011; Veijola et al., 2014). It should also be recognized that lower grey matter volumes are also seen in the prodrome to psychosis prior to antipsychotic treatment (Pantelis et al., 2003), suggesting at least some of the structural changes cannot be explained by drug effects. The reductions in brain volume associated with dopamine antagonist treatment have not been shown to be associated with cognitive impairment. Nevertheless, further work is required to address this controversy and determine the significance of the structural brain changes seen in schizophrenia.

References

Adams CE, Fenton MK, Quraishi S, David AS (2001). Systematic meta-review of depot antipsychotic drugs for people with schizophrenia. *Br J Psychiatry*, 179, 290–299.

Arranz MJ, Rivera M, Munro JC (2011). Pharmacogenetics of response to antipsychotics in patients with schizophrenia. *CNS Drugs*, 25(11), 933–939.

Ashok AH, Marques TR, Jauhar S, et al. (2017). The dopamine hypothesis of bipolar affective disorder: the state of the art and implications for treatment. *Mol Psychiatry*, 22(5), 666–679.

Bagnall AM, Jones L, Ginnelly L, et al. (2003). A systematic review of atypical antipsychotic drugs in schizophrenia. *Health Technol Assess*, 7(13), 1–193.

Beck K, McCutcheon R, Bloomfield MAP, et al. (2014). The practical management of refractory schizophrenia – the Maudsley Treatment Review and Assessment Team service approach. *Acta Psychiatr Scand*, 130(6), 427–438.

Beresford R, Ward A (1987). Haloperidol decanoate. A preliminary review of its pharmacodynamic and pharmacokinetic properties and therapeutic use in psychosis. *Drugs*, 33(1), 31–49.

Bleakley S (2012). Identifying and reducing the risk of antipsychotic drug interactions. *Prog Neurol Psychiatry*, 16(2), 20–24.

Bolden C, Cusack B, Richelson E (1992). Antagonism by antimuscarinic and neuroleptic compounds at the five cloned human muscarinic cholinergic receptors expressed in Chinese hamster ovary cells. *J Pharmacol Exp Ther*, 260(2), 576–580.

Brugger SP, Howes OD (2017). Heterogeneity and homogeneity of regional brain structure in schizophrenia: a meta-analysis. *JAMA Psychiatry*, 74(11), 1104–1111.

Buckley PF, Schooler NR, Goff DC, et al. (2016). Comparison of injectable and oral antipsychotics in relapse rates in a pragmatic 30-month schizophrenia relapse prevention study. *Psychiatr Serv*, 67(12), 1370–1372.

Bymaster FP, Calligaro DO, Falcone JF, et al. (1996). Radioreceptor binding profile of the atypical antipsychotic olanzapine. *Neuropsychopharmacology*, 14, 87–96.

Carbon M, Kane MJ, Leucht S, Correll CU (2018). Tardive dyskinesia risk with first- and second-generation antipsychotics in comparative randomized controlled trials: a meta-analysis. *World Psychiatry*, 17(3), 330–340. doi:10.1002/wps.20579.

Carlsson A, Lindqvist M (1963). Effect of chlorpromazine or haloperidol on formation of 3-methoxytyramine and normetanephrine in mouse brain. *Acta Pharmacol Toxicol (Copenh)*, 20(2), 140–144.

Cipriani A, Barbui C, Salanti G, et al. (2011). Comparative efficacy and acceptability of antimanic drugs in acute mania: a multiple-treatments meta-analysis. *Lancet*, 378(9799), 1306–1315.

Correll CU (2010). From receptor pharmacology to improved outcomes: individualising the selection, dosing, and switching of antipsychotics. *Eur Psychiatry*, 25(Suppl 2), S12–S21. doi:10.1016/S0924-9338(10)71701-6.

Correll CU, Citrome L, Haddad PM, et al. (2016). The use of long-acting injectable antipsychotics in schizophrenia: evaluating the evidence. *J Clin Psychiatry*, 77(Suppl 3), 1–24.

Creese I, Burt D, Snyder S (1976). Dopamine receptor binding predicts clinical and pharmacological potencies of antischizophrenic drugs. *Science*, 192(4238), 481–483.

Davidson M, Saoud J, Staner C, et al. (2017). Efficacy and safety of MIN-101: a 12-week randomized, double-blind, placebo-controlled trial of a new drug in development for the treatment of negative symptoms in schizophrenia. *Am J Psychiatry*, 174(12), 1195–1202.

Davies DL, Shepherd M (1955). Reserpine in the treatment of anxious and depressed patients. *Lancet*, 269(6881), 117–120.

Dold M, Aigner M, Lanzenberger R, Kasper S (2015). Antipsychotic augmentation of serotonin reuptake inhibitors in treatment-resistant obsessive-compulsive disorder: an update meta-analysis of double-blind, randomized, placebo-controlled trials. *Int J Neuropsychopharmacol*, 18(9), pyv047.

Douglas IJ, Smeeth L (2008). Exposure to antipsychotics and risk of stroke: self controlled case series study. *BMJ*, 337, a1227.

Dzahini O, Singh N, Taylor D, Haddad PM (2018). Antipsychotic drug use and pneumonia:

systematic review and meta-analysis. *J Psychopharmacol*, 32(11), 1167–1181.

Emsley R, Medori R, Koen L, et al. (2008). Long-acting injectable risperidone in the treatment of subjects with recent-onset psychosis: a preliminary study. *J Clin Psychopharmacol*, 28(2), 210–213.

Fallon P, Dursun S, Deakin B (2012). Drug-induced supersensitivity psychosis revisited: characteristics of relapse in treatment-compliant patients. *Ther Adv Psychopharmacol*, 2(1), 13–22.

Frampton JE (2010). Olanzapine long-acting injection: a review of its use in the treatment of schizophrenia. *Drugs*, 70(17), 2289–2313.

González-Blanco L, Greenhalgh AMD, Garcia-Rizo C, et al. (2016). Prolactin concentrations in antipsychotic-naïve patients with schizophrenia and related disorders: a meta-analysis. *Schizophr Res*, 174(1), 156–160.

Goodwin GM, Haddad PM, Ferrier IN, et al. (2016). Evidence-based guidelines for treating bipolar disorder: revised third edition recommendations from the British Association for Psychopharmacology. *J Psychopharmacol*, 30(6), 495–553.

Grace AA, Gomes FV (2019). The circuitry of dopamine system regulation and its disruption in schizophrenia: insights into treatment and prevention. *Schizophr Bull*, 45(1), 148–157. doi:10.1093/schbul/sbx199.

Graff-Guerrero A, Mizrahi R, Agid O, et al. (2009). The dopamine D2 receptors in high-affinity state and D3 receptors in schizophrenia: a clinical [11C]-(+)-PHNO PET study. *Neuropsychopharmacology*, 34(4), 1078–1086.

Graff-Guerrero A, Mamo D, Shammi C, et al. (2013). The effect of antipsychotics on the high-affinity state of D2 and D3 receptors: a positron emission tomography study with [11c]-(+)-PHNO. *Arch Gen Psychiatry*, 66(6), 606–615.

Grossman I, Sullivan PF, Walley N, et al. (2008). Genetic determinants of variable metabolism have little impact on the clinical use of leading antipsychotics in the CATIE study. *Genet Med*, 10(10), 720–729.

Haddad PM, Anderson IM (2002). Antipsychotic-related QTc prolongation, torsade de pointes and sudden death. *Drugs*, 62(11), 1649–1671.

Haddad PM, Correll CU (2018). The acute efficacy of antipsychotics in schizophrenia: a review of recent meta-analyses. *Ther Adv Psychopharmacol*, 8(11), 303–318.

Haddad PM, Wieck A (2004). Antipsychotic-induced hyperprolactinaemia: mechanisms, clinical features and management. *Drugs*, 64, 2291–2314.

Hedges D, Jeppson K, Whitehead P (2003). Antipsychotic medication and seizures: a review. *Drugs Today (Barc)*, 39(7), 551–557.

Heres S, Hamann J, Kissling W, Leucht S (2006). Attitudes of psychiatrists toward antipsychotic depot medication. *J Clin Psychiatry*, 67(12), 1948–1953.

Hirsch SR, Gaind R, Rohde PD, Stevens BC, Wing JK (1973). Outpatient maintenance of chronic schizophrenic patients with long-acting fluphenazine: double-blind placebo. *Br Med J*, 1(5854), 633–637.

Ho BC, Andreasen NC, Ziebell S, Pierson R, Magnotta V (2011). Long-term antipsychotic treatment and brain volumes: a longitudinal study of first-episode schizophrenia. *Arch Gen Psychiatry*, 68(2), 128–137.

Horvitz-Lennon M, Mattke S, Predmore Z, Howes OD (2017). The role of antipsychotic plasma levels in the treatment of schizophrenia. *Am J Psychiatry*, 174(5), 421–426.

Howes OD, Kapur S (2014). A neurobiological hypothesis for the classification of schizophrenia: type a (hyperdopaminergic) and type b (normodopaminergic). *Br J Psychiatry*, 205, 1–3.

Howes OD, McCutcheon R. (2017). Inflammation and the neural diathesis-stress hypothesis of schizophrenia: a reconceptualization. *Transl Psychiatry*, 7(2), e1024. doi:10.1038/tp.2016.278.

Howes OD, Kambeitz J, Kim E, et al. (2012). The nature of dopamine dysfunction in schizophrenia and what this means for treatment. *Arch Gen Psychiatry*, 69(8), 776–786.

Howes O, McCutcheon R, Stone J (2015). Glutamate and dopamine in schizophrenia: an update for the 21(st) century. *J Psychopharmacol*, 29(2), 97–115.

Howes OD, McCutcheon R, Agid O, et al. (2017a). Treatment-resistant schizophrenia: Treatment Response and Resistance in Psychosis (TRRIP) working group consensus guidelines on diagnosis and terminology. *Am J Psychiatry*, 174(3), 216–229.

Howes OD, McCutcheon R, Owen MJ, Murray RM (2017b). The role of genes, stress, and dopamine in the development of schizophrenia. *Biol Psychiatry*, 81(1), 9–20.

Jauhar S, Veronese M, Rogdaki M, et al. (2017). Regulation of dopaminergic function: an [18 F]-DOPA PET apomorphine challenge study in humans. *Transl Psychiatry*, 7(2), e1027. doi:10.1038/tp.2016.270.

Johnsen E, Kroken RA, Abaza M, Olberg H, Jørgensen HA (2008). Antipsychotic-induced hyperprolactinemia: a cross-sectional survey. *J Clin Psychopharmacol*, 28(6), 686–690. doi:10.1097/JCP.0b013e31818ba5d8.

Johnson DAW (2009). Historical perspective on antipsychotic long-acting injections. *Br J Psychiatry*, 195(52), S7–S12.

Kane JM, Detke HC, Naber D, et al. (2010). Olanzapine long-acting injection: a 24-week, randomized, double-blind trial of maintenance treatment in patients with schizophrenia. *Am J Psychiatry*, 167(2), 181–189.

Kapur S (1998). A new framework for investigating antipsychotic action in humans: lessons from PET imaging. *Mol Psychiatry*, 3(2), 135–140.

Kapur S, Seeman P (2000). Antipsychotic agents differ in how fast they come off the dopamine D2 receptors. Implications for atypical antipsychotic action. *J Psychiatry Neurosci*, 25(2), 161–166.

Kapur S, Seeman P (2001). Does fast dissociation from the dopamine D2 receptor explain the action of atypical antipsychotics?: a new hypothesis. *Am J Psychiatry*, 158(3), 360–369.

Kapur S, Zipursky RB, Remington G, et al. (1998). 5-HT2 and D2 receptor occupancy of olanzapine in schizophrenia: a PET investigation. *Am J Psychiatry*, 155(7), 921–928.

Kapur S, Zipursky RB, Remington G (1999). Clinical and theoretical implications of 5-HT2 and D2 receptor occupancy of clozapine, risperidone, and olanzapine in schizophrenia. *Am J Psychiatry*, 156(2), 286–293.

Kapur S, Zipursky R, Jones C, Remington G, Houle S (2000). Relationship between dopamine D2 occupancy, clinical response, and side effects: a double-blind PET study of first-episode schizophrenia. *Am J Psychiatry*, 157(4), 514–520.

Kebabian JW, Calne DB (1979). Multiple receptors for dopamine. *Nature*, 277(5692), 93–96.

Kim B, Lee SH, Choi TK, et al. (2008). Effectiveness of risperidone long-acting injection in first-episode schizophrenia: in naturalistic setting. *Prog Neuropsychopharmacol Biol Psychiatry*, 32 (5), 1231–1235. doi:10.1016/j.pnpbp.2008.03.012.

King C, Voruganti LNP (2002). What's in a name? The evolution of the nomenclature of antipsychotic drugs. *J Psychiatry Neurosci*, 27(3), 168–175.

Kirson NY, Weiden PJ, Yermakov S, et al. (2013). Efficacy and effectiveness of depot versus oral antipsychotics in schizophrenia: synthesizing results across different research designs. *J Clin Psychiatry*, 74(6), 568–575.

Kisely S, Sawyer E, Robinson G, Siskind D (2015). A systematic review and meta-analysis of the effect of depot antipsychotic frequency on compliance and outcome. *Schizophr Res*, 166(1–3), 178–186.

Kishimoto T, Robenzadeh A, Leucht C, et al. (2014). Long-acting injectable vs oral antipsychotics for relapse prevention in schizophrenia: a meta-analysis of randomized trials. *Schizophr Bull*, 40(1), 192–213.

Kwentus J, Riesenberg RA, Marandi M, et al. (2012). Rapid acute treatment of agitation in patients with bipolar I disorder: a multicenter, randomized, placebo-controlled clinical trial with inhaled loxapine. *Bipolar Disord*, 14(1), 31–40. doi:10.1111/j.1399-5618.2011.00975.x.

Laborit H, Huguenard P, Alluaume R (1952). Un noveau stabilisateur végétatif (le 4560 RP). *La Presse Médicale*, 60, 206–208.

Lambert M, Conus P, Eide P, et al. (2004). Impact of present and past antipsychotic side effects on attitude toward typical antipsychotic treatment and adherence. *Eur Psychiatry*, 19(7), 415–422.

Lesem MD, Tran-Johnson TK, Riesenberg RA, et al. (2011). Rapid acute treatment of agitation in individuals with schizophrenia: multicentre, randomised, placebo-controlled study of inhaled loxapine. *Br J Psychiatry*, 198(1), 51–58. doi:10.1192/bjp.bp.110.081513.

Leucht S, Pitschel-Walz G, Abraham D, Kissling W (1999). Efficacy and extrapyramidal side-effects of the new antipsychotics olanzapine, quetiapine, risperidone, and sertindole compared to conventional antipsychotics and placebo. A meta-analysis of randomized controlled trials. *Schizophr Res*, 35(1), 51–68.

Leucht S, Busch R, Kissling W, Kane JM (2007). Early prediction of antipsychotic nonresponse among patients with schizophrenia. *J Clin Psychiatry*, 68(3), 352–360.

Leucht S, Corves C, Arbter D, et al. (2009). Second-generation versus first-generation antipsychotic drugs for schizophrenia: a meta-analysis. *Lancet*, 373(9657), 31–41.

Leucht S, Hierl S, Kissling W, Dold M, Davis JM (2012a). Putting the efficacy of psychiatric and general medicine medication into perspective: review of meta-analyses. *Br J Psychiatry*, 200(2), 97–106.

Leucht S, Tardy M, Komossa K, et al. (2012b). Maintenance treatment with antipsychotic drugs for schizophrenia. *Cochrane Database Syst Rev*, (5), CD008016.

Leucht S, Cipriani A, Spineli L, et al. (2013). Comparative efficacy and tolerability of 15 antipsychotic drugs in schizophrenia: a multiple-treatments meta-analysis. *Lancet*, 382(9896), 951–962.

Leucht S, Leucht C, Huhn M, et al. (2017). Sixty years of placebo-controlled antipsychotic drug trials in acute schizophrenia: systematic review, Bayesian meta-analysis, and meta-regression of efficacy predictors. *Am J Psychiatry*, 174(10), 927–942.

Lieberman JA, 3rd (2004). Managing anticholinergic side effects. *Prim Care Companion J Clin Psychiatry*, 6(Suppl 2), 20–23.

Lindström L, Lindström E, Nilsson M, Höistad M (2017). Maintenance therapy with second generation antipsychotics for bipolar disorder – a systematic review and meta-analysis. *J Affect Disord*, 213, 138–150. doi:10.1016/j.jad.2017.02.012.

Mallikaarjun S, Kane JM, Bricmont P, et al. (2013). Pharmacokinetics, tolerability and safety of aripiprazole once-monthly in adult schizophrenia: an open-label, parallel-arm, multiple-dose study. *Schizophr Res*, 150(1), 281–288.

Maneeton N, Maneeton B, Woottiluk P, et al. (2016). Quetiapine monotherapy in acute treatment of generalized anxiety disorder: a systematic review and meta-analysis of randomized controlled trials. *Drug Des Devel Ther*, 10, 259–276. doi:10.2147/DDDT.S89485.

Marder SR, Hubbard JW, Van Putten T, Midha KK (1989). Pharmacokinetics of long-acting injectable neuroleptic drugs: clinical implications. *Psychopharmacology*, 98(4), 433–439.

Mauri MC, Volonteri LS, Colasanti A, et al. (2007). Clinical pharmacokinetics of atypical antipsychotics: a critical review of the relationship between plasma concentrations and clinical response. *Clin Pharmacokinet*, 46(5), 359–388.

McCutcheon R, Beck K, Bloomfield MA, et al. (2015). Treatment resistant or resistant to treatment? Antipsychotic plasma levels in patients with poorly controlled psychotic symptoms. *J Psychopharmacol*, 29(8), 892–897.

McCutcheon R, Beck K, D'Ambrosio E, et al. (2017). Antipsychotic plasma levels in the assessment of poor treatment response in schizophrenia. *Acta Psychiatr Scand*, 137(1), 39–46.

McCutcheon R, Beck K, Jauhar S, Howes OD (2018). Defining the locus of dopaminergic dysfunction in schizophrenia: a meta-analysis and test of the mesolimbic hypothesis. *Schizophr Bull*, 44(6), 1301–1311.

McCutcheon RA, Abi-Dargham A, Howes OD (2019). Schizophrenia, dopamine and the striatum: from biology to symptoms. *Trends Neurosci*, 42(3), 205–220.

Meltzer HY, Matsubara S, Lee J-C (1989). Classification of typical and atypical antipsychotic drugs on the basis of dopamine. *J Pharmacol Exp Ther*, 251(1), 238–246.

Minzenberg MJ, Poole JH, Benton C, Vinogradov S (2004). Association of anticholinergic load with impairment of complex attention and memory in schizophrenia. *Am J Psychiatry*, 161(1), 116–124.

Murphy BP, Chung Y-C, Park T-W, McGorry PD (2006). Pharmacological treatment of primary negative symptoms in schizophrenia: a systematic review. *Schizophr Res*, 88(1–3), 5–25.

Murray RM, Quattrone D, Natesan S, et al. (2016). Should psychiatrists be more cautious about the long-term prophylactic use of antipsychotics? *Br J Psychiatry*, 209(5), 361–365.

Nyberg S, Farde L, Eriksson L, Halldin C, Eriksson B (1993). 5-HT2 and D2 dopamine receptor occupancy in the living human brain. *Psychopharmacology*, 110(3), 265–272.

Oehl M, Hummer M, Fleischhacker WW (2000). Compliance with antipsychotic treatment. *Acta Psychiatr Scand*, 102, 83–86.

Olianas MC, Maullu C, Onali P (1997). Effects of clozapine on rat striatal muscarinic receptors coupled to inhibition of adenylyl cyclase activity and on the human cloned m4 receptor. *Br J Pharmacol*, 122(3), 401–408.

Ortiz-Orendain J, Castiello-de Obeso S, Colunga-Lozano LE, et al. (2017). Antipsychotic combinations for schizophrenia. *Cochrane Database Syst Rev*, (6), CD009005. doi:10.1002/14651858.CD009005.pub2.

Pantelis C, Velakoulis D, McGorry PD, et al. (2003). Neuroanatomical abnormalities before and after onset of psychosis: a cross-sectional and longitudinal MRI comparison. *Lancet*, 361(9354), 281–288.

Park EJ, Amatya S, Kim MS, et al. (2013). Long-acting injectable formulations of antipsychotic drugs for the treatment of schizophrenia. *Arch Pharm Res*, 36(6), 651–659.

Parsons B, Allison DB, Loebel A, et al. (2009). Weight effects associated with antipsychotics: a comprehensive database analysis. *Schizophr Res*, 110(1–3), 103–110.

Pelonero AL, Levenson JL, Pandurangi AK (1998). Neuroleptic malignant syndrome: a review. *Psychiatr Serv*, 49(9), 1163–1172.

Perreault ML, Hasbi A, Alijaniaram M, et al. (2010). The dopamine D1-D2 receptor heteromer localizes in dynorphin/enkephalin neurons: increased high affinity state following amphetamine and in schizophrenia. *J Biol Chem*, 285(47), 36625–36634.

Ravyn D, Ravyn V, Lowney R, Nasrallah HA (2013). CYP450 pharmacogenetic treatment strategies for antipsychotics: a review of the evidence. *Schizophr Res*, 149(1–3), 1–14.

Ronaldson KJ (2017). Cardiovascular disease in clozapine-treated patients: evidence, mechanisms and management. *CNS Drugs*, 31(9), 777–795.

Rummel-Kluge C, Komossa K, Schwarz S, et al. (2010). Head-to-head comparisons of metabolic side effects of second generation antipsychotics in the treatment of schizophrenia: a systematic review and meta-analysis. *Schizophr Res*, 123(2–3), 225–233.

Sachs GS, Nierenberg AA, Calabrese JR, et al. (2007). Effectiveness of adjunctive antidepressant treatment for bipolar depression. *N Engl J Med*, 356, 1711–1722. doi:10.1056/NEJMoa064135.

Samara MT, Dold M, Gianatsi M, et al. (2016). Efficacy, acceptability, and tolerability of antipsychotics in treatment-resistant schizophrenia: a network meta-analysis. *JAMA Psychiatry*, 73(3), 199–210.

Seeman P (2001). Antipsychotic drugs, dopamine receptors, and schizophrenia. *Clin Neurosci Res*, 1(1–2), 53–60.

Seeman P (2011). All roads to schizophrenia lead to dopamine supersensitivity and elevated dopamine D2High receptors. *CNS Neurosci Ther*, 17(2), 118–132.

Seeman P (2012). Dopamine agonist radioligand binds to both D2High and D2Low receptors, explaining why alterations in D2High are not detected in human brain scans. *Synapse*, 66(1), 88–93.

Seeman P, Chau-Wong M, Tedesco J, Wong K (1975). Brain receptors for antipsychotic drugs and dopamine: direct binding assays. *Proc Natl Acad Sci U S A*, 72(11), 4376–4380.

Sepede G, De Berardis D, Gambi F, et al. (2006). Olanzapine augmentation in treatment-resistant panic disorder: a 12-week, fixed-dose, open-label trial. *J Clin Psychopharmacol*, 26(1), 45–49.

Shen WW (1999). A history of antipsychotic drug development. *Compr Psychiatry*, 40, 407–414.

Siskind D, McCartney L, Goldschlager R, Kisely S (2016). Clozapine v. first- and second-generation antipsychotics in treatment-refractory schizophrenia: systematic review and meta-analysis. *Br J Psychiatry*, 209(5), 385–392.

Slifstein M, van de Giessen E, Van Snellenberg J, et al. (2015). Deficits in prefrontal cortical and extrastriatal dopamine release in schizophrenia: a positron emission tomographic functional magnetic resonance imaging study. *JAMA Psychiatry*, 72(4), 316–324.

Soderberg MM, Dahl ML (2013). Pharmacogenetics of olanzapine metabolism. *Pharmacogenomics*, 14(11), 1319–1336.

Soldin OP, Mattison DR (2009). Sex differences in pharmacokinetics and pharmacodynamics. *Clin Pharmacokinet*, 48(3), 143–157.

Spielmans GI, Berman MI, Linardatos E, et al. (2013). Adjunctive atypical antipsychotic treatment for major depressive disorder: a meta-analysis of depression, quality of life, and safety outcomes. *PLoS Med*, 10(3), e1001403.

Spina E, de Leon J (2007). Metabolic drug interactions with newer antipsychotics: a comparative review. *Basic Clin Pharmacol Toxicol*, 100(1), 4–22.

Stein G, Wilkinson G (eds.) (2007). *Seminars in General Adult Psychiatry*, 2nd ed. London: Royal College of Psychiatrists.

Taylor D (2009). Psychopharmacology and adverse effects of antipsychotic long-acting injections: a review. *Br J Psychiatry*, 195(52), S13–S19.

Tiihonen J, Haukka J, Taylor M, et al. (2011). A nationwide cohort study of oral and depot antipsychotics after first hospitalization for schizophrenia. *Am J Psychiatry*, 168(6), 603–609.

Tiihonen J, Mittendorfer-Rutz E, Majak M, et al. (2017). Real-world effectiveness of antipsychotic treatments in a nationwide cohort of 29 823 patients with schizophrenia. *JAMA Psychiatry*, 74(7), 686–693.

Veijola J, Guo JY, Moilanen JS, et al. (2014). Longitudinal changes in total brain volume in schizophrenia: relation to symptom severity, cognition and antipsychotic medication. *PLoS One*, 9(7), e101689.

Weiden PJ, Schooler NR, Weedon JC, et al. (2009). A randomized controlled trial of long-acting injectable risperidone vs continuation on oral atypical antipsychotics for first-episode schizophrenia patients: initial adherence outcome. *J Clin Psychiatry*, 70(10), 1397–1406. doi:10.4088/JCP.09m05284yel.

Weinberger DR (1987). Implications of normal brain development for the pathogenesis of schizophrenia. *Arch Gen Psychiatry*, 44(7), 660–669.

Wijkstra J, Lijmer J, Burger H, et al. (2015). Pharmacological treatment for psychotic depression. *Cochrane Database Syst Rev*, (7), CD004044.

Wu CS, Wang SC, Yeh IJ, Liu SK (2016). Comparative risk of seizure with use of first- and second-generation antipsychotics in patients with schizophrenia and mood disorders. *J Clin Psychiatry*, 77(5), e573–e579.

Young SL, Taylor M, Lawrie SM (2015). 'First do no harm.' A systematic review of the prevalence and management of antipsychotic adverse effects. *J Psychopharmacol*, 29(4), 353–362.

Zeng XP, Le F, Richelson E (1997). Muscarinic m4 receptor activation by some atypical antipsychotic drugs. *Eur J Pharmacol*, 321(3), 349–354.

Zhang ZJ, Yao ZJ, Liu W, Fang Q, Reynolds GP (2004). Effects of antipsychotics on fat deposition and changes in leptin and insulin levels. Magnetic resonance imaging study of previously untreated people with schizophrenia. *Br J Psychiatry*, 184, 58–62.

Zhu Y, Li C, Huhn M, et al. (2017). How well do patients with a first episode of schizophrenia respond to antipsychotics: a systematic review and meta-analysis. *Eur Neuropsychopharmacol*, 27(9), 835–844. doi:10.1016/j.euroneuro.2017.06.011.

Zohar J, Stahl S, Moller H-J, et al. (2015). A review of the current nomenclature for psychotropic agents and an introduction to the Neuroscience-based Nomenclature. *Eur Neuropsychopharmacol*, 25(12), 2318–2325.

Chapter 10

Clozapine

Richard Drake

10.1 Introduction and Brief History

Clozapine is a dopamine receptor antagonist that blocks a range of other monoamine receptors and may have some effects on the glutamatergic system. There is evidence that it has better efficacy and effectiveness than other dopamine antagonists in treating schizophrenia that has failed to respond to other dopamine receptor antagonists. It appears to reduce impulsive behaviours such as violence (Frogley et al., 2011), self-harm (Meltzer et al., 2003) and substance misuse (Lalanne et al., 2016) and to have mood-stabilizing properties (Chang et al., 2006). In the UK it is licensed for three indications: (i) treatment-resistant schizophrenia; (ii) for treating schizophrenia when other antipsychotics have led to severe neurological adverse reactions; and (iii) treating psychosis associated with Parkinson's disease where standard treatment has failed (electronic Medicines Compendium, 2019).

Having been first synthesized in 1958 and marketed in 1972 (Crilly, 2007) it was soon linked to fatal agranulocytosis and withdrawn from several markets. German-speaking psychiatrists continued to use it occasionally, as it developed a reputation for treating schizophrenia resistant to other treatments (Healy, 1997). Its peculiar efficacy in this situation was first investigated definitively in a classic randomized, double-blind, controlled trial in the late 1980s (Kane et al., 1988). Participants who failed to respond to an initial course of haloperidol were then allocated to treatment with either chlorpromazine or clozapine at identical doses, with significantly more responding to the experimental drug. Since then it has been approved for use against 'treatment-resistant' schizophrenia in a range of countries and it is now listed by the World Health Organization (WHO) as an Essential Medicine (WHO, 2017).

Since it has placebo-level motor adverse effects it also has a niche treating those with Parkinson's disease and psychosis (Chang & Fox, 2016). These features have also led to its suggested use treating those with tardive dyskinesia and those with a history of neuroleptic malignant syndrome (it appears to have a relatively low risk of causing either disorder, though it has been linked to cases of each).

Apart from agranulocytosis, as an antagonist at a broad range of receptors, it has a broad range of adverse effects. Many are common and some are potentially lethal, including constipation, metabolic disorders, hypotension, seizures, myocarditis and ventricular arrhythmia (Electronic Medicines Compendium, 2019). This makes it a tricky drug to prescribe safely, since staff across a service should be confident in identifying and dealing with or seeking help for a multitude of adverse effects, often easily addressed or at least not serious; but sometimes dangerous. Its dose is initially titrated slowly to avoid adverse effects, and enhanced monitoring is required then, as many of the adverse effects are more severe or probable.

Clozapine is a dibenzodiazepine with a rich pharmacology (Table 10.1) but is not a potent D_2 antagonist, having the lowest affinity of clinically used dopamine antagonists apart from quetiapine. Its low affinity for the D_2 receptor and hence the relative ease with which physiological dopamine can dislodge it has been linked to its low propensity for Parkinsonian adverse effects and akathisia, though since quetiapine has an even lower affinity but lacks its unique efficacy profile it is unlikely that this accounts for clozapine's specific efficacy. Many peculiar properties have been posited as responsible for this efficacy only later to be rejected; others are not yet supported by consistent and strong enough evidence to drive a consensus on its mode of action. These include: relatively high affinity as an antagonist at D_3 (Gross et al., 2013), D_4 (Lahti et al., 1993) or D_1 receptors (where it may be a weak partial agonist; Potkin et al., 2003); relatively high affinity at α_2-adrenoceptors (Brosda et al., 2014); relatively high affinity at 5-$HT_{2A/C}$ 5-HT_6, or 5-HT_7 receptors (Miyamoto et al., 2012). Its main metabolite, norclozapine or *N*-desmethylclozapine, is pharmacologically active and has higher affinity for dopamine receptors but there is no evidence that it is responsible for its unique efficacy either (Mendoza &

Table 10.1 Clozapine and norclozapine monoamine receptor affinities: low K_i indicates high affinity (Roth & Driscol, 2013; Selent et al., 2008)

Receptor	Clozapine affinity (K_i)	Norclozapine affinity (K_i)
D_1	266.5	14.3
D_2	157.0	101.4
D_3	269.1	193.5
D_4	26.4	63.9
$5\text{-}HT_{1A}$	123.7	13.9
$5\text{-}HT_{2A}$	5.4	10.9
$5\text{-}HT_3$	241.0	272.2
$5\text{-}HT_7$	18.0	60.1
α_{1A}	1.6	104.8
α_{2A}	37.0	137.6
M_1	6.2	67.6
M_4	15.3	169.9
H_1	1.1	3.4

Lindenmayer, 2009). In fact, it may be an important cause of metabolic adverse effects, so some have advocated using fluvoxamine to reduce the metabolism of clozapine to norclozapine for this reason (Polcwiartek & Nielsen, 2016) though this risks toxicity (see pharmacokinetics, below) and no benefit is yet well evidenced.

Clozapine reduces glutamate and serine reuptake and increases glutamate exocytosis in rat models, increasing peri-synaptic glutamate concentrations in rats (Tanahashi et al., 2012) and humans (Melkersson et al., 2015); there is evidence that some of these changes are specific to clozapine or to treatment resistance (Demjaha et al., 2014; Goldstein et al., 2015). Animal evidence indicates that clozapine may interact with interneuronal $GABA_B$ receptors (O'Connor & O'Shea, 2015; Wu et al., 2011), which have a putative role in schizophrenia. It is an agonist at M_4 muscarinic receptors which may have cognitive benefits but may cause sialorrhoea (Rogers & Shramko, 2000). Both the cholinergic agonism and glutamate/GABA effects may explain clozapine's propensity to produce seizures.

Given that its clinical potency appears related to D_2 affinity and its therapeutic levels to D_2 occupancy at peak concentrations (though PET evidence is mixed, this may be because occupancy at therapeutic levels is brief; Seeman, 2014), it appears that D_2 antagonism is at least an important element of its antipsychotic action.

10.2 Efficacy in Schizophrenia

Clozapine's efficacy in schizophrenia is most studied in those described as 'treatment resistant'. Though this has been defined variously, most trials involve patients who suffer substantial residual psychotic symptoms after at least two other dopamine antagonists have been tried. A recent statement from the Treatment Response and Resistance in Psychosis consensus group (Howes et al., 2017) emphasized the importance of considering adherence, adequate duration and dose (e.g. over six weeks at Summary of Product Characteristics (SPC) or *British National Formulary* (BNF) midpoint for oral, four months for long-acting injectable (LAI) medication) in future research, but this is a reasonable clinical standard too.

Most meta-analyses confirm clozapine to have better efficacy than other dopamine antagonists, with a standardized effect size of about 0.49 in a meta-analysis of trials that compared different dopamine antagonists with haloperidol (Davis et al., 2003; cf. Bagnall et al., 2003), and better than others at standardized effect size 0.88 in a network meta-analysis of efficacy against placebo (Leucht et al., 2013). A more recent meta-analysis by Siskind et al. (2016) analyzed data from 21 randomized controlled trials (RCTs) and found that clozapine was superior to other antipsychotics for positive symptoms in both the short and long term (see Figure 10.1). Superiority for total symptoms and negative symptoms was only seen in the short term. A further meta-analysis reported on the response rate with clozapine (Siskind et al., 2017). The individual RCTs included in the analysis adopted different definitions of response but all required a reduction of at least 20% in overall symptoms as assessed by either the Positive and Negative Syndrome Scale (PANSS) or the Brief Psychiatric Rating Scale (BPRS). Overall, 40% who had failed to respond to non-clozapine antipsychotics responded to clozapine. The response rate was higher in trials that lasted more than three months compared with those that were shorter.

Nonetheless, another recent network meta-analysis in people with treatment-resistant schizophrenia (Samara et al., 2016) found no evidence of superior efficacy for clozapine when all trials were pooled, and in Lobos et al.'s (2010) Cochrane review evidence was inconsistent. In response there has been scrutiny of these studies' methodological limitations and interpretation. Essentially, network meta-analyses like Samara and colleagues use Bayesian statistical techniques within a set of trials that compare different agents to each other in different combinations (e.g. clozapine with placebo, risperidone with placebo, risperidone with clozapine, haloperidol with clozapine etc). The effect of each agent compared with the others is used to construct an overall ranking of its performance – rather like ranking sports teams as they play each other in a league. Network meta-analysis assumes that the patient groups used in the various combinations of trials are comparable; if clozapine is compared to chlorpromazine in first-episode patients who respond to any agent well, but chlorpromazine to risperidone and clozapine to risperidone in very refractory patients who respond specifically to clozapine, the system of comparisons begins to fail and the matrix of comparisons is said to be 'poorly conditioned'. Just like predicting the results for teams playing in different leagues purely on the basis of the few clubs that are promoted or demoted, and their performance in the league they had left, the chances of a 'shock' result are increased. This appears to have been an issue in the analyses by Samara et al. (2016) and Lobos et al. (2010) as both analyses included studies that loosely defined treatment resistance. Even when trials have comparable samples, they may all recruit samples that fail to demonstrate the effect of an agent with specific value for other groups of patients. For example, if all trial samples are in their first episode perhaps any drug would work and furthermore, they would show equivalent efficacy. Conversely, if studies are conducted in all 'ultra-treatment resistant' groups, perhaps no dopamine antagonist will work. Finally, in Samara et al. and Lobos et al.'s papers the quality of many trials was questionable, with high attrition and low clozapine doses.

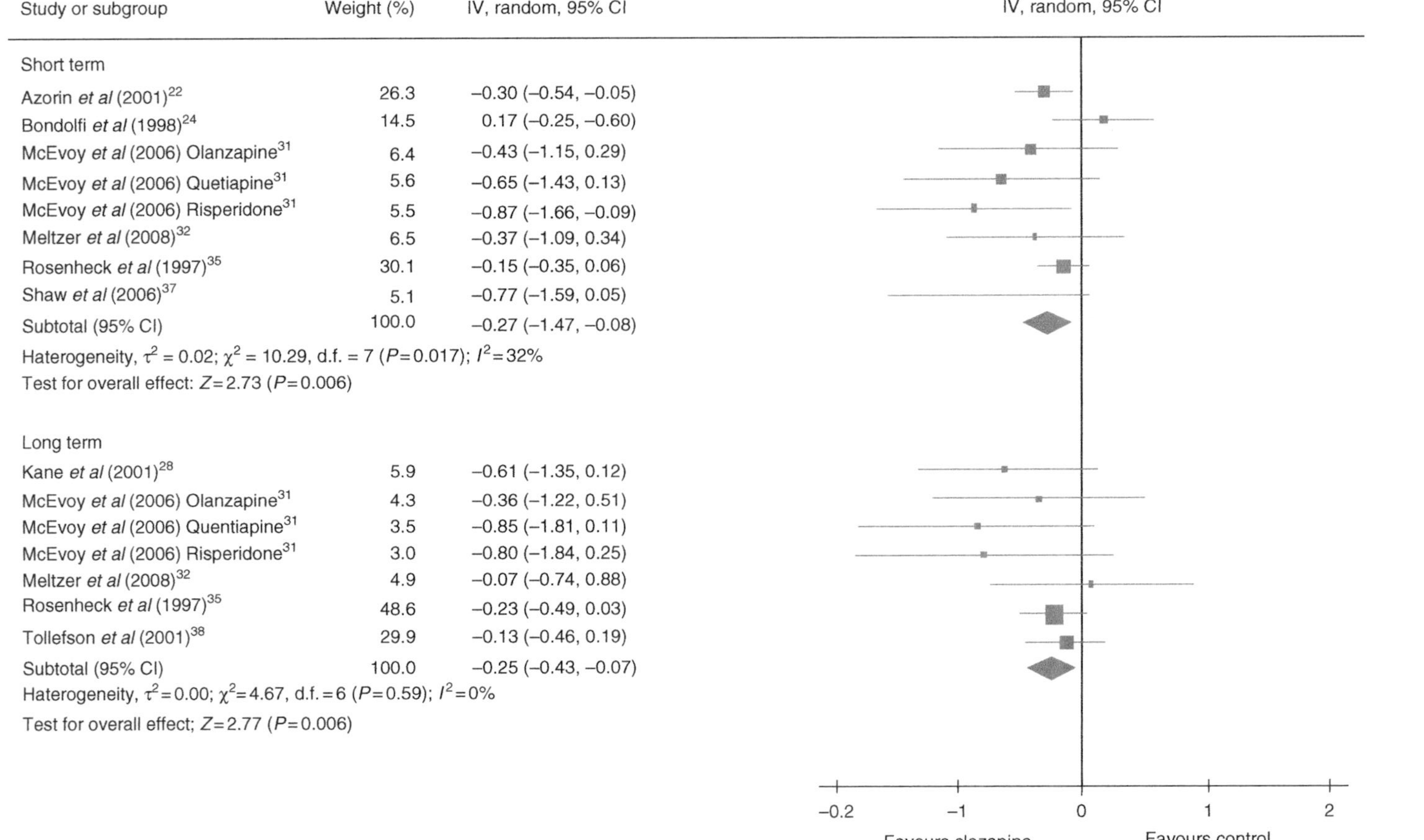

Figure 10.1 Change in positive symptoms in patients with treatment-resistance schizophrenia treated with clozapine in meta-analysis by Siskind et al. (2016). Reproduced with permission from Siskind et al. (2016) The British Journal of Psychiatry 209, 385–392. SMD = standardized mean difference.

Clozapine's efficacy in treatment-resistant schizophrenia is largely against psychotic symptoms. Its efficacy against primary negative symptoms (i.e. those not secondary to psychosis or medications' adverse effects) has not been convincingly demonstrated. Nevertheless, clozapine has benefit in schizophrenia beyond the treatment of psychotic symptoms. There is evidence that it reduces self-harm in comparison with olanzapine (Meltzer et al., 2003). The trial that showed this (International Suicide Prevention Trial or InterSePT) was not conducted primarily in treatment-refractory patients. In the United States clozapine is approved not only for treatment-resistant schizophrenia but also for reducing suicidal behaviour in patients with schizophrenia or schizoaffective disorder. There is also evidence that clozapine can reduce violence (Frogley et al., 2011) and relapse into substance misuse (Lalanne et al., 2016). These 'anti-impulsive' effects may reflect its serotonergic (likely 5-HT_{1A} agonist) action. The cognitive profile of most antipsychotic drugs depends on their non-dopaminergic mechanisms of action and clozapine is no exception (Meltzer, 2013) – there is some evidence that it can improve executive function, shifting cognitive set and planning, at least compared with most other antipsychotic drugs, that fits with its activity at M_4, perhaps frontal 5-HT_2, 5-HT_7 and D_2 receptors. As predicted by its M_1 antagonism it worsens learning and long-term memory tasks, and its sedation is liable to prove a problem, e.g. with attentional tasks.

10.3 At What Stage Should Clozapine Be Used in Schizophrenia?

Most schizophrenia treatment guidelines recommend that clozapine is offered to patients who have not responded adequately to trials of at least two different antipsychotic drugs. In the UK, the National Institute for Health and Care Excellence (NICE) (2014) recommends that at least one of the drug trials is with a non-clozapine second-generation antipsychotic. In clinical practice, clozapine is underused; rates of use vary markedly between countries and most eligible patients experience long delays before starting a trial of clozapine (Howes et al., 2012). This partly reflects clinicians' attitudes and knowledge about clozapine and in some countries limitations within services can act as a barrier to the prescribing and monitoring of clozapine.

Studies have examined clozapine's place in the algorithm of schizophrenia treatment. Lieberman's group (2003) found that it was a little more efficacious than chlorpromazine in first-episode psychosis. Agid et al.'s (2011) elegant study of first-episode treatment in Toronto examined its effectiveness third line. It first compared olanzapine or risperidone as first-line agents for six weeks: 75% responded with a symptom reduction of at least one point on the CGI (Clinical Global Impression) – the difference between moderate and mild illness – or a comparable drop in BPRS score. Then the same agents were studied as second line for six weeks. Seventeen per cent of this group, 4% of the original sample, responded at this stage to whichever drug they did not get first line. Those who had not responded adequately (20% of the original sample) then started clozapine: 75% of them responded. This is better than typical proportions responding in more chronic illness. This does suggest that starting clozapine earlier in the course of schizophrenia is better, something consistent with evidence from Yoshimura et al. (2017) who found that the later the initiation of clozapine, the worse the eventual residual symptoms (their analysis suggested a cut-off three years after identifying treatment resistance).

Otherwise, stratifying to predict response is difficult (Suzuki et al., 2011b). There is preliminary evidence that those who respond well to other dopamine antagonists have excessive dopamine synthesis and striatal release (on PET scanning to detect ^{19}FluroDOPA), while those who require clozapine have abnormal glutamate metabolism (as indicated by anterior cingulate glutamate signalling on magnetic resonance spectroscopy; e.g. Demjaha et al., 2014; Mouchliantis et al., 2016). However, these are small studies and it still is unclear if any differences in metabolism detected arise from causes of differences in responsiveness or consequences of differences in other unstudied processes.

Early studies suggested that clozapine's benefits might take six months or even a year to become apparent but Fabrazzo et al.'s (2002) study of serum levels indicated that improvements in psychosis occurred soon (a month or two) after therapeutic levels were reached, though finding the right dose took months in some cases. Recommendations regarding the optimal duration of a trial of clozapine in treatment-resistant schizophrenia vary. The British Association of Psychopharmacology recommends continuing clozapine for three to six months before judging its effectiveness (Barnes et al., 2011). If there has been no response after this time one should consider switching to a drug with a lower risk of side effects.

10.4 Effectiveness in Treatment-Resistant Schizophrenia

If efficacy is a measure of an agent's performance against its intended target in the most favourable circumstances, effectiveness aims to describe the overall value of an agent in more typical circumstances. Trials investigating effectiveness tend to recruit patients less selectively than efficacy trials and use outcomes that reflect the overall utility of an agent, such as time to discontinuation or quality of life, rather than a measure close to the mechanism of action of the agent, such as severity of psychosis for dopamine antagonists. The open Clinical Antipsychotic Trials of Intervention Effectiveness (CATIE) (McEvoy et al., 2006) and blind-rated Cost Utility of the Latest Antipsychotic Drugs in Schizophrenia Study (CUtLASS) (Lewis et al., 2006) clozapine studies were RCTs comparing clozapine's effectiveness to other second-generation dopamine antagonists in treatment-resistant schizophrenia. Both found that clozapine performed better and CUtLASS also found evidence of superior cost utility (Davies et al., 2007).

Tiihonen's group has conducted national case register studies of clozapine treatment in schizophrenia. These showed, broadly, that those started on clozapine across Finland (Tiihonen et al., 2011) and Sweden (Tiihonen et al., 2017) were less likely to experience treatment failure over any given period than those started on other oral agents. Though (given the absence of random allocation) the groups being started on clozapine were likely different in unmeasured ways to those started on other agents, it seems likely that those starting clozapine had more refractory illness and would on the whole otherwise be expected to relapse *more* quickly than most other groups. If so, then the relative protection from clozapine was meaningful. Another paper (FIN11 study) found that clozapine was associated with a significantly lower mortality than any other antipsychotics during an 11-year follow-up (Tiihonen et al., 2009).

The Tiihonen studies also allow a comparison of the superiority of clozapine and LAI antipsychotics to non-clozapine oral antipsychotics. The Finnish and Swedish populations included those starting various LAIs; with all LAIs the risk of treatment failure compared with oral antipsychotics was reduced by about 20–30% (Tiihonen et al., 2011, 2017). The size of this effect was similar to that of clozapine versus other oral antipsychotics. Clearly, the samples being treated with clozapine and those with LAIs likely had different characteristics since these were both observational studies; clozapine will largely be prescribed to those with treatment resistance and LAI for those who have shown adherence problems with oral antipsychotics. Nevertheless, the results indicate that clozapine and LAIs have a similar magnitude of superiority to other oral antipsychotics in terms of reducing overall treatment failure, albeit almost certainly in different populations.

A secondary analysis of the CUtLASS data was consistent with this finding (Barnes et al., 2013). It compared those who had taken LAI first-generation dopamine antagonists before entering the trial and then switched to oral formulation, to those who remained on oral medications before and after allocation. Those previously on LAIs benefitted less from being in the trial: their symptoms started lower than those on oral drugs before the trial and ended higher. A further analysis compared a switch from LAIs to clozapine versus a switch from LAIs to another oral antipsychotic. There was a big difference in the effects of switching from LAIs to oral drugs depending on adherence. If participants' adherence was poor the difference in improvement after switching off LAI was about 0.4 in terms of standardized effect size (7 points mean difference in PANSS score), while clozapine was not significantly better as the oral replacement than any other drug. If their adherence was good then switching from LAI to oral had no significant effect, while in this group switching to clozapine, rather than another drug, improved total symptom score by effect size 0.5 (9 PANSS points). In other words, it appears from naturalistic studies that the benefit of clozapine in preventing relapse and improving symptoms is of a similar scale to the benefit of being on an injectable rather than an oral drug; but of a different kind. It is due to better efficacy in those who are adherent, while LAIs produce better adherence to agents with typical efficacy. Unless poor adherence can be addressed, switching from LAI to clozapine may bring no persistent improvement.

10.5 Clozapine Augmentation in Schizophrenia

The Treatment Response and Resistance in Psychosis group (Howes et al., 2017) suggested that for research purposes a positive response to clozapine monotherapy is at least 20–25% improvement in symptom scores on a validated instrument (PANSS or BPRS) over at least six weeks at 350 ng/ml. Howes and colleagues argued that this should be sustained for another six weeks and that adherence should be good (over 80% of doses). They accepted that in some circumstances symptom remission and no more than mild impairment in social function is a better target. There are good arguments for using a validated scale to detect potentially small improvements over months: Hampson et al. (2011) also mention the KGV scale (Krawiecka et al., 1977). The KGV item scores are quick to complete after standard clinical assessments and (experience suggests) more reliable with minimal training than the BPRS and PANSS. In those whose illness fails to adequately respond to clozapine it is common clinical practice to add another drug to clozapine to try and improve symptoms. This is often referred to as clozapine augmentation. The approach may also be used in those with disabling or distressing residual symptoms, even if they have responded. Clozapine augmentation may involve adding a second antipsychotic or a non-antipsychotic medication but in both cases the evidence to support this practice is weak and inconsistent (Barber et al., 2017; Correll et al., 2017; Galling et al., 2017; Sommer et al., 2012; Veerman et al., 2014). Augmentation with an antipsychotic is however part of NICE clinical guidance (NICE, 2014). A recent narrative review of meta-analytic evidence concluded that there was insufficient evidence to recommend any augmentation strategy (second antipsychotic or another drug) in those who have only partially responsed to clozapine (Haddad & Correll, 2018). The authors recommended that if clozapine was augmented then it should be undertaken as an individual trial in that person and if there is no improvement apparent after an appropriate period then the augmentation agent should be withdrawn. If this is not done the patient is at risk of additional side effects for no benefit.

Amisulpride, risperidone and aripiprazole are the commonest drugs used to augment clozapine; there is little direct evidence for haloperidol or other first-generation agents other than sulpiride (Sommer et al., 2012). However, with all these drugs predictors of efficacy are not well understood, doses are uncertain and safety data limited, so it is important to discontinue such drugs if there is no clear response (e.g. 25% reduction in symptom scores). The combined equivalent dose also often exceeds guidelines for totals (e.g. combined dose >100% BNF doses; or 900 mg chlorpromazine equivalents) so enhanced 'high dose' monitoring for cardiac side effects may be needed (e.g. see Royal College of Psychiatrists' guidance on use of high-dose antipsychotics, Barnes et al., 2014). Clozapine augmentation can increase the risk of other side effects depending on the added drug. For example, amisulpride increases risk of arrhythmia and sexual dysfunction, risperidone has similar but lesser effects and might increase risk of agranulocytosis. Aripiprazole has many adverse effects but these often antagonize clozapine's: insomnia and sedation, weight gain and anorexia; neither raises prolactin much and aripiprazole will do little to worsen metabolic effects or cardiac risk.

As already stated, there is no consistent evidence from the many small trials of non-antipsychotic agents as adjunctives to clozapine (Sommer et al., 2012). Two meta-analyses found a small effect for the adjunctive glutamatergic agent lamotrigine (Tiihonen et al., 2009; Zheng et al., 2017), but the few trials are inconsistent (Sommer et al., 2012); similarly for aspirin, *N*-acetylcysteine and oestrogen (Sommer et al., 2014). Findings for valproate (Zheng et al., 2017) and topiramate are even less consistent (e.g. Galling et al., 2017; Sommer et al., 2012) and depend on low-quality trials. Electroconvulsive therapy is evidenced in the short term (Lally et al., 2016) but there are no long-term RCTs. A recently published trial (the Focusing on Clozapine Unresponsive Symptoms (FOCUS) trial) investigated the efficacy of cognitive behavioural therapy (CBT) for clozapine-resistant schizophrenia (Morrison et al., 2019). CBT was not superior to treatment as usual on total PANSS symptoms at 21 months, the primary outcome. However, CBT was superior to treatment as usual on total PANSS symptoms at nine months (i.e. end of treatment).

10.6 Clozapine in Other Psychiatric Disorders

A small amount of observational data supports the use of clozapine in treatment-resistant mania (Li et al., 2015). One small randomized study supports its benefit compared with treatment as usual in treatment-refractory bipolar disorder (Suppes et al., 1999). Its apparent mood-stabilizing properties may partly reflect its serotonergic effects. Clozapine also reduces arousal, both directly by antagonising noradrenaline at α_1-adrenoceptors and by sedative effects (including H_1, M_1 and 5-HT_2 antagonism). It is sometimes used (usually in low doses where 5-HT_2 antagonism is more important than other effects) to treat severe emotionally unstable personality disorder (Beri & Boydell, 2014). It is important to note that the use of clozapine in bipolar disorder and in severe emotionally unstable personality disorder represents off-label use in both the UK and USA.

10.7 Adverse Effects

10.7.1 Agranulocytosis

There is evidence of autoimmune processes induced by clozapine and causing a range of inflammatory adverse effects. For example, agranulocytosis has been hypothesized to be due to interaction of oxidated clozapine metabolites with cell surface proteins in bone marrow. These proteins are posited to become *haptenes* and hence trigger an autoimmune response to what the immune system identifies as a novel compound (Regen et al., 2017). Bone marrow activity is consequently greatly impaired and those cells with the fastest turnover, granulocytes, disappear from circulation first. Similar mechanisms may underlie myocarditis, cardiomyopathy, pericardial effusion and very rarely pancreatitis, nephritis, coagulopathy, or even pneumonia. These inflammations may be mediated by eosinophils, though eosinophilia alone is often benign (Roberts et al., 2011). Being autoimmune, these processes do not depend directly on clozapine dose and are most likely to occur early in the course of clozapine treatment.

Agranulocytosis can allow otherwise trivial bacterial infections such as streptococcal tonsillitis to progress to lethal sepsis, so patients should be warned to report pyrexia as a possible indication of agranulocytosis and bacterial infection. Approaching 1% of those prescribed clozapine will develop agranulocytosis, 70% within the first 18 weeks (electronic Medicines Compendium, 2019). To mitigate these risks the drug is now prescribed in the UK (as elsewhere) on a weekly basis for the first 18 weeks, then 2 weekly up to 1 year and then 4 weekly if white cell counts were stable throughout, with new tablets not being dispensed until a normal neutrophil count is confirmed by full blood count (electronic Medicines Compendium, 2019). In the event that white cell count drops below 3.5×10^9 per litre and neutrophil below 2.0×10^9 per litre an 'amber' warning is issued and further close monitoring required – white cell counts below 3.0 and neutrophils below 1.5×10^9 per litre are described as 'red' and lead to immediate cessation of prescription and dispensing. Agranulocytosis appears to cause an overall risk of death of 18 per 100 000 people prescribed the drug, mostly during the first few weeks (Regen et al., 2017). The risk can be exacerbated by co-prescribing bone marrow depressants, e.g. most psychotropic medications. Such agents can prolong any periods of agranulocytosis, which would otherwise be short given the relatively rapid elimination of the drug. Eosinophilia above 3×10^9 per litre should also trigger discontinuation (electronic Medicines Compendium, 2019).

10.7.2 Myocarditis and Cardiomyopathy

Autoimmune myocarditis is commonest during the third and fourth weeks of prescription and almost always associated with raised troponin and sometimes raised erythrocyte sedimentation rate (ESR) and eosinophilia too (Ronaldson et al., 2010). Transient tachycardia (from the noradrenaline receptor blockade in peripheral arteries leading to postural hypotension – see below) or transient mild pyrexia without other adverse effects (probably caused by changes in cytokines, e.g. interleukin 6; Kluge et al., 2009) are also common at about three to four weeks but though their appearance should raise a degree of concern, classically myocarditis also presents with breathlessness, palpitations and heart failure. The risk of myocarditis appears to have been relatively high during surveillance in Australia, but it is not clear if differing titration practice or other factors affect the relative risk in other countries (Ronaldson et al., 2012). Cardiomyopathy also occurs with longer-term use, often around 12 months, and presents with heart failure.

10.7.3 Other Cardiovascular Adverse Events

Risk of long QTc and torsade de pointes increases with clozapine serum level, as well as with electrolyte disturbances and genetic vulnerability (Lambiase et al., 2019). It is likely that like other dopamine antagonists it increases risk of sudden cardiac death and stroke in the first weeks of prescription. All patients should have an ECG before commencing treatment and ideally again within the first week of reaching therapeutic levels, as well as if other cardiotoxic drugs, such as a second dopamine antagonist, are initiated; and regularly if high combined doses of dopamine antagonists are maintained. A range of arrhythmias is recognized, including transient atrial tachycardia during titration.

All dopamine antagonists appear to be associated with several-fold increased risks of sudden cardiac death, myocardial infarction and cerebrovascular accidents in the weeks after initial prescription (Huang et al., 2017; Wu et al., 2013, 2015). These risks may decrease to insignificance after two to three months.

10.7.4 Hypotension and Titration

Hypotension is common in the first month after starting clozapine. It tends to reduce in severity over time on clozapine but can remain an impediment. It is dose dependent, caused mainly by α_1-adrenoceptor antagonism. The SPC for clozapine specifies that doses of clozapine are titrated upwards from 12.5 mg mane to therapeutic doses over a few weeks (electronic Medicines Compendium, 2019) because of the risk of seizures, myocarditis (Ronaldson et al., 2012) and hypotension (previously noted in about 10% with circulatory collapse in perhaps 1 per 3000). Any titration scheme must balance adverse effects against delay in reaching a therapeutic concentration of medication. More rapid schemes have been evaluated (Ifteni et al., 2014) on this basis, though there is not as yet sufficient evidence to provide good data on their relative risks and merits. Schemes often fail to distinguish smokers and non-smokers, young and old, or men and women, which can cause problems as serum levels for any given dose vary substantially between these groups. Rostami-Hodjegan and colleagues (2004) provide nomograms comparing concentrations and doses in different groups on the basis of national UK data. These can be useful in estimating what dose might be sufficient to achieve 350 ng/ml with low risk of toxicity as a target at the end of titration. Persistent hypotension can be ameliorated by prescribing fludrocortisone (Testani, 1994). Incidentally, clozapine can also be associated with hypertension (Norman et al., 2017).

10.7.5 Seizures

The risk of seizure increases above 600 ng/ml and particularly above 1000 ng/ml. Clozapine historically has been considered a relatively epileptogenic medication (electronic Medicines

Compendium, 2019), though the risk is probably less in current practice given that serum levels are routinely monitored in most developed countries.

10.7.6 Sedation

This is a common problem at therapeutic concentrations, often being disruptive even with chronic use, and worsens with toxicity, with a risk of fatal respiratory depression (Perdigues et al., 2016). This risk is exacerbated by incautious co-prescription of benzodiazepines or other sedatives, e.g. during titration. It is multifactorial, given clozapine's antagonism of 5-HT_2, H_1, α_1 and M_1 receptors. Minimizing dose and prescribing aripiprazole have been tried.

10.7.7 Abnormal Gastrointestinal Motility

Constipation is common with clozapine treatment and multifactorial – muscarinic and dopamine antagonism are both important (Shirazi et al., 2016). It should be treated assertively (Cohen, 2017), e.g. by improving diet, hydration, prescription of bulking or osmotic agents (e.g. ispaghula husk, lactulose, macrogol; though there is concern that in severe constipation they may worsen gut paralysis), and further courses of stimulants (e.g. senna) or stimulant stool softeners (e.g. bisacodyl, docusate), even strong laxatives and enemas if necessary. Some advocate routine laxatives (Cohen, 2017). The risk of paralytic ileus, often a consequence of toxic serum levels, is absolutely small but relatively high (maybe 30 deaths per 100 000 people prescribed; Nielsen & Meyer, 2012). Clozapine can also cause nausea.

10.7.8 Antimuscarinic Effects

Other antimuscarinic adverse effects include urinary retention, altered focal distance (affecting glasses and contact lenses) and blurred vision, dry mouth and eyes, gum disease and dental decay, and persistent tachycardia. At high concentrations an atropine-like psychosis can develop with features of delirium. Urinary adverse effects can include nocturnal enuresis, sometimes unreported, which is worsened by severe nocturnal sedation. This can often be addressed by altering the timing, as well as the overall dose, of clozapine.

10.7.9 Sialorrhoea

Sialorrhoea and difficulty swallowing saliva is common. It is often worse at night, when serum levels are high because most people take the majority of their dose in the evening because of sedation. Some alleviate drooling using a towel on their pillow but it can still be an embarrassment in the day. Antagonists at muscarinic receptors, e.g. pirenzepine (a relatively selective $M_{1/4}$ antagonist) 25–50 mg OD-TDS, are often prescribed but can worsen constipation and other adverse effects. Chewing hyoscine hydrobromide 300 μg maximizes its local compared to systemic effects and glycopyrrolate does not cross the blood–brain barrier to cause central adverse effects. Other drugs trialled to treat salivary problems include lofexidine, an α_{2A}-adrenoceptor agonist that can cause depression; and amisulpride, a selective D_2 and D_3 antagonist. Again, sialorrhoea may become more severe during toxic events.

10.7.10 Hepatic Toxicity

Raised liver function test values can occur and if they exceed threefold above normal limits necessitate discontinuation. Clozapine can be cautiously prescribed to those with stable liver impairment, though liver function should be monitored.

10.7.11 Metabolic Effects

Clozapine has a range of metabolic effects that it shares with other second-generation dopamine antagonists, though generally it has them more severely. It affects orexin and ghrelin levels and directly affects hypothalamic 5-HT_2 and H_1 receptors, consequently inducing hunger (sometimes severe) and preventing satiation, even despite elevated leptin levels (Holt & Peveler, 2009). Dopamine antagonists also have direct metabolic effects that are more marked in those drugs with 5-HT_2 antagonism, e.g. they can exert a toxic effect on pancreatic β-cell function in the islets of Langerhans. One consequence is a particular propensity for rapid early weight gain. This rises rapidly within three to six months and the effect tails off gradually over years (Novick et al., 2009). Another is a risk of type II diabetes mellitus that can occur even without obesity and in the early phase of prescription – surveillance in Western Australia suggested the prevalence was 17%, though oddly the relative risk was only 1.5 (95% confidence interval 0.6–3.5) in those who were first-degree relatives of diabetics, and 7.2 (1.6–32.2) in the rest (Foley et al., 2015). Yet further metabolic effects include hypertriglyceridaemia and hypercholesterolaemia. The prevalence of full metabolic syndrome (insulin resistance, central obesity, hypertension) varies in surveys but most patients have some features and perhaps 29% meet criteria (Koponen et al., 2010). The combination of these risk factors, which potentiate one another, in those who are often sedentary smokers leads to substantial increases in long-term cardiovascular disease risk. Conversely, the fact that risk factors potentiate each other means that mitigating even a single risk factor can have appreciable benefits in reducing risk. Chapter 21 provides a detailed review of weight gain and metabolic side effects seen with antipsychotics.

10.7.12 Sexual Adverse Effects

More potent D_2 antagonists, including risperidone and amisulpride, are often associated with hyperprolactinaemia which can cause a range of symptoms including irregular periods, galactorrhoea and sexual dysfunction (Haddad & Wieck, 2004). Clozapine does not elevate serum prolactin but still has some association with sexual dysfunction. This is because there are many mechanisms by which drugs can cause sexual dysfunction other than by hyperprolactinaemia (Park et al., 2012). A 'dirty' drug such as clozapine is likely to affect the delicate series of responses involved in sexual and reproductive health in several ways. Histamine receptor antagonism can impair arousal through sedation, D_2 receptor antagonism can reduce libido by inhibiting motivation and reward, both cholinergic receptor antagonism and α-adrenergic receptor antagonism can reduce peripheral vasodilation, resulting in erectile dysfunction in men and decreased vaginal lubrication in women. The naturalistic SOHO study suggests that perhaps 33% will experience some erectile dysfunction (Lambert et al., 2005). Amenorrhoea and erectile dysfunction commonly worsen when a second antipsychotic is co-prescribed.

10.7.13 Obsessive-Compulsive Symptoms

Clozapine, even more than other 5-HT_2 antagonist second-generation dopamine antagonists, shows an association with the development of obsessions and compulsions. Treatments include dose reduction, aripiprazole augmentation, selective serotonin reuptake inhibitors (SSRIs), and perhaps CBT or clomipramine (Laroche & Gaillard, 2016).

10.7.14 Pneumonia

Clozapine, in common with other antipsychotics, is associated with an increased risk of pneumonia in observational studies (Dzahini et al., 2018; Stoecker et al., 2017). The risk appears higher with clozapine than with other agents. The association with pneumonia has been demonstrated for clozapine use in people with bipolar disorder (Yang et al., 2013) and schizophrenia (Kuo et al., 2013) and in both studies the risk was dose related. In a further study, clozapine re-exposure was linked to a greater risk for recurrent pneumonia than the risk of baseline pneumonia with initial clozapine treatment (Hung et al., 2016). The risk of pneumonia with antipsychotics appears highest early in treatment. The methodological weaknesses of observational studies, including being unable to control for all relevant confounders, mean they cannot prove causality. On the other hand, plausible mechanisms exist by which clozapine and other antipsychotics could increase the risk of aspiration pneumonia. It is recommended that patients prescribed clozapine and other antipsychotics are monitored for signs of chest infection and appropriate treatment commenced if there is evidence of infection.

10.7.15 Monitoring for Adverse Effects

Clozapine's adverse effect profile makes it important to monitor for adverse effects during treatment with closer monitoring being required during the initial period of dose titration. A range of investigations, beyond neutrophil monitoring, is recommended before and during prescription (Cohen et al., 2012; electronic Medicines Compendium, 2019; CG178, NICE, 2014; Remington et al., 2016) depending on local and national guidelines. These include fasting lipids and glucose, liver function, ECG and electrolytes, weight, body mass index (BMI), heart rate, blood pressure and C-reactive protein (CRP). QTc should be checked before starting treatment and arguably at the end of titration, with daily lying and standing blood pressure, pulse and temperature initially and then weekly during titration. Some would argue for weekly ESR/CRP and troponin until week 6. Weight, pulse and blood pressure should probably be assessed monthly and fasting glucose and lipids, liver function test at the same time for the first 3 months; thereafter every 6 to 12 months. In addition, patients need to be asked systematically about common adverse effects including sialorrhoea, constipation and sedation. The Glasgow Antipsychotic Side-effects Scale for Clozapine (GASS-C) is a reliable and valid scale that allows a systematic assessment of the subjectively unpleasant side effects of clozapine (Hynes et al., 2015).

10.8 Pharmacokinetics

Clozapine is well absorbed whether or not taken with food. It does not form a stable solution or suspension in water, though the tablets can be crushed and administered with liquid in those with questionable adherence. It is 95% protein bound in serum (Mauri et al., 2007). Forty per cent to 70% of the drug is removed by first-pass metabolism, mainly metabolized by cytochrome P450 isoenzyme 1A2 (electronic Medicines Compendium, 2019; Mauri et al., 2007). This is greatly induced by the aromatic hydrocarbons in tobacco smoke (but not by nicotine) and perhaps caffeine and carbamazepine; and inhibited by co-administration of theophylline, ciprofloxacin, hypericum (St John's wort), oral contraceptives and fluvoxamine (which can increase levels 10-fold). Consequently, smokers require higher doses of clozapine and dose reduction if they stop smoking. As with almost all other dopamine antagonists a mixture of isoenzymes contributes to metabolism, including for clozapine, as well as 1A2, 3A3/4, 2C, 2D6 and 2E1. Agents that induce or inhibit these may have variable effects too, depending in part on the expression of the various alleles of the genes coding for them (e.g. 2D6); for instance, fluoxetine.

Peak concentration occurs around 2 hours after ingestion and once-daily dosing appears to be sufficient. Half-life estimates vary (9–17 hours; Mauri et al., 2007) but it is probably around 14 hours during steady state; the half-life of norclozapine is longer. Serum levels can be assayed and are taken at trough, i.e. just before the next dose is due (24 hours) or at least 12 hours after the last one.

Metabolism is slower for women, perhaps those of East Asian descent (Suzuki et al., 2011b), and perhaps begins to decrease after 40 years of age; but is clearly lower in those over 65 (Ismail et al., 2012). As metabolism is reduced so doses at least 30% (or in some models 50%) lower are appropriate, and slower titration than for younger patients (Bowskill et al., 2012).

10.8.1 Serum Monitoring

Monitoring serum levels reduces risk of toxicity and increases the chance of reaching efficacious levels. It is also a way to check adherence. Serum levels appear to vary in a linear relationship with dose for most individuals, with about 20% variation from time to time (Mauri et al., 2007). At the higher doses however some individuals may find that their metabolizing enzymes saturate and kinetics shift from 'first order' (with an exponential decay after a dose, described by 'half-life', because like most drugs at therapeutic levels there are sufficient enzymes to remove half *any* amount of the drug in a given period) to 'zero order' kinetics (the saturated system can only remove the same amount of drug and no more, as with alcohol). In that situation elimination slows and serum levels can suddenly increase disproportionately (Couchman et al., 2010). Serum level might increase even without further medication if toxicity halts gut motility and more clozapine returns from the intestinal lumen to the circulation.

10.8.2 Therapeutic Threshold

There is evidence that concentrations between 250 and 420 ng/ml are therapeutic, with 350 ng/ml generally quoted as the target as there is some evidence that response is three times more likely above this limit than below it (Suzuki et al., 2011b). This implies that a significant minority of patients will respond to levels below 350 ng/ml and hence patients who respond to the initial trial of clozapine without problematic adverse effects do not routinely require levels, unless it is to establish a baseline in case of later non-adherence or changes in smoking or co-prescription.

There have been suggestions that levels above 600 ng/ml can reduce efficacy, as antimuscarinic adverse effects worsen psychotic symptoms, and that levels above this (and perhaps particularly above thresholds of 750 ng/ml or 1000 ng/ml) disproportionately increase the risk of seizures. Nonetheless, there are those who advocate cautious trials of >1000 ng/ml on an anecdotal basis in ultra-treatment-resistant illness.

There have been suggestions that those of East Asian (e.g. Korean or Chinese) descent may require both lower serum levels (e.g. 200 ng/ml; Xiang et al., 2006) and lower doses to achieve typical levels (Suzuki et al., 2011b).

Few patients over 50 have been included in trials and serum thresholds for this group are uncertain, though in one trial of over 55-year-olds 300 mg/day was well tolerated (see review by Suzuki et al., 2011a). There are suggestions that efficacy is reduced and risk of neutropenia increased in those over 65 years.

10.8.3 Toxicity

Overall toxicity appears to increase with serum concentration – adverse effects correlate weakly with levels and are twice as common above 350 ng/ml as below (Yusufi et al., 2007). Severe toxicity (e.g. concentration >1000 ng/ml) can occur due to excessive increases in dose, variable adherence (as tolerance is lost on restarting the drug, or doses are increased in those with poor response or low serum levels and this is combined with closer monitoring and better compliance) or alterations in environmental agents such as tobacco smoke or other drugs. Those who stop smoking need to decrease dose over the next two weeks: first enzyme down-regulation and turnover reduces the capacity to metabolize; then serum levels rise to a new (potentially toxic) steady state. This is often heralded by an increase in adverse effects. It is likely to be true for cannabis smokers too. There have been suggestions that metabolic changes during inflammatory episodes can increase serum levels, perhaps by reducing metabolism or due to interactions with treatments for the inflammatory disorder (Pfuhlmann et al., 2009).

After episodes of toxicity there is no well-evidenced procedure and a wide range of individual circumstances will determine the likely best course for an individual patient. Serum assays are of limited use since levels are dynamic and assays take time to come back. It can be more useful to rely on adverse effects as an immediate bioassay. Certain theoretical considerations apply in most cases.

Untreated toxicity can kill. If patients display severe and/or increasing adverse effects; have indications of cardiotoxicity (e.g. palpitations and breathlessness, ECG changes) or seizure risk (e.g. myoclonic jerks); or serum levels are likely to still increase (e.g. they are constipated and unable to eliminate clozapine that recirculates from the gut) then the situation is more urgent than if patients have been stable at the current levels and display only mild adverse effects. Older patients (e.g. over 65) are more vulnerable.

During any intervention it is critical to monitor the patient's clinical state frequently. ECG is required if possible. Lying and standing blood pressure, pulse and temperature can be monitored several times daily for the first 24–72 hours, then at least once daily (usually twice) for the next week. Lying and standing comparison may give better warning of α_1 toxicity than simple blood pressure. If clinicians are concerned about the risk of seizure, they can start valproate 400 mg twice a day (some do this as a routine) but it is best to avoid benzodiazepines if possible due to their risk of sedation. Constipation is an important risk to monitor and treat during and after episodes of toxicity. If the patient is severely toxic, clearly has serum levels of approaching 2000 ng/ml or more, has co-morbidity or is deteriorating then the risk of serious adverse events is high and admission for medical treatment is very likely necessary.

The easiest practical approach to bringing serum levels down is to stop clozapine. It is important to remember that elimination may be slowed if metabolism becomes saturated, as described above, so it can be easy to misunderstand the time course of serum levels. The option least likely to cause toxicity is to stop the drug for 48–72 hours and then re-titrate.

However, relatively rapid elimination and slow return to therapeutic levels could provoke an immediate relapse as there is sometimes a rebound psychosis. If the patient does not appear too toxic on initial examination (no marked increase in adverse effects, lying and standing blood pressure normal, no severe tachycardia, no myoclonic jerks, a normal ECG and even EEG) and/or levels are available and are not too high then one might instead stop for 24–36 hours. *If* metabolism is unsaturated (and kinetics first order) that will reduce levels 3- to 30-fold. One needs to reassess what the level may then be (e.g. any evidence of improvements in adverse effects; if side effects are still greater than those the patient normally experiences during clozapine treatment then the serum levels probably remain dangerously high). If adverse effects are no worse than normal, including pulse, lying and standing blood pressure and constipation, one might start on about half the maintenance dose (sometimes much lower, e.g. after smoking stops) and continue at that level for two to three days. If the patient still appears to have their usual level of adverse effects at that point one might return by increments to the previous dose, provided the reason for toxicity no longer applies.

In the event that a patient has become toxic after stopping an enzyme inducer (e.g. smoking) then a new maintenance dose may be more suitable as the target instead. Rostami-Hodjegan et al.'s (2004) nomograms can help determine a suitable dose, but a rule of thumb is to reduce to 60% of the previous dose. The situation after stopping smoking can be particularly complex – if the prescriber knows about the change in smoking status within a couple of days then simply reducing the maintenance dose to 60% of the original and repeating serum levels after a week or two may be enough.

10.8.4 Adherence Monitoring

Serum monitoring can also indicate level of adherence. Dopamine antagonist serum levels usually provide a snapshot, from which it can be difficult to infer adherence unless doses and concomitant drugs remain the same in successive assays and the concentration falls. With clozapine, norclozapine levels are also assayed. The median ratio is 1.3 and though this varies between individuals it varies much less within each individual. Since norclozapine has a longer half-life than clozapine and the ratio of the two should stay the same in most circumstances (even if doses are altered somewhat), a fall in the ratio indicates that adherence over the few days preceding the assay (rather than the night before) might not have been the same as in the past. However, if concentrations increase then a high clozapine:norclozapine ratio can instead warn of saturation of metabolism; or that this was not a trough level.

10.9 Rechallenge and Continuation

Given the lack of pharmacological alternatives (and the reality that interventions such as cognitive behavioural therapy for psychosis (CBTp), family intervention, occupational rehabilitation and cognitive remediation, each with reasonable evidence of efficacy, are not panaceas) it is often attractive to return to clozapine for some of those with severe refractory illness even after they have had to stop treatment due to toxicity, serious adverse effects or a co-morbid physical illness, especially if they have had a good response previously (Manu et al., 2012; Nielsen et al., 2013).

There is now reasonable evidence that about half of those with previous neutropenia sufficient to trigger a 'red' warning may be able to restart the drug (e.g. Manu et al., 2018), even if the SPC warns against it (electronic Medicines Compendium, 2019). This is particularly true when the patient is of African or Asian descent – serum neutrophil norms are usually Eurocentric and patients from other racial groups can suffer 'benign ethnic neutropenia', i.e. relatively low but normal neutrophil counts. In that case if a haematologist can identify this and recommend safe, lower limits (see also Meyer et al., 2015) then pharmaceutical monitoring services are generally willing to provide the drug again. Granulocyte colony stimulating factor (GCSF) or lithium have been used to boost neutrophil counts, though it is not clear that lithium prevents agranulocytosis. Restarting after agranulocytosis is more hazardous and much less successful (Manu et al., 2018).

The situation is less certain with other adverse events (Manu et al., 2018). There is scanty evidence that some people can tolerate reintroduction of clozapine after myocarditis. The same may be true after uncomplicated myocardial infarction or stroke, if these were not associated with the initiation of the drug (indicating lack of causation). Stroke may increase the risk of seizure, but even after generalized seizures patients can often tolerate the drug again with valproate cover, despite the slightly enhanced risk of neutropenia. In people who have experienced pneumonia with clozapine treatment, it seems there is a higher risk of a further episode of pneumonia with challenge compared with the risk with initial treatment (Hung et al., 2016). Patients and clinicians need to consider this risk in making decisions.

10.10 Summary

Clozapine is unique in terms of its greater efficacy compared with other antipsychotics in treatment-resistant schizophrenia (Siskind et al., 2016). For many patients the reduction or elimination of distressing psychotic symptoms and the improved quality of life are considerable. National observational data show that among a wide range of antipsychotics clozapine is associated with one of the lowest rates of treatment failure (Tiihonen et al., 2011, 2017). Such data also show that over the long term clozapine is associated with reduced mortality compared with other antipsychotics and no treatment.

Clozapine can cause a wide range of adverse effects which at the most serious are potentially fatal. Monitoring of the mental state, screening for side effects and regular haematological testing are important parts of treatment. A community psychiatric nurse or other professional working as a care coordinator alongside the psychiatrist, to help monitor patients prescribed clozapine, plus a dedicated hospital-based pharmacist for clozapine are the norm in UK psychiatric services and some other countries. Often follow-up involves attendance at dedicated clozapine clinics. Such integrated working can improve the quality of treatment for patients.

It is unfortunate that clozapine remains underused in treatment-resistant schizophrenia in many countries and that many people experience a long delay before being offered a trial of clozapine. Clozapine also has an important role in treating psychosis associated with Parkinson's disease where other treatments have failed (electronic Medicines Compendium, 2019). There are limited data, largely non-randomized, that suggest that off-label use of clozapine may be of benefit in conditions other than schizophrenia. Perhaps the data are more supportive in refractory mania and difficult to treat bipolar disorder (Li et al., 2015; Suppes et al., 1999). The mechanism that underlies clozapine unique efficacy remains unclear and warrants further research.

References

Agid O, Arenovich T, Sajeev G, et al. (2011). An algorithm-based approach to first-episode schizophrenia: response rates over 3 prospective antipsychotic trials with a retrospective data analysis. *J Clin Psychiatry*, 72, 1439–1444.

Bagnall AM, Jones L, Ginnelly L, et al. (2003). A systematic review of atypical antipsychotic drugs in schizophrenia. *Health Technol Assess*, 7(13), 1–193.

Barber S, Olotu U, Corsi M, Cipriani A (2017). Clozapine combined with different antipsychotic drugs for treatment-resistant schizophrenia. *Cochrane Database Syst Rev*, (3), CD006324.

Barnes TR; Schizophrenia Consensus Group of the British Association for Psychopharmacology (2011). Evidence-based guidelines for the pharmacological treatment of schizophrenia: recommendations from the British Association for Psychopharmacology. *J Psychopharmacol*, 25, 567–620.

Barnes TRE, Drake RJ, Dunn G, et al. (2013). The effect of prior treatment with long-acting injectable antipsychotic drugs on randomised, clinical trial treatment outcomes. *Br J Psychiatry*, 203(3), 215–220.

Barnes TRE, Dye S, Ferrier N, et al. (2014). *Consensus Statement on High-Dose Antipsychotic Medication*. College Report CR190. London: Royal College of Psychiatrists.

Beri A, Boydell J (2014). Clozapine in borderline personality disorder: a review of the evidence. *Ann Clin Psychiatry*, 26(2), 139–144.

Bowskill S, Couchman L, MacCabe JH, Flanagan RJ (2012). Plasma clozapine and norclozapine in relation to prescribed dose and other factors in patients aged 65 years and over: data from a therapeutic drug monitoring service, 1996–2010. *Hum Psychopharmacol*, 27(3), 277–283.

Brosda J, Jantschak F, Pertz HH (2014). Alpha2-adrenoceptors are targets for antipsychotic drugs. *Psychopharmacology*, 231(5), 801–812.

Chang A, Fox SH (2016). Psychosis in Parkinson's disease: epidemiology, pathophysiology, and management. *Drugs*, 76(11), 1093–1118.

Chang JS, Ha KS, Young Lee K, Sik Kim Y, Min Ahn Y (2006). The effects of long-term clozapine add-on therapy on the rehospitalization rate and the mood polarity patterns in bipolar disorders. *J Clin Psychiatry*, 67(3), 461–467.

Cohen D (2017). Clozapine and gastrointestinal hypomotility. *CNS Drugs*, 31(12), 1083–1091.

Cohen D, Bogers JP, van Dijk D, Bakker B, Schulte PF (2012). Beyond white blood cell monitoring: screening in the initial phase of clozapine therapy. *J Clin Psychiatry*, 73(10), 1307–1312.

Correll CU, Rubio JM, Inczedy-Farkas G, et al. (2017). Efficacy of 42 pharmacologic cotreatment strategies added to antipsychotic monotherapy in schizophrenia: systematic overview and quality appraisal of the meta-analytic evidence. *JAMA Psychiatry*, 74, 675–684.

Couchman L, Morgan EL, Spencer EP, Flanagan RJ (2010). Plasma clozapine, norclozapine, and the clozapine:norclozapine ratio in relation to prescribed dose and other factors: data from a therapeutic drug monitoring service, 1993–2007. *Ther Drug Monit*, 32, 438–447.

Crilly J (2007). The history of clozapine and its emergence in the US market: a review and analysis. *Hist Psychiatry*, 18(1), 39–60.

Davies LM, Lewis S, Jones PB, et al.; CUtLASS team (2007). Cost-effectiveness of first- v. second-generation antipsychotic drugs: results from a randomised controlled trial in schizophrenia responding poorly to previous therapy. *Br J Psychiatry*, 191, 14–22.

Davis JM, Chen N, Glick ID (2003). A meta-analysis of the efficacy of second-generation antipsychotics. *Arch Gen Psychiatry*, 60(6), 553–564.

Demjaha A, Egerton A, Murray RM, et al. (2014). Antipsychotic treatment resistance in schizophrenia associated with elevated glutamate levels but normal dopamine function. *Biol Psychiatry*, 75(5), e11–e13.

Dzahini O, Singh N, Taylor D, Haddad PM (2018). Antipsychotic drug use and pneumonia:

systematic review and meta-analysis. *J Psychopharmacol*, 32(11), 1167–1181.

electronic Medicines Compendium (2019). Summary of Product Characteristics: Clorazil. Mylan. Last updated 6 June 2019. Available at: www.medicines.org.uk/emc/product/10290/smpc (last accessed 4.10.19).

Fabrazzo M, La Pia S, Monteleone P, et al. (2002). Is the time course of clozapine response correlated to the time course of clozapine plasma levels? A one-year prospective study in drug-resistant patients with schizophrenia. *Neuropsychopharmacology*, 27(6), 1050–1055.

Foley DL, Mackinnon A, Morgan VA, et al. (2015). Effect of age, family history of diabetes, and antipsychotic drug treatment on risk of diabetes in people with psychosis: a population-based cross-sectional study. *Lancet Psychiatry*, 2(12), 1092–1098.

Frogley C, Taylor D, Dickens G, Picchioni M (2011). A systematic review of the evidence of clozapine's anti-aggressive effects. *Int J Neuropsychopharmacol*, 15(9), 1351–1371.

Galling B, Roldán A, Hagi K, et al. (2017). Antipsychotic augmentation vs. monotherapy in schizophrenia: systematic review, meta-analysis and meta-regression analysis. *World Psychiatry*, 16(1), 77–89.

Goldstein ME, Anderson VM, Pillai A, Kydd RR, Russell BR (2015). Glutamatergic neurometabolites in clozapine-responsive and -resistant schizophrenia. *Int J Neuropsychopharmacol*, 18(6), 117.

Gross G, Wicke K, Drescher KU (2013). Dopamine D3 receptor antagonism – still a therapeutic option for the treatment of schizophrenia. *Naunyn Schmiedebergs Arch Pharmacol*, 386(2), 155–166.

Haddad PM, Correll CU (2018). The acute efficacy of antipsychotics in schizophrenia: a review of recent meta-analyses. *Ther Adv Psychopharmacol*, 8(11), 303–318.

Haddad PM, Wieck A (2004). Antipsychotic-induced hyperprolactinaemia: mechanisms, clinical features and management. *Drugs*, 64, 2291–2314.

Hampson M, Killaspy H, Mynors-Wallis L, Meier R (2011). Outcome measures recommended for use in adult psychiatry. Occasional Paper OP78. London: Royal College of Psychiatrists. Available at: www.rcpsych.ac.uk/files/pdfversion/OP78x.pdf (last accessed 11.8.17).

Healy D (1997). *The Psychopharmcologists: Interviews by David Healy*. New York: Chapman and Hall.

Holt RIG, Peveler RC (2009). Obesity, serious mental illness and antipsychotic drugs. *Diabetes Obes Metabol*, 11, 665–679.

Howes OD, Vergunst F, Gee S, et al. (2012). Adherence to treatment guidelines in clinical practice: study of antipsychotic treatment prior to clozapine initiation. *Br J Psychiatry*, 201, 481–485.

Howes OD, McCutcheon R, Agid O, et al. (2017). Treatment resistant schizophrenia: Treatment Response and Resistance in Psychosis (TRRIP) working group consensus guidelines on diagnosis and terminology. *Am J Psychiatry*, 174(3), 216–229.

Huang KL, Fang CJ, Hsu CC, et al. (2017). Myocardial infarction risk and antipsychotics use revisited: a meta-analysis of 10 observational studies. *J Psychopharmacol*, 31(12), 1544–1555. doi:10.1177/0269881117714047.

Hung GC, Liu HC, Yang SY, et al. (2016). Antipsychotic reexposure and recurrent pneumonia in schizophrenia: a nested case-control study. *J Clin Psychiatry*, 77, 60–66.

Hynes C, Keating D, McWilliams S, et al. (2015). Glasgow Antipsychotic Side-effects Scale for Clozapine – development and validation of a clozapine-specific side-effects scale. *Schizophr Res*, 168(1–2), 505–513.

Ifteni P, Nielsen J, Burtea V, et al. (2014). Effectiveness and safety of rapid clozapine titration in schizophrenia. *Acta Psychiatr Scand*, 130, 25–29.

Ismail Z, Wessels AM, Uchida H, et al. (2012). Age and sex impact clozapine plasma concentrations in inpatients and outpatients with schizophrenia. *Am J Geriatr Psychiatry*, 20(1), 53–60.

Kane JM, Honigfield G, Singer J, Meltzer HY (1988). Clozapine for the treatment-resistant schizophrenic: a double-blind comparison with chlorpromazine. *Arch Gen Psychiatry*, 45, 789–796.

Kluge M, Schuld A, Schacht A, et al. (2009). Effects of clozapine and olanzapine on cytokine systems are closely linked to weight gain and drug-induced fever. *Psychoneuroendocrinology*, 34(1), 118–128.

Koponen HJ, Hakko HH, Saari KM, et al. (2010). The prevalence and predictive value of individual criteria for metabolic syndrome in schizophrenia: a Northern Finland 1966 Birth Cohort Study. *World J Biol Psychiatry*, 11(2 Pt 2), 262–267.

Krawiecka M, Goldberg D, Vaughan M. (1977). A standardised psychiatric assessment scale for rating chronic psychiatric patients. *Acta Psychiatr Scand*, 55, 299–308.

Kuo CJ, Yang SY, Liao YT, et al. (2013). Second-generation antipsychotic medications and risk of pneumonia in schizophrenia. *Schizophr Bull*, 39, 648–657.

Lahti RA, Evans DL, Stratman NC, Figur LM (1993). Dopamine D4 versus D2 receptor selectivity of dopamine receptor antagonists: possible therapeutic implications. *Eur J Pharmacol*, 236(3), 483–486.

Lalanne L, Lutz PE, Trojak B, et al. (2016). Medications between psychiatric and addictive disorders. *Prog Neuropsychopharmacol Biol Psychiatry*, 65, 215–223.

Lally J, Tully J, Robertson D, et al. (2016). Augmentation of clozapine with electroconvulsive therapy in treatment resistant schizophrenia: a systematic review and meta-analysis. *Schizophr Res*, 171(1–3), 215–224.

Lambert M, Haro JM, Novick D, et al. (2005). Olanzapine vs. other antipsychotics in actual out-patient settings: six months tolerability results from the European Schizophrenia Out-patient Health Outcomes study. *Acta Psychiatr Scand*, 111(3), 232–243.

Lambiase PD, de Bono JP, Schilling RJ, et al. (2019). British Heart Rhythm Society clinical practice guidelines on the management of patients developing QT prolongation on antipsychotic medication. *Arrhythm Electrophysiol Rev*, 8(3), 161–165.

Laroche DG, Gaillard A (2016). Induced obsessive compulsive symptoms (OCS) in schizophrenia patients under atypical 2 antipsychotics (AAPs): review and hypotheses. *Psychiatry Res*, 246, 119–128.

Leucht S, Cipriani A, Spijeli L, et al. (2013). Comparative efficacy and tolerability of 15 antipsychotic drugs in schizophrenia: a multiple-treatments meta-analysis. *Lancet*, 382, 951–962.

Lewis SW, Barnes TR, Davies L, et al. (2006). Randomized controlled trial of effect of prescription of clozapine versus other second-generation antipsychotic drugs in resistant schizophrenia. *Schizophr Bull*, 32(4), 715–723.

Li XB, Tang YL, Wang CY, et al. (2015). Clozapine for treatment-resistant bipolar disorder: a systematic review. *Bipolar Disord*, 17, 235–247.

Lieberman JA, Phillips M, Gu H, et al. (2003). Atypical and conventional antipsychotic drugs in treatment-naive first-episode schizophrenia: a 52-week randomized trial of clozapine vs chlorpromazine. *Neuropsychopharmacology*, 28(5), 995–1003.

Lobos CA, Komossa K, Rummel-Kluge C, et al. (2010). Clozapine versus other atypical antipsychotics for schizophrenia. *Cochrane Database Syst Rev*, (11), CD006633.

Manu P, Sarpal D, Muir O, Kane JM, Correll CU (2012). When can patients with potentially life-threatening adverse effects be rechallenged with clozapine? A systematic review of the published literature. *Schizophr Res*, 134(2–3), 180–186.

Manu P, Lapitskaya Y, Shaikh A, Nielsen J (2018). Clozapine rechallenge after major adverse effects: clinical guidelines based on 259 cases. *Am J Ther*, 25(2), e218–e223.

Mauri MC, Volonteri LS, Colasanti A, et al. (2007). Clinical pharmacokinetics of atypical antipsychotics: a critical review of the relationship between plasma concentrations and clinical response. *Clin Pharmacokinet*, 46(5), 359–388.

McEvoy JP, Lieberman JA, Stroup TS, et al.; CATIE Investigators (2006). Effectiveness of clozapine versus olanzapine, quetiapine, and risperidone in patients with chronic schizophrenia who did not respond to prior atypical antipsychotic treatment. *Am J Psychiatry*, 163(4), 600–610.

Melkersson K, Lewitt M, Hall K (2015). Higher serum concentrations of tyrosine and glutamate in schizophrenia patients treated with clozapine, compared to in those treated with conventional antipsychotics. *Neuro Endocrinol Lett*, 36(5), 465–480.

Meltzer HY (2013). Update on typical and atypical antipsychotic drugs. *Annu Rev Med*, 64, 393–406.

Meltzer HY, Alphs L, Green AI, et al.; International Suicide Prevention Trial Study Group (2003). Clozapine treatment for suicidality in schizophrenia. *Arch Gen Psychiatry*, 60, 82–91.

Mendoza MC, Lindenmayer JP (2009). *N*-desmethylclozapine: is there evidence for its antipsychotic potential? *Clin Neuropharmacol*, 32(3), 154–157.

Meyer N, Gee S, Whiskey E, et al. (2015). Optimizing outcomes in clozapine rechallenge following neutropenia: a cohort analysis. *J Clin Psychiatry*, 76(11), e1410–e1416.

Miyamoto S, Miyake N, Jarskog LF, Fleischhacker WW, Lieberman JA (2012). Pharmacological treatment of schizophrenia: a critical review of the pharmacology and clinical effects of current and future therapeutic agents. *Mol Psychiatry*, 17(12), 1206–1227.

Morrison AP, Pyle M, Gumley A, et al. (2019). Cognitive-behavioural therapy for clozapine-resistant schizophrenia: the FOCUS RCT. *Health Technol Assess*, 23(7), 1–144.

Mouchlianitis E, Bloomfield MA, Law V, et al. (2016). Treatment-resistant schizophrenia patients show elevated anterior cingulate cortex glutamate compared to treatment-responsive. *Schizophr Bull*, 42(3), 744–752.

National Institute for Health and Care Excellence (NICE) (2014). *Psychosis and schizophrenia in adults: prevention and management*. Clinical guideline [CG178]. London: National Institute for Health and Care Excellence. Available at: www.nice.org.uk/guidance/cg178 (last accessed 4.10.19).

Nielsen J, Meyer JM (2012). Risk factors for ileus in patients with schizophrenia. *Schizophr Bull*, 38(3), 592–598.

Nielsen J, Correll CU, Manu P, Kane JM (2013). Termination of clozapine treatment due to medical reasons: when is it warranted and how can it be avoided? *J Clin Psychiatry*, 74(6), 603–613.

Norman SM, Sullivan KM, Liu F, et al. (2017). Blood pressure and heart rate changes during clozapine treatment. *Psychiatr Q*, 88(3), 545–552.

Novick D, Haro JM, Perrin E, Suarez D, Texeira JM (2009). Tolerability of outpatient antipsychotic treatment: 36-month results from the European Schizophrenia Outpatient Health Outcomes (SOHO) study. *Eur Neuropsychopharmacol*, 19(8), 542–550.

O'Connor WT, O'Shea SD (2015). Clozapine and GABA transmission in schizophrenia disease models: establishing principles to guide treatments. *Pharmacol Ther*, 150, 47–80.

Park YW, Kim Y, Lee JH (2012). Antipsychotic-induced sexual dysfunction and its management. *World J Mens Health*, 30(3), 153–159.

Perdigues SR, Quecuti RS, Mane A, et al. (2016). An observational study of clozapine induced sedation and its pharmacological management. *Eur Neuropsychopharmacol*, 26(1), 156–161.

Pfuhlmann B, Hiemke C, Unterecker S, et al. (2009). Toxic clozapine serum levels during inflammatory reactions. *J Clin Psychopharmacol*, 29(4), 392–394.

Polcwiartek C, Nielsen J (2016). The clinical potentials of adjunctive fluvoxamine to clozapine treatment: a systematic review. *Psychopharmacology*, 233(5), 741–750.

Potkin SG, Basile VS, Jin Y, et al. (2003). D1 receptor alleles predict PET metabolic correlates of clinical response to clozapine. *Mol Psychiatry*, 8, 109–113.

Regen F, Herzog I, Hahn E, et al. (2017). Clozapine-induced agranulocytosis: evidence for an immune-mediated mechanism from a patient-specific in-vitro approach. *Toxicol Appl Pharmacol*, 316, 10–16.

Remington G, Lee J, Agid O, et al. (2016). Clozapine's critical role in treatment resistant schizophrenia: ensuring both safety and use. *Expert Opin Drug Saf*, 15(9), 1193–1203.

Roberts CE, Mortenson LY, Merrill DB, et al. (2011). Successful rechallenge with clozapine after eosinophilia. *Am J Psychiatry*, 168(11), 1147–1151.

Rogers DP, Shramko JK (2000). Therapeutic options in the treatment of clozapine-induced sialorrhea. *Pharmacotherapy*, 20(9), 1092–1095.

Ronaldson KJ, Taylor AJ, Fitzgerald PB, et al. (2010). Diagnostic characteristics of clozapine-induced myocarditis identified by an analysis of 38 cases and 47 controls. *J Clin Psychiatry*, 71(8), 976–981.

Ronaldson KJ, Fitzgerald PB, Taylor AJ, et al. (2012). Rapid clozapine dose titration and concomitant sodium valproate increase the risk of myocarditis with clozapine: a case-control study. *Schizophr Res*, 141(2–3), 173–178.

Rostami-Hodjegan A, Amin AM, Spencer EP, et al. (2004). Influence of dose, cigarette smoking, age, sex, and metabolic activity on plasma clozapine concentrations: a predictive model and nomograms to aid clozapine dose adjustment and to assess compliance in individual patients. *J Clin Psychopharmacol*, 24(1), 70–78.

Roth BL, Driscol J (2013). PDSP Ki Database. Psychoactive Drug Screening Program (PDSP). University of North Carolina at Chapel Hill and the United States National Institute of Mental Health. Retrieved 10.10.13 from 'Archived copy'. Archived from the original on 8.11.13. Retrieved 25.11.13.

Samara MT, Dold M, Gianatsi M, et al. (2016). Efficacy, acceptability, and tolerability of antipsychotics in treatment-resistant schizophrenia: a network meta-analysis. *JAMA Psychiatry*, 73(3), 199–210.

Seeman P (2014). Clozapine, a fast-off-D2 antipsychotic. *ACS Chem Neurosci*, 5, 24–29.

Selent J, Lopez L, Sanz F, Pastor M (2008). Multi-receptor binding profile of clozapine and olanzapine: a structural study based on the new β2 adrenergic receptor template. *ChemMedChem*, 3, 1194–1198.

Shirazi A, Stubbs B, Gomez L, et al. (2016). Prevalence and predictors of clozapine-associated constipation: a systematic review and meta-analysis. *Int J Mol Sci*, 17(6), 863.

Siskind D, McCartney L, Goldschlager R, Kisely S (2016). Clozapine v. first- and second-generation antipsychotics in treatment refractory schizophrenia: systematic review and meta-analysis. *Br J Psychiatry*, 209(5), 385–392.

Siskind D, Siskind V, Kisely S (2017). Clozapine response rates among people with treatment-resistant schizophrenia: data from a systematic review and meta-analysis. *Can J Psychiatry*, 62(11), 772–777.

Sommer IE, Begemann MJ, Temmerman A, Leucht S (2012). Pharmacological augmentation strategies for schizophrenia patients with insufficient response to clozapine: a quantitative literature review. *Schizophr Bull*, 38(5), 1003–1011.

Sommer IE, van Westrhenen R, Begemann MJH, et al. (2014). Efficacy of anti-inflammatory agents to improve symptoms in patients with schizophrenia: an update. *Schizophr Bull*, 40(1), 181–191.

Stoecker ZR, George WT, O'Brien JB, et al. (2017). Clozapine usage increases the incidence of pneumonia compared with risperidone and the general population: a retrospective comparison of clozapine, risperidone, and the general population in a single hospital over 25 months. *Int Clin Psychopharmacol*, 32(3), 155–160.

Suppes T, Webb A, Paul B, et al. (1999). Clinical outcome in a randomized 1-year trial of clozapine versus treatment as usual for patients with treatment-resistant illness and a history of mania. *Am J Psychiatry*, 156, 1164–1169.

Suzuki T, Remington G, Uchida H, et al. (2011a). Mangement of schizophrenia in late life with antipsychotic medications. A qualitative review. *Drugs Aging*, 28(12), 961–980.

Suzuki T, Uchida H, Watanabe K, Kashima H (2011b). Factors associated with response to clozapine in schizophrenia: a review. *Psychopharmacol Bull*, 44(1), 32–60.

Tanahashi S, Yamamura S, Nakagawa M, Motomura E, Okada M (2012). Clozapine, but not haloperidol, enhances glial D-serine and L-glutamate release in rat frontal cortex and primary cultured astrocytes. *Br J Pharmacol*, 165(5), 1543–1555.

Testani M Jr (1994). Clozapine-induced orthostatic hypotension treated with fludrocortisone. *J Clin Psychiatry*, 55(11), 497–498.

Tiihonen J, Lönnqvist J, Wahlbeck K, et al. (2009). 11-year follow-up of mortality in patients with schizophrenia: a population-based cohort study (FIN11 study). *Lancet*, 374(9690), 620–627.

Tiihonen J, Haukka J, Taylor M, et al. (2011). A nationwide cohort study of oral and depot antipsychotics after first hospitalization for schizophrenia. *Am J Psychiatry*, 168(6), 603–609.

Tiihonen J, Mittendorfer-Rutz E, Majak M, et al. (2017). Real-world effectiveness of antipsychotic treatments in a nationwide cohort of 29 823 patients with schizophrenia. *JAMA Psychiatry*, 74(7), 686–693.

Veerman SR, Schulte PF, Begemann MJ, de Haan L (2014). Non-glutamatergic clozapine augmentation strategies: a review and meta-analysis. *Pharmacopsychiatry*, 47(7), 231–8.

World Health Organization (WHO) (2017). *WHO Model Lists of Essential Medicines*, 20th list, 24.1. Geneva: World Health Organization. Available at: www.who.int/medicines/publications/essentialmedicines/en/ (last accessed 9.8.17).

Wu CS, Wang SC, Gau SSF, Tsai HJ, Cheng YC (2013). Association of stroke with the receptor-binding profiles of antipsychotics – a case-crossover study. *Biol Psychiatry*, 73, 414–421.

Wu CS, Tsai YT, Tsai HJ (2015). Antipsychotic drugs and the risk of ventricular arrhythmia and/or sudden cardiac death: a nation-wide case-crossover study. *J Am Heart Assoc*, 4(2), e001568.

Wu Y, Blichowski M, Daskalakis ZJ, et al. (2011). Evidence that clozapine directly interacts on the GABAB receptor. *Neuroreport*, 22(13), 637–641.

Xiang YQ, Zhang ZJ, Weng YZ, et al. (2006). Serum concentrations of clozapine and norclozapine in the prediction of relapse of patients with schizophrenia. *Schizophr Res*, 83(2–3), 201–210.

Yang SY, Liao YT, Liu HC, et al. (2013). Antipsychotic drugs, mood stabilizers, and risk of pneumonia in bipolar disorder: a nationwide case-control study. *J Clin Psychiatry*, 74, e79–e86.

Yoshimura B, Yada Y, So R, Takaki M, Yamada N (2017). The critical treatment window of clozapine in treatment-resistant schizophrenia: secondary analysis of an observational study. *Psychiatry Res*, 250, 65–70.

Yusufi B, Mukherjee S, Flanagan R, et al. (2007). Prevalence and nature of side effects during clozapine maintenance treatment and the relationship with clozapine dose and plasma concentration. *Int J Psychopharmacol*, 22, 238–243.

Zheng W, Xiang YT, Yang XH, Xiang YQ, de Leon J (2017). Clozapine augmentation with antiepileptic drugs for treatment-resistant schizophrenia: a meta-analysis of randomized controlled trials. *J Clin Psychiatry*, 78(5), e498–e505.

Lithium

Allan H. Young and Dilveer S. Sually

11.1 History

Lithium is the third element in the periodic table. It was discovered just over 200 years ago in the mineral petalite by the Swedish chemist Arfwedson, and later separated by others (Cogen 2006; Weeks & Larson, 1937). It was initially named lithion (Greek for stone).

In the nineteenth century medicine focused on the potential usefulness of clearing excess urate from the body to treat a variety of illnesses, including psychiatric ailments. Karl Lange and then, in 1894, his brother Fritz Lange individually authored clinical monographs promoting the use of lithium (Cogen, 2006). In 1946, John Cade conducted animal-based laboratory experiments testing first lithium urate and then lithium carbonate which led to the clinical studies and the publication of the seminal paper in 1949 which reported a case series illustrating the beneficial effect of lithium in treating mania (Cade, 1949).

However, Cade's paper coincided with concern over the risks of lithium chloride as a substitute for table salt (sodium chloride) in the United States for people with cardiovascular problems (Cogen, 2006). Moreover, in the 1960s, the clinical use of lithium was questioned by two prominent figures at the Maudsley Hospital – Aubrey Lewis, Professor of Psychiatry and Head of the Maudsley, and his colleague, Michael Shepherd. Notwithstanding these criticisms, the work of other psychiatrists, including Baastrup, Coppen, Gershon, Hartigan, Kline, Maggs, Rice and Schou, led to lithium becoming established in clinical practice as the first 'mood stabilizer' (Cogen, 2006). Despite this, for several reasons, the use of lithium has declined (Young, 2014). Malhi et al. (2009) discuss the factors that have reduced the clinical use of lithium, despite its established effectiveness. One is a lack of potential commercial gain because lithium is a naturally occurring element and not a patentable drug. Another is that there are biases in research created by designs employing lithium as a standard and searching for improvement on the use of lithium, or only exposing patients to novel agents if they have responded poorly to existing treatment, but not conversely observing the response to lithium after a poor response to a novel treatment.

Despite such obstacles, lithium has retained international recognition as the 'gold standard' mood stabilizer and an established adjunct in the treatment of affective disorders, a fact evident from a comparison of nine different national guidelines and two world guidelines (Malhi et al., 2017).

11.2 Mechanism(s) of Action

A complete understanding of the mechanism(s) of action of lithium has not yet been reached although various candidates have been proposed (see Malhi et al., 2013 for a comprehensive review). Putative mechanisms for lithium's effects include effects on neurotransmitter release, neurotransmitter receptors, second messenger cascades and gene expression. It is also now recognized that lithium is a neuroprotective agent that preserves the function of neurons and neuronal circuits (Jope & Nemeroff, 2016). Lithium also promotes the creation of new neurons (neurogenesis) in the hippocampus, important for learning, memory and stress responses (Hanson et al., 2011).

11.2.1 Neurotransmission

Lithium attenuates dopaminergic neurotransmission and animal work specifically suggests that decreased dopamine release may mediate the mood-stabilizing action of lithium (Ferrie, 2005).

Lithium also has an inhibitory effect on postsynaptic excitation related to *N*-methyl-D-aspartate (NMDA) through actions on presynaptic glutamate receptors (Wakita et al., 2015) and an inhibitory postsynaptic effect on NMDA receptors.

Lithium has been shown to increase plasma and cerebrospinal fluid levels of gamma-aminobutyric acid (GABA) in humans (Brunello & Tascedda, 2003), and the GABA increase induced by lithium leads to NMDA receptor down-regulation (Ghasemi & Dehpour, 2011).

11.2.2 Cellular Signalling Second Messenger Systems

Animal studies show lithium affects phosphoinositide signalling leading to changes in gene expression and behaviour. Machado-Vieira et al. (2015) found remission of depressive episodes amongst bipolar disorder I and II patients correlated with the metabolic ratio of myoinositol and creatine in the anterior cingulate cortex.

Lithium blocks the activity of the enzyme glycogen synthase kinase (GSK3). This enzyme has a role in activating metabolic sequences which lead to the death of cells (Beurel & Jope, 2006), a process which may become abnormally activated in neurodegenerative disorders such as Alzheimer's disease or Parkinson's disease (Jope & Nemeroff, 2016) which has supported the notion that lithium may be beneficial in these disorders. Through inhibition of GSK3β, lithium has been shown to indirectly inhibit protein kinase C (PKC) (Malhi et al., 2013). Inhibition of PKC supports neuronal repair after dopaminergic excitation. One transcription factor inhibited by GSK3 is CREB which would otherwise enable expression of brain-derived neurotrophic factor (BDNF) (Beurel et al., 2015). Lithium's inhibition of GSK therefore promotes the expression of BDNF.

11.2.3 Effects on Brain Structure

The Malhi and Outhred (2016) review speculatively links the lithium-related increase in hippocampal volume seen in patients with bipolar disorder (Hajek et al., 2012, 2014) with lithium's effect of reducing the risk of dementia in psychiatric patients (Kessing et al., 2008, 2010), and cites studies linking lithium exposure to beneficial effects on grey and white matter tracts.

11.2.4 Circadian Rhythms

Malhi and Outhred (2016) cite several papers which tie together successful treatment for bipolar disorder and synchronization of the circadian rhythm (processes repeated over approximately 24 hours) through the effect of lithium on the expression of proteins coded for by 'clock genes', which modulate circadian rhythms.

11.3 Pharmacokinetics

Lithium can be prescribed in tablet or liquid form. Peak serum levels occur 2 to 3 hours after ingestion. The distribution phase occurs over 5 to 7 hours. Lithium is not bound to serum proteins and there is no hepatic first-pass metabolism. It is excreted unchanged, mostly by the kidneys.

It is standard practice to measure serum lithium levels 12 hours after the last dose when monitoring lithium levels in a patient, or for comparing lithium blood levels between patient groups. As lithium is usually taken at night this means blood levels are usually checked the following morning.

The half-life of lithium in plasma is between 10 and 24 hours, and most patients will be at a steady-state lithium level between 5 and 7 days after initiating lithium/a change in dose/lithium preparation. Once a day dosing is preferred (see below).

Because of lithium's narrow therapeutic index and because different preparations of lithium have different rates of absorption, a change in dose or a change in preparation requires more closer monitoring of serum blood levels and vigilance for adverse effects, reverting to the schedule used when initiating lithium.

11.4 Therapeutic Uses

11.4.1 Augmentation of Antidepressants in Unipolar Depression

The British Association for Psychopharmacology (BAP) evidence-based guidelines for treating depressive orders with antidepressants (Cleare et al., 2015) recommend lithium and quetiapine as first choice agents for augmenting the existing antidepressant. Lithium augmentation of antidepressants is likely more effective at a lithium serum level of 0.6–1.0 mmol/L (Bauer et al., 2013). Bauer et al. (2013) highlight two key problems with lithium augmentation evidence: (i) many studies had used lithium to augment tricyclic antidepressants (TCAs) as the initial antidepressant, but TCAs are no longer widely used; and (ii) many of the studies considered in their review had small samples and/or were not considered methodologically robust. Nevertheless, their review showed a response rate ranging from 20% to 100%, with most studies showing a response rate of more than 50%. Lithium is used in combination with antidepressants and L-tryptophan to treat severe resistant depression in the 'Newcastle' cocktail (Barker et al., 1987).

11.4.2 Prophylaxis of Unipolar Depression

Meta-analyses support the efficacy of lithium in the maintenance treatment of unipolar depression (Abou-Saleh et al., 2017). Cipriani et al. (2006) analyzed eight randomized controlled trials (RCTs; n = 475) and found lithium was significantly superior to antidepressants in preventing relapses that required hospitalization. Recent population-level studies support the clinical trials (Tiihonen et al., 2017).

Abou-Saleh et al. (2017) propose lithium prophylaxis in unipolar depression if a patient suffers two depressive episodes in five years; or in line with the recommendation of Bauer and Gitlin (2016) after one episode if the episode is severe and there is a strong suicide risk; with indefinite treatment if there is adherence and adverse events are not problematic, particularly if a bipolar background is suspected.

The issue of the optimum lithium level for maintenance treatment in major depression has not yet been determined, but a level of 0.6–0.8 mmol/L would be reasonable.

11.4.3 Acute Treatment of Mania

Lithium is effective in the acute treatment of mania but is not used often as a first-line treatment in this indication. A recent network meta-analysis ranked it as less efficacious than dopamine antagonists (Cipriani et al., 2011). However, if a patient is already taking lithium as a maintenance agent and breakthrough manic symptoms occur, then it may be appropriate to increase the dose of lithium, i.e. optimize treatment. This would be the case if symptoms were relatively mild, there were no signs of toxicity, the patient confirmed their recent adherence to lithium and a recent lithium level showed scope to increase the dose, i.e. a dose increase is unlikely to lead to an elevation of the lithium level into the toxic range. An alternative course of action would be to augment the current dose of lithium with a dopamine antagonist.

There is a strong evidence base to support the combination of dopamine antagonist and either lithium or valproate in the treatment of mania (Goodwin et al., 2016). However, most of the trials adopted a methodology in which a dopamine antagonist was added in those already taking lithium or valproate rather than vice versa.

11.4.4 Maintenance Treatment of Bipolar Disorder

The BAP guideline recommends lithium as the first-line maintenance agent in bipolar disorder (Goodwin et al., 2016). A meta-analysis confirmed the efficacy of lithium in comparison with placebo and alternative drug treatments (Severus et al., 2018). In this meta-analysis, seven RCTs compared lithium with placebo. Lithium was more effective than placebo in preventing overall mood episodes, manic episodes and depressive episodes. Lithium's efficacy was greater in preventing relapse at the manic than the depressive pole. Seven studies compared lithium with anticonvulsants. Lithium was superior to anticonvulsants in preventing mania but not in terms of prevention of overall mood episodes or depressive episode (Severus et al., 2018). The largest trial of lithium maintenance treatment in bipolar disorder was reported by Weisler et al. (2011). This confirmed the superiority of lithium monotherapy compared with placebo in preventing both manic and depressive relapses. It is notable that this result was obtained despite the study not having an enriched design for lithium response in either bipolar depression or mania. A post-hoc analysis of the data showed that those with a lithium level of >0.6 mmol/L had a lower rate of relapse compared with those with lower lithium levels (Nolen et al., 2019). Observational data from Denmark show that bipolar patients who start lithium early in the course of their illness (i.e. following first psychiatric contact or a single manic/mixed episode) have a higher likelihood of achieving a very good outcome compared with those who start treatment later (Kessing et al., 2014).

An anonymized UK database of real-world primary care prescribing (Hayes et al., 2016a) prospectively analyzed data from 5089 bipolar patients prescribed monotherapy maintenance treatment: lithium (n = 1505), olanzapine (n = 1366), valproate (n = 1173) and quetiapine (n = 1075). With at least three months of monotherapy, the subsequent stopping of medication or addition of another mood stabilizer/antipsychotic/antidepressant or benzodiazepine was considered a failure of monotherapy. It was found that monotherapy failure in 75% of each cohort occurred by 2.05 years for lithium monotherapy, 1.13 years for olanzapine monotherapy, 0.98 years for valproate monotherapy and 0.76 years for quetiapine monotherapy. Thus, lithium appeared to be more successful as a monotherapy maintenance treatment than valproate, olanzapine or quetiapine.

11.5 Key Interactions

Drugs which reduce lithium excretion, so raising lithium serum levels, include: non-steroidal anti-inflammatory drugs (NSAIDs), angiotensin-converting enzyme (ACE) inhibitors, aldosterone antagonists, angiotensin II receptor antagonists, loop diuretics, potassium-sparing diuretics, thiazides and thiazide-related diuretics. Lithium levels usually rise within 10 days of taking thiazide diuretics and can increase from 25% to 400% (Taylor et al., 2015).

11.6 Key Adverse Effects at Therapeutic Plasma Levels (0.6–1.0 mmol/L)

Most adverse effects are related to dose, and therefore the serum/plasma level. Adverse effects include mild gastrointestinal upset, fine tremor, polyuria and polydipsia, a metallic taste and aggravation of skin conditions such as acne and psoriasis (Taylor et al., 2015). Other examples include cardiac side effects, nephrogenic diabetes insipidus, extrapyramidal side effects, vertigo, cognitive deficits, reduced thyroid and parathyroid function, sexual dysfunction and weight gain (*British National Formulary*, BNF, 2017).

Lithium treatment leads to a risk of hypothyroidism and more rarely hyperthyroidism. Hypothyroidism is treated with thyroxine, and thyroid function tests (TFTs) usually return to normal when lithium is stopped (Taylor et al., 2015).

11.7 Lithium Toxicity

Toxicity particularly occurs at a serum level above 1.5 mmol/L although it can occur with serum levels in the therapeutic range (Bell et al., 1993). Symptoms include increasing diarrhoea, vomiting, anorexia, polyuria, ataxia, blurred vision, weakness, tinnitus, coarse tremor, muscle twitching, irritability and agitation. Drowsiness, seizures, psychosis and coma may occur (Malhi et al., 2009) and arrhythmias (including fatal ones) can uncommonly occur (Baird-Gunning et al., 2017).

Symptoms reflect three categories of lithium poisoning: acute (due to an overdose and has the lowest risk of neurotoxicity); chronic – the most common (due to intake exceeding excretion over a prolonged period and has the highest risk of neurotoxicity); and acute-on-chronic (Baird-Gunning et al., 2017). Although a complex problem, lithium poisoning can be successfully managed – current mortality from cases of lithium poisoning in Australia, Canada, UK and USA ranges from 0% to 1% (Baird-Gunning et al., 2017). Management should be tailored to the pattern and cause, address the manifestations/risks of toxicity at presentation and factors for recurrence.

11.8 Reduction in Suicide Risk

The lifetime risk of suicide for people with a mood disorder is between 6% and 15%, the greater risk being for those with major depressive disorder (Department of Mental Health, World Health Organization, 2000).

Ahrens and Müller-Oerlinghausen (2001) found that suicide reduction in affective disorder patients was not just through a reduction in the number of depressive episodes severe enough to require hospitalization, but that lithium also had a statistically significant independent anti-suicide effect. Cipriani et al. (2013) conducted a meta-analysis of 48 RCTs comparing lithium with placebo or a psychopharmacological comparator to investigate whether lithium had a specific preventative effect on the outcomes of suicide, self-harm and death from any cause in unipolar and bipolar disorders. The minimum duration of lithium treatment for inclusion was >12 weeks. A pool of 6674 participants was analysed: 4246 patients contributed to analyses of suicide or deliberate self-harm; and 2515 participants contributed to the analysis of all-cause mortality. The comparators were amitriptyline, carbamazepine, valproate (including divalproex), sertraline, fluoxetine, olanzapine, fluvoxamine, imipramine, lamotrigine, mianserin, maprotiline, nortriptyline, phenelzine, quetiapine and thyroid hormone. Sixty per cent of included studies had less than 100 participants.

Lithium reduced the risk of death and suicide by over 60% compared with placebo. However, the difference in risk of suicides or deaths from any cause between lithium and each active treatment was not statistically significant.

Hayes et al. (2016b) used a UK database of National Health Service (NHS) primary care prescribing. The researchers analyzed longitudinal cohort data covering a 19-year period for 6671 patients prescribed lithium (n = 2148), valproate (n =

1670), olanzapine (n = 1477) and quetiapine (n = 1376). The prescription of lithium was associated with a significantly lower rate of self-harm than valproate, olanzapine and quetiapine; and this was postulated to be due to better mood control or a specific effect of lithium on aggressive or impulsive behaviour. However, although observed suicide rates were lowest in the lithium group Hayes et al. (2016b) found no statistically significant difference compared with valproate, olanzapine and quetiapine.

Song et al. (2017) used within-individual analyses of longitudinal data linking five national registers in Sweden to include health, causes of death and migration for 51 535 bipolar patients from 2005 to 2013. Lithium was compared with valproate. A total of 10 648 suicide-related events occurred in 4643 people. The number of people eligible for within-individual analyses was 4405. The suicide rate was significantly lower, by 14%, on lithium compared with off lithium. Valproate was not found to significantly reduce the suicide rate.

11.9 Practicalities When Prescribing Lithium

11.9.1 Tests Before Commencing Treatment

National Institute for Health and Care Excellence (NICE, 2014) guidelines advise the following tests prior to initiating lithium therapy: ECG (if indicated by cardiovascular disease or risk factors for it); urea and electrolytes (U&Es), creatinine and estimated glomerular filtration rate (because lithium is almost entirely excreted in urine); thyroid function tests (TFTs); calcium and weight.

11.9.2 Monitoring

NICE (2014) recommend measuring lithium levels every week until stabilized, then every three months for the first year and every six months thereafter (or to continue measurement every three months if the patient is in a higher risk group, e.g. at risk of impaired renal/thyroid function; elderly; taking medications with risk of interaction with lithium; last lithium level was 0.8 mmol/L or higher).

Once the patient and their serum lithium has been stabilized, lithium levels should be monitored every three months, and TFT and U&Es measured every six months. More frequent testing of the lithium plasma level, renal function and thyroid function should be carried out for those prescribed interacting drugs, the elderly, or those with chronic kidney disease (Taylor et al., 2015).

The need to observe monitoring parameters for patient safety cannot be emphasized strongly enough. A systematic review of local and national audits of lithium monitoring and the impact of shared care between primary and secondary providers on lithium monitoring in the UK and Ireland over 25 years found that there has been some overall improvement in adherence to guidelines, such as BNF and NICE guidelines, but found that there was still room for improvement in the performance of both aspects, and a continuing need for recent audit (Aubrey et al., 2017).

The lithium content in a prescribed dose varies between different formulations. For example, 546 mg of lithium citrate contains 6.0 mmol of lithium, whereas 400 mg of lithium carbonate contains 10.8 mmol of lithium (Shelley, 2004). Because of the narrow therapeutic window of lithium and variable lithium content and bioavailability between different preparations, a change in lithium preparation requires the same frequency of monitoring as when initiating treatment.

Lithium should be started with a single evening dose. A steady lithium serum level is expected to be achieved five to seven days after initiating lithium or changing the formulation, or size, or timing of lithium doses. Once a steady lithium level has been achieved, a once-daily dose in the evening should be continued.

A blood sample for a serum lithium level should be drawn 12 hours after the last dose of lithium and the next dose of lithium should be after the level has been inspected by a psychiatrist and the appropriate next dose determined.

11.9.3 Lithium Rebound

Sudden stoppage of lithium is associated with high rates of relapse into mania (Mander & Loudon, 1988) and this seems to generalize into clinical practice (Franks et al., 2008). Goodwin, in an intriguing thought experiment, explored the consequences of this and concluded that for the poorly adherent the outcomes with lithium maintenance outweigh any benefits (Goodwin, 1994). Figure 11.1 neatly illustrates this.

Withdrawal should be done gradually over a period of at least four weeks to avoid relapse to mania, a depressive episode or increased suicide risk; and caution taken to

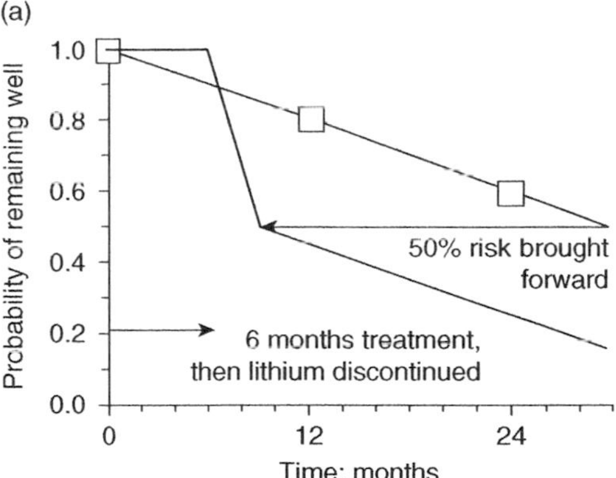

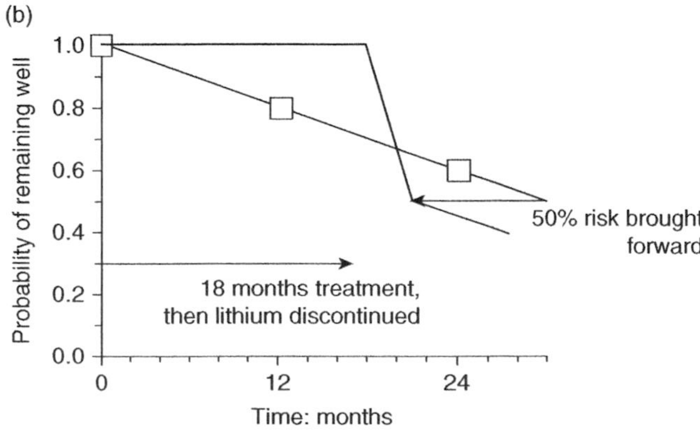

Figure 11.1 The graphs show the effects of lithium discontinuation assuming a 50% risk of recurrence within the subsequent three months. The time of discontinuation is after (a) 6 months or (b) 18 months. Lines without symbols show the effect of stopping. The control risk in first-episode bipolar patients not treated with lithium is taken from Mander and Laudon (1988) (□). The left directed horizontal arrows show how discontinuation brings forward the time of 50% recurrence in either case.

avoid immediately withdrawing monitoring and to retain patient contact with support services (Goodwin et al., 2016).

If short-term treatment for mania is being withdrawn then both antimanic and antidepressant drugs should be withdrawn together, and withdrawal of antidepressants should be tapered over four weeks as per British Association for Psychopharmacology guidelines for depression (Goodwin et al., 2016).

11.9.4 Education for Patients

The BAP 2016 guidelines (Goodwin et al., 2016) recommend developing a treatment plan in a 'flexible alliance' with patients and their next of kin. Include information on managing lifestyle, for example, to avoid deleterious factors on mood episode control, such as poor sleep or excessive alcohol or caffeine intake, and provide information on support groups.

The timescale for therapeutic effects to emerge varies widely with the indication and the dose: 6–10 days in acute mania (Gershon et al., 2009; Grandjean & Aubry, 2009); after 6–8 weeks in bipolar depression (Gershon et al., 2009; Grandjean & Aubry, 2009); and after 2 months in depression (Can et al., 2014). Discussing this with patients and next of kin may help manage expectations, and thereby encourage adherence.

Patients and their carers/next of kin should be informed on recognizing toxic effects.

Patients should be advised to maintain an adequate fluid intake and be wary of dehydration through excess sweating in hot climates, vigorous exercise or a fever; and the need to consult their doctor if experiencing vomiting or diarrhoea (NICE, 2014).

Patients should be given a written lithium information pack (contains patient information booklet, lithium alert card and a record book for tracking serum-lithium concentration), and there is an information leaflet for those whose lithium preparation is changing (BNF, 2017). Contact details of their care team should be provided and details of peer support groups should also be considered.

Patients should be advised to avoid use of over-the-counter NSAIDs such as ibuprofen (NICE, 2014).

11.9.5 Special Populations

Pregnancy: Lithium is teratogenic, particularly in the first trimester and is associated with congenital heart defects and floppy baby syndrome. Management requires a dialogue between patient and the medical team and an understanding and balancing of risks and benefits. Fifty-two per cent of women who discontinued lithium during pregnancy relapsed, and 70% of the women who remained stable after stopping lithium during pregnancy relapsed during the post-partum period (Viguera et al., 2000).

Lactation: On the one hand, lithium has a narrow therapeutic index and is present in breast milk at a relatively high proportion to the maternal serum level; and on the other hand, women are at high risk of relapse to mania or depression after birth. Therefore, an informed decision on breastfeeding is advised (Goodwin et al., 2016).

Elderly: NICE (2014) and BAP (2016) guidelines (Goodwin et al., 2016) concur on aiming for a therapeutic lithium serum level at the lower end of the range 0.4–0.6 mmol/L and cautious dose titration. Age-related factors include decreased renal function (on which lithium clearance is dependent) and increased risk of polypharmacy.

11.10 Conclusion

Lithium remains an important and useful medicine which, when used with expert care, will benefit many patients greatly.

Dr Sually dedicates this chapter to his parents Mr Ram Singh Sually and Mrs Rani Kaur Sually.

References

Abou-Saleh MT, Müller Oerlinghausen B, Coppen AJ (2017). Lithium in the episode and suicide prophylaxis and in augmenting strategies in patients with unipolar depression. *Int J Bipolar Disord*, 5, 11.

Ahrens B, Müller-Oerlinghausen B (2001). Does lithium exert an independent antisuicidal effect? *Pharmacopsychiatry*, 34(4), 132–136.

Aubrey RE, Scott L, Cassidy E (2017). Lithium monitoring patterns in the United Kingdom and Ireland: can shared care agreements play a role in monitoring quality? A systematic review. *Ir J Psychol Med*, 34, 127–140.

Baird-Gunning J, Lea-Henry T, Hoegberg LCG, Gosselin S, Roberts DM (2017). Lithium poisoning. *J Intensive Care Med*, 32, 249–263.

Barker WA, Scott J, Eccleston D (1987). The Newcastle chronic depression study: results of a treatment regime. *Int Clin Psychopharmacol*, 2(3), 261–272.

Bauer M, Gitlin M (2016). *The Essential Guide to Lithium Treatment*. Berlin: Springer International Publishing AG.

Bauer M, Dell'osso L, Kasper S, et al. (2013). Extended-release quetiapine fumarate (quetiapine XR) monotherapy and quetiapine XR or lithium as add-on to antidepressants in patients with treatment-resistant major depressive disorder. *J Affect Disord*, 151, 209–219.

Bell AJ, Cole A, Eccleston D, Ferrier IN (1993). Lithium neurotoxicity at normal therapeutic levels. *Br J Psychiatry*, 162, 689–692.

Beurel E, Jope RS (2006). The paradoxical pro- and anti-apoptotic actions of GSK3 in the intrinsic and extrinsic apoptosis signaling pathways. *Prog Neurobiol*, 79(4), 173–189.

Beurel E, Grieco SF, Jope RS (2015). Glycogen synthase kinase-3 (GSK3): regulation, actions, and diseases. *Pharmacol Ther*, 148, 114–131.

BNF (2017). *British National Formulary*. London: NICE.

Brunello N, Tascedda F (2003). Cellular mechanisms and second messengers: relevance to the psychopharmacology of bipolar disorders. *Int J Neuropsychopharmacol*, 6, 181–189.

Cade JF (1949). Lithium salts in the treatment of psychotic excitement. *Med J Aust*, 2, 349–352.

Can A, Schulze TG, Gould TD (2014). Molecular actions and clinical pharmacogenetics of lithium therapy. *Pharmacol Biochem Behav*, 123, 3–16.

Cipriani A, Smith K, Burgess S, et al. (2006). Lithium versus antidepressants in the long-term treatment of unipolar affective disorder. *Cochrane Database Syst Rev*, (4), CD003492.

Cipriani A, Barbui C, Salanti G, et al. (2011). Comparative efficacy and acceptability of antimanic drugs in acute mania: a multiple-treatments meta-analysis. *Lancet*, 378, 1306–1315.

Cipriani A, Hawton K, Stockton S, Geddes JR (2013). Lithium in the prevention of suicide in mood disorders: updated systematic review and meta-analysis. *BMJ*, 346, f3646.

Cleare A, Pariante CM, Young AH, et al. (2015). Evidence-based guidelines for treating depressive disorders with antidepressants: a revision of the 2008 British Association for Psychopharmacology guidelines. *J Psychopharmacol*, 29, 459–525.

Cogen PH, Whybrow PC (2006). Lithium: a fascinating element in neuropsychiatry. In M Bauer, P Grof, B Muller-Oerlinghausen, eds., *Lithium in Psychiatry: The Comprehensive Guide*. London: Informa Healthcare.

Ferrie L, Young AH, McQuade R (2005). Effect of chronic lithium and withdrawal from chronic lithium on presynaptic dopamine function in the rat. *J Psychopharmacol*, 19(3), 229–234.

Franks M, Macritchie KA, Mahmood T, Young AH (2008). Bouncing back: is the bipolar rebound phenomenon peculiar to lithium? A retrospective naturalistic study. *J Psychopharmacol*, 22(4), 452–456. doi:10.1177/0269881107085238.

Gershon S, Chengappa KN, Malhi GS (2009). Lithium specificity in bipolar illness: a classic agent for the classic disorder. *Bipolar Disord*, 11(Suppl 2), 34–44.

Ghasemi M, Dehpour AR (2011). The NMDA receptor/nitric oxide pathway: a target for the therapeutic and toxic effects of lithium. *Trends Pharmacol Sci*, 32, 420–434.

Goodwin GM (1994). Recurrence of mania after lithium withdrawal. Implications for the use of lithium in the treatment of bipolar affective disorder. *Br J Psychiatry*, 164(2), 149–152.

Goodwin GM, Haddad PM, Ferrier IN, et al. (2016). Evidence-based guidelines for treating bipolar disorder: revised third edition recommendations from the British Association for Psychopharmacology. *J Psychopharmacol*, 30, 495–553.

Grandjean EM, Aubry JM (2009). Lithium: updated human knowledge using an evidence-based approach. Part II: Clinical pharmacology and therapeutic monitoring. *CNS Drugs*, 23, 331–349.

Hajek T, Cullis J, Novak T, et al. (2012). Hippocampal volumes in bipolar disorders: opposing effects of illness burden and lithium treatment. *Bipolar Disord*, 14, 261–270.

Hajek T, Bauer M, Simhandl C, et al. (2014). Neuroprotective effect of lithium on hippocampal volumes in bipolar disorder independent of long-term treatment response. *Psychol Med*, 44, 507–517.

Hanson ND, Nemeroff CB, Owens MJ (2011). Lithium, but not fluoxetine or the corticotropin-releasing factor receptor 1 receptor antagonist R121919, increases cell proliferation in the adult dentate gyrus. *J Pharmacol Exp Ther*, 337, 180–186.

Hayes JF, Marston L, Walters K, et al. (2016a). Lithium vs. valproate vs. olanzapine vs. quetiapine as maintenance monotherapy for bipolar disorder: a population-based UK cohort study using electronic health records. *World Psychiatry*, 15, 53–58.

Hayes JF, Pitman A, Marston L, et al. (2016b). Self-harm, unintentional injury, and suicide in bipolar disorder during maintenance mood stabilizer treatment: a UK population-based electronic health records study. *JAMA Psychiatry*, 73(6), 630–637. doi:10.1001/jamapsychiatry.2016.0432.

Jope RS, Nemeroff CB (2016). Lithium to the rescue. *Cerebrum*, 2016, cer-02-16.

Kessing LV, Sondergard L, Forman JL, Andersen PK (2008). Lithium treatment and risk of dementia. *Arch Gen Psychiatry*, 65, 1331–1335.

Kessing LV, Forman JL, Andersen PK (2010). Does lithium protect against dementia? *Bipolar Disord*, 12, 87–94.

Kessing LV, Vradi E, Andersen PK (2014). Starting lithium prophylaxis early v. late in bipolar disorder. *Br J Psychiatry*, 205(3), 214–220. doi:10.1192/bjp.bp.113.142802.

Machado-Vieira R, Gattaz WF, Zanetti MV, et al. (2015). A longitudinal (6-week) 3T (1)H-MRS study on the effects of lithium treatment on anterior cingulate cortex metabolites in bipolar depression. *Eur Neuropsychopharmacol*, 25, 2311–2317.

Malhi GS, Outhred T (2016). Therapeutic mechanisms of lithium in bipolar disorder: recent advances and current understanding. *CNS Drugs*, 30, 931–949.

Malhi GS, Adams D, Berk M (2009). Is lithium in a class of its own? A brief profile of its clinical use. *Aust N Z J Psychiatry*, 43, 1096–1104.

Malhi GS, Tanious M, Das P, Coulston CM, Berk M (2013). Potential mechanisms of action of lithium in bipolar disorder. Current understanding. *CNS Drugs*, 27(2), 135–153. doi:10.1007/s40263-013-0039-0.

Malhi GS, Gessler D, Outhred T (2017). The use of lithium for the treatment of bipolar disorder: recommendations from clinical practice guidelines. *J Affect Disord*, 217, 266–280.

Mander AJ, Loudon JB (1988). Rapid recurrence of mania following abrupt discontinuation of lithium. *Lancet*, 2(8601), 15–17.

National Institute for Health and Care Excellence (NICE) (2014). *Bipolar disorder: assessment and management*. Clinical Guidelines [CG185]. London: National Institute for Health and Care Excellence.

Nolen WA, Licht RW, Young AH, et al.; Task Force on the treatment with lithium (2019). What is the optimal serum level for lithium in the maintenance treatment of bipolar disorder? A systematic review and recommendations from the ISBD/IGSLI Task Force on treatment with lithium. *Bipolar Disord*, 21(5), 394–409. doi:10.1111/bdi.12805.

Severus E, Bauer M, Geddes J (2018). Efficacy and effectiveness of lithium in the long-term treatment of bipolar disorders: an update 2018. *Pharmacopsychiatry*, 51(5), 173–176. doi:10.1055/a-0627-7489.

Shelley R (2004). Affective disorders: 2. Lithium and anticonvulsants. In DJ King, ed., *Seminars in Psychopharmacology*, 2nd ed. London: Royal College of Psychiatrists.

Song J, Sjölander A, Joas E, et al. (1917). Suicidal behavior during lithium and valproate treatment: a within-individual 8-year prospective study of 50,000 patients with bipolar disorder. *Am J Psychiatry*, 174(8), 795–802. doi:10.1176/appi.ajp.2017.16050542.

Taylor D, Paton C, Kapur S (2015). *The Maudsley Prescribing Guidelines in Psychiatry*, 12th ed. Hoboken: Wiley Blackwell.

Tiihonen J, Tanskanen A, Hoti F, et al. (2017). Pharmacological treatments and risk of readmission to hospital for unipolar depression in Finland: a nationwide cohort study. *Lancet Psychiatry*, 4(7), 547–553. doi:10.1016/S2215-0366(17)30134-7.

Viguera AC, Nonacs R, Cohen LS, et al. (2000). Risk of recurrence of bipolar disorder in pregnant and nonpregnant women after discontinuing lithium maintenance. *Am J Psychiatry*, 157, 179–184.

Wakita M, Nagami H, Takase Y, et al. (2015). Modifications of excitatory and inhibitory transmission in rat hippocampal pyramidal neurons by acute lithium treatment. *Brain Res Bull*, 117, 39–44.

Weeks ME, Larson ME (1937). J.A. Arfwedson and his services to chemistry. *J Chem Educ*, 14, 403–407.

Weisler RH, Nolen WA, Neijber A, Hellqvist A, Paulsson B; Trial 144 Study Investigators (2011). Continuation of quetiapine versus switching to placebo or lithium for maintenance treatment of bipolar I disorder (Trial 144: a randomized controlled study). *J Clin Psychiatry*, 72(11), 1452–1464. doi:10.4088/JCP.11m06878. Erratum in: *J Clin Psychiatry* 2014, 75(3), 290.

World Health Organization (2000). *Preventing Suicide: A Resource for General Physicians*. Available at: www.who.int/mental_health/media/en/56.pdf (last accessed 22.8.19).

Young AH (2014). Lithium and suicide. *Lancet Psychiatry*, 1(6), 483–484. doi:10.1016/S2215-0366(14)70320-7.

Anticonvulsants for Mental Disorders: Valproate, Lamotrigine, Carbamazepine and Oxcarbazepine

Peter S. Talbot

12.1 Introduction

Several anticonvulsants are licensed and used in the treatment of bipolar disorder. However, anticonvulsant activity does not automatically confer benefits for mood disorders on a drug. The anticonvulsant drugs with the strongest evidence for effectiveness in bipolar disorder are valproate, lamotrigine and carbamazepine. Furthermore, the relative effectiveness of these drugs for the different phases of bipolar illness (mania or depression, and acute or maintenance treatment) differs, and none of them has a pattern of effectiveness across the three phases equivalent to lithium. This chapter will describe the basic and clinical psychopharmacology for each of these drugs in turn, as it relates to their use and effectiveness in mental disorders. It is not the aim of this chapter to cover their use in epilepsy. The evidence for the effectiveness of other anticonvulsants in bipolar disorder, including oxcarbazepine, topiramate and gabapentin, is much weaker, and they have no licensed indications for use in mental disorders in the UK at present. They are included here but described more briefly. The information on 'Clinical indications' for valproate, lamotrigine and carbamazepine refers to their UK licences. Licences can vary between countries and readers should consult the marketing approval relevant to their country of practice before prescribing. Drugs can sometimes be of benefit outside their licensed indications but such use must be guided by the evidence base (see Chapter 6 for a discussion of off-label prescribing).

12.2 Valproate

12.2.1 Introduction

Valproate is often used as a generic term to refer to valproic acid, sodium valproate (the sodium salt of the acid) and valproate semisodium (a coordination complex of valproic acid and sodium valproate in a 1:1 molar relationship). More correctly, valproate is the conjugate base in all these salts and the pharmacologically active moiety. Valproate semisodium is also known as divalproex sodium (divalproate) in the USA.

Valproic acid (2-propylpentanoic acid) is a branched-chain fatty acid derived from valeric acid which is naturally produced by the perennial flowering plant valerian (*Valeriana officinalis*). It was first synthesized by Burton in 1882, but there was no known clinical use until its anticonvulsant properties were fortuitously discovered by Eymard in France in 1962 while using it as a solvent for preclinical drug testing (Löscher, 1999). It was introduced into clinical practice for epilepsy in 1967 and is used worldwide as a major anticonvulsant drug for all forms of epilepsy. Subsequently, it was shown to be effective in bipolar disorder and in the prevention of migraine headaches.

The antimanic efficacy of sodium valproate and valproate semisodium was shown in studies undertaken in Europe and the USA in the 1980s and 1990s, and valproate semisodium was approved by the US Food and Drug Administration (FDA) for the acute treatment of mania in 1995 (Lempérière, 2001). Valproate semisodium (Depakote) was licensed for the treatment of acute mania in the UK in 2001.

12.2.2 Psychiatric Indications

In the UK, Depakote (valproate semisodium) and Episenta (sodium valproate prolonged release) are the only available valproate preparations licensed for use in bipolar disorder, for the following therapeutic indications (*British National Formulary*, BNF, 2019):

- Treatment of manic episode in bipolar disorder when lithium is contraindicated or not tolerated.
- The continuation of treatment after manic episode could be considered in patients who have responded (to Depakote or sodium valproate) for acute mania.

12.2.3 Mechanism of Action

Valproate has a wide range of immediate and long-term biochemical and genomic effects (Rosenberg, 2007). However, their relative contributions, if any, to the therapeutic benefits of valproate, and whether these differ between epilepsy, bipolar disorder and migraine prophylaxis, remain unclear. Valproate acutely increases brain levels of the inhibitory neurotransmitter gamma-aminobutyric acid (GABA) and reduces neuronal excitability via the blockade of voltage-gated Na^+ channels. With longer-term use, changes are seen in other systems, including the glucocorticoid, serotonin (5-HT) (Nugent et al., 2013) and dopamine neurotransmitter systems; inositol metabolism and protein kinase C activity; the Wnt/β-catenin cell signalling pathway; brain lipids and their metabolism; and activation of the extracellular signal-related kinase (ERK) pathway resulting in increases in trophic and protective factors such as brain-derived neurotrophic factor (BDNF) and the anti-apoptotic factor, B-cell lymphoma-2 (Bcl-2) (Chen et al., 2006; Nishino et al., 2012; Rosenberg, 2007). This increase in trophic factors may be particularly relevant to valproate's mechanism of action in bipolar disorder, as chronic treatment with valproate has been shown to ameliorate the reduction in volume and number of neurons and glia in discrete brain areas found by brain imaging and post-mortem studies in patients with bipolar disorder (Drevets, 2000; Rajkowska, 2000). Valproate has the ability to alter the expression of various genes relevant to neuropsychiatric disorders, through the enhancement of activator protein 1 binding to DNA and the inhibition of class I histone deacetylases (HDACs) (Rosenberg, 2007). Valproate's HDAC inhibition has also sparked great interest in its potential use in cancer therapy.

12.2.4 Pharmacokinetics

With oral dosing valproate is rapidly absorbed, reaching peak plasma concentration in approximately 3–5 hours (Carrigan et al., 1990). Rates of absorption may vary depending on the formulation (liquid, solid, sprinkle), although these differences are unlikely to be clinically significant with chronic use. Administration with food delays the time to peak plasma concentration (T_{max}) by about 4 hours but does not modify the extent of absorption. With chronic dosing, steady state is achieved in three to four days. At therapeutic doses valproate is highly bound to plasma proteins (80–95%) and the concentration in brain (approximately 7–28% of plasma concentration) is related to the free valproate level in plasma (Klotz & Antonin, 1977; Vajda et al., 1981). Elimination from plasma is relatively slow, with a biological half-life of 9–16 hours. In the elderly, drug clearance and protein binding are generally reduced and dose reductions may be necessary based on the best balance of tolerability and clinical response.

Almost all valproate metabolism occurs in the liver, and at least 10 metabolites have been identified (Peterson & Naunton, 2005). Up to 50% is metabolized by glucuronidation and excreted in the urine, while β-oxidation in the mitochondria accounts for around 40%. Oxidation by cytochrome P450 (CYP) enzymes (CYP2C9, CYP2A6 and to a lesser extent CYP2B6) is a minor route (~10%). Very little valproate (<3%) is excreted unchanged in the urine (Ghodke-Puranik et al., 2013).

12.2.5 Adverse Effects

12.2.5.1 Adverse Effects Unrelated to Pregnancy

Valproate is associated with a wide range of adverse effects which are summarized in Table 12.1 (for further details see electronic Medicines Compendium, 2019a). The most common adverse effects include gastrointestinal symptoms (particularly nausea), tremor, sleepiness (somnolence) and weight gain. Many adverse effects are dose dependent and can be minimized by dose adjustments. Gastrointestinal side effects frequently occur at the start of treatment, but they usually disappear after a few days without discontinuing treatment and can often be overcome by taking valproate with or after food.

Clinically significant weight gain occurs in about a third of patients, more commonly in women than men. It can be substantial and has been associated with a range of metabolic disturbances, particularly hyperinsulinaemia and insulin resistance, hyperleptinaemia and leptin resistance (Belcastro et al., 2013). In women with bipolar disorder, use of valproate is also associated with higher rates of polycystic ovary syndrome, menstrual disorder and hyperandrogenism (hirsutism, virilism, acne, male pattern alopecia and/or androgen increase) (Zhang et al., 2016).

Alopecia (hair loss) is common but is usually transient and regrowth normally begins within six months, although the hair may become curlier than previously. Other kinds of hair disorder are less common, and include abnormal hair texture, hair colour changes and abnormal hair growth.

Increased liver enzymes are common, particularly early in treatment, and may be transient. However, severe liver damage, including hepatic failure which is sometimes fatal, has been very rarely reported. In practice, this is of more relevance to the use of valproate for epilepsy than bipolar disorder, as severe liver damage is particularly seen in children under the age of three years and those with severe seizure disorders, organic brain disease, and in patients with congenital metabolic defects such as mitochondrial disorders. Valproate is contraindicated in some of these disorders, including those associated with mitochondrial polymerase gamma (POLG) and Twinkle mutations (Tomson et al., 2016). Nevertheless, valproate is contraindicated in all patients with active liver disease, and in patients with a personal or family history of drug-induced severe hepatic dysfunction. Acute pancreatitis is another serious idiosyncratic reaction, and in rare cases can be fatal.

Valproate can cause haematological disorders, most commonly thrombocytopenia and anaemia. Blood abnormalities tend to be dose related and usually occur with a serum valproate level greater than 100 mg/L (Acharya & Bussel, 2000; Vasudev et al., 2010). Haematological indices usually normalize if valproate is reduced in dose; drug discontinuation is rarely required. Valproate has been associated with a reduction in blood fibrinogen and/or an increase in prothrombin time. This is usually asymptomatic. Spontaneous bruising or bleeding should lead to withdrawal of valproate while the cause is clarified.

Table 12.1 Adverse effects associated with valproate

Very common (≥1/10)	Common (≥1/100)	Uncommon (≥1/1000)	Rare (≥1/10 000) or very rare (<1/10 000)
• Nausea • Tremor • Weight gain	• Liver function abnormalities • Vomiting and diarrhoea • Gum swelling • Stomatitis • Somnolence • Memory impairment • Headache • Nystagmus • Confusional state • Hallucinations • Hyponatraemia • Anaemia • Thrombocytopenia • Hypersensitivity • Hair loss, usually transient • Nail and nail bed disorders • Dysmenorrhoea	• Pancreatitis, sometimes fatal • Ataxia • Parkinsonism • Paraesthesia • Syndrome of inappropriate secretion of ADH (SIADH) • Hyperandrogenism • Pancytopenia • Leucopenia • Angioedema • Rash • Hair disorder • Amenorrhoea • Vasculitis • Renal failure • Decreased bone mineral density • Pleural effusion • Peripheral oedema	• Reversible dementia associated with reversible cerebral atrophy • Hyperammonaemia • Obesity • Hypothyroidism • Bone marrow failure • Serious rashes • Male infertility • Polycystic ovaries • Gynaecomastia • Systemic lupus erythematosus • Coagulation abnormalities

Adapted from electronic Medicines Compendium (2019a).

12.2.5.2 Adverse Effects Related to Pregnancy and Breastfeeding

Valproate exposure is a major risk to the intrauterine development of children, and no safe dose has been identified (Wieck & Jones, 2018). Congenital neural tube defects in the offspring of mothers taking valproate were first reported in the early 1980s (Bjerkedal et al., 1982; Robert & Guibaud, 1982). Subsequently, evidence accumulated for a teratogenic effect on a wider range of organ systems (Tanoshima et al., 2015) and that the teratogenic risk increases with increasing drug dosage (Vajda et al., 2013). Rates reported for major malformations range from approximately 7% to 14% (Angus-Lepan & Liu, 2018). A large population-based case-control study found significant associations between exposure to valproate monotherapy in the first trimester and spina bifida, atrial septal defect, cleft palate, hypospadias, polydactyly, craniosynostosis and limb reduction (Jentink et al., 2010). For spina bifida, exposure to valproate increased the risk by 12–16 times, while for the other malformations the elevation was between two and seven times. The risks of congenital malformations are even higher when valproate is used with one or more other antiepileptic drugs in polytherapy (Meador et al., 2008).

Neurodevelopmental problems occur in up to 30–40% of children exposed to valproate in utero, including delayed walking and talking, memory problems, difficulty with speech and language, and lower intellectual ability (Bromley et al., 2014; Cummings et al., 2011; Meador et al., 2008; Thomas et al., 2008; Veroniki et al., 2017b). Poor school performance persists through primary and lower secondary school (Elkjaer et al., 2018). Children exposed to valproate in utero are also at three to five times higher risk of having autism (Christensen et al., 2013) and may be more likely to develop symptoms of attention deficit hyperactivity disorder (Cohen et al., 2011, 2013). This spectrum of harm suggests that the risk to the developing fetus is not limited to the first trimester (Wieck & Jones, 2018). While a dose effect for valproate has been reported, with doses above approximately 800–1000 mg daily particularly associated with a poorer cognitive outcome in children, no safe dose has been identified (Bromley et al., 2014). Like congenital malformations, the risk of mental and motor developmental problems from polypharmacy is even higher than for monotherapy (Thomas et al., 2008).

The teratogenic and neurodevelopmental risks associated with valproate are likely to arise through multiple mechanisms, with their relative contributions potentially varying across gestational stages and different abnormalities (Lloyd, 2013; Ornoy, 2009). Vitamin B_9 (folate) is vital for normal RNA and DNA synthesis and DNA methylation, and earlier studies focused on the role of valproate in interfering with folate metabolism to alter the concentrations of specific folate metabolites in the embryo (Wegner & Nau, 1992). However, this is now thought to play only a partial role in valproate teratogenicity, and folate supplementation during pregnancy does not eliminate the risks associated with valproate. Other mechanisms with potentially greater contributions include increased oxidative stress to the developing embryo imposed by intermediate metabolites of valproate; demethylation of DNA through valproate's action as a potent HDAC inhibitor resulting in changes in embryonic/fetal gene expression and inhibition of cell proliferation; and mechanisms contributing to the accumulation of valproate in the fetal circulation at a higher concentration than in maternal blood.

Nevertheless, only a proportion of pregnancies exposed to valproate result in children with birth defects (approximately 10% of cases) or neurodevelopmental abnormalities (up to 30–40% of cases) indicating the existence of individual susceptibility factors. These may potentially include genetic factors which contribute to interindividual variation in folic acid metabolism, DNA methylation and valproate metabolism (Tomson et al., 2016), as well as environmental factors such as maternal age, alcohol consumption, smoking, lifestyle and possible environmental carcinogens (Lloyd, 2013).

Because of the major risks, in February 2018 the Pharmacovigilance Risk Assessment Committee of the European Medicines Agency recommended new restrictions and measures to avoid exposure of babies to valproate in utero. These measures include a ban on the use of valproate for bipolar disorder or migraine during pregnancy, and a ban on treating epilepsy during pregnancy unless there is no other effective treatment available. In addition, valproate is now contraindicated in girls and women of childbearing potential unless the 'pregnancy prevention programme' is followed. This includes:

- an assessment of their potential for becoming pregnant
- pregnancy tests before starting and during treatment
- counselling about the risks of valproate and the need for effective contraception throughout treatment
- a review of ongoing treatment by a specialist at least annually
- a new risk acknowledgement form that patients and prescribers will go through every year.

Valproate packaging will also now carry a visual warning, patients will be given a warning card with every prescription and pharmacists will be required to discuss the risks every time they dispense valproate to women of childbearing potential (European Medicines Agency, 2018).

There is a paucity of data on valproate excretion in breast milk. However, the infant/maternal ratio of serum drug concentration seems to be lower in valproate exposure compared with other anticonvulsants used in psychiatry. The incidence of adverse events in infants exposed to valproate via breast milk is reported to be very low (Uguz & Sharma, 2016). Nevertheless, haematological disorders have occurred in breastfed infants of treated women, and the manufacturer advises to decide whether or not to breastfeed based on the balance of risks and benefits (electronic Medicines Compendium, 2019a).

12.2.6 Drug Interactions

Pharmacokinetic drug interactions can occur when another drug acts to alter valproate's plasma protein binding, hepatic metabolism or both. In addition, valproate can act to alter the protein binding and metabolism of other drugs.

Valproate is highly bound (80–95%) to plasma proteins, predominantly albumin. Only the free (non-bound) fraction of a drug in plasma is available to cross membranes, is pharmacologically active and is available to be metabolized and cleared. Changes to protein binding will therefore alter the free fraction of a drug, and using two highly protein-bound drugs at the same time may affect the free fraction of each through competition for protein binding sites resulting in mutual displacement. Indeed, for highly protein-bound drugs, small reductions in the large bound fraction give rise to large fractional increases in free drug. In most cases, this increase in free fraction has only transient or limited pharmacological effects, as the extra free drug is metabolized. However, if the addition of a second drug increases the free fraction of the first *and* inhibits its metabolism, this can lead to dramatic increases of the free *concentration* of the first drug and a significant risk of toxicity. This is the case with **aspirin**, which both displaces and inhibits the metabolism of valproate. An eightfold increase in free valproate concentration, and clinical toxicity, has been reported when as little as 325 mg/day of aspirin was added for a patient taking valproate (Sandson et al., 2006). Valproate increases the free **phenytoin** concentration by the same mechanism of displacement of protein binding and metabolic inhibition.

The free fraction of valproate is also increased in situations when **serum albumin is low**, such as in the elderly and pathological states such as liver failure, renal failure and malnutrition. Caution is needed in these situations, and valproate is contraindicated with a personal or family history of severe hepatic dysfunction. In cases of potential valproate toxicity due to drug interactions or low albumin, clinical management will be better informed by measuring serum-*free* valproate concentration in addition to the total concentration routinely reported by laboratories.

The major elimination pathway for valproate is hepatic metabolism, predominantly by glucuronidation and β-oxidation. Valproate levels can therefore be altered by a range of drugs that inhibit, induce or act as competitive substrates for these metabolic pathways. In contrast, drugs that are inhibitors of cytochrome P450 are expected to have only a minor effect on valproate clearance because cytochrome P450-mediated microsomal oxidation is a relatively minor secondary metabolic pathway for valproate (Fleming & Chetty, 2005). Moreover, valproate is a broad metabolic inhibitor, both of its own metabolism and that of other drugs, so will act to increase levels of a range of other drugs. The most clinically important interactions with other psychotropic drugs are included in Table 12.2.

In particular, as **lamotrigine** is commonly prescribed in bipolar disorder, clinicians should be aware that doses of lamotrigine need to be significantly reduced if it is co-prescribed with valproate. A useful rule of thumb is to reduce the lamotrigine dose by 50% and be vigilant for rashes. Monitoring of serum levels may be useful (see Lamotrigine section, below). Because of the wide range of potential interactions between valproate and other drugs, both psychotropic and non-psychotropic, clinicians are advised to consult an authoritative prescribing reference such as the BNF before initiating valproate for a patient taking general medical drugs or co-prescribing for a patient taking valproate.

Valproate usually has no enzyme inducing effect, so does not accelerate the metabolism of other drugs. It does not reduce the efficacy of oestrogen/progestogen-containing **hormonal contraception**, including the oral contraceptive pill. Nevertheless, several small studies have found that valproate decreases the plasma concentration of olanzapine (summarized in Vella & Mifsud, 2014). The reduction is usually modest but can be associated with clinical deterioration in some cases. The mechanism of this pharmacokinetic interaction remains uncertain but may involve the up-regulation of CYP3A4 (a minor metabolic pathway of olanzapine) and a reduction of olanzapine bioavailability by up-regulation of P-glycoproteins at a gastrointestinal level.

Table 12.2 Pharmacokinetic interactions of valproate with other psychotropic drugs

Valproate levels increased by	Valproate levels decreased by	Valproate increases levels of	Valproate decreases levels of	Other interactions
• SSRIs, especially fluoxetine • Moclobemide • Venlafaxine • Modafinil • Chlorpromazine	• Carbamazepine • Phenytoin • Hormonal contraceptives	• Lamotrigine • Carbamazepine (active metabolites) • Phenytoin (free fraction) • Barbiturates • Tricyclic antidepressants (particularly clomipramine) • Bupropion • Lorazepam • Paliperidone • Quetiapine • Donepezil	• Olanzapine	• Increased risk of neutropenia when used with olanzapine or quetiapine • Topiramate increases risk of toxicity when given with valproate • May potentiate effect of other psychotropics such as antipsychotics, MAOIs, antidepressants and benzodiazepines

MAOIs, monoamine oxidase inhibitors; SSRIs, selective serotonin reuptake inhibitors.
Adapted from electronic Medicines Compendium (2019a); Fleming and Chetty (2005); Taylor et al. (2015); Vella and Mifsud (2014).

12.2.7 Clinical Use of Valproate

12.2.7.1 Evidence for Effectiveness

The great majority of clinical trials of valproate in mental disorders have used valproate semisodium (Depakote; divalproex). In bipolar disorder, valproate is effective to varying degrees in all illness phases – acute mania, acute depression and maintenance. It is included among first-line treatments for acute mania and maintenance treatment of bipolar I disorder in national and international guidelines (for example, Goodwin et al., 2016; Yatham et al., 2018). For acute antimanic efficacy, network meta-analyses rank D_2 receptor antagonists/partial agonists (antipsychotics) and lithium ahead of valproate, but the differences are not great and for men valproate has modest tolerability advantages over lithium and some antipsychotics (Cipriani et al., 2011; Yildiz et al., 2015). For maintenance treatment, randomized controlled trial (RCT) evidence for valproate is weak, but good long-term naturalistic data strongly support its efficacy in reducing total relapses in bipolar I disorder.

The data on its relative effectiveness in manic and depressive relapse are somewhat confusing. Current guidelines advocate using lithium as initial monotherapy above other maintenance treatments due to its superior evidence for prevention of new episodes (both mania and depression), greater evidence base documenting the risks of prolonged exposure, and its efficacy in reducing the risk of suicide. For acute bipolar depressive episodes, valproate has some evidence for effectiveness in reducing depressive symptoms and improving the chances of both response and remission (Bond et al., 2010; Smith et al., 2010). However, the average effect size and the evidence base are small, and a larger, more convincing RCT is needed to establish efficacy (Goodwin et al., 2016). In recent guidelines valproate is included among second-line treatments for bipolar I depression and third-line treatments for bipolar II depression and maintenance (Yatham et al., 2018).

In major depressive disorder ('unipolar' depression) several small open studies and case reports have found benefits of antidepressant augmentation with valproate in resistant depression (Davis et al., 2000; Ghabrash et al., 2016). However, recent RCT evidence for such a role is lacking (Cleare et al., 2015).

In schizophrenia, valproate has an established use for prophylaxis of clozapine-induced myoclonic jerks and seizures. However, there is no convincing evidence that it is of benefit as an adjunct to antipsychotics for reduction of core symptoms in treatment-resistant schizophrenia. Although open trials reported a small improvement in total psychopathology with the addition of valproate to dopamine antagonists, no significant improvement is found in RCTs or studies beyond four weeks duration (Tseng et al., 2016; Wang et al., 2008). Aggression scores were lower in patients receiving valproate, but the evidence quality was very low. Further randomized, blinded studies are necessary before any clear recommendation can be made, and on current evidence no single co-treatment strategy, let alone valproate, can be recommended for patients with schizophrenia (Correll et al., 2017).

The use of valproate has been studied for potential symptom reduction in personality disorders. There is modest evidence that valproate is superior to placebo for outpatient men with recurrent impulsive aggression, for impulsively aggressive adults with cluster B personality disorders (antisocial, borderline, histrionic and narcissistic) and for youths with conduct disorder (Citrome & Volavka, 2011; Huband et al., 2010). In borderline personality disorder (BPD), valproate was superior to placebo for interpersonal problems and depression, but not for impulsivity or suicidal thoughts (Stoffers et al., 2010). Nevertheless, the evidence base is very small, and the current National Institute for Health and Care Excellence (NICE) guidelines in the UK do not recommend drug treatment for BPD (NICE, 2009).

A small double-blind RCT in generalized anxiety disorder found valproate monotherapy superior to placebo (Aliyev & Aliyev, 2008), but larger RCTs are needed before conclusions can be drawn.

12.2.7.2 Starting, Monitoring and Stopping Valproate

Baseline full blood count (FBC) and liver function tests (LFTs) should be checked before starting valproate, after six months treatment and when symptoms of liver or blood disorders occur (Sie, 2014). The Summary of Product Characteristics (SPC) recommends checking FBC, bleeding time and coagulation tests before starting valproate or before surgery, and in case of spontaneous bruising or bleeding. Weight or body mass index (BMI) should also be measured before initiation and regularly monitored.

In addition to the well-recognized increased risk of manic relapse following the abrupt withdrawal of lithium, there is some preliminary naturalistic evidence to suggest that abrupt withdrawal of valproate and some other maintenance medications in bipolar disorder (carbamazepine, antipsychotics and antidepressants) is also associated with increased risk of relapse into a mood episode, particularly mania or hypomania (Franks et al., 2008). In the absence of better evidence, if valproate is to be withdrawn it should be done slowly over at least four weeks.

12.2.7.3 Serum Levels

In the UK, clinical biochemistry laboratories quote a reference range for trough (12-hour post-dose for once-daily dosing; pre-dose for twice-daily dosing) total serum valproate in the 50–100 mg/L range based on recommendations for the treatment of epilepsy. However, the therapeutic range for bipolar disorder is unclear, and neither dose–concentration nor concentration–effect relationships are well defined. Clinical trials in bipolar disorder have used a therapeutic range within 50–125 mg/L, and this has become generally accepted. For the treatment of acute mania, one study found a linear relationship between serum valproate concentration and response and that efficacy was significantly greater than placebo only at levels above approximately 70 mg/L (Allen et al., 2006). Best response was achieved when levels were above 94 mg/L. However, most other studies in acute mania have not been as clear-cut as this, and correlations between valproate levels and both therapeutic and adverse effects are generally weak within the 50–125 mg/L range (Haymond & Ensom, 2010). Nevertheless, the studies do suggest that some patients may benefit from levels in the 100–125 mg/L range, and that a strict adherence to an upper limit of 100 mg/L may disadvantage them. The optimum therapeutic range in the maintenance phase is unknown, but a level below 50 mg/L is unlikely to be effective, between 50 and 100 mg/L is probably optimal and 100–125 mg/L may confer benefit in some cases.

Nausea, vomiting and sedation are commoner with levels >125 mg/L, though common side effects have all been reported at much lower levels. Routine monitoring of valproate levels does not seem warranted, but may be helpful in individual cases complicated by potential drug–drug interactions impacting on valproate levels, poor clinical response or suspected non-compliance (Haymond & Ensom, 2010).

12.3 Lamotrigine

12.3.1 Introduction

Lamotrigine is a phenyltriazine compound which was synthesized as one of a sequence of folic acid antagonists based on evidence dating from the mid-1960s that folate was proconvulsant (Brodie, 1992). Human Phase I studies started in the early 1980s, and it was first approved for the treatment of epilepsy in 1990 in Ireland and in the UK in 1991 (Yasam et al., 2016). For epilepsy it is used worldwide to treat partial seizures, primary and secondary tonic-clonic seizures, seizures associated with Lennox–Gastaut syndrome, and typical absence seizures in children and adolescents. Based on early reports of improved mood and communicativeness in patients taking it for epilepsy, lamotrigine started to be used off-licence in the early 1990s for individual patients with bipolar disorder. It showed promising results in a number of open-label trials, before being commercially developed in a large programme of RCTs (Weisler et al., 2008).

12.3.2 Psychiatric Indications

Lamotrigine is currently licensed in the UK at doses up to 200 mg/day for prevention of depressive episodes in patients with bipolar I disorder who experience predominantly depressive episodes.

12.3.3 Mechanism of Action

Lamotrigine inhibits voltage-gated sodium channels, which reduces neuronal excitability and reduces the presynaptic release of excitatory amino acid neurotransmitters such as glutamate and aspartate (Leach et al., 1986). These effects are likely to contribute to its anticonvulsant properties. In contrast, its mechanism of action in bipolar disorder has not been established. Inhibition of voltage-gated sodium channels is likely to be important, with potential contributions from blockade of L-, N- and P-type voltage-gated calcium channels and weak 5-HT_3 receptor antagonism. Lamotrigine is also a weak inhibitor of dihydrofolate reductase, the enzyme that reduces dihydrofolic acid to tetrahydrofolic acid. The unexpected clinical trial finding that folate impairs the effectiveness of lamotrigine in bipolar depression (Geddes et al., 2016) raises the conjecture that the tetrahydrofolate synthesis pathway may be implicated in lamotrigine's mechanism of antidepressant action (Goodwin et al., 2016), although a pharmacokinetic effect of folate to reduce lamotrigine absorption is an alternative possibility (Geddes et al., 2016).

12.3.4 Pharmacokinetics

After oral dosing in healthy humans, lamotrigine is rapidly and completely absorbed with negligible first-pass metabolism. Bioavailability approaches 100% and is not strongly affected by food intake. T_{max} is approximately 2–3 hours post-dose in healthy volunteers (Brodie, 1992). Protein binding, which is primarily to albumin, is approximately 55%, and lamotrigine is not expected to undergo clinically significant interactions with other drugs through competition for protein binding sites. Mean elimination half-life is approximately 26 hours. Metabolism is predominantly by glucuronidation in the liver to the pharmacologically inactive 2-*N*-glucuronide conjugate, followed by excretion in the urine. Approximately 70% of the oral dose is recovered in the urine of which 10% is unchanged lamotrigine and 90% is the 2-*N*-glucuronide metabolite. Lamotrigine does not induce its own metabolism to a clinically significant extent, and does not inhibit or induce the hepatic metabolism of other drugs (Cohen et al., 1987; Drugbank, 2019a; Ramsay et al., 1991).

12.3.5 Adverse Effects

With the exception of rare serious rash (see below), lamotrigine is generally well tolerated in bipolar disorder and has a favourable side-effect profile (Bowden et al., 2004). In clinical practice, rates of compliance with lamotrigine are high and significantly better than for lithium (Seo et al., 2011) and other anticonvulsants (Chung et al., 2007). The most common adverse effects are headache, nausea and mild rash. It is not generally associated with sexual dysfunction, weight gain, marked sedation, cognitive impairment or withdrawal symptoms (Bowden et al., 2004; Reid et al., 2013). A range of adverse effects found in clinical trials of bipolar disorder and clinical experience are listed in Table 12.3, ranked by frequency.

12.3.5.1 Rash

Mild skin rashes are common (8–10%) with lamotrigine, including morbilliform (i.e. looks like measles) rash, urticaria and erythema multiforme (Reid et al., 2013). More serious rashes are fortunately rare, but include severe mucocutaneous reactions such as Stevens–Johnson syndrome (SJS) and toxic epidermal necrolysis (TEN) which are

Table 12.3 Adverse effects associated with lamotrigine

Very common (≥1/10)	Common (≥1/100)	Uncommon (≥1/1000)	Rare (≥1/10 000) or very rare (<1/10 000)
• Headache • Skin rash (non-serious)	• Nausea • Dry mouth • Dizziness • Aggression, irritability • Agitation • Somnolence • Arthralgia and back pain		• Serious skin rashes, including Stevens–Johnson syndrome • Hypersensitivity syndrome • Lupus-like reactions • Haematological abnormalities • Confusion, hallucinations, tics • Unsteadiness, movement disorders • Conjunctivitis • Hepatic dysfunction

Taken from electronic Medicines Compendium (2019b).

associated with high levels of pain, systemic illness and (particularly for TEN) mortality. In adults receiving lamotrigine for bipolar and other mood disorders, the rate of serious rash is reported as 0.08% (1 in 1233 subjects) for monotherapy and 0.13% (2 in 1538 subjects) for lamotrigine as adjunctive therapy (Seo et al., 2011). The risk of serious rash is highest in the first six weeks of treatment, and is reduced by slow dose titration and adjustment of the dosing schedule for pharmacokinetic interactions with valproate and enzyme inducing drugs such as carbamazepine (BNF, 2019). These schedules should be rigorously adhered to, and restarted if the patient misses more than five consecutive days of lamotrigine.

Based on the prior literature and a case series of 27 patients receiving lamotrigine rechallenge after an initial rash, Aiken and Orr (2010) have proposed a rating scale for dermatological drug eruptions as a guide for clinical judgement in the event of a lamotrigine rash (Box 12.1). This is based on the presence or absence of six non-benign clinical features.

They propose the following treatment algorithm for managing a rash:

For a benign rash (absence of any of the six features; i.e. a score of 0)

- Dose titration can be reduced a step (e.g. lowering the dose by 25–50 mg) with close clinical monitoring until the rash resolves. After resolution of the rash, the titration can be continued if a higher dose is still clinically necessary.
- If dose reduction does not resolve the rash, stop lamotrigine.
- If lamotrigine remains clinically indicated, wait for at least four weeks after the rash has resolved and consider reintroducing lamotrigine using very-low-dose titration (see below).

For a moderate rash (score of 1 or 2)

- Stop lamotrigine.
- If lamotrigine remains clinically indicated, wait for at least four weeks after the rash has resolved and consider reintroducing lamotrigine using very-low-dose titration (see below).

Box 12.1 Rating scale for dermatological drug eruptions

Clinical feature	Present	Absent
• Exfoliation or erythroderma	3	0
• Purpura, tenderness or blistering	1	0
• Facial or mucous membrane involvement	1	0
• Lymphadenopathy	1	0
• Haematological abnormalities (e.g. eosinophilia) or elevated transaminase enzymes	1	0
• Constitutional symptoms (fever, malaise, arthralgia, meningism, pharyngitis, cough)	1	0

Scoring: add the scores for each item above (range = 0–8)

Adapted from Aiken and Orr (2010).

For a severe rash (score of 3 or more)

- Stop lamotrigine.
- Data do not support the safety of reintroduction.

The SPC recommends that lamotrigine is not restarted in patients who have discontinued due to rash unless the potential benefit clearly outweighs the risk. However, where appropriate, reintroduction of lamotrigine after at least four weeks has high (~80%) rates of success (Aiken & Orr, 2010; Serrani Azcurra, 2013), and in the Aiken and Orr case series no patients developed SJS or TEN. For very-low-dose titration, they advise restarting with 5 mg daily (or every other day for patients also on valproate) for 14 days, then increasing the daily dose by 5 mg every 14 days until 25 mg/day is reached. Thereafter the standard schedule can be followed (Aiken & Orr, 2010).

12.3.5.2 Cognitive Function

Lamotrigine appears to have a better cognitive profile than a number of other anticonvulsants and medications used in bipolar disorder (Dias et al., 2012). It has no negative effects on attention, concentration, information processing, complex visual-motor processing, verbal learning and fluency, and short- or long-term memory in healthy adults and patients with epilepsy, and can have positive effects on cognitive function (Hurley, 2002) including self-report ratings in bipolar I patients whether or not they were receiving concomitant valproate, antidepressants or antipsychotics (Kaye et al., 2007).

12.3.5.3 Adverse Effects Related to Pregnancy and Breastfeeding

Large studies have suggested that in utero exposure to lamotrigine is not associated with a substantial increase in the risk for major congenital malformations, including oral clefts (Hernandez-Diaz et al., 2012; Molgaard-Nielsen & Hviid, 2011; Veroniki et al., 2017a), although the risk may possibly increase with doses above 400 mg/day (Campbell et al., 2014). Nor does lamotrigine appear to be associated with significant neurodevelopmental delay (Cummings et al., 2011). Nevertheless, this does not imply a complete absence of risk, and if lamotrigine is considered necessary during pregnancy the lowest possible therapeutic dose is recommended. The risks of lamotrigine should be weighed against the risks associated with deterioration of bipolar disorder control. Due to pharmacokinetic changes in serum concentration of lamotrigine over the course of pregnancy and in the immediate post-partum period, doses should be adjusted on the basis of serum levels to maintain the same level as before pregnancy.

Lamotrigine is excreted in breast milk, and infant serum levels can reach up to 50% of maternal serum levels, making the theoretical risk of life-threatening rashes a concern. However, among a limited group of exposed infants no adverse effects have been seen (electronic Medicines Compendium, 2019b).

12.3.6 Drug Interactions

Lamotrigine does not inhibit or induce the metabolism of other drugs. However, other drugs can act to induce or inhibit the glucuronidation of lamotrigine, thereby decreasing or increasing the serum levels of lamotrigine to a clinically significant extent (Table 12.4).

Table 12.4 Effects of other drugs on the glucuronidation of lamotrigine

Serum lamotrigine levels increased by	Serum lamotrigine levels decreased by	Serum lamotrigine levels unchanged by
• Valproate	• Carbamazepine • Phenytoin • Primidone • Phenobarbital • Rifampicin • Oestrogen/progestogen combination • Lopinavir/ritonavir • Atazanavir/ritonavir	• Lithium • Bupropion • Olanzapine • Aripiprazole • Pregabalin • Oxcarbazepine • Gabapentin • Levetiracetam • Topiramate • Zonisamide

Adapted from electronic Medicines Compendium (2019b).

Most importantly perhaps for routine psychiatric practice, **valproate** *inhibits* the glucuronidation of lamotrigine and doubles its elimination half-life (Ramsay et al., 1991). If valproate and lamotrigine are to be co-prescribed, the dose of lamotrigine should be reduced by 50% and serum levels of lamotrigine monitored if necessary (refer to the BNF for details of dose adjustments).

In contrast, a number of drugs *induce* (increase) the glucuronidation of lamotrigine, including **hormonal contraception,** several other **anticonvulsants, rifampicin** and **antiretroviral drugs.** This induction will act to shorten the half-life and reduce serum levels of lamotrigine, potentially reducing its efficacy and requiring the dose of lamotrigine to be increased to compensate.

A number of other anticonvulsants and commonly used psychotropic drugs neither induce nor inhibit glucuronidation, including pregabalin, lithium, bupropion, olanzapine and aripiprazole (Table 12.4). Lamotrigine is not metabolized by cytochrome P450 enzymes, and interactions between lamotrigine and drugs metabolized by cytochrome P450 enzymes are unlikely to occur.

The combination of lamotrigine with a wide range of other drugs that can have central nervous system depressant effects might affect the ability to perform skilled tasks such as driving.

12.3.7 Clinical Use of Lamotrigine

12.3.7.1 Evidence for Effectiveness

Lamotrigine has an important role in reducing the risk of relapse of depression in bipolar disorder but it is less effective against manic relapse (Geddes et al., 2016; Goodwin et al., 2004). Consequently, it usually needs to be combined with a more effective agent preventing recurrence of mania. Lamotrigine is not effective as an acute antimanic agent (Cipriani et al., 2011; Yildiz et al., 2015). Lamotrigine in monotherapy shows some efficacy in the acute treatment of bipolar depression but its effect is modest (Geddes et al., 2009). Lamotrigine appears more effective in treating acute bipolar depression when combined with lithium (van der Loos et al., 2009) or quetiapine (Geddes et al., 2016). An advantage of lamotrigine is its very low risk of inducing a switch to mania (Taylor et al., 2014). National and international guidelines recommend lamotrigine among first- or second-line treatments for acute episodes of depression in bipolar I and bipolar II disorder, and for maintenance in bipolar I and II, particularly when depression is the major burden (for example, Goodwin et al., 2016; Yatham et al., 2018). In acute bipolar depression, the need for slow titration may be a limitation when speed of action is a priority. However, lamotrigine's good tolerability is an advantage and it warrants being used more frequently.

In contrast to bipolar depression, lamotrigine appears to be less effective in treating unipolar depression. Augmentation of an antidepressant with lamotrigine 50–200 mg/day was not found to be significantly better than placebo on meta-analysis (Zhou et al., 2015). Nevertheless, because of the need for slow titration, short-term treatment trials may not be the optimum design to assess the effectiveness of lamotrigine and other authors have appraised its potential benefits in unipolar depression more favourably (Solmi et al., 2016). Larger and longer RCTs are needed of lamotrigine at optimum doses for an adequate duration.

In schizophrenia, several small trials have investigated the addition of lamotrigine to clozapine and non-clozapine antipsychotics for suboptimal response. When added to non-clozapine antipsychotics, improvements in total, positive and negative symptoms of medium to large effect size have been reported. However, other studies have shown either no benefit or minor benefit. Furthermore, the supportive studies had methodological limitations and their quality was not considered high enough to warrant recommending augmentation with lamotrigine over antipsychotic monotherapy for clinical care guidelines (Correll et al., 2017). For augmentation of clozapine for treatment-resistant schizophrenia, lamotrigine did not outperform placebo and cannot be recommended on current meta-analytic evidence (Correll et al., 2017).

In BPD, earlier small and relatively short-term trials of lamotrigine had suggested benefits for anger and impulsivity (Lieb et al., 2010; Stoffers et al., 2010). However, a recent, much larger (n = 276), 52-week, placebo-controlled RCT found no benefits of lamotrigine for overall borderline psychopathology or a range of secondary outcomes including depressive symptoms, deliberate self-harm, social functioning, health-related quality of life, or resource use and costs (Crawford et al., 2018). On current evidence, therefore, the use of lamotrigine in people with BPD is not recommended.

Several small studies and case reports have investigated lamotrigine for post-traumatic stress disorder (PTSD), obsessive-compulsive disorder and panic disorder. While some individual patients have benefitted, particularly for PTSD, the data are too sparse to draw overall conclusions (Mula et al., 2007; Reid et al., 2013).

12.3.7.2 Starting, Monitoring and Stopping Lamotrigine

As mentioned above, lamotrigine must be introduced slowly in order to minimize the risk of serious skin rashes, and dose adjustments are necessary for patients also taking valproate or enzyme inducing drugs. Serum concentration monitoring is not usually warranted, and a therapeutic range has not been established although a trough concentration of 2.5–15 mg/L has been suggested (Taylor et al., 2015). Monitoring is, however, advised to guide dose adjustments if lamotrigine is prescribed during pregnancy and the puerperium. For stopping lamotrigine, the SPC indicates that clinical trials found no increase in adverse events following abrupt termination of lamotrigine compared with placebo. It is therefore suggested that patients may terminate lamotrigine without a step-wise dose reduction.

The SPC recommends that prescribers should assess the need for escalation to a maintenance dose when restarting lamotrigine in patients who have stopped or interrupted treatment for any reason. The greater the time period since the previous dose, the more consideration should be given to gradually building the dose back up to the previous maintenance dose. If the period during which lamotrigine has not been taken exceeds five half-lives, the SPC recommends adopting the appropriate titration schedule that would be used when lamotrigine is first commenced. The half-life of lamotrigine can vary between individuals and be significantly affected by co-prescribed medication (e.g. reduced by carbamazepine and extended by valproate). When prescribed as a monotherapy in healthy individuals, the mean half-life for lamotrigine is approximately 26 hours and so five half-lives will correspond to approximately five days.

12.4 Carbamazepine

12.4.1 Introduction

Carbamazepine is a dibenzazepine derivative and chemically related to the tricyclic antidepressants, particularly imipramine. It was synthesized by Walter Schindler at the Swiss company J. R. Geigy in 1953 as a possible competitor for the recently introduced antipsychotic chlorpromazine (Brodie, 2010). The first study in epilepsy was carried out in 1963, and it was licensed for use in epilepsy in the UK in 1965 and in the USA in 1968. It is used worldwide as an anticonvulsant for generalized tonic-clonic and partial seizures. It is not usually effective in absences (petit mal) and myoclonic seizures. It is also used for pain in trigeminal neuralgia and diabetic neuropathy, and as adjunctive treatment in acute alcohol withdrawal.

Based on observations of beneficial psychotropic effects in patients with epilepsy, carbamazepine was investigated in bipolar mania in the early 1970s in pioneering parallel work by Takezaki and Hanaoka, and Okuma, in Japan, where lithium was not yet available (Okuma & Kishimoto, 1998). Early open trials found significant acute antimanic and prophylactic efficacy (Okuma et al., 1973; Takezaki & Hanaoka, 1971). The first report outside Japan was by Ballenger and Post (1978, 1980) in bipolar patients who had not responded favourably to lithium. They found both antimanic and antidepressant benefits of carbamazepine in a small double-blind placebo-controlled trial (Ballenger & Post, 1978). However, it was not until 2005 that carbamazepine was approved for bipolar disorder in the USA.

Carbamazepine is not commonly used in the UK any more, particularly due to its pharmacokinetic interactions with a wide range of other medications and its adverse effect profile in longer-term use. However, it remains important to know about as it still has a place in the antimanic and maintenance treatment of patients with bipolar disorder who have not adequately responded to lithium and other first-line treatments.

12.4.2 Psychiatric Indications

In the UK, carbamazepine is licensed for prophylaxis of bipolar disorder unresponsive to lithium.

12.4.3 Mechanism of Action

Carbamazepine inhibits sustained repetitive neuronal firing by blocking voltage-gated sodium channels in their inactivated state. This effect in the trigeminal nucleus is believed to underlie its effects on pain. Seizure control may be due to reduction of post-tetanic potentiation of synaptic transmission in the spinal cord. Its mechanisms in bipolar disorder are not well understood, but blockade of voltage-gated sodium channels is likely to contribute. Other mechanisms may include reduced release of the excitatory neurotransmitter glutamate; actions via dopamine D_2 and glutamate NMDA (*N*-methyl-D-aspartate) receptors to down-regulate the arachidonic acid cascade, with neuroprotective effects including increased BDNF and Bcl-2; effects on adenosine receptors, adenylate cyclase and protein kinase C activity; and effects on monoamine neurotransmitter systems including noradrenaline reuptake inhibition (Drugbank, 2019b; Rapoport et al., 2009).

12.4.4 Pharmacokinetics

Following oral dosing, carbamazepine is well absorbed and bioavailability is around 80%. T_{max} is not significantly affected by food, and varies from 1.5 to 12 hours depending on whether suspension, conventional tablets or extended-release tablets are taken. Plasma protein binding is 70–85%. Variable transport of carbamazepine, particularly across the blood–brain barrier, may contribute to the variability in its pharmacodynamic effect. After a single dose, initial elimination half-life values range from 25 to 65 hours. With repeated dosing this falls to 12–17 hours as carbamazepine induces its own metabolism. Dose increases are therefore necessary to maintain serum levels. The degree of auto-induction is dose dependent but is usually complete after three to five weeks of treatment. Carbamazepine is almost completely metabolized in the liver with only around 3% of the drug excreted unchanged. Hepatic metabolism is principally by CYP3A4 to the active metabolite carbamazepine-10,11-epoxide, which is equipotent to carbamazepine as an anticonvulsant. Some hepatic glucuronidation may also occur. Carbamazepine-10,11-epoxide is further metabolized by epoxide hydrolase. Approximately 75% of the carbamazepine dose is excreted in the urine and 25% in the faeces (Drugbank, 2019b; Thorn et al., 2011).

12.4.5 Adverse Effects

12.4.5.1 Adverse Effects Unrelated to Pregnancy

Carbamazepine has a wide range of adverse effects, and while tolerability is usually good during acute use for bipolar mania it may be problematic in longer-term use. Common initial side effects of carbamazepine include nausea and vomiting, dizziness, diplopia, drowsiness, dry mouth, headaches and ataxia. Weight gain is less than with lithium or valproate. Other important but less common adverse effects are included in Table 12.5.

East and Southeast Asian populations, and people genetically related to them, have a higher prevalence of the HLA allele *B*1502* (10–15%) compared with Whites (1–2%), conferring a 10-fold to 25-fold higher incidence of carbamazepine-induced SJS and TEN (Locharernkul et al., 2011). Genotyping is necessary before starting carbamazepine in these populations, including people from China, Thailand, Malaysia and the Philippines. The incidence of carbamazepine-induced SJS/TEN is approximately 1 to 6

Table 12.5 Important adverse effects associated with carbamazepine

Adverse effects
• Teratogenicity in pregnancy, though lower risk than valproate
• Serious dermatological reactions, including SJS and TEN, especially in the first eight weeks of therapy. The risk is particularly high in Asian populations with a higher prevalence of the *HLA-B*1502* allele (see below).
• Leucopenia and thrombocytopenia
• Bone marrow suppression with agranulocytosis and aplastic anaemia (1 in 20 000)
• Raised liver enzymes, particularly gamma glutamyl transferase
• Hypersensitivity syndrome
• Mild anticholinergic activity, so use in patients with raised intraocular pressure and urinary retention requires caution
• Hyponatraemia
• Small increased risk of suicidal ideation and behaviour
• Confusion or agitation in older patients

Adapted from Drugbank (2019b).

per 10 000 new users in countries with mainly White populations. The prevalence of *HLA-B*1502* is also very low (~1%) in African, Hispanic, Japanese and Korean populations (Drugbank, 2019b).

12.4.5.2 Adverse Effects Related to Pregnancy and Breastfeeding

Carbamazepine is teratogenic and prenatal exposure increases the risk of major and minor congenital malformations, particularly cleft palate, neural tube defects, hypospadias and cardiovascular defects, though the risk is lower than for valproate (Hernandez-Diaz et al., 2012; Veroniki et al., 2017a). Carbamazepine is excreted in breast milk (about 25–60% of serum levels), and there are some case reports of adverse effects in infants (cholestatic hepatitis, hepatic dysfunction, seizure-like activity, drowsiness, irritability, hyperexcitability, poor suckling). However, studies have found that exposure to carbamazepine is not associated with impaired development or IQ at the age of three years (Taylor et al., 2015). The manufacturer advises that the benefits of breastfeeding should be weighed against the very small possibility of adverse effects occurring in the infant, and that mothers may breastfeed provided the infant is observed for possible adverse reactions.

12.4.6 Drug Interactions

Carbamazepine has a wide range of clinically important pharmacokinetic interactions with other drugs, and clinicians are advised to consult an authoritative prescribing reference such as the BNF before initiating treatment or co-prescribing for patients taking it. Interactions arise from two main mechanisms. Firstly, carbamazepine acts to induce the hepatic metabolism of many other drugs, thereby lowering their serum levels and potentially their clinical effectiveness unless the dose is adjusted. Secondly, other drugs can induce or inhibit the metabolism of carbamazepine and/or its active epoxide metabolite, thereby decreasing or increasing their serum levels, respectively. These mechanisms are addressed in turn below.

Carbamazepine potently stimulates the synthesis of (induces) CYP3A4 and a wide range of other oxidative and conjugating enzymes, with the result that for very many lipid and non-lipid drugs their metabolism is increased and their duration of action decreased. In addition to inducing its own metabolism (see Pharmacokinetics, above), this includes anticoagulants, cytotoxics, analgesics, antiretrovirals, glucocorticoids, statins, antihypertensives, oral contraceptives, psychoactive drugs, immunosuppressants and other anticonvulsants (Brodie et al., 2013). This effect to reduce serum levels of many **antidepressants**, **antipsychotics**, **anxiolytics**, some **cholinesterase inhibitors**, **methadone**, and **other psychotropics**, and the need for compensatory dose adjustments and serum monitoring, is among the main reasons for the decline in the use of carbamazepine in recent years. In clinical practice for mental disorders, drug combinations with carbamazepine are better avoided where possible, and its use is less complicated in monotherapy or with drugs lacking hepatic metabolism such as lithium. Even then, however, drug interactions may occur, and the combination with lithium is predicted to increase the risk of neurotoxicity. Carbamazepine will also induce the metabolism of **L-thyroxine** prescribed for hypothyroidism, necessitating close monitoring of thyroid function and dose increases. The effectiveness of **hormonal contraception** may also be reduced, requiring counselling, potential dose increases and alternative contraception.

Carbamazepine is principally metabolized by CYP3A4 to carbamazepine-10,11-epoxide, which in turn is detoxified by epoxide hydrolase. Co-administration of inhibitors or inducers of CYP3A4 or epoxide hydrolase with carbamazepine can increase or decrease serum levels of carbamazepine and/or the epoxide metabolite. Similarly, discontinuation of a CYP3A4 inducer may increase carbamazepine serum concentrations. These interactions may induce adverse effects, impair drug effectiveness, and necessitate dose changes and/or monitoring of serum levels. The list of drugs interacting by these mechanisms is extensive. The most important interactions with psychotropic drugs commonly used in psychiatric practice are listed in Table 12.6. For interactions with other drugs, clinicians should consult the BNF or SPC, which can be found online (electronic Medicines Compendium, 2019c).

Table 12.6 Psychotropic and anticonvulsant drugs affecting the metabolism of carbamazepine

Psychotropic and anticonvulsant drug effects on metabolism of carbamazepine		
Drugs that *raise* carbamazepine serum levels	**Drugs that *raise* serum levels of carbamazepine-10,11-epoxide**	**Drugs that *decrease* carbamazepine serum levels**
• Fluoxetine • Fluvoxamine • Paroxetine • Trazodone • Olanzapine • Vigabatrin	• Quetiapine • Valproate • Primidone	• Oxcarbazepine • Phenobarbital • Phenytoin

Adapted from electronic Medicines Compendium (2019c).

Carbamazepine is structurally similar to tricyclic antidepressants and concerns have been raised regarding the safety of combining it with monoamine oxidase inhibitors (MAOIs). The SPC states that carbamazepine is contraindicated in combination with MAOIs and that MAOIs should be discontinued for a minimum of two weeks before starting carbamazepine. Nevertheless, the combination has been tried in refractory depression in a small number of patients and was reported to be well tolerated (Ketter et al., 1995).

12.4.7 Clinical Use of Carbamazepine

12.4.7.1 Evidence for Effectiveness

Carbamazepine has good evidence as an antimanic agent, with efficacy broadly comparable with that of antipsychotics and lithium, and slightly better than valproate (Cipriani et al., 2011; Yildiz et al., 2015). However, due to safety and tolerability concerns, treatment guidelines recommend it among second-line antimanic treatments when first-line options have failed, or in combination with lithium or valproate among third-line treatments in more resistant mania (Goodwin et al., 2016; Yatham et al., 2018). Certain clinical features may modestly predict antimanic response to carbamazepine, including a history of head trauma, co-morbid anxiety and substance abuse, mood-incongruent delusions, and a lack of history of bipolar disorder in first-degree relatives (Yatham et al., 2018). For maintenance treatment in bipolar I disorder, it is protective against manic relapse but less effective than lithium and poorly protective against depressive relapse. It is recommended as an option when a range of first-line options have been ineffective, and there is some evidence that it may be more effective than lithium in patients with bipolar II disorder, schizoaffective disorder, and who do not have the classical pattern of episodic euphoric mania (Kleindienst & Greil, 2000). As acute treatment for bipolar depression, the evidence is poor and recommendations either omit carbamazepine (Goodwin et al., 2016) or relegate it to patients with bipolar I depression who fail to respond to multiple first- and second-line agents (Yatham et al., 2018). It does not appear to be effective for depression in bipolar II disorder.

On current RCT evidence, carbamazepine is not effective in reducing core symptoms of schizophrenia, either in monotherapy or when combined with an antipsychotic (Correll et al., 2017; Leucht et al., 2014). There is a small amount of evidence to suggest it may be beneficial in unipolar depression as monotherapy (Zhang et al., 2008) or when combined with lithium (Kramlinger & Post, 1989), but in a small open-label study it did not augment the antidepressant efficacy of mirtazapine (Schule et al., 2009). Pharmacokinetic effects of carbamazepine to reduce the serum concentrations of a wide range of other drugs are a particular problem, and large well-conducted RCTs which control for drug serum levels are required. Carbamazepine is not recommended for unipolar depression in current guidelines.

Carbamazepine has evidence for effectiveness as adjunctive treatment in alcohol withdrawal syndrome (Hammond et al., 2015). For BPD, no significant benefits of carbamazepine have been found in well-controlled trials (Stoffers et al., 2010). Good evidence for an effect on aggression and associated impulsivity is lacking (Huband et al., 2010).

12.4.7.2 Starting, Monitoring and Stopping Carbamazepine

Before starting carbamazepine, urea and electrolytes, FBC and LFTs should be checked, and repeated after six months. Weight or BMI should also be measured at baseline and monitored during treatment. Guidelines recommend that sodium levels should be measured at least annually due to the risk of hyponatraemia (Yatham et al., 2018). Before starting, patients from high-risk Asian populations (see Adverse Effects, above) should be genotyped for the *HLA-B*1502* allele, which confers a high risk for SJS and TEN with carbamazepine (Locharernkul et al., 2011). Serum trough levels of 7–12 mg/L are suggested for bipolar disorder (Taylor et al., 2015), although there is no established relationship between efficacy and serum levels. Serum level monitoring should be carried out 2–4 weeks after a dose increase to check that the desired level is still being maintained (Taylor et al., 2015), routinely every 6–12 months (Yatham et al., 2018), and when clinically indicated to check for treatment adherence or to make sure levels are not in the toxic range . As carbamazepine induces the metabolism of many other drugs, patients on carbamazepine and other medications should have serum levels of all psychotropic medications monitored, particularly when clinical response is poor, in case dose adjustments are necessary. Similarly, carbamazepine may impair the effectiveness of hormonal contraception and women of childbearing potential should be advised to use alternative contraceptive methods.

Given preliminary evidence that abrupt withdrawal of carbamazepine may increase the risk of relapse in bipolar disorder, particularly of mania or hypomania (Franks et al., 2008), in the absence of better evidence carbamazepine should be withdrawn slowly over at least four weeks.

12.5 Oxcarbazepine and Eslicarbazepine

12.5.1 Introduction

Oxcarbazepine is a structural derivative of carbamazepine, by adding an extra oxygen atom to the benzylcarboxamide group. It is not a metabolite of carbamazepine. The structural change helps reduce the risk of bone marrow toxicity and the strength of induction of hepatic metabolism associated with carbamazepine. Oxcarbazepine is a prodrug with little intrinsic activity itself, and is metabolized to the active 10-monohydroxy metabolite. The 10-monohydroxy metabolite has been named licarbazepine, and its active S enantiomer has been developed and marketed as eslicarbazepine acetate. Oxcarbazepine and eslicarbazepine are licensed and effective for the treatment of partial seizures with or without secondarily generalized tonic-clonic seizures.

12.5.2 Psychiatric Indications

Oxcarbazepine and eslicarbazepine are not licensed in the UK for any psychiatric indication. However, they are sometimes used off-licence as an alternative to carbamazepine in the acute treatment of mania and the prevention of manic relapse though the supporting evidence is poor (see later on in chapter for a discussion of the evidence).

12.5.3 Mechanism of Action, Pharmacokinetics and Adverse Effects

The mechanism of action of oxcarbazepine and eslicarbazepine is considered to be the same as carbamazepine. In comparison with carbamazepine, oxcarbazepine and eslicarbazepine induce hepatic metabolic enzymes (mainly CYP3A4, CYP3A5 and UDP-glucuronyl transferases) only weakly. Nevertheless, the induction is not negligible and oxcarbazepine/eslicarbazepine can reduce the serum levels and effectiveness of other drugs including hormonal contraceptives and the many psychotropic drugs metabolized via CYP3A4. In addition, strong inhibitors of CYP3A4 such as fluoxetine and paroxetine may inhibit the metabolism of oxcarbazepine/eslicarbazepine and increase their serum levels and adverse effects. Oxcarbazepine and eslicarbazepine inhibit CYP2C19 so have the potential to increase serum levels and adverse effects of CYP2C19 substrates such as escitalopram.

The range of possible adverse effects reported for oxcarbazepine is similar to carbamazepine. Dizziness, nausea, somnolence, diplopia, fatigue and benign rash are quite common (>5%), but are usually mild or moderate and occur early in dose titration. Rare adverse effects include hypersensitivity, serious skin reactions (SJS, TEN), hyponatraemia and reports of suicidal ideation and behaviour. Genotyping for *HLA-B*1502* allele, which increases the risk of SJS/TEN, remains necessary for at-risk populations.

12.5.4 Clinical Use of Oxcarbazepine and Eslicarbazepine

Oxcarbazepine and eslicarbazepine are not licensed for treating bipolar or any other mental disorder, and clear evidence for antimanic or prophylactic effectiveness in bipolar disorder is lacking. Because of its structural similarity to carbamazepine and weaker induction of hepatic metabolism, oxcarbazepine has been thought of as a safer version of carbamazepine and indications for carbamazepine have tended to be applied to oxcarbazepine by extrapolation (Goodwin et al., 2016). It has been recommended as an alternative to carbamazepine among third-line combination treatments for acute mania in adults but requires further evaluation (Yatham et al., 2018). It is not an effective treatment in children and adolescents with bipolar disorder (Wagner et al., 2006). Eslicarbazepine does not appear to be an effective antimanic agent, but preliminary evidence suggests some support for efficacy in prevention (Grunze et al., 2015). More data are needed before it can be considered a useful alternative to established medications.

12.6 Other Anticonvulsants: Topiramate and Gabapentin

The evidence base for the use of other anticonvulsants is sparse, and none is licensed in the UK for any mental disorder. Topiramate has been added to antipsychotics for suboptimal response in schizophrenia, and reductions have been reported in total psychopathology and positive symptoms. However, the quality of the data and the size of the effect do not warrant its recommendation as a strategy in clinical practice (Correll et al., 2017). Topiramate and gabapentin are not effective for the treatment of acute mania in bipolar disorder (Yatham et al., 2018), but may be beneficial in bipolar patients with co-morbid alcohol misuse (Azorin et al., 2010; Perugi et al., 2002). There are no controlled data to support a recommendation for topiramate in bipolar maintenance treatment (Yatham et al., 2018), but a small placebo-controlled trial found some benefits of adjunctive topiramate for mania with obsessive-compulsive symptoms (Sahraian et al., 2014). Gabapentin does not seem to be effective in refractory bipolar or unipolar depression (Frye et al., 2000), but may have some usefulness for maintenance in patients who remain unwell despite a range of other treatments (Vieta et al., 2006). Gabapentin may also have some benefits in anxiety disorders, particularly social phobia and generalized anxiety disorder (Mula et al., 2007). However, a clear role for topiramate and gabapentin in psychiatric practice is not apparent from the current evidence, and they are not commonly used.

References

Acharya S, Bussel JB (2000). Hematologic toxicity of sodium valproate. *J Pediatr Hematol Oncol*, 22(1), 62–65.

Aiken CB, Orr C (2010). Rechallenge with lamotrigine after a rash: a prospective case series and review of the literature. *Psychiatry*, 7, 27–32.

Aliyev NA, Aliyev ZN (2008). Valproate (depakine-chrono) in the acute treatment of outpatients with generalized anxiety disorder without psychiatric comorbidity: randomized, double-blind placebo-controlled study. *Eur Psychiatry*, 23, 109–114.

Allen MH, Hirschfeld RM, Wozniak PJ, Baker JD, Bowden CL (2006). Linear relationship of valproate serum concentration to response and optimal serum levels for acute mania. *Am J Psychiatry*, 163, 272–275.

Angus-Lepan H, Liu R (2018). Weighing the risks of valproate in women who could become pregnant. *BMJ*, 361, k1596.

Azorin JM, Bowden CL, Garay RP, et al. (2010). Possible new ways in the pharmacological treatment of bipolar disorder and comorbid alcoholism. *Neuropsychiatr Dis Treat*, 6, 37–46.

Ballenger JC, Post RM (1978). Therapeutic effects of carbamazepine in affective illness: a preliminary report. *Commun Psychopharmacol*, 2, 159–175.

Ballenger JC, Post RM (1980). Carbamazepine in manic-depressive illness: a new treatment. *Am J Psychiatry*, 137, 782–790.

Belcastro V, D'Egidio C, Striano P, Verrotti A (2013). Metabolic and endocrine effects of valproic acid chronic treatment. *Epilepsy Res*, 107, 1–8.

Bjerkedal T, Czeizel A, Goujard J, et al. (1982). Valproic acid and spina bifida. *Lancet*, 2, 1096.

BNF (2019). *British National Formulary* (online). London: BMJ Group and Pharmaceutical Press. Available at: www.medicinescomplete.com (last accessed 13.8.19).

Bond DJ, Lam RW, Yatham LN (2010). Divalproex sodium versus placebo in the treatment of acute bipolar depression: a systematic review and meta-analysis. *J Affect Disord*, 124, 228–234.

Bowden CL, Asnis GM, Ginsberg LD, et al. (2004). Safety and tolerability of lamotrigine for bipolar disorder. *Drug Saf*, 27, 173–184.

Brodie MJ (1992). Lamotrigine. *Lancet*, 339, 1397–1400.

Brodie MJ (2010). Antiepileptic drug therapy the story so far. *Seizure*, 19, 650–655.

Brodie MJ, Mintzer S, Pack AM, et al. (2013). Enzyme induction with antiepileptic drugs: cause for concern? *Epilepsia*, 54, 11–27.

Bromley R, Weston J, Adab N, et al. (2014). Treatment for epilepsy in pregnancy: neurodevelopmental outcomes in the child. *Cochrane Database Syst Rev*, (10), CD010236.

Campbell E, Kennedy F, Russell A, et al. (2014). Malformation risks of antiepileptic drug monotherapies in pregnancy: updated results from the UK and Ireland Epilepsy and Pregnancy Registers. *J Neurol Neurosurg Psychiatry*, 85, 1029–1034.

Carrigan PJ, Brinker DR, Cavanaugh JH, Lamm JE, Cloyd JC (1990). Absorption characteristics of a new valproate formulation: divalproex sodium-coated particles in capsules (Depakote Sprinkle). *J Clin Pharmacol*, 30, 743–747.

Chen PS, Peng GS, Li G, et al. (2006). Valproate protects dopaminergic neurons in midbrain neuron/glia cultures by stimulating the release of neurotrophic factors from astrocytes. *Mol Psychiatry*, 11, 1116–1125.

Christensen J, Gronborg TK, Sorensen MJ, et al. (2013). Prenatal valproate exposure and risk of autism spectrum disorders and childhood autism. *JAMA*, 309, 1696–1703.

Chung S, Wang N, Hank N (2007). Comparative retention rates and long-term tolerability of new antiepileptic drugs. *Seizure*, 16, 296–304.

Cipriani A, Barbui C, Salanti G, et al. (2011). Comparative efficacy and acceptability of antimanic drugs in acute mania: a multiple-treatments meta-analysis. *Lancet*, 378, 1306–1315.

Citrome L, Volavka J (2011). Pharmacological management of acute and persistent aggression in forensic psychiatry settings. *CNS Drugs*, 25, 1009–1021.

Cleare A, Pariante CM, Young AH, et al.; Members of the Consensus Meeting (2015). Evidence-based guidelines for treating depressive disorders with antidepressants: a revision of the 2008 British Association for Psychopharmacology guidelines. *J Psychopharmacol*, 29, 459–525.

Cohen AF, Land GS, Breimer DD, et al. (1987). Lamotrigine, a new anticonvulsant: pharmacokinetics in normal humans. *Clin Pharmacol Ther*, 42, 535–541.

Cohen MJ, Meador KJ, Browning N, et al. (2011). Fetal antiepileptic drug exposure: motor, adaptive, and emotional/behavioral functioning at age 3 years. *Epilepsy Behav*, 22, 240–246.

Cohen MJ, Meador KJ, Browning N, et al.; NEAD study group (2013). Fetal antiepileptic drug exposure: adaptive and emotional/behavioral functioning at age 6 years. *Epilepsy Behav*, 29, 308–315.

Correll CU, Rubio JM, Inczedy Farkas G, et al. (2017). Efficacy of 42 pharmacologic cotreatment strategies added to antipsychotic monotherapy in schizophrenia: systematic overview and quality appraisal of the meta-analytic evidence. *JAMA Psychiatry*, 74, 675–684.

Crawford MJ, Sanatinia R, Barrett B, et al. (2018). Lamotrigine for people with borderline personality disorder: a RCT. *Health Technol Assess*, 22, 1–68.

Cummings C, Stewart M, Stevenson M, Morrow J, Nelson J (2011). Neurodevelopment of children exposed in utero to lamotrigine, sodium valproate and carbamazepine. *Arch Dis Child*, 96, 643–647.

Davis LL, Ryan W, Adinoff B, Petty F (2000). Comprehensive review of the psychiatric uses of valproate. *J Clin Psychopharmacol*, 20, 1S–17S.

Dias VV, Balanza-Martinez V, Soeiro-de-Souza MG, et al. (2012). Pharmacological approaches in bipolar disorders and the impact on cognition: a critical overview. *Acta Psychiatr Scand*, 126, 315–331.

Drevets WC (2000). Neuroimaging studies of mood disorders. *Biol Psychiatry*, 48, 813–829.

Drugbank (2019a). Lamotrigine. Available at: www.drugbank.ca/drugs/DB00555 (last accessed 6.8.19).

Drugbank (2019b). Carbamazepine. Available at: www.drugbank.ca/drugs/DB00564 (last accessed 6.8.19).

electronic Medicines Compendium (2019a). Summary of Product Characteristics: Depakote. SANOFI. Available at: www.medicines.org.uk/emc/product/6113/smpc (last accessed 6.8.19).

electronic Medicines Compendium (2019b). Summary of Product Characteristics: Lamotrigine. Accord Healthcare Limited. Available at: www.medicines.org.uk/emc/product/6091/smpc (last accessed 6.8.19).

electronic Medicines Compendium (2019c). Summary of Product Characteristics: Carbamazepine. Novartis Pharmaceuticals UK Ltd. Available at: www.medicines.org.uk/emc/product/1040/smpc (last accessed 6.8.19).

Elkjaer LS, Bech BH, Sun Y, Laursen TM, Christensen J (2018). Association between prenatal valproate exposure and performance on standardized language and mathematics tests in school-aged children. *JAMA Neurol*, 19, 19.

European Medicines Agency (2018). New measures to avoid valproate exposure in pregnancy endorsed. Press release, 23 March 2018. Available at: www.ema.europa.eu/docs/en_GB/document_library/Press_release/2018/03/WC500246391.pdf (last accessed 22.8.19).

Fleming J, Chetty M (2005). Psychotropic drug interactions with valproate. *Clin Neuropharmacol*, 28, 96–101.

Franks M, Macritchie KA, Mahmood T, Young AH (2008). Bouncing back: is the bipolar rebound phenomenon peculiar to lithium? A retrospective naturalistic study. *J Psychopharmacol*, 22, 452–456.

Frye MA, Ketter TA, Kimbrell TA, et al. (2000). A placebo-controlled study of lamotrigine and gabapentin monotherapy in refractory mood disorders. *J Clin Psychopharmacol*, 20, 607–614.

Geddes JR, Calabrese JR, Goodwin GM (2009). Lamotrigine for treatment of bipolar depression: independent meta-analysis and meta-regression of individual patient data from five randomised trials. *Br J Psychiatry*, 194, 4–9.

Geddes JR, Gardiner A, Rendell J, et al.; CEQUEL Investigators and Collaborators (2016). Comparative evaluation of quetiapine plus lamotrigine combination versus quetiapine monotherapy (and folic acid versus placebo) in bipolar depression (CEQUEL): a 2 × 2 factorial randomised trial. *Lancet Psychiatry*, 3, 31–39.

Ghabrash MF, Comai S, Tabaka J, et al. (2016). Valproate augmentation in a subgroup of patients with treatment-resistant unipolar depression. *World J Biol Psychiatry*, 17, 165–170.

Ghodke-Puranik Y, Thorn CF, Lamba JK, et al. (2013). Valproic acid pathway: pharmacokinetics and pharmacodynamics. *Pharmacogenet Genomics*, 23, 236–241.

Goodwin GM, Bowden CL, Calabrese JR, et al. (2004). A pooled analysis of 2 placebo-controlled 18-month trials of lamotrigine and lithium maintenance in bipolar I disorder. *J Clin Psychiatry*, 65, 432–441.

Goodwin GM, Haddad PM, Ferrier IN, et al. (2016). Evidence-based guidelines for treating bipolar disorder: revised third edition recommendations from the British Association for Psychopharmacology. *J Psychopharmacol*, 30, 495–553.

Grunze H, Kotlik E, Costa R, et al. (2015). Assessment of the efficacy and safety of eslicarbazepine acetate in acute mania and prevention of recurrence: experience from multicentre, double-blind, randomised phase II clinical studies in patients with bipolar disorder I. *J Affect Disord*, 174, 70–82.

Hammond CJ, Niciu MJ, Drew S, Arias AJ (2015). Anticonvulsants for the treatment of alcohol withdrawal syndrome and alcohol use disorders. *CNS Drugs*, 29, 293–311.

Haymond J, Ensom MH (2010). Does valproic acid warrant therapeutic drug monitoring in bipolar affective disorder? *Ther Drug Monit*, 32, 19–29.

Hernandez-Diaz S, Smith CR, Shen A, et al.; North American AED Pregnancy Registry (2012). Comparative safety of antiepileptic drugs during pregnancy. *Neurology*, 78, 1692–1699.

Huband N, Ferriter M, Nathan R, Jones H (2010). Antiepileptics for aggression and associated impulsivity. *Cochrane Database Syst Rev*, (2), CD003499.

Hurley SC (2002). Lamotrigine update and its use in mood disorders. *Ann Pharmacother*, 36, 860–873.

Jentink J, Loane MA, Dolk H, et al.; EUROCAT Antiepileptic Study Working Group (2010). Valproic acid monotherapy in pregnancy and major congenital malformations. *N Engl J Med*, 362, 2185–2193.

Kaye NS, Graham J, Roberts J, Thompson T, Nanry K (2007). Effect of open-label lamotrigine as monotherapy and adjunctive therapy on the self-assessed cognitive function scores of patients with bipolar I disorder. *J Clin Psychopharmacol*, 27, 387–391.

Ketter TA, Post RM, Parekh PI, Worthington K (1995). Addition of monoamine oxidase inhibitors to carbamazepine: preliminary evidence of safety and antidepressant efficacy in treatment-resistant depression. *J Clin Psychiatry*, 56(10), 471–475.

Kleindienst N, Greil W (2000). Differential efficacy of lithium and carbamazepine in the prophylaxis of bipolar disorder: results of the MAP study. *Neuropsychobiology*, 42(Suppl 1), 2–10.

Klotz U, Antonin KH (1977). Pharmacokinetics and bioavailability of sodium valproate. *Clin Pharmacol Ther*, 21, 736–743.

Kramlinger KG, Post RM (1989). The addition of lithium to carbamazepine. Antidepressant efficacy in treatment-resistant depression. *Arch Gen Psychiatry*, 46, 794–800.

Leach MJ, Marden CM, Miller AA (1986). Pharmacological studies on lamotrigine, a novel potential antiepileptic drug: II. Neurochemical studies on the mechanism of action. *Epilepsia*, 27, 490–497.

Lempérière T (2001). Brief history of the development of valproate in bipolar disorders. *Encephale*, 27, 365–372.

Leucht S, Helfer B, Dold M, Kissling W, McGrath J (2014). Carbamazepine for schizophrenia. *Cochrane Database Syst Rev*, (5), CD001258.

Lieb K, Vollm B, Rucker G, Timmer A, Stoffers JM (2010). Pharmacotherapy for borderline personality disorder: Cochrane systematic review of randomised trials. *Br J Psychiatry*, 196, 4–12.

Lloyd KA (2013). A scientific review: mechanisms of valproate-mediated teratogenesis. *Biosci Horizons*, 6, hzt003-hzt03.

Locharernkul C, Shotelersuk V, Hirankarn N (2011). Pharmacogenetic screening of carbamazepine-induced severe cutaneous allergic reactions. *J Clin Neurosci*, 18, 1289–1294.

Löscher W (1999). The discovery of valproate. In W Löscher, ed., *Valproate*. Basel: Birkhäuser Basel, pp. 1–3.

Meador K, Reynolds MW, Crean S, Fahrbach K, Probst C (2008). Pregnancy outcomes in women with epilepsy: a systematic review and meta-analysis of published pregnancy registries and cohorts. *Epilepsy Res*, 81, 1–13.

Molgaard-Nielsen D, Hviid A (2011). Newer-generation antiepileptic drugs and the risk of major birth defects. *JAMA*, 305, 1996–2002.

Mula M, Pini S , Cassano GB (2007). The role of anticonvulsant drugs in anxiety disorders: a critical review of the evidence. *J Clin Psychopharmacol*, 27, 263–272.

National Institute for Health and Clinical Excellence (NICE) (2009). *Borderline personality disorder: recognition and management*. Clinical guideline [CG78]. London: National Institute for Health and Care Excellence. Available at: www.nice.org.uk/guidance/cg78 (last accessed 22.8.19).

Nishino S, Ohtomo K, Numata Y, et al. (2012). Divergent effects of lithium and sodium valproate on brain-derived neurotrophic factor (BDNF) production in human astrocytoma cells at therapeutic concentrations. *Prog Neuropsychopharmacol Biol Psychiatry*, 39, 17–22.

Nugent AC, Carlson PJ, Bain EE, et al. (2013). Mood stabilizer treatment increases serotonin type 1A receptor binding in bipolar depression. *J Psychopharmacol*, 27, 894–902.

Okuma T, Kishimoto A (1998). A history of investigation on the mood stabilizing effect of carbamazepine in Japan. *Psychiatry Clin Neurosci*, 52, 3–12.

Okuma T, Kishimoto A, Inoue K, Matsumoto H, Ogura A (1973). Anti-manic and prophylactic effects of carbamazepine (Tegretol) on manic depressive psychosis. A preliminary report. *Folia Psychiatr Neurol Jpn*, 27, 283–297.

Ornoy A (2009). Valproic acid in pregnancy: how much are we endangering the embryo and fetus? *Reprod Toxicol*, 28, 1–10.

Perugi G, Toni C, Frare F, et al. (2002). Effectiveness of adjunctive gabapentin in resistant bipolar disorder: is it due to anxious-alcohol abuse comorbidity? *J Clin Psychopharmacol*, 22, 584–591.

Peterson GM, Naunton M (2005). Valproate: a simple chemical with so much to offer. *J Clin Pharm Ther*, 30, 417–421.

Rajkowska G (2000). Postmortem studies in mood disorders indicate altered numbers of neurons and glial cells. *Biol Psychiatry*, 48, 766–777.

Ramsay RE, Pellock JM, Garnett WR, et al. (1991). Pharmacokinetics and safety of lamotrigine (Lamictal) in patients with epilepsy. *Epilepsy Res*, 10, 191–200.

Rapoport SI, Basselin M, Kim HW, Rao JS (2009). Bipolar disorder and mechanisms of action of mood stabilizers. *Brain Res Rev*, 61, 185–209.

Reid JG, Gitlin MJ, Altshuler LL (2013). Lamotrigine in psychiatric disorders. *J Clin Psychiatry*, 74, 675–684.

Robert E, Guibaud P (1982). Maternal valproic acid and congenital neural tube defects. *Lancet*, 2, 937.

Rosenberg G (2007). The mechanisms of action of valproate in neuropsychiatric disorders: can we see the forest for the trees? *Cell Mol Life Sci*, 64, 2090–2103.

Sahraian A, Bigdeli M, Ghanizadeh A, Akhondzadeh S (2014). Topiramate as an adjuvant treatment for obsessive compulsive symptoms in patients with bipolar disorder: a randomized double blind placebo controlled clinical trial. *J Affect Disord*, 166, 201–205.

Sandson NB, Marcucci C, Bourke DL, Smith-Lamacchia R (2006). An interaction between aspirin and valproate: the relevance of plasma protein displacement drug-drug interactions. *Am J Psychiatry*, 163, 1891–1896.

Schule C, Baghai TC, Eser D, Nothdurfter C, Rupprecht R (2009). Lithium but not carbamazepine augments antidepressant efficacy of mirtazapine in unipolar depression: an open-label study. *World J Biol Psychiatry*, 10, 390–399.

Seo HJ, Chiesa A, Lee SJ, et al. (2011). Safety and tolerability of lamotrigine: results from 12 placebo-controlled clinical trials and clinical implications. *Clin Neuropharmacol*, 34, 39–47.

Serrani Azcurra DJ (2013). Lamotrigine rechallenge after a skin rash. A combined study of open cases and a meta-analysis. *Rev Psiquiatr Salud Ment*, 6, 144–149.

Sie M (2014). Mood stabilisers in the management of bipolar affective disorder. *Prog Neurol Psychiatry*, 18, 22–32.

Smith LA, Cornelius VR, Azorin JM, et al. (2010). Valproate for the treatment of acute bipolar depression: systematic review and meta-analysis. *J Affect Disord*, 122, 1–9.

Solmi M, Veronese N, Zaninotto L, et al. (2016). Lamotrigine compared to placebo and other agents with antidepressant activity in patients with unipolar and bipolar depression: a comprehensive meta-analysis of efficacy and safety outcomes in short-term trials. *CNS Spectr*, 21, 403–418.

Stoffers J, Vollm BA, Rucker G, et al. (2010). Pharmacological interventions for borderline personality disorder. *Cochrane Database Syst Rev*, (6), CD005653.

Takezaki H, Hanaoka M (1971). The use of carbamazepine (Tegretol) in the control of manic depressive psychosis and other manic depressive states. *Saishin Igaku*, 13, 1310–1318 (in Japanese).

Tanoshima M, Kobayashi T, Tanoshima R, et al. (2015). Risks of congenital malformations in offspring exposed to valproic acid in utero: a systematic review and cumulative meta-analysis. *Clin Pharmacol Ther*, 98, 417–441.

Taylor DM, Cornelius V, Smith L, Young AH (2014). Comparative efficacy and acceptability of drug treatments for bipolar depression: a multiple-treatments meta-analysis. *Acta Psychiatr Scand*, 130, 452–469.

Taylor D, Paton C, Kapur S (2015). *The Maudsley Prescribing Guidelines in Psychiatry*, 12th ed. Hoboken: Wiley Blackwell.

Thomas SV, Ajaykumar B, Sindhu K, et al. (2008). Motor and mental development of infants exposed to antiepileptic drugs in utero. *Epilepsy Behav*, 13, 229–236.

Thorn CF, Leckband SG, Kelsoe J, et al. (2011). PharmGKB summary: carbamazepine pathway. *Pharmacogenet Genomics*, 21, 906–910.

Tomson T, Battino D, Perucca E (2016). Valproic acid after five decades of use in epilepsy: time to reconsider the indications of a time-honoured drug. *Lancet Neurol*, 15, 210–218.

Tseng PT, Chen YW, Chung W, et al. (2016). Significant effect of valproate augmentation therapy in patients with schizophrenia: a meta-analysis study. *Medicine*, 95, e2475.

Uguz F, Sharma V (2016). Mood stabilizers during breastfeeding: a systematic review of the recent literature. *Bipolar Disord*, 18, 325–333.

Vajda FJ, Donnan GA, Phillips J, Bladin PF (1981). Human brain, plasma, and cerebrospinal fluid concentration of sodium valproate after 72 hours of therapy. *Neurology*, 31, 486–487.

Vajda FJ, O'Brien TJ, Graham JE, Lander CM, Eadie MJ (2013). Dose dependence of fetal malformations associated with valproate. *Neurology*, 81, 999–1003.

Vasudev K, Keown P, Gibb I, McAllister-Williams RH (2010). Hematological effects of valproate in psychiatric patients: what are the risk factors? *J Clin Psychopharmacol*, 30(3), 282–285.

van der Loos ML, Mulder PG, Hartong EG, et al.; LamLit Study Group (2009). Efficacy and safety of lamotrigine as add-on treatment to lithium in bipolar depression: a multicenter, double-blind, placebo-controlled trial. *J Clin Psychiatry*, 70, 223–231.

Vella T, Mifsud J (2014). Interactions between valproic acid and quetiapine/olanzapine in the treatment of bipolar disorder and the role of therapeutic drug monitoring. *J Pharmacy Pharmacol*, 66, 747–759.

Veroniki AA, Cogo E, Rios P, et al. (2017a). Comparative safety of anti-epileptic drugs during pregnancy: a systematic review and network meta-analysis of congenital malformations and prenatal outcomes. *BMC Med*, 15, 95.

Veroniki AA, Rios P, Cogo E, et al. (2017b). Comparative safety of antiepileptic drugs for neurological development in children exposed during pregnancy and breast feeding: a systematic review and network meta-analysis. *BMJ Open*, 7, e017248.

Vieta E, Manuel Goikolea J, Martinez-Aran A, et al. (2006). A double-blind, randomized, placebo-controlled, prophylaxis study of adjunctive gabapentin for bipolar disorder. *J Clin Psychiatry*, 67, 473–477.

Wagner KD, Kowatch RA, Emslie GJ, et al. (2006). A double-blind, randomized, placebo-controlled trial of oxcarbazepine in the treatment of bipolar disorder in children and adolescents. *Am J Psychiatry*, 163, 1179–1186. Erratum in: *Am J Psychiatry* 2006, 163(10), 1843.

Wang Y, Xia J, Helfer B, Li C, Leucht S (2008). Valproate for schizophrenia. *Cochrane Database Syst Rev*, (3), CD004028.

Wegner C, Nau H (1992). Alteration of embryonic folate metabolism by valproic acid during organogenesis: implications for mechanism of teratogenesis. *Neurology*, 42, 17–24.

Weisler RH, Calabrese JR, Bowden CL, et al. (2008). Discovery and development of lamotrigine for bipolar disorder: a story of serendipity, clinical observations, risk taking, and persistence. *J Affect Disord*, 108, 1–9.

Wieck A, Jones S (2018). Dangers of valproate in pregnancy. *BMJ*, 361, k1609.

Yasam VR, Jakki SL, Senthil V, et al. (2016). A pharmacological overview of lamotrigine for the treatment of epilepsy. *Expert Rev Clin Pharmacol*, 9, 1533–1546.

Yatham LN, Kennedy SH, Parikh SV, et al. (2018). Canadian Network for Mood and Anxiety Treatments (CANMAT) and International Society for Bipolar Disorders (ISBD) 2018 guidelines for the management of patients with bipolar disorder. *Bipolar Disord*, 20, 97–170.

Yildiz A, Nikodem M, Vieta E, Correll CU, Baldessarini RJ (2015). A network meta-analysis on comparative efficacy and all-cause discontinuation of antimanic treatments in acute bipolar mania. *Psychol Med*, 45, 299–317.

Zhang L, Li H, Li S, Zou X (2016). Reproductive and metabolic abnormalities in women taking valproate for bipolar disorder: a meta-analysis. *Eur J Obstet Gynecol Reprod Biol*, 202, 26–31.

Zhang ZJ, Tan QR, Tong Y, et al. (2008). The effectiveness of carbamazepine in unipolar depression: a double-blind, randomized, placebo-controlled study. *J Affect Disord*, 109, 91–97.

Zhou X, Ravindran AV, Qin B, et al. (2015). Comparative efficacy, acceptability, and tolerability of augmentation agents in treatment-resistant depression: systematic review and network meta-analysis. *J Clin Psychiatry*, 76, e487–e498.

Drugs to Treat Attention Deficit Hyperactivity Disorder (ADHD)

Ulrich Müller-Sedgwick and
Jane A. Sedgwick-Müller

13.1 Introduction

The aim of this chapter is to enable psychiatrists and nurses to safely prescribe medication for treating attention deficit hyperactivity disorder (ADHD) so that patients across the lifespan get optimal benefits from these medications. In the chapter, we summarize the evidence base for the pharmacological treatment of ADHD and relevant guideline recommendations for prescribing ADHD medications in the UK.

There is good evidence from randomized controlled trials (RCTs) and meta-analyses for the efficacy of stimulants (amphetamines and methylphenidate) and non-stimulant medications (atomoxetine, bupropion and guanfacine) in treating ADHD. There is some evidence for treating ADHD with co-morbid substance use disorder (SUD), but not for other common co-morbid conditions such as depression, anxiety, personality disorders, bipolar affective disorder or neurodevelopmental conditions (e.g. autism spectrum disorder, Tourette syndrome). The optimal clinical management of non-complicated ADHD and ADHD with co-morbid mental and physical health problems requires careful selection and titration of medication as part of a shared decision-making (SDM) process with ongoing psychoeducation.

Service models and prescribing for specific populations (*preschool children, university students, athletes, men who have sex with men, women, certain females, faith groups and older adults*) are illustrated. Considerations are also given to placebo effects, practicalities of dose titration and the non-prescribed use of stimulant medications.

13.2 History of Drugs Used to Treat ADHD

Amphetamines and methylphenidate are some of the oldest central nervous system (CNS) medications still in use and prescribed in contemporary psychiatry. *Amphetamine* was first synthesized in 1887 in Berlin by the Romanian chemist, Lazăr Edeleanu. Smith, Kline and French (SKF) then patented amphetamine in 1932 and marketed it as a Benzedrine Inhaler, a nasal decongestant, in a capped tube with 325 mg of base racemic amphetamine that a person could inhale every hour as needed. It was sold over the counter until concerns of abuse led SKF to cease production in 1949, and in 1959, the US Food and Drug Administration (FDA) made the product a prescription only item (Jackson, 1971). The first case series on the beneficial effects of Benzedrine in children with ADHD-like symptoms was published by Charles Bradley in 1936. These coincidental findings heralded the modern era of pharmacological treatments for ADHD.

Methylphenidate was first synthesized in 1944 in Basel by the Argentinean chemist Leandro Panizzon, who named it Ritalin (after his wife Rita). The positive effects of methylphenidate on ADHD-like symptoms in children were first reported by Keith Conners in the 1960s. The first double-blind placebo trial of treatment in 15 adults with ADHD was published by Wood et al. (1976). In 2002, the first non-stimulant for treating ADHD, *atomoxetine* (Strattera), was approved by the FDA.

Prescriptions of ADHD medication have increased in most industrialized countries over the last 30 years, perhaps with overprescribing in some parts of the USA (Taylor, 2017). In the UK, however, ADHD continues to be underdiagnosed and undertreated; less than 2% of children and less than 0.1% of adults (19–45 years) were on prescribed ADHD medication in 2015, up from 'virtually zero' for adults in 1990 (Renoux et al., 2016).

13.3 Pharmacology and Mechanisms of Action

Stimulants and non-stimulants used to treat ADHD act on dopamine (DA) and/or noradrenaline (NA) neurotransmission, either as reuptake inhibitors, presynaptic releasers or receptor agonists. The pharmacokinetics of these agents are either short-acting (immediate release, IR), or medium- to long-acting (modified/extended release, MR or XL) (see Table 13.1). The role of DA and NA in causing ADHD is not fully understood. However, ADHD medications are designed to activate the brainstem arousal system and cortical networks, to produce a stimulant effect and improve cognitive function. Methylphenidate blocks the reuptake of DA and NA in presynaptic neurons, thereby increasing the release of these monoamines into the synaptic space. Amphetamines have a similar mechanism of action to methylphenidate with additional presynaptic release of DA and NA and inhibition of serotonin reuptake (Heal et al., 2013). Lisdexamfetamine is a prodrug that is broken down into active dexamfetamine when binding to red blood cells, resulting in slow onset of action and lower abuse potential, even when injected (Faraone, 2018).

Non-stimulants, such as atomoxetine, bupropion or guanfacine, are used to treat ADHD when stimulants cannot be tolerated, or when patients are not responding to them. Atomoxetine is a selective NA reuptake inhibitor, bupropion a DA and NA reuptake inhibitor and guanfacine a selective agonist of the α_2-adrenergic receptor. The advantages of non-stimulants over stimulants are their 24-hour effects, minimal potential for abuse and not being scheduled as controlled substances (British Association for Psychopharmacology, 2016; Canadian ADHD Resource Alliance, 2018).

Stimulants (amphetamines and methylphenidate), unlike most other pharmacological agents used in psychiatry, start having an effect a few hours after ingesting them and take full effect after one week of titration. Non-stimulants, however, have a much slower onset of action and dose titration can take more than six weeks.

13.4 Legal Status and Licensing of Drugs for Treating ADHD

This section refers to the legal and licensing status within the UK for drugs used to treat ADHD at the time this chapter was revised (2019). In the UK, amphetamines and methylphenidate are controlled 'class B' substances. Possession without a prescription carries a prison sentence of up to 5 years or an unlimited fine, or both; supplying carries a

Table 13.1 Medicines to treat ADHD in adults (products available in the UK)

Substance	Product name	UK licence for ADHD	Caps./tabs. per box	Available dosages (mg)	Starting dose (mg)	Titration duration[a]	BNF limit (mg)	Duration of action (hours)	Costs[b] per box in £ (maximum)
First-line stimulants (NICE, 2018)									
Lisdexamfetamine	Elvanse Adult (Elvanse)	adults only (C&A only)	28 capsules	30, 50, 70 (20, 30, 40, 50, 60, 70)	30 (20)	6 weeks	70	8–14	83.16 (83.16)
Methylphenidate ER (OROS)	Concerta XL	continuation licence	30 tablets	18, 27, 36, 54	10	6 weeks	108	8–12	73.62
Methylphenidate ER	Delmosart XL Matoride XL Xaggitin XL Xenidate XL	C&A only	30 (28, 100) tablets	17, 27, 36, 54 18, 36, 54 18, 27, 36, 54 18, 27, 36, 54	18	6 weeks	54	8–12	36.81 36.80 36.80 36.79
Methylphenidate ER	Equasym XL	C&A only	30 capsules	10, 20, 30	10	6 weeks	60	8–10	35.00
Methylphenidate ER	Medikinet XL	full licence	30 capsules	5, 10, 20, 30, 40, 50, 60	10 (5)	6 weeks	80	6–8	67.32
Methylphenidate IR	NP Medikinet Ritalin Tranquilyn	C&A only	30 (20, 28, 40) tablets	5, 10, 20 5, 10, 20 10 5, 10, 20	5–10 TDS (or BD)	6 weeks	100	3–5	9.28–10.92 10.92 6.68 10.92
Other stimulants (third line or not recommended by NICE, 2018)									
Caffeine[c]	Pro-Plus etc.	(food supplement)	48 tablets	50	50–100 BD or TDS	n/a	n/a (400)	1–3	(3.99)
Dexamfetamine	Amfexa NP	C&A only	30 tablets 28 tablets OS	5, 10, 20 5 150, 500 ml	5 (2.5) BD		60	4–6	79.56 24.75 114.49

Table 13.1 (cont.)

Substance	Product name	UK licence for ADHD	Caps./tabs. per box	Available dosages (mg)	Starting dose (mg)	Titration duration[a]	BNF limit (mg)	Duration of action (hours)	Costs[b] per box in £ (maximum)
Modafinil[c]	NP, Provigil	(narcolepsy)	30 tablets	100, 200 100, 200	100 (50)		400	10–16	9.12 105.21
Non-stimulants									
Atomoxetine	Strattera	full licence	7 capsules/ 28 capsules OS	10, 18, 25, 40, 60, 80, 100 300 ml	40 (10)		120	24	13.28 /70.79 85.00
Bupropion ER	Zyban	(smoking cessation)	60 tablets	150	150 (75)		300	12	41.76
Guanfacine[c]	Intuniv	C&A only	28 tablets	1, 2, 3, 4	1	6 weeks	7	24	76.16

[a] As recommended by NICE (2018), [b] BNF (2018), [c] not recommended by NICE (2018). BD, twice daily; C&A, child & adolescents; ER/IR, extended/immediate release; NP, non-proprietary; OS, oral solution; TDS: three times daily.

prison sentence of up to 14 years or an unlimited fine, or both (*Misuse of Drugs Act* 1971 (c. 38): Schedule 2: Controlled Drugs). The import of stimulants is illegal in some countries, even for personal use and patients should contact the embassy (or high commission) for country-specific advice and carry relevant documentation (copy of clinic letter and/or prescription).

Atomoxetine, dexamfetamine, lisdexamfetamine and methylphenidate are licensed for the treatment of ADHD in the UK; atomoxetine (Strattera® since 2013), lisdexamfetamine (Elvanse Adult® since 2015) and methylphenidate (Medikinet XL® since 2018) have full licences for treating adults. Concerta XL® (and similar generic brands) had transitional licences at the time of preparing this book (2018). Prescriptions for dexamfetamine (various brands), methylphenidate IR (various brands) and Equasym XL® are 'off-label' for adults but recommended by the National Institute for Health and Care Excellence (NICE, 2018) and the *British National Formulary* (BNF), which has dose limits for adults (for more details see Table 13.1). The Royal College of Psychiatrists (RCPsych) Psychopharmacology Committee has released updated guidelines on the *Use of licensed medicines for unlicensed applications in psychiatric practice* (Boilson et al., 2017). Online versions of the latest summaries of product characteristics (SPCs) are available on the following webpage: www.medicines.org.uk/emc.

Mixed amphetamine salts (e.g. Adderall®, which is popular in the USA) are not licensed in the UK (or elsewhere in Europe) though can be imported and used on a named-patient basis; the high cost for this, however, makes National Health Service (NHS) prescribing difficult to justify, if there are less expensive alternatives. Dexmethylphenidate is only licensed in the USA and Switzerland (Kooij et al. 2018). Guanfacine is only licensed for children and adolescents with ADHD, but not for adults. In the UK, bupropion (Zyban®) is only licensed for smoking cessation and is used 'off-label' for treating depression and ADHD. Dexamfetamine (Amfexa and non-proprietary), methylphenidate IR (Medikinet®, Ritalin®, Tranquilin® and non-proprietary) and Equasym XL® are recommended by NICE (2018) and the BNF but prescribed off-label (for more details see Table 13.1). Off-label prescribing and informed consent from patients should be clearly documented.

Modafinil is not licensed for the treatment of ADHD in any country. Methamphetamine is not licensed in the UK, but is available as a prescription drug in some other countries (e.g. Hong Kong, USA). Caffeine can be classified as a CNS stimulant; it is legal and unregulated in the UK, available as coffee/tea, added to drinks or over the counter in tablets (e.g. Pro Plus®). Cannabinoids (medicinal cannabis) are not recommended by any ADHD guidelines; though there has been a positive Phase II study of oromucosal spray (Sativex®) in the UK (Cooper et al., 2017).

13.5 Writing Prescriptions for Stimulants in the UK

Medicines may be prescribed by 'brand' (proprietary) or 'generic' (recommended International Non-proprietary Name, rINN) name. Methylphenidate MR preparations contain both IR and MR methylphenidate (see Table 13.1). The purpose of having mixed-release forms is to get an early effect soon after the medicine is taken and to maintain this effect throughout the day. The proportion of IR and MR methylphenidate differs between brands; different preparations may not have the same clinical effect and brand-name prescribing is explicitly recommended (UK Medicines Information, 2017).

Specific rules need to be followed when prescribing stimulants that are classified as controlled drugs in the UK. These rules include the following:

- The prescription must give the total quantity of the preparation in both words and figures.
- Medications can only be prescribed for 30 days (exemptions need to be explained on prescriptions, e.g. longer absence abroad).
- Special FP10PCD prescription forms ('pink form') need to be used for prescribing in private practice (prescription pads and six-digit prescriber identification number for qualified prescribers can be obtained from local Clinical Commissioning Groups).

For more details see the Pharmaceutical Service Negotiating Committee (PSNC) webpage: https://psnc.org.uk/dispensing-supply/dispensing-controlled-drugs.

13.6 Shared Decision Making/Psychoeducation

Medication should not be prescribed to patients without first explaining the benefits, the potential side effects and alternative treatment options including no treatment. Frameworks that conceptualize this clinical practice are: *shared decision making* (SDM) and *psychoeducation*. SDM is a process that places the patient (and their family/carers) at the centre of decisions that are made about their treatment and care. This means the prescriber explores medication options, risks and benefits together with the patient before a shared decision is made to prescribe. Slade (2017) lists essential elements of the SDM process as follows:

- define and explain the healthcare problem
- present options
- discuss benefits/risks/costs
- clarify patient values/preferences
- discuss patient ability/self-efficacy
- present what is known and make recommendations
- clarify the patient's understanding
- make (or explicitly defer) a decision.

Communicating like this, in a patient-centred manner, is associated with increases in service-user satisfaction, adherence with treatment and better health outcomes (Coulter & Collins, 2011).

Psychoeducation is the provision of information and advice about ADHD to service users. This is recommended by NICE (2018) as the first step in the treatment of ADHD. Provision of information from clinicians regarding ADHD and treatment options is a strong predictor for service-user satisfaction (Solberg et al., 2019). Prescribers should talk to their patients (and family members) about ADHD, listen to their concerns and provide them with oral and written information about stimulant and non-stimulant medications. We recommend the following *webpages and internet sources* for educational materials on ADHD:

- Choice and Medication (www.choiceandmedication.org – branded versions of patient information leaflets (PILLs) with NHS trust logo available).
- Royal College of Psychiatrists (www.rcpsych.org – Adult ADHD leaflet, Scottish Adult ADHD guideline etc.).
- The Canadian ADHD Resource Alliance (www.caddra.ca – free registration, questionnaires and information leaflets).
- UK Adult ADHD Network (www.ukaan.org – for professionals).

NICE (2018) also recommends environmental modifications before starting the pharmacological treatment of ADHD. Some questions to ask patients in this regard are:

- Is there anything that helps you to concentrate better?
- Do you drink coffee, tea, coke or energy drinks? If yes, how much caffeine per day?
- Where do you get your thrills or highs from (for neurobiological minded patients: Where do you get your bursts of noradrenaline and dopamine from)?
- Have you ever taken a stimulant like cocaine? If yes, what were the effects that you noticed? (Patients with ADHD describe 'paradoxical' calming effects.)

Dopamine release is associated with activities promising reward (e.g. gambling, sex, romantic love, professional success), while *noradrenaline* is associated with novelty and stress (e.g. thrill seeking, deadline stress, fear of failure). Successful treatment of ADHD with stimulants may reduce thrill- and high-seeking activities (e.g. watching online porn, dangerous driving) and recreational substance use (e.g. drinking excessive amounts of coffee). This should be conceptualized and explained. Multimodal approaches are often required to effectively manage and/or treat ADHD. These approaches include both the use of medication as well as non-pharmacological interventions (e.g. parent and teacher training, cognitive behavioural therapies (CBT), mindfulness, coaching).

13.7 Efficacy of Drug Treatment

Systematic reviews and meta-analyses of RCTs consistently demonstrate the efficacy and safety of stimulants (amphetamines and methylphenidate) and non-stimulants (atomoxetine and bupropion) in the treatment of ADHD across the lifespan. A recent debate about controversial findings and interpretation of meta-analyses of RCTs with methylphenidate in children and adolescents with ADHD highlighted the wide range of available evidence and the need for methodological improvements (Cortese, 2018). RCTs are often performed on highly selected study patients with no or little co-morbidity and the duration can be for a couple of weeks only.

A *meta-review* of 40 systematic reviews and meta-analyses relevant to the pharmacological and non-pharmacological treatment of ADHD in adults addressed clinically relevant questions that face healthcare practitioners in daily decision making about treatments (De Crescenzo et al., 2017). Key findings that emerged from this review are as follows:

- Overall, pharmacological treatments are significantly more efficacious than placebo but are less well accepted and tolerated.
- Drugs that are more efficacious than placebo are methylphenidate (IR and XL); dextroamphetamine, lisdexamfetamine, mixed amphetamine salts and atomoxetine. *There is no difference in efficacy between atomoxetine and methylphenidate XL.*

- Effect sizes for efficacy versus placebo are higher for amphetamines than for methylphenidate or atomoxetine.
- There are no published meta-analytically based hierarchies on the efficacy and acceptability of all available ADHD drugs in adults.
- There is no evidence from systematic reviews/meta-analyses on the efficacy of multimodal treatment in adults.

Guanfacine MR has been shown to be effective in children and adolescents with ADHD (Ruggiero et al., 2014). Morning and evening dosing of guanfacine MR are equally effective (Newcorn et al., 2013) and sedative effects do not drive the improvement of inattentive and hyperactive/impulsive symptoms (Huss et al., 2019). A RCT in adults, where guanfacine MR was added on to stimulant medication, found no difference compared with a placebo add-on (Butterfield et al., 2016). A positive RCT of monotherapy with guanfacine MR in adult Japanese patients was presented at a conference in April 2019 (Iwanami et al., 2019).

Cortese et al. (2018) published the most comprehensive comparative evaluation of 133 RCTs (81 in children and adolescents, 51 in adults and 1 in both). The efficacy meta-analysis in children and adolescents with ADHD included 21 placebo-controlled RCTs with atomoxetine, 9 with methylphenidate, 6 with amphetamines and 6 with guanfacine. All drugs were superior to placebo. For the efficacy analysis in adults, 11 RCTs with atomoxetine, 11 with methylphenidate and 5 with amphetamines (mixed amphetamine salts or lisdexamfetamine) were included. In adults (based on clinicians' ratings), amphetamines (effect size −0.79), methylphenidate (−0.49), bupropion (−0.46) and atomoxetine (−0.45), but not modafinil (0.16), were better than placebo (see Figure 13.1). With respect to tolerability – amphetamines, atomoxetine, methylphenidate and modafinil in adults were less well tolerated than placebo. There are very few head-to-head studies comparing stimulants and non-stimulants in adults. Only two RCTs with lisdexamfetamine in adults were included in this meta-analysis and the authors did '*not feel confident at this stage to recommend lisdexamfetamine over other amphetamines for adults*' (p. 9).

13.8 New Drugs on the ADHD Portfolio

In the last 10 years we have seen considerable investment in RCTs of new and established ADHD medications. New preparations of stimulants such as chewable tablets, oral solutions, triple-bead capsules with longer duration of action and capsules with daytime release that can be taken in the evening are on the way to the US market (Cortese et al., 2017). Innovative medications are now often first being investigated in adults with ADHD, because informed consent is easier to obtain. According to information published on ClinicalTrials.gov and news on company webpages, Phase III trials of metadoxine (Alcobra) and vortioxetine (Lundbeck), a multimodal serotonin reuptake inhibitor/serotonin receptor agent (Biederman et al., 2019), were negative. Most drugs in development for ADHD continue to focus on enhancing DA and NA (e.g. centanafadine, fasoracetam, dasotraline, mazindol, molindone and viloxazine). These substances are being tested in Phase II and III trials and may enter the market. Mechanisms of action and side-effect profiles/contraindications of these substances overlap with those of medications already available (Caye et al., 2019).

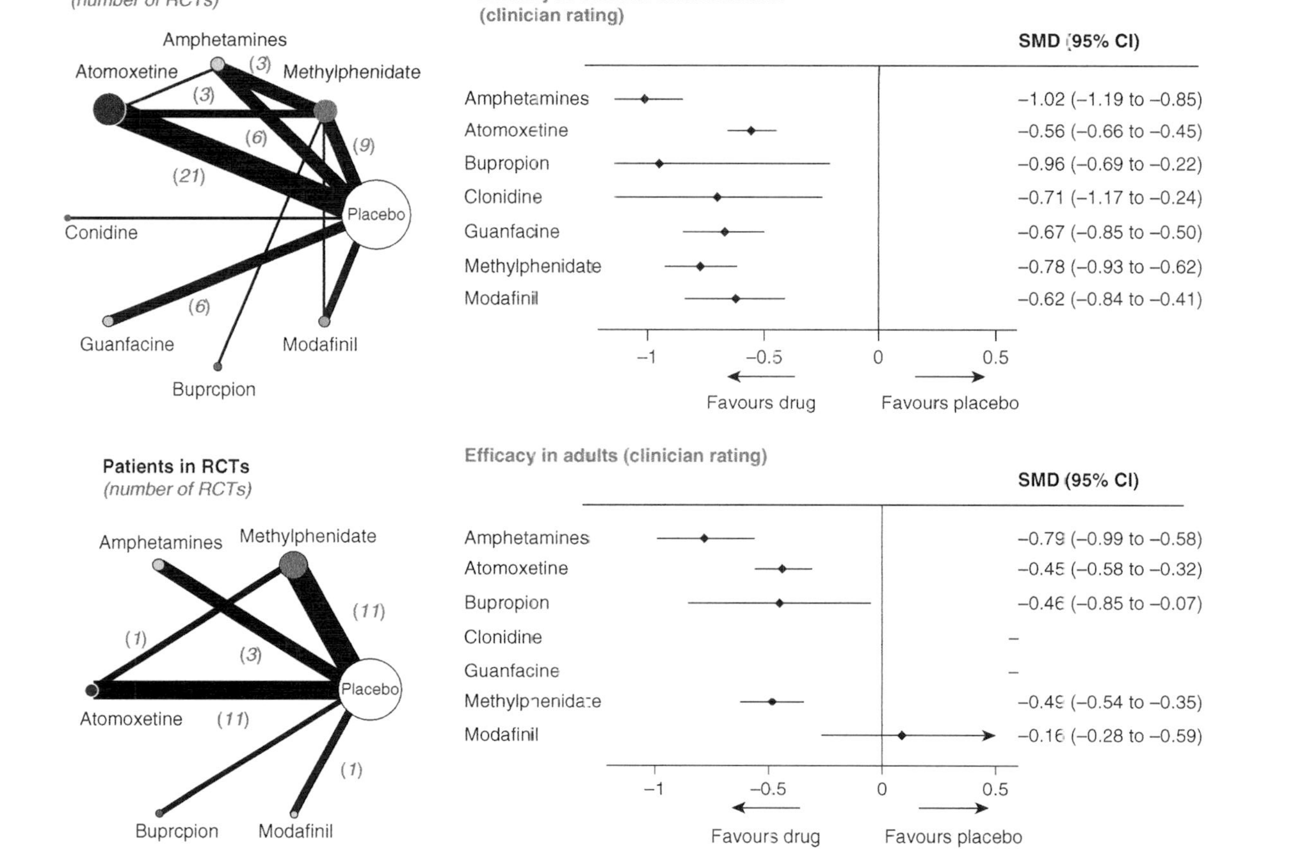

Figure 13.1 Network meta-analyses of medications to treat ADHD (Cortese et al., 2018). Left: Number of patients and RCTs selected for meta-analyses in children and adolescents (upper panel) and adults (lower panels); right: Forrest plot of efficacy rated by clinicians (no RCTs for clonidine and guanfacine in adults were included).

Only one pharmacological agent, dasotraline, has made it from a positive clinical trial to an FDA (licence) application for adults with ADHD in the USA; a negative response letter was issued by the FDA in August 2018 asking for more clinical data (see Sunovion webpage). Dasotraline is a stereoisomer of desmethyl-sertraline, which blocks DA and NA transporters and has a long half-life of 47–77 hours. Once-daily doses of 4 mg and 8 mg reduced ADHD symptoms significantly more than placebo in a 5-week RCT in adults; insomnia got worse after dasotraline compared with placebo (Koblan et al., 2015). A 6-week RCT in children (6–12 years) with ADHD found that 4 mg (but not 2 mg) of dasotraline were superior to placebo (Findling et al., 2019).

13.9 Longer-Term Use of Medications

The National Institute of Mental Health (NIMH) Collaborative Multimodal Treatment of ADHD (MTA) study of 579 children with combined type ADHD and 258 classmate controls was originally designed to compare the effects of medication management, intensive behavioural treatment (parent, child and school components with therapist involvement gradually reduced over time), the combination of both and treatment as usual. Over the 14 months of the RCT medication management (alone or in combination with behavioural treatment) was superior. In the longer term high baseline severity, lower IQ and lower household income in childhood were the main predictors for poor functional outcomes in adulthood (Roy et al., 2017). Extended use of medication throughout childhood was associated with lower height in adulthood, but not with reduction of symptom severity in adulthood (Swanson et al., 2017). The longest RCT of methylphenidate in adults with ADHD lasted 12 months and was part of a four-arm psychotherapy versus pharmacotherapy study that could not demonstrate a benefit of the combination of methylphenidate (titrated and monitored by experts in adult ADHD) with group CBT (Philipsen et al., 2015).

Longer-term use of prescribed stimulants has been investigated in cohort and registry studies. In these studies, cohorts of adults with ADHD have been followed up for up to 6 years (Edvinsson & Ekselius, 2018a, 2018b). Adherence to medication after one year was down to 40–60%, but this is still higher than in similar studies in children. Psychosocial outcomes are generally better when adults with ADHD stay on prescribed medication. In one Dutch cohort study, women and higher educated patients were more likely to discontinue treatment (Bijlenga et al., 2017). High dropout rates from 20% to 50% within the first year of treatment was also observed in one Danish study, especially when appointments were missed (Soendergaard et al., 2016). A one-year clinical audit from Norway in 232 patients (164 on medication) demonstrates that psychiatric co-morbidity and side effects were related to lower effectiveness and more frequent termination of stimulants and atomoxetine; the Adult ADHD Symptoms Rating Scale (ASRS) was used to document symptom improvement over time (Fredriksen et al., 2014).

Pharmaco-epidemiological studies from Sweden, Denmark and Taiwan have investigated real life effects of ADHD medication (see meta-analysis of Chang et al., 2019). Patients with a diagnosis of ADHD had higher risks of criminal offending (Lichtenstein et al., 2012), sexually transmitted infection (Chen et al., 2018), road traffic accidents (Chang et al., 2014) and other physical injuries (Man et al., 2017) that were all reduced when patients were on prescribed ADHD medication. Similar studies found that ADHD medication was associated with a reduced long-term risk for depression and reduced rates of concurrent depression; within-individual analysis suggested that occurrence of depression was 20% less common during periods when patients received ADHD medication compared with periods when they did not (Chang et al., 2016).

13.10 Placebo Effects in RCTs and Clinical Practice

Most RCTs of ADHD medications show considerable placebo effects (in adults and children/adolescents). Placebo effects are stronger in trials where a formal programme of psychoeducation was delivered (e.g. Rösler et al., 2009) and relatively negligible in trials where only medication was prescribed to patients with severe forms of ADHD (Ginsberg & Lindefors, 2012). Placebo effects can be reduced by using a placebo lead-in period and excluding high placebo responders from the subsequent trial (Adler et al., 2009). Placebo effects in RCTs of ADHD medications submitted to the FDA for approval have increased over time (Khan et al., 2017).

Prescribers need to be aware of placebo effects and the 'honeymoon' effect, which is observed as extreme improvement during the first weeks of treatment and these effects are often not sustained. Most patients learn to differentiate real effects of stimulants from additional placebo (and nocebo) effects.

13.11 Adverse Effects of ADHD Medicines and Monitoring

It is well known that both stimulants and non-stimulants used in the treatment of ADHD are associated with a range of adverse effects (for a summary see Table 13.2). These adverse effects are generally reported as mild, self-limiting and well tolerated (Graham et al., 2011). They include cardiovascular effects (*increased blood pressure typically 5–10 mmHg and heart rate*). NICE (2018) recommends that '*before starting medication for ADHD, people with ADHD should have a full assessment, which should include: . . . baseline pulse and blood pressure . . ., a cardiovascular assessment [and] an electrocardiogram (ECG) if the treatment may affect the QT interval*'. The NICE 2018 guideline clearly states, '*do not offer routine blood tests (including liver function tests) or ECGs to people taking medication for ADHD unless there is a clinical indication*'. Concerns have been raised about extreme adverse effects such as cardiac death. But it seems to be so uncommon that a very large number of patients will be needed to detect if the risk is more than the base rate of cardiac death in the general population (Graham & Coghill, 2008).

Other typical side effects are neurological effects (*headache, dizziness, insomnia*); psychiatric effects (*nervousness, anxiety/mood*); and gastroenterological effects (*dry mouth, abdominal pain/discomfort, nausea, vomiting, poor appetite*). Patients tend to report nausea/vomiting, abdominal pain and headache in the first weeks of commencing treatment. Typically, these effects reduce appetite and can result in weight loss. These effects tend to remit in the evening, leading some patients to experience rebound binge eating, which can result in weight gain. If stimulants are taken too late in the day, they can interfere with sleep. Both guanfacine and atomoxetine, however, have sedating effects and can aid sleep at night (British Association for Psychopharmacology, 2014).

Table 13.2 Common side effects associated with drugs used to treat ADHD

	Dexamfetamine/ Lisdexamfetamine	Methylphenidate IR/ER	Atomoxetine	Bupropion	Guanfacine ER
Increased blood pressure + heart rate	++	++	+	+	–
Palpitations	+	+			
Headache	++	++	+	+	++
Reduced appetite	++	++	+		+
Nausea/vomiting/stomach ache	+	+	++	+	++
Diarrhoea	+	+			
Constipation			+		+
Dry mouth	+	+	++		
Insomnia	+				+
Irritability/mood changes		+ (1)			+
Tics	+	+	–		
Cough/nasopharyngitis	+	+			
Erectile dysfunction/reduced libido		+	++	–	–
Epileptic seizures				+	
Urinary incontinence					+
Sedation	–		+		++

IR/ER = immediate/extended release, (1) end of dose phenomenon.

In 2005, the Committee for Safety of Medicines (CSM) issued guidance following reports of rare but severe hepatic disorders associated with the use of atomoxetine. This guidance advised discontinuation with no future use of atomoxetine in patients with laboratory evidence of liver injury. It seems to be a rare adverse effect; therefore, routine liver function tests in patients prescribed atomoxetine have not been recommended. Clinicians should still be vigilant in spotting early signs of hepatic disorders (e.g. persistent and unexplained malaise, jaundice, dark urine or itching).

The potential for psychiatric adverse effects (e.g. suicidal ideation, mania or psychosis) means that all patients should be monitored for signs of depression, suicidal thoughts or behaviour and referred for appropriate treatment if necessary. A pharmaco-epidemiological study of 337 919 adolescents and young adults (13–25 years) with ADHD from the USA found a risk of stimulant-related onset of psychosis of 1:500 for amphetamines and 1:1000 for methylphenidate (Moran et al., 2019).

Immediate-release amphetamines have a higher potential for abuse. Administration over prolonged periods of time can lead to tolerance and dependence. Attention should be paid to patients who could malinger with ADHD to obtain dexamfetamine (or methylphenidate IR) for non-therapeutic uses or for distribution to others (diversion). Dexamfetamine should not be prescribed as first-line medication. Misuse can cause adverse psychiatric and cardiovascular effects, including sudden death.

There is uncertainty about whether ADHD medications can permanently change neurotransmitter levels or receptor density in the brain. So far, treatment with stimulants for decades in disorders such as narcolepsy have not revealed any problematic signals of altered brain functioning (Thorpy, 2015) and there are no clinical reports of long-term use of ADHD drugs being associated with cognitive malfunction or brain damage (Graham et al., 2011). Novel techniques of investigation (e.g. pharmacogenomics, repeated monitoring of bloods levels and neuroimaging) certainly have potential to yield new insights into how the brain responds to ADHD medications in the short and long term.

For most clinicians, the benefits of treatment versus cost/risks are likely to influence their prescribing practice. The European Medicines Agency (EMA) review of the safety of medicines containing methylphenidate has concluded that their benefits outweigh the risks associated with cardiovascular, cerebrovascular and psychiatric safety and long-term effects (EMEA, 2009). As with all medicines, prescribing clinicians will be responsible for ongoing monitoring of efficacy and potential adverse effects.

13.12 Prescribing Recommendations in ADHD Guidelines

There are a wide range of ADHD guidelines with recommendations for the assessment and management of ADHD in adults. These guidelines are based on the best available evidence or expert consensus. The authors recommend the following British and international guidelines for prescribers in the United Kingdom (see Seixas et al., 2012 for methodological evaluations):

- British Association for Psychopharmacology (BAP, 2006/2014)
- National Institute for Health and Care Excellence (NICE, 2008/2018)
- European Network Adult ADHD/EPA Special interest group (ENAA, 2010/2019)
- Royal College of Psychiatrists in Scotland (Boilson et al., 2017)
- Canadian ADHD Resource Alliance (CADDRA, 2018).

Table 13.3 Factors to be considered in the selection of the first medication treatment for ADHD

Effectiveness	Stimulants are the most effective class	Prefer stimulants for moderate to severe cases
Adverse effects	Non-stimulants (especially atomoxetine) have different profile of adverse effects	Prefer non-stimulants in case of intolerance to stimulants or when specific adverse effects are a special concern
Duration of action	Modified-release formulations of stimulants last for 8–12 hours (in most patients)	Atomoxetine has 24-hour efficacy, including evening and night hours; consider atomoxetine when the effect is desired for more than one segment of the day
Abuse potential	Immediate-release stimulants have theoretical abuse liability	Non-stimulants (or MR stimulants) might be an option when abuse is a relevant concern
Time to onset of effect	Stimulants have immediate onset/offset of action	Prefer stimulants when immediate onset/predicted offset is needed
Patient (and carer) preferences	Patients (and carers) might have personal opinions on existing options	Consider patient (and carer) preferences, provide evidence-based information

Modified from Caye et al. (2019).

The 2018 NICE guidelines refer to the diagnosis and treatment of ADHD in children, young people and adults. Recommendations in NICE guidelines are the gold standard for the NHS. The following new recommendations for the treatment of ADHD have been added to NICE (2018) (compared to NICE, 2008):

- Cardiac examination (including auscultation) of every patient (this can be difficult to organize for patients under mental health services)
- *Children aged 5 and over and young people*: First-line methylphenidate (short or long acting) if ADHD symptoms are causing persistent significant impairment in at least one domain and after parent training, group-based support and environmental modifications
- *Adults*: Lisdexamfetamine (or methylphenidate) first-line after environmental modications. If no benefit after 6 weeks, switch to methylphenidate (or lisdexamfetamine)
- Dexamfetamine if a patient responds to lisdexamfetamine but cannot tolerate the longer effect profile
- Atomoxetine if stimulants are not tolerated or contraindicated
- Top-up with IR stimulants if required

- Slower titration time in patients with co-morbidities
- Do not offer guanfacine or modafinil to adults with ADHD [recommendation for guanfacine may change when results of RCT in adult are published]
- Shared decision making [with patient and family members]
- Referral to tertiary service [if first- and second-line treatments do not work and for discussion of complex cases]

13.13 Personalized Drug Selection, Titration and Dose Regimens

Several factors need to be considered for the personalized selection of the first medication or alternative medication if the first choice does not work or is not tolerated (Table 13.3). Treatment sequences have not been evaluated in clinical research. Most guidelines recommend stimulants as first-line medication across the lifespan. Coghill et al. (2019) suggest questions like the following before switching to another medication:

- Have I titrated properly?
- Is the dose too low/too high?
- Should I titrate up to the maximum dose?
- Is this medication working well throughout the day?
- Have I got good enough collateral information (family, school/college/working place)?
- Are all parties in agreement about the effects of the medication?
- Are we targeting the right symptoms?
- Is there a behavioural explanation for the drug 'wearing off' (e.g. fatigue, conflicts at home)?
- Is the medication working but effects limited by side effects?
- Have I missed any co-morbidity?
- Does the initial diagnosis have to be re-evaluated?

Published RCTs of stimulants tend to use relatively fast titration regimens with one to three dose increases per week over a period of three days to six weeks (Müller-Sedgwick et al., 2018). NICE (2018) recommend six-week trials up to 'an adequate dose' of lisdexamfetamine and methylphenidate in line with the BNF; slower dose titration and more frequent monitoring are recommended for patients with co-morbidities. Most ADHD clinics in the UK titrate patients slower than within six weeks and often book patients for four-weekly follow-up appointments. There are pros and cons of fast versus slow titration of stimulant and more research is needed. Shared decision making (SDM) is important at all stages of medication management (Kooij, 2012). Table 13.4 lists a series of questions that clinician and patient should answer if results are suboptimal at the end of the titration process (Coghill et al., 2019).

NICE (2018) explicitly recommends the 'topping-up' of long-acting stimulants with short-acting stimulants: '*Think about using immediate- and modified-release preparations of stimulants to optimise effect (for example, a modified-release preparation of methylphenidate in the morning and an immediate-release preparation of*

Table 13.4 Questions you should ask before changing to another drug (Coghill et al., 2019)

- Have I titrated properly?
- Is the patient at the maximum dose?
- Is this drug/preparation working well at any times during the day?
- Have I got good enough information from school?
- Are parents and school in agreement about the effects of the drug?
- Am I targeting the right symptoms?
- Is there a behavioural explanation for the drug 'wearing off'?
- What else is going on in patient's life/family life?
- Is the medication working but effects limited by side effects?
- Have I missed any co-morbidity?
- Is the diagnosis right?

methylphenidate at another time of the day to extend the duration of effect).' The cost of (short-acting) dexamfetamine is 10–20 times higher than short-acting methylphenidate and this makes topping-up of lisdexamfetamine with dexamfetamine a relatively expensive dosing regimen.

13.14 Adherence to Medication, Drug Holidays and Flexible Dosing

The updated ADHD guidelines from NICE (2018) recommend that people with ADHD must be encouraged to use the following strategies to support adherence with treatment:

- *Be responsible for their own health, including taking medication as needed*
- *Follow instructions about how to take their medication using picture or written format. These instructions will include information on dose, duration, adverse effects and dosage schedule.*
- *Take medication as part of their daily routine (e.g. before meals or after brushing teeth)*
- *Use visual reminders to take medication (e.g. apps, alarms, clocks, pill dispensers, or notes on a fridge)*
- *Attend peer support groups (for both the person with ADHD and their families and/or carers).*

'Drug holidays' or breaks in taking medication are recommended for children and adolescents with ADHD to improve overall compliance with prescribed stimulants (Graham et al., 2011). One RCT randomized children with ADHD to receive seven days of methylphenidate or five days of methylphenidate + two days of placebo on weekends; weekend holidays during methylphenidate administration reduce the side effects of insomnia and appetite suppression without a significant increase in symptoms, either on weekends or in the first school day after them (Martins et al., 2004). Drug holidays may help to reduce problems related to tolerance. In his latest review, Taylor (2019) states that '*if tolerance is indeed significant for some treated people, then our attention should shift in research to understanding the mechanisms. In the meantime, it would be logical for clinical practice to include "holidays" from the drugs to allow the brain to recover its responsiveness*' (p. 3). Drug holidays are therefore not only recommended for children and adolescents, but also for adults with ADHD.

Table 13.5 Pros and cons of flexible dosing of stimulants

Pro (benefits of flexible dosing)	Con (risks/disadvantages of flexible dosing)
• Widely practised/patient choice • Not all days are the same • Fexible dosing requires good insight and understanding (of strengths/ weaknesses and of medication effects) • May reduce risk of tolerance/addiction • Lower prescribing costs (less waste)	• Suboptimal effects • Increased risk of poor adherence • No evidence from clinical trials that flexible dosing works better than fixed dosing regimens • Higher risk of overdosing (?) • Non-efficient use of coping strategies/ relapse into dysfunctional patterns of behaviour

Flexible, as needed, dosing and *pro re nata* (PRN) prescribing of stimulants can be used if patients take their medication only on working days, at a lower dose or not at all during the weekend or holidays. A recent survey among university students in Canada revealed that 'flexible dosing' was common among students with ADHD and that they used higher doses of their prescribed stimulants during the week than on weekends (Gould & Doucette, 2018). The authors' clinical experience is that flexible dosing of stimulants seems to be widely practised by university students and adults with ADHD; this is often what a patient decides or prefers to do. However, patients need to have very good knowledge and understanding of the effects and side effects of stimulant medications. Part of the SDM process is about listening to patients (and parents) and being mindful of treatment options or outcomes that patients are seeking. This may include a conversation about the pros and cons of drug holidays and flexible dosing (Table 13.5). The non-stimulant atomoxetine cannot be used flexibly and needs to be re-titrated after discontinuation.

Flexible dosing is a controversial topic amongst clinicians and there are no RCTs that support the flexible use of stimulants in adults. Lower doses as well as poor adherence in clinical trials tend to produce suboptimal effects and lower effect sizes (Caisley & Müller, 2012). Flexible dosing may reduce the risk of tolerance and could lower prescribing costs by lengthening prescribing intervals (e.g. a 30-day prescription could last 6 weeks). Therefore, more research is needed to understand why patients use their stimulant medication flexibly and what are the risks and benefits of this kind of dosing regimen in different groups of patients.

13.15 Annual Review of Medication

Most ADHD clinics in the UK are organized as assessment and dose titration clinics. After titration prescribing is often handed over to general practitioners (GPs) under shared-care agreements; in other countries (USA, Germany) most patients are seen by practice-based paediatricians or psychiatrists. NICE (2008/2018) recommends an annual review of ADHD medication by a '*healthcare professional with training and expertise in managing ADHD*' to make a shared decision about whether the medication should be continued. This review should include a comprehensive assessment of the following (*taken verbatim from the guideline*):

- Preference of the adult with ADHD (and their family or carers as appropriate)
- Benefits, including how well the current treatment is working throughout the day
- Adverse *effects*
- Clinical need and whether medication has been optimized
- Impact on education and employment
- Effects of missing a dose, planned dose reductions or periods of no treatment
- Effect of medication on existing or mental health, physical health or neurodevelopmental conditions
- Need for support and type of support.

Keeping all diagnosed patients registered with an adult ADHD clinic results in ever growing caseloads (and waiting lists). The authors' impression is that patients, who have been stable on their ADHD medication for more than one year, could be reviewed more cost-efficiently in primary care.

13.16 Treating ADHD with Co-morbid Disorders

ADHD often comes along with other mental and physical health conditions, most frequently depression, anxiety, sleep problems, personality and SUD, specific learning and social communication disabilities (Figure 13.2). In clinical samples of adults with ADHD there is a higher prevalence of co-morbidities, with estimates at 50–75% (Kessler et al., 2006). Many core symptoms of ADHD can also be non-specific symptoms of other neurodevelopmental or mental health disorders, which can impede proper recognition and treatment of ADHD. Co-morbid disorders can impact on a patient's insight, response to and adherence to treatment (Kooji et al., 2012). Prescribing clinicians should routinely assess ADHD and associated co-morbid disorders, and vice versa, because this maximizes the efficacy of pharmacotherapies.

Treatment plans should aim to address both ADHD and associated co-morbidities, with the order of prescribing dependent on the type and severity of the co-morbid disorder. General practice stipulates that severe psychiatric disorders should be treated first. This includes inpatients with major depressive disorders, mania or SUD. Afterwards, the diagnosis and treatment for ADHD can be considered.

13.16.1 Anxiety and Depression

The pharmacological treatment of ADHD with co-morbid anxiety can be a clinical challenge. Symptoms of anxiety and resulting avoidance behaviour are confounded and overlap with ADHD symptoms. Stimulants and non-stimulants like atomoxetine have side effects associated with hypertension, palpitations, nausea and dizziness, which are especially problematic in patients with anxiety disorders.

Atomoxetine has some evidence for treatment of ADHD with co-morbid social anxiety (Adler et al., 2009) and bupropion is licensed as an antidepressant in many countries. Very low initial doses of stimulants (e.g. 2.5 mg/half a 5 mg tablet of methylphenidate IR, or 5 mg Medikinet XL® – the smallest dose available for methylphenidate

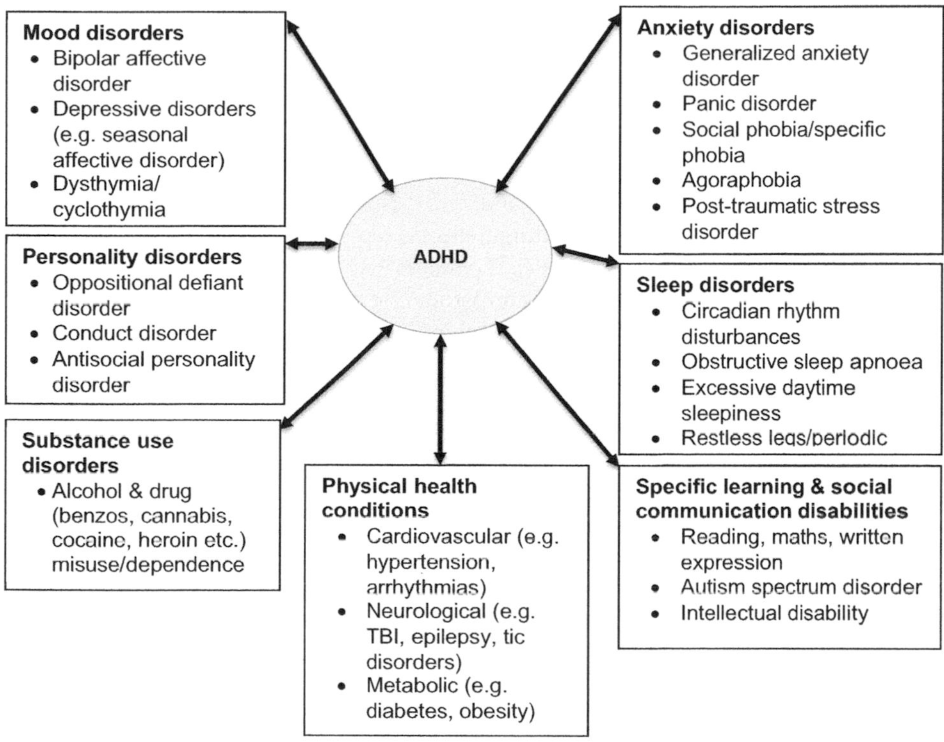

Figure 13.2 Co-morbidities in ADHD (adapted from Kooij et al., 2012). TBI, traumatic brain injury.

ER, or 20 mg of lisdexamfetamine – please note that this dose is only licensed for children and adolescents in the UK) can be used in this population; however, this strategy has yet to be tested in rigorous clinical trials.

No RCTs have explicitly evaluated pharmacological treatments in adults with ADHD and depressive disorders. Patients with milder forms of depression and anxiety are not excluded in most clinical trials of ADHD. One open-label add-on study in children and adolescents with ADHD and depression reported treatment with fluoxetine (n = 127) or placebo (n = 46) for 8 weeks followed by add-on of atomoxetine (ATX) for 5 weeks. At the end of the study 66% of patients on fluoxetine + ATX, and 58% on placebo + ATX had a reduction in ADHD and depressive symptoms (98% after fluoxetine + ATX and 80% after placebo + ATX) (Kratochvil et al., 2005). In a small case series in adults (n = 17) 80% demonstrated improvements in ADHD and depressive symptoms when treated with venlafaxine, compared with 88% of patients treated with combined stimulant and antidepressant and 33% of patients treated with just a stimulant (Hornig-Rohan & Amsterdam, 2002).

Most experts recommend treating co-morbid depression and anxiety first, and then reassessing ADHD-related symptoms to create an effective treatment plan, while others suggest deferring the treatment of anxiety and depressive disorder until after treating ADHD symptoms, as the co-morbid symptoms may resolve once the ADHD is treated (Kooij et al., 2010; Philipsen et al., 2008).

13.16.2 Bipolar Disorder

Even though around 20% of people with bipolar disorder (BD) may have co-morbid ADHD, there are very limited data about treatment responses in this population, especially among adults. While there is evidence for a positive association between methylphenidate and BD among patients taking mood stabilizers, there is also a higher risk of triggering a manic (or hypomanic) episode when initiating methylphenidate in patients with BD not taking a mood stabilizer. It is therefore advisable for prescribing clinicians to rule out BD before initiating monotherapy with a stimulant medication for ADHD symptoms (Viktorin et al., 2017). If patients with milder forms of BD (i.e. no clear manic episode, or no previous hospital admission) are not compliant with, or opposed to, a mood stabilizer then the risk of treatment-emergent mania needs to be clearly documented.

Children and adolescents with ADHD and co-morbid BD have been successfully treated with mixed amphetamine salts, after their mania was stabilized with sodium valproate (Scheffer et al., 2005). A staged approach, initially using a mood stabilizer, when treating patients with ADHD and BD is advisable (Scheffer, 2007).

In one open-label study, atomoxetine was effective in treating children and adolescents with ADHD and BD, also taking a mood stabilizer or antipsychotic (Bahali et al., 2009; Chang et al., 2005). Although there are no comparable studies in adults, when used with caution, stimulants and atomoxetine may be safe and effective for adults with ADHD and BD who are also taking a mood stabilizer.

Based on the evidence so far, treating adults with ADHD and BD only with ADHD medications in the absence of a mood stabilizer is not advisable. Scheffer (2010) recommends the following regimen:

- Ascertain a clear diagnosis of co-morbid ADHD and BD.
- Treat BD first (the more serious condition) with lithium or another mood stabilizer (quetiapine or lamotrigine); avoid lithium and valproate in women of childbearing potential.
- Add ADHD medication (stimulant or atomoxetine), if symptoms of ADHD continue to be troubling after mood stabilization.

13.16.3 Personality Disorders

It can be difficult to ascertain if an adult with ADHD has a borderline personality disorder (BPD)/emotionally unstable personality disorder or antisocial personality disorder, because symptoms of either condition could be an artefact of the symptoms that overlap between them (Philipsen et al., 2008). Long-term psychotherapy (e.g. dialectical behaviour therapy or schema therapy) is usually indicated for people with BPD, but it may also be useful for adults with ADHD and BPD (Philipsen et al., 2007).

There are case reports of successful use of methylphenidate in the treatment of ADHD and BDP (Hooberman & Stern, 1984; van Reekum & Links, 1994). In one open-label study, Golubchik et al. (2008) used methylphenidate for 12 weeks to treat 14 adolescent females with ADHD and BPD. Significant improvements in ADHD symptoms, BPD severity, aggressive and self-injurious behaviours were observed. In another study with 12 adolescent females with ADHD and BPD, methylphenidate was also found to 'attenuate smoking behaviour' (Golubchik et al., 2009).

Both ADHD and BPD are characterized by impulsivity; a behaviour which could involve the serotonergic and noradrenergic systems (Dalley & Rosier, 2012). In some studies, pharmacological agents that affect these systems (e.g. selective serotonin reuptake inhibitors (SSRIs) and atypical antipsychotics) were found to reduce impulsivity in BPD. They might do the same in ADHD, given that serotonergic dysfunction has also been reported (Stoffers et al., 2010). Clonidine, an α_2-adrenoreceptor agonist like guanfacine, has been reported to reduce impulsivity and hyperactivity in children and adolescents with ADHD, as well as attenuating aversive inner tension, urges to self-harm, dissociative symptoms and suicidal ideation in female patients with BPD (Philipsen et al., 2004).

Pharmacological treatments for adults with ADHD and BPD have yet to be investigated in large-scale RCTs. This makes it difficult to predict treatment outcomes for individual patients. Clinical experience indicates that if core symptoms of ADHD are treated and improve, some patients with co-morbid personality disorders can become less distressed, show less mood instability, become more functional in their day-to-day lives and have better impulse control. This treatment response is not the same for all patients with ADHD and personality disorders (Asherson et al., 2014). However, given the potential benefits, it remains advisable to treat ADHD in patients with co-morbid personality disorders.

13.16.4 Substance Use Disorder

There is increasing evidence from meta-analyses of cohort studies that ADHD medication does not increase the risk of substance use (Humphreys et al., 2013). The latest meta-analysis of RCTs in patients with ADHD + co-morbid substance use disorder (SUD) showed good effects of stimulants (amphetamines and methylphenidate) and non-stimulants (atomoxetine and bupropion) on ADHD symptoms; however, there were no effects on co-morbid substance use or time of abstinence (Cunill et al., 2015).

There are only two newer RCTs (published after this meta-analysis) that have positive effects on both domains. In a multi-centre study from Sweden, 54 incarcerated men with ADHD and amphetamine dependence were randomized to receive either methylphenidate (Concerta XL®) or placebo and weekly CBT. The men who were treated with high doses (up to 180 mg) of methylphenidate and CBT had significantly higher proportions of negative-drug urine screens and better retention in treatment in comparison with the placebo group (Konstenius et al., 2014). Another RCT demonstrated that treatment with extended-release mixed amphetamine salts (compared with placebo) increased urine-confirmed abstinence among patients with co-occurring ADHD and cocaine dependence; re-analysis of the data showed that abstinence is most likely preceded by improvement in ADHD symptoms, which tends to occur early with medication treatment (Levin et al., 2015, 2018).

A recent *European consensus statement* makes the following recommendations (Crunelle et al., 2018):

- *Consider adequate medical treatment of both ADHD and SUD.*
- *Always consider a combination of psychotherapy and pharmacotherapy.*

- *Integrate the ADHD and other psychiatric comorbidity treatment with SUD treatment as soon as possible.*
- *Psychotherapy, preferentially targeting the combination of ADHD and SUD, should be considered.*
- *Long-acting methylphenidate, extended-release amphetamines [e.g. lisdexamfetamine in Europe], and atomoxetine are effective in the treatment of comorbid ADHD and SUD, and up-titration to higher dosages may be considered in some patients. The abuse potential is limited with slow onset acting [slow onset] agents.*
- *Caution and careful clinical management is needed to prevent abuse and diversion of prescribed stimulants.*

NICE (2018) recommends cautious prescribing of '*stimulants for ADHD if there is a risk of diversion for cognitive enhancement or appetite suppression*' and makes one of the few **do not** recommendations: '*Do not offer immediate-release stimulants that can be easily injected or insufflated [snorted] if there is a risk of stimulant misuse or diversion.*'

13.16.5 Sleep Problems

Based on systematic reviews and meta-analyses, ADHD is significantly associated with both subjective and objective insomnia. Although diagnosis relies on observations made while patients are awake, the prevalence of sleep disturbances in individuals with ADHD is reported to be in the range 25–55%. The interrelationship between ADHD and sleep problems is complicated by the use of ADHD medications, which can impair sleep in some patients (Spruyt & Gozal, 2011), but paradoxically can also improve sleep in others by inducing a calming effect on the wandering mind (Jerome, 2001). The recommendation is that primary sleep disorders should be ruled out before initiating stimulant treatment. Behavioural interventions targeted at improving sleep, starting with advice on sleep hygiene, may be of benefit to some patients and should form part of the multimodal ADHD management plan (Cortese et al., 2013; Graham et al., 2011; Wolraich et al., 2011).

Treatment of insomnia with melatonin has some evidence for children, but not for adults with ADHD (Kooij, 2013). In the UK, long-acting melatonin is licensed as Circadin® and can be prescribed 'off-label' for insomnia in patients under 55 years. Z-drugs (zopiclone, zolpidem) should not be prescribed in the longer term. Mirtazapine, a sedating antidepressant, is interesting for patients with ADHD + depression + insomnia, who are at risk of losing weight on stimulants. For more detailed advice see the BAP consensus statement on evidence-based treatment of insomnia (Wilson et al., 2010).

13.16.6 Autism Spectrum Disorder

Autism spectrum disorder (ASD) is frequently co-morbid with ADHD. Reports estimate that around 20% of patients in a typical adult ADHD clinic have co-morbid ASD and 40% of patients in a typical adult autism clinic have co-morbid ADHD (Gillberg et al., 2009). So far, no RCTs have been completed in adults with ASD + ADHD (Howes et al., 2018). The authors of a recent BAP guideline on ASD recommend cautiously following the BAP (2014) guidelines for treating ADHD. However, there is now emerging evidence of positive treatment effects with methylphenidate, atomoxetine and guanfacine for targeting ADHD symptoms in children and adolescents with ASD. Some antipsychotics, especially partial antagonists such as aripiprazole, may also be helpful in treating hyperactivity symptoms in ASD; however, no study has examined the effects of these medications on ADHD symptoms as a primary outcome. Moreover, the use of antipsychotics should be limited to severe behavioural disruption due to significant side-effect concerns with this medication class (Ameis et al., 2018).

13.16.7 Intellectual disability

The assessment of ADHD in patients with intellectual disability (ID) is more difficult, because often it has to rely more on documentation of behavioural problems observed by carers and clinicians specialized in the assessment of ID. Adults with ADHD + ID often present with challenging behaviour that can respond (at least partially) to ADHD medication (Perera, 2018). However, no RCTs have been performed in this co-morbid group of patients and published cases are mainly in children and adolescents, which makes conclusions for adults with ADHD + ID hard to draw (Tarrant et al., 2018). Nevertheless, people with ID tend to be more sensitive to side effects of psychiatric medications (RCPsych, 2017). BAP (2014) is the only guideline with specific consensus-based recommendations for the clinical management of patients with ADHD + ID as follows:

- Treatment is effective, albeit with reduced efficacy and increased side effects, ID, IQ (intelligence) and neuro-disability should be no barrier to treatment

  Services are needed for adults who do not come under the care of adult LD teams
  Drug treatment needs to be started at lowest dose and increased slowly
- Increased monitoring is likely to be required [and] may present logistical difficulties.

The Royal College of Psychiatrists (RCPsych) supports bi-annual meetings of the peer group ADHD in ID under the umbrella of the Neurodevelopmental Psychiatry Special Interest Group (NDPSIG, see RCPsych webpage for details).

13.16.8 Binge Eating, Obesity and Diabetes

ADHD patients with high levels of impulsivity tend to binge and comfort eat. Screening of eating disorder (ED) patients revealed that those with high levels of ADHD symptoms have worse outcomes after one year (Svedlund et al., 2018). There is meta-analytic evidence for increased levels of obesity in individuals with ADHD; which is somewhat counterintuitive for those with hyperactivity. This effect is small in children and moderate in adults (Nigg et al., 2016). Adolescents and young adults with ADHD were more likely than non-ADHD controls to develop type 2 diabetes mellitus in later life (Chen et al., 2018).

The pharmacological treatment of ADHD symptoms can improve control over eating/bingeing/purging and improve outcomes in patients with ADHD + ED (Ioannidis et al., 2014) and help patients with ADHD + obesity to improve their diet and lose weight (Cortese & Tessari, 2017). If ADHD medication helps patients with ADHD + diabetes to become more organized, they will find it easier to adhere to complex diets and medication regimens, which results in better metabolic control and long-term outcomes (Nylander et al., 2018).

13.16.9 Cardiovascular Co-morbidities

Hypertension is a frequent problem in patients over 40 and should be treated following established guidelines. SDM is very important as patients need to understand the risk of having untreated hypertension. Patients should also take responsibility for monitoring their own blood pressure, reducing risk factors for hypertension and engage with treatment for their hypertension. Guanfacine ER may have a niche indication for patients with treatment-resistant hypertension, but further research is needed. NICE (2018) recommends a *referral for a cardiology opinion* before starting medication for ADHD if any of the following apply (taken verbatim):

- History of congenital heart disease or previous cardiac surgery
- History of sudden death in a first-degree relative under 40 years suggesting a cardiac disease
- Shortness of breath on exertion compared with peers
- Fainting on exertion or in response to fright or noise
- Palpitations that are rapid, regular and start and stop suddenly (fleeting occasional bumps are usually ectopic and do not need investigation)
- Chest pain suggesting cardiac origin
- Signs of heart failure
- A murmur heard on cardiac examination
- Blood pressure that is classified as hypertensive for adults.

In the authors' experience, hypertension and palpitations that are related to the disorganized and stressful lifestyle of many adults with ADHD tend to benefit from treatment with ADHD medication, as often it makes patients feel calmer and more in control of their life.

13.16.10 Neurological Conditions

ADHD can co-occur with other neurodevelopmental conditions such as Tic disorders/ Tourette syndrome. Stimulants can make pre-existing tics worse and atomoxetine or/and aripiprazole are pharmacological strategies for the management of those patients (Ogundele & Ayyah, 2018).

ADHD patients have a higher risk of traffic and sports accidents and may present with ADHD and traumatic brain injury (TBI). Milder forms of TBI can mimic ADHD and lead to deterioration of inattentive and hyperactive/impulsive symptoms. ADHD medications can theoretically lower the threshold for epileptic seizures in patients with post-traumatic epilepsy (Park et al., 2018).

Other forms of epilepsy can co-occur with ADHD. No studies or reviews on adults with ADHD + epilepsy have been published; however, the same challenges exist as in the treatment of children. Sedating side effects of antiepileptic drugs can be confounded with inattentive symptoms of ADHD. Methylphenidate is effective, without a significant increase of seizure risk, although data are still limited, with few controlled trials (Verrotti et al., 2018).

13.17 ADHD in Specific Populations

The term 'specific populations' refers to certain groups of people across the lifespan that have distinctive needs, which must be considered when prescribing ADHD medication within an SDM and psychoeducational framework. Seven specific groups: *preschool children, university students, athletes, men who have sex with men, women, faith groups* and *older adults* are discussed in more detail.

13.17.1 Preschool Children (Under Five Years)

Rates of ADHD diagnoses in preschoolers are lower than for school-aged children, but they have been rising in most countries, especially in the USA, where two- to five-year-old children with ADHD and behavioural problems are frequently medicated. Early identification and multimodal treatment can yield lasting benefits and alter the often adverse trajectory of the disorder (Halperin & Marks, 2019). For children with ADHD under five years seen by NHS services in the UK, NICE (2018) recommends an ADHD-focused group parent-training as first-line intervention and make a clear statement: '*Do not offer medication for ADHD for any child under 5 years without a second specialist opinion from an ADHD service with expertise in managing ADHD in young children (ideally a tertiary service).*'

13.17.2 University Students

The new Canadian guideline seems to be the only guideline with recommendations for the management of ADHD in people with 'intellectual giftedness' (CADDRA, 2018). In a recent review of the literature, Sedgwick (2018) found hardly any studies investigated the efficacy of treating ADHD in students in relation to learning at university and the extent to which practitioners considered the unique demands of university life when prescribing ADHD medication regimens was not known.

There is some research which shows that university students with ADHD who take medication report improvements in note taking, scores on tests and writing output (Advokat et al., 2011). A small RCT tested the efficacy of lisdexamfetamine within a sample of 24 university students diagnosed with ADHD. The drug was administered over five weeks in three different doses and as placebo. The drug resulted in reductions in ADHD symptoms with improvements reported in task management, planning, organization, use of study skills and working memory (DuPaul et al., 2012). A pharmaco-epidemiological study from Sweden showed that young people with ADHD had better scores in standardized university entrance exams when they were taking prescribed ADHD medication compared with those patients not on ADHD medication (Lu et al., 2017).

In our experience, most students are quick learners and understand the concept of ADHD. After psychoeducation, students tend to understand how ADHD symptoms can impact on their functioning at university. In most cases their symptoms respond well to relatively low doses of stimulants.

It has also been observed that a substantial number of university students do not take their medication as prescribed (Rabiner et al., 2009). When and how much stimulant medication is taken seems to depend on what academic tasks need to be completed within a certain time frame (DeSaints et al., 2008). These observations suggest that further research is needed to investigate the PRN use of stimulants amongst university students with ADHD (Greely et al., 2008), especially in view of the high rates of non-medical use of stimulant medications observed within this population.

13.17.3 Athletes

Professional sports can be an ideal niche for people with ADHD. The list of Olympic medal winners who 'came out' with their ADHD diagnosis has grown over the last decade. However, professional athletes may need cardiovascular monitoring including ECG and echocardiogram if there is a history or family history of cardiovascular problems. Stimulants are banned substances in most competitive sports and often there are doping screening programmes (McArdle, 2016). Prescribing practitioners can check the UK Anti-Doping webpage (www.ukad.org.uk) for an up-to-date list of banned substances. Stimulants are banned in most sports for training and competition, although atomoxetine is more widely accepted. UK Anti-Doping (UKAD) has issued an *ADHD Therapeutic Use Exemption* (TUE) *Policy* that details the following requirements:

- bespoke ADHD TUE application form (same for initial and annual renewal)
- psychiatric assessment report (adult ADHD assessment)
- copy of diagnostic schedule (DIVA 2.0, CAADID, ACE+)
- copy of rating scales (ADHD-RS, AISRS, ASRS, BAARS-IV)
- signed by medical practitioner and patient.

In our opinion, TUE certificates should be issued by doctors that are employed by or work for the athlete's sports club, as they are better placed to understand specific rules and regulations. ADHD specialists and GPs can charge a fee if they are requested to complete and sign TUE application forms.

13.17.4 Men Who Have Sex with Men

Methamphetamine is a potent CNS stimulant that (as 'crystal' or 'ice') is also a substance of abuse but it has long been a medicine and has a valid licence (FDA approval) in the USA as Desoxyn® for the treatment of ADHD. In the UK (and elsewhere in Europe), a trend in 'chemsex' is being observed mostly among men who have sex with men (MSM), in which psychoactive drugs like methamphetamine are intentionally being used to facilitate promiscuous sex.

Chemsex typically involves multiple sex partners. Main drugs of choice, often used in combination, are mephedrone, gamma-hydroxybutyrate (GHB), gamma-butyrolactone (GBL) and crystallized (crystal) methamphetamine ('Tina'), which usually is 'slammed' (intravenously injected) (Bourne et al., 2015). The effects of methamphetamine, alertness, exhilaration, enhanced sexual disinhibition, desire, arousal, pleasure and a surge of energy, can enable users to engage in sexual activity continuously for several hours or even days (Lorvick et al., 2012; Melendez-Torres et al., 2016).

In 2009–10, it was estimated that around 14–53 million people worldwide had used methamphetamine at least once in the previous year and that it was the second most used substance, exceeded only by cannabis. The use of, and dependence on, methamphetamine is now a serious public health concern (Galbraith, 2015; Gonzales et al., 2010; WHO, 2011). For instance, the use of crystallized methamphetamine by MSM has been linked with the spread of sexually transmitted infections, including HIV (human immunodeficiency virus) (Centers for Disease Control and Prevention, 2007; Gonzales et al., 2010; Halkitis et al., 2016). Such associations, however, could also be related to other factors such as high prevalence of HIV among MSM, high-risk sexual behaviours and the sharing of injection equipment (Bourne et al., 2015; WHO, 2011).

For prescribing clinicians, we advise sensitive enquiries about the sexual behaviour/practices of both female and male patients with ADHD. This should include questions about chemsex and/or the use of crystallized methamphetamine to facilitate sexual activity. Crystallized methamphetamine has high addiction and dependence liabilities. It requires due consideration as a co-morbid SUD when treating ADHD, especially in patients who engage in high-risk sexual behaviours. Atomoxetine may be the safer option for treatment of ADHD symptoms in this population and it reduces symptoms continuously, not just during daytime as stimulants do.

Another important point to note is that ADHD medications are not reported in the SPC as a contraindication for pre-exposure prophylaxis (PrEP) medicine that contains tenofovir and emtricitabine. PrEP can be taken daily to prevent HIV in high-risk groups (e.g. MSM, sex workers, intravenous drug users) (Eakle et al., 2018; Reyniers et al., 2017; Stein et al., 2014).

13.17.5 Women

NICE (2018) raises awareness about how ADHD is commonly diagnosed in boys, whereas in girls it may be a 'hidden disorder', at least until adulthood, when the male/female gender ratio tends to get closer to 1:1. Anxiety, depression, bipolar and eating disorders seem to co-occur more frequently with ADHD in females, whereas SUD, hypertension, obesity/type 2 diabetes tend to be co-morbidities more frequently associated with ADHD in males (Chen et al., 2018; Williamson & Johnson, 2015). For prescribing practitioners, female-specific issues may arise due to the menstrual cycle, pregnancy and breastfeeding.

ADHD symptoms and related functional impairments tend to become more salient for girls during puberty. Oestrogen levels rise, then fluctuate during the menstrual cycle (*up during the luteal phase then down during the follicular phase*), decline perimenopause and remain low post-menopause. Oestrogen is known to interact with different neurotransmitter systems including DA, NA and serotonin (Shanmugan & Epperson, 2014). DA seems to exert a potent effect as a neuromodulator, and oestrogen is thought to have a special role in regulating its synthesis, release, reuptake and turnover at the synaptic level (Tritsch & Sabatini, 2012).

Oestrogen/DA interactions are indeed highly complex and not well understood, but the theory is that low or high oestrogen levels also *equate* to high or low DA levels (Chavez et al., 2010). Prescribing clinicians should consider the oestrous cycle when determining optimal doses of ADHD medication. When oestrogen levels are high during the luteal phase, females may need to reduce their dose of ADHD medication, and when oestrogen levels are low during the follicular phase, they may need to increase it (Nussbaum, 2012; Quinn, 2005).

During pregnancy oestrogen levels rise and then rapidly fall post-partum. Pregnancy and breastfeeding are part of the oestrous cycle. No controlled studies on the use of ADHD medication during pregnancy or while breastfeeding were found. However, Diav-Citrin et al. (2016) conducted a prospective, comparative, multi-centre observational study that evaluated the risk of major congenital malformations post-partum in 382 women who took methylphenidates during pregnancy (almost 90% took the drug in the first trimester).

Although the findings revealed a higher rate of miscarriages and elective terminations, suggesting further research about this, it seemed that taking methylphenidates during pregnancy did not increase the risk of major congenital malformations.

Bolea-Alamanac et al. (2013) reviewed evidence about the risks of taking methylphenidate during pregnancy and while breastfeeding, and no adverse effects on child development were reported. The default position for prescribing practitioners seems to be to stop non-essential pharmacological treatments during pregnancy and breastfeeding. However, in ADHD this could present significant risks, especially post-partum when oestrogen rapidly declines. Prescribing physicians can continue to be mindful, but it is probably best to consider the circumstances of individual patients on a case-by-case basis, using the model of SDM (i.e. shared decision making).

13.17.6 Faith Groups

The pharmacological treatment of ADHD can be more difficult when patients strictly adhere to religious or cultural rules. Stimulants are a daytime medication and *Muslim* patients may want to stop taking their stimulant medication during Ramadan, especially when religious fasting starts early in the morning during summer months. Switching medication to atomoxetine, which can be taken after sunset, could be a pragmatic solution (see Ramadan information leaflets on Choice & Medication webpage). *Jewish* patients often ask about Kosher ADHD medication. This is a problem that is difficult to solve, especially outside Israel. Therefore, Jewish patients with ADHD should be advised to consult their Rabbi for advice. Patients, who adhere to a strict *Vegan* diet, may have issues with capsules that contain gelatine. Ingredients of all licensed ADHD medication can be checked in SPCs, which are available on the eMC webpage (www.medicines.org.uk/emc). It is worth noting that Concerta XL tablets do not contain gelatine.

13.17.7 Older Adults

ADHD can persist into older age; however, epidemiological studies indicate that the prevalence of ADHD symptoms appears to decline to 1.0–2.8% in patients over 65 years (Torgersen et al., 2016). No RCTs of ADHD medication have been completed in patients over 50, a small number of case series reported good response in patients aged 50 to 65 years (summarized in Torgersen et al., 2016, Table 2). Pharmacological treatment with ADHD medication is limited by higher rate of cardiological co-morbidity (high blood pressure, coronary heart disease, atrial fibrillation etc.) in elderly people (Kooij et al., 2016). Blood pressure and ECG monitoring, liaison with cardiologists (or experienced primary care physicians) and slower dose titration are recommended. Wandering in elderly patients with ADHD and mild cognitive impairment/dementia may respond to ADHD medication, but clinical trials are lacking.

13.18 ADHD and Driving

Adults with ADHD have higher rates of road traffic accidents and citations for road traffic offences. ADHD medication improves attention and makes driving safer (Surman et al., 2017). In some countries (e.g. the Netherlands) it is a requirement for drivers with a diagnosis of ADHD to take their medicine when driving (Kooij, 2013). The authors recommend asking and documenting if patients have a driving licence and if they have points on their licence before prescribing ADHD medication. In the UK, the Driver & Vehicle Licensing Agency (DVLA) updated advice on their webpage (www.gov.uk/adhd-and-driving) and guidance for doctors in March 2019: car and motorcycle drivers 'may be able to drive but must notify DVLA if [their ADHD] affects the ability to drive safely', bus and lorry drivers 'may be able to drive but must notify the DVLA'. The DVLA guidance states that a diagnosis of ADHD is not in itself a bar to licensing and that when reaching a decision the 'DVLA considers factors such as the level of impulsivity [and the person's] awareness of the impacts of behaviours on self and others' (DVLA, 2019, p. 84).

13.19 Stimulants for 'Off-Label' Indications

Stimulants have been investigated in a range of psychiatric, neurological and other conditions that come along with cognitive deficits, apathy or fatigue. Most studies did not evaluate patients for the presence of ADHD. The following indications for stimulants (and atomoxetine) are emerging, but all 'off-label':

- augmentation of antidepressants in depression (McIntyre et al., 2017)
- apathy in dementia (Padala et al., 2018; Ruthirakuhan et al., 2018)
- fatigue and opioid-induced sedation in cancer and transplantation patients (Andrew et al., 2018; Tomlinson et al., 2018)
- cognitive deficits/apathy after traumatic brain injury (Iaccarino et al., 2018)
- Aphasia/other cognitive deficits after stroke (Müller, 2008).

Drugs to treat ADHD were evaluated in RCTs in patients with schizophrenia with no beneficial effects on negative symptoms. Atomoxetine and amphetamines may improve cognitive deficits in schizophrenia (Solmi et al., 2018). This remains controversial and the risk of triggering a psychotic episode has to be closely monitored – as with any DA-enhancing medication.

13.20 Non-Medical Use of Stimulants

The misuse and diversion of ADHD stimulants is a relevant issue for prescribing practitioners. The non-medical use of stimulants occurs when these medications are not used for purposes of treating symptoms of ADHD. This may include recreational use, but increasingly the concern is about healthy individuals using ADHD stimulant medications to enhance their work and/or academic performance. This behaviour is conceptualized within neuroscience literature as *pharmacological cognitive enhancement* (PCE), *neuro-enhancement* or *cosmetic pharmacology* (Dietz et al., 2016; Sahakian & Morein-Zamir, 2015). Methylphenidate and modafinil are common PCEs, but other preparations such as dexamphetamine, atomoxetine and guanfacine have also been used by healthy individuals to improve memory, alertness and concentration (Husain & Mehta, 2011).

Evidence for PCE and/or the effectiveness of stimulants when used by healthy individuals does need to be interpreted cautiously, because some studies have produced null results, as well as task-specific impairments (Advokat, 2010). Also the impact of prior poor sleep as a predictor of effect has not routinely been evaluated. While certain professional groups may be susceptible to PCE use (i.e. bankers, surgeons, lawyers) (Cederström, 2016; Sugden et al., 2012), the phenomenon is usually investigated among college (or university) students, who coin stimulant medications used for the purposes of enhancing academic performance as 'study drugs', 'smart drugs', 'brain dope' or 'academic steroids'. Prevalence estimates for the use of 'smart drugs' is between 5% and 35% for college students in North American (Wilens et al., 2008), and between 0.8% and 16% for university students in Switzerland and Germany (Castaldi et al., 2012; Maier et al., 2013; Ott & Biller-Andorno, 2014).

Practitioners may be concerned that university students malinger with ADHD to get a prescription for stimulants. Malingering can be difficult to detect and often depends on the skills and expertise of the practitioner undertaking the assessment. More so, concerns about malingering, especially amongst university students in the UK and elsewhere in Europe, could result in a failure to recognize and treat ADHD within this population. Perhaps it is worth considering the findings of the first national online survey of 'PCE' use among 877 UK university students, who were mostly enrolled within a Russell Group University. The authors concluded that university students in the UK were resilient to PCE use, due to the low prevalence rates that were reported in the survey (Singh et al., 2014). We therefore recommend that if a patient's potential for misuse or diversion becomes of concern to a prescribing practitioner, then they should consider prescribing a non-stimulant medication, which lacks potential for abuse/misuse.

13.21 ADHD Medication Clinics

The initiation and titration of ADHD medication requires clinical expertise (trained psychiatrist and/or nurse prescriber), arrangements for funding (ADHD clinic, primary care or private), prescribing (hospital pharmacy, FP10 or 'pink' private prescription form) and dispensing (hospital or other any pharmacy) of ADHD medication. ADHD clinics should be equipped to measure blood pressure, weight and height (for BMI calculation). Clinics can run daily or just weekly but should be able to offer follow-up appointments within one to five weeks. ADHD medication clinics can be streamlined like clinics for patients on clozapine or depot (injectable long-acting) antipsychotics. The authors recommend regular audits of prescribing patterns and frequent attenders (i.e. patients that need more than 5 or 10 follow-up appointments for titration or re-titration).

Ideally, diagnostic assessments for ADHD and prescribing of ADHD medication should become part of general adult psychiatry. The following *service models* are used to manage adults with ADHD in the UK:

- specialist (stand-alone service for adults with ADHD)
- integrated (i.e. part of secondary care adult mental health services)
- neurodevelopmental (ADHD + ASD, adult only or lifespan)
- clinic for university students (mixed models)
- forensic service (as part of specialist service or integrated)
- primary care (non-complicated patients only)
- private sector (prescribing often taken over by NHS primary care).

The *Five Year Forward View for Mental Health* (NHS England, 2016) listed an (lifespan) ADHD pathway for 2018/19, but no extra funding has been released so far. Specialist services are an ideal setting for service improvement projects and clinical audits. Guideline recommendations will only improve clinical outcomes if they are implemented in clinical practice. The first published audit of NICE (2008) recommendations showed (Magon et al., 2015). The national *Prescribing Observatory Mental Health*

(POMH-UK) audited the prescribing of ADHD medication in children/adolescents and adults in 2013 (n = 1313 adults with ADHD) and 2015 (n = 1443 adults) with a focus on recommended monitoring of blood pressure/pulse and weight (POMH-UK, 2015).

13.22 Nurse Prescribing

ADHD is an ideal area for specialist nurse prescribing. Nurses with a background in mental health nursing or child and adolescent/paediatric nursing can specialize in prescribing ADHD medication. The programme of study to become a non-medical prescriber (NMP) within the UK is rigorous and involves a combination of taught curricula and practice-based learning. Prescribing is a complex skill that is high risk and error prone, with many influencing factors (Cope et al., 2016). A Community Practitioner Nurse Prescriber (CPNP) can only prescribe from the Nurse Prescriber Formulary, which does not list any ADHD medication. Therefore, only Nurse Independent Prescribers (NIP), who have successfully completed an NMC (Nursing and Midwifery Council) Independent Nurse Prescribing Course will be able to prescribe 'any medicine provided it is in their competency to do so. This includes medicines and products listed in the BNF, unlicensed medicines and all controlled drugs.' Supplementary prescribing is a form of prescribing that can be undertaken by non-medical health professionals after a doctor (or independent prescriber) has made a diagnosis and drawn up a clinical management plan for the patient (see information on the webpage of the Royal College of Nursing (RCN): www.rcn.org.uk/get-help/rcn-advice/nurse-prescribing). NMPs/NIPs will need specialist training and ongoing clinical supervision by a named psychiatrist.

13.23 Specialist Training

Specialist Adult ADHD services are an ideal learning environment, where doctors and nurses can be trained to become specialists. The UK Adult ADHD Network (UKAAN) recommends three days of adult ADHD-specific workshops or symposia and the management of 20 patients under supervision of an adult ADHD expert. Prescribers of ADHD medication should have in-depth knowledge (and understanding) of relevant guideline recommendations (Bolea-Alamañac et al., 2014; NICE, 2018) and available medications (Table 13.1). Difficult cases should be presented and discussed in supervision, in CPD peer group meetings or at local/regional adult ADHD peer group meetings. Documented case-based discussions (CBD) are a key element of annual appraisal and revalidation of psychiatrists in the UK.

Acknowledgements and Disclosures

We would like to acknowledge collegial support from the members of the Executive Committee of the UK Adult ADHD Network (www.UKAAN.org) under direction of our mentor and friend Professor Philip Asherson. We finalized this book chapter while on summer holiday and therefore also thank our hosts at Paliochori Studios.

UM-S has received advisory board and speaker honoraria from Shire (2014–15, 2017–18), Heptares (2014–14) and Eli Lilly (2012, 2015), UKAAN (UK Adult ADHD Network, since 2011), BAP (British Association for Psychopharmacology, since 2010) and NHS trusts (outside London and East Anglia). JS-M is receiving an educational grant from the

Royal College of Nursing (RCN) Foundation for a contribution towards PhD tuition and conference fees and has received speaker honoraria from Shire (2017–18) and UKAAN (UK Adult ADHD Network, since 2016).

References

Adler L, Wilen T, Zhang S, et al. (2009). Retrospective safety analysis of atomoxetine in adult ADHD patients with or without comorbid alcohol abuse and dependence. *Am J Addict*, 18(5), 393–401.

Advokat C (2010). What are the cognitive effects of stimulant medications? Emphasis on adults with attention-deficit/hyperactivity disorder (ADHD). *Neurosci Biobehav Rev*, 34(8), 1255–1266.

Advokat C, Lane SM, Luo C (2011). College students with and without ADHD: comparison of self-report of medication usage, study habits, and academic achievement. *J Atten Disord*, 15, 656–666.

Ameis SH, Szatmari P (2012). Imaging-genetics in autism spectrum disorder: advances, translational impact and future directions. *Front Psychiatry*, 3(46), 1–13.

Ameis SH, Kassee C, Corbett-Dick P, et al. (2018). Systematic review and guide to management of core and psychiatric symptoms in youth with autism. *Acta Psychiatr Scand*, 138, 379–400.

American Psychiatric Association (APA) (1980). *Diagnostic and Statistical Manual of Mental Disorders*, 3rd ed. Arlington, VA: American Psychiatric Association.

American Psychiatric Association (APA) (2013). *Diagnostic and Statistical Manual of Mental Disorders*, 5th ed. Arlington, VA: American Psychiatric Association.

Andrew BN, Guan NC, Jaafar NRN (2018). The use of methylphenidate for physical and psychological symptoms in cancer patients: a review. *Curr Drug Targets*, 19(8), 877–887.

Asherson P, Young AH, Eich-Höchli D, et al. (2014). Differential diagnosis, comorbidity and treatment of attention-deficit/hyperactivity disorder in relation to bipolar disorder or borderline personality disorder in adults. *Curr Med Res Opin*, 30(8), 1657–1672.

Biederman J, Lindsten A, Sluth LB, et al. (2019). Vortioxetine for attention deficit hyperactivity disorder in adults: a randomized, double-blind, placebo-controlled, proof-of-concept study. *J Psychopharmacol*, 33(4), 511–521.

Bijlenga D, Kulcu S, van Gellecum T, Eryigit Z, Kooij JJS (2017). Persistence and adherence to psychostimulants, and psychological well-being up to 3 years after specialized treatment of adult attention-deficit/hyperactivity disorder: a naturalistic follow-up study. *J Clin Psychopharmacol*, 37(6), 689–696.

Boilson M, Shah P and Royal College of Psychiatrists in Scotland special interest group in ADHD (2017). *ADHD in Adults: Good Practice Guidelines*, London: The Royal College of Psychiatrists.

Bolea-Alamanac BM, Green A, Verma G, Maxwell P, Davies SJC (2013). Methylphenidate use in pregnancy and lactation: a systematic review of evidence. *Br J Clin Pharmacol*, 77(1), 96–101.

Bolea-Alamañac B, Nutt DJ, Adamou M, et al. (2014). Evidence-based guidelines for the pharmacological management of attention deficit hyperactivity disorder: update on recommendations from the British Association for Psychopharmacology. *J Psychopharmacol*, 28(3), 179–203.

Bonell CP, Hickson FC, Weatherburn P, Reid DS (2010). Methamphetamine use among gay men across the UK. *Int J Drug Policy*, 21(3), 244–246.

Bourne A, Reid D, Hickson F, Torres-Rueda S, Weatherburn P (2015). Illicit drug use in sexual settings ('chemsex') and HIV/STI transmission risk behaviour among gay men in south London: findings from a qualitative study. *Sex Transm Infect*, 91(8), 564–568.

Brook DW, Brook JS, Zhang C, Koppel J (2010). Association between attention-deficit/hyperactivity disorder in adolescence and substance use disorders in adulthood. *Arch Pediatr Adolesc Med*, 164(10), 930–934.

Butterfield ME, Saal J, Young B, Young JL (2016). Supplementary guanfacine hydrochloride as a treatment of attention deficit hyperactivity disorder in adults: a double blind, placebo-controlled study. *Psychiatry Res*, 236, 136–141.

Caisley H, Müller U (2012). Adherence to medication in adults with attention deficit hyperactivity disorder and *pro re nata* dosing of psychostimulants: a systematic review. *Eur Psychiatry*, 27, 343–349.

Canadian ADHD Resource Alliance (CADDRA) (2018). *Canadian ADHD Practice Guidelines*, 4th ed. Toronto: CADDRA. Available at: www.caddra.ca/canadian-adhd-practice-guidelines (last accessed 15.8.18).

Castaldi S, Gelatti U, Orizio G, et al. (2012). Use of cognitive enhancement medication among Northern Italian university students. *J Addict Med*, 6, 112–117.

Caye A, Swanson JM, Coghill D, Rohde LA (2019). Treatment strategies for ADHD: an evidence-based guide to select optimal treatment. *Mol Psychiatry*, 24, 390–408.

Cederström C (2016). Like it or not 'smart drugs' are coming to the office. *Harvard Business Review*. Available at: https://hbr.org/2016/05/like-it-or-not-smart-drugs-are-coming-to-the-office (last accessed 1.11.18).

Centers for Disease Control and Prevention (CDC) (2007). *Methamphetamine Use and Risk for HIV/AIDS*. Available at: file:///C:/Users/K1517101/Downloads/cdc_11778_DS1.pdf (last accessed 1.8.18).

Chan E, Fogler JM, Hammerness PG (2016). Treatment of attention-deficit/hyperactivity disorder in adolescents: a systematic review. *JAMA*, 315, 1997–2008.

Chang Z, Lichtenstein P, D'Onofrio BM, Sjölander A, Larsson H (2014). Serious transport accidents in adults with attention-deficit/hyperactivity disorder and the effect of medication: a population-based study. *JAMA Psychiatry*, 71, 319–325.

Chang Z, D'Onofrio BM, Quinn PD, Lichtenstein P, Larsson H (2016). Medication for attention-deficit/hyperactivity disorder and risk for depression: a nationwide longitudinal cohort study. *Biol Psychiatry*, 80, 916–922.

Chang Z, Ghirardi L, Quinn PD, et al. (2019). Risks and benefits of ADHD medication on behavioral and neuropsychiatric outcomes: a qualitative review of pharmacoepidemiology studies using linked prescription databases. *Biol Psychiatry* [Epub ahead of print] doi:doi.org/10.1016/j.biopsych.2019.04.009.

Chavez C, Hollaus M, Scarr E, et al. (2010). The effect of estrogen on dopamine and serotonin receptor and transporter levels in the brain: an autoradiography study. *Brain Res*, 1321, 51–59.

Chen Q, Hartman CA, Haavik J, et al. (2018). Common psychiatric and metabolic comorbidity of adult attention-deficit/hyperactivity disorder: a population-based cross-sectional study *PLoS One*, 13(9), e0204516.

Coghill D, Chen W, Silva D (2019). Organizing and delivering treatment for ADHD. In LA Rohde, JK Buitelaar, M Gerlach, SV Faraone, eds., *The World Federation of ADHD Guide*, pp. 93–109. [open access pdf and e-book: http://cpo-media.net/ADHD/2019/ebook/HTML/93/].

Cooper RE, Williams E, Seegobin S, et al. (2017). Cannabinoids in attention-deficit/hyperactivity disorder: a randomised-controlled trial. *Eur Neuropsychopharmacol*, 27, 795–808.

Cope LC, Abuzour AS, Tully MP (2016). Nonmedical prescribing: where are we now? *Ther Adv Drug Saf*, 7(4), 165–172.

Cortese S (2018). Are the effects of methylphenidate uncertain? *Ir J Psychol Med*, 35, 163–167.

Cortese S, Tessari L (2017). Attention-deficit/hyperactivity disorder (ADHD) and obesity: update 2016. *Curr Psychiatry Rep*, 19(1), 4.

Cortese S, Brown TE, Corkum P, et al. (2013). Assessment and management of sleep problems in youths with attention-deficit/hyperactivity disorder. *J Am Acad Child Adolesc Psychiatry*, 52, 784–796.

Cortese S, D'Acunto G, Konofal E, Masi G, Vitiello B (2017). New formulations of methylphenidate for the treatment of attention-deficit/hyperactivity disorder: pharmacokinetics, efficacy, and tolerability. *CNS Drugs*, 31, 149–160.

Cortese S, Adamo N, Del Giovane C, et al. (2018). Comparative efficacy and tolerability of medications for attention-deficit hyperactivity disorder in children, adolescents, and adults: a systematic review and network meta-analysis. *Lancet Psychiatry*, 5, 727–738.

Coulter A, Collins A (2011). *Making shared decision-making a reality: no decision about me, without me*. London: The King's Fund.

Crunelle CL, van den Brink W, Moggi F, et al.; ICASA consensus group, Matthys F (2018). International consensus statement on screening, diagnosis and treatment of substance use disorder patients with comorbid attention deficit/hyperactivity disorder. *Eur Addict Res*, 24(1), 43–51.

Cunill R, Castells X, Tobias A, Capellà D (2015). Pharmacological treatment of attention deficit hyperactivity disorder with co-morbid drug dependence. *J Psychopharmacol*, 29, 15–23.

Dalley JW, Roiser JP (2012). Dopamine, serotonin and impulsivity. *Neuroscience*, 215, 42–58.

De Crescenzo F, Cortese S, Adamo N, Janiri L (2017). Pharmacological and non-pharmacological treatment of adults with ADHD: a meta-review. *Evid Based Ment Health*, 20, 4–11.

DeSaints AD, Webb EM, Noar SM (2008). Illicit use of prescription ADHD medications on a college campus: a multimethodological approach. *J Am Coll Health*, 75, 315–324.

Diav-Citrin O, Shechtman S, Arnon J, et al. (2016). Methylphenidate in pregnancy: a multicentre, prospective, comparative, observational study. *J Clin Psychiatry*, 77(9), 1176–1181.

Díaz-Román A, Mitchell R, Cortese S (2018). Sleep in adults with ADHD: systematic review and meta-analysis of subjective and objective studies. *Neurosci Biobehav Rev*, 89, 61–71.

Dietz P, Soyka M, Franke AG (2016). Pharmacological neuroenhancement in the field of economics: poll results from an online survey. *Front Psychol*, 7(520), 1–8.

Driver & Vehicle Licensing Agency (DVLA) (2019). *Assessing fitness to drive: a guide for medical professionals*. Available at: www.gov.uk/government/publications/ assessing-fitness-to-drive-a-guide-for-medical-professionals (last accessed 1.04.19).

DuPaul GJ, Weyandt LL, Rossi JS, et al. (2012). Double-bind, placebo-controlled, crossover study of the efficacy and safety of lisdexamfetamine dimesylate in college students with ADHD. *J Atten Disord*, 16, 202–220.

Eakle R, Mbogua J, Mutanha N, Ress H (2018). Exploring acceptability of oral PrEP prior to implementation among female sex workers in South Africa. *J Int AIDS Soc*, 21, e25081.

Edvinsson D, Ekselius L (2018a). Long-term tolerability and safety of pharmacological treatment of adult attention-deficit/ hyperactivity disorder: a 6-year prospective naturalistic study. *J Clin Psychopharmacol*, 38(4), 370–375.

Edvinsson D, Ekselius L (2018b). Six-year outcome in subjects diagnosed with attention-deficit/hyperactivity disorder as adults. *Eur Arch Psychiatry Clin Neurosci*, 268(4), 337–347.

Faraone SV (2018). The pharmacology of amphetamine and methylphenidate: relevance to the neurobiology of attention-deficit/ hyperactivity disorder and other psychiatric comorbidities. *Neurosci Biobehav Rev*, 87, 255–270.

Findling RL, Adler LA, Spencer TJ, et al. (2019). Dasotraline in children with attention-deficit/ hyperactivity disorder: a six-week, placebo-controlled, fixed-dose trial. *J Child Adolesc Psychopharmacol*, 29(2), 80–89.

Fredriksen M, Dahl AA, Martinsen EW, et al. (2014). Effectiveness of one-year pharmacological treatment of adult attention-deficit/hyperactivity disorder (ADHD): an open-label prospective study of time in treatment, dose, side-effects and comorbidity. *Eur Neuropsychopharmacol*, 24, 1873–1884.

Galbraith N (2015). The methamphetamine problem. *BJPsych Bull*, 39, 218–220.

Gillberg C, Gillberg IC, Rasmussen P, et al. (2004). Co-existing disorders in ADHD: implications for diagnosis and intervention. *Eur Child Adolesc Psychiatry*, 13(Suppl 1), 80–92.

Gillies GE, McArthur S (2010). Estrogen actions in the brain and the basis for differential action in men and women: a case for sex-specific medicines. *Pharmacol Rev*, 62(2), 155–198.

Ginsberg Y, Lindefors N (2012). Methylphenidate treatment of adult male prison inmates with attention-deficit hyperactivity disorder: randomised double-blind placebo-controlled trial with open-label extension. *Br J Psychiatry*, 200(1), 68–73.

Golubchik P, Sever J, Zalsman G, Weizman A (2008). Methylphenidate in the treatment of female adolescents with cooccurrence of attention deficit/hyperactivity disorder and borderline personality disorder: a preliminary open-label trial. *Int Clin Psychopharmacol*, 23(4), 228–231.

Gonzales R, Mooney L, Rawson RA (2010). The methamphetamine problem in the United States. *Annu Rev Public Health*, 31, 385–398.

Gould ON, Doucette C (2018). Self-management of adherence to prescribed stimulants in college students with ADD/ADHD. *J Atten Disord*, 22, 349–355.

Graham J, Coghill D (2008). Adverse effects of pharmacotherapies for attention-deficit hyperactivity disorder: epidemiology, prevention and management. *CNS Drugs*, 22(3), 213–237.

Graham J, Banaschewski T, Buitelaar J, et al. (2011). European guidelines on managing adverse effects of medication for ADHD. *Eur Child Adolesc Psychiatry*, 20(1), 17–37.

Greely H, Sanakian B, Harris J, et al. (2008). Towards responsible use of cognitive-enhancing drugs by the healthy. *Nature*, 456, 702–705.

Halkitis PN (2010). Reframing HIV prevention for gay men in the United States. *Am Psychol*, 65(8), 752–763.

Halkitis PN, Levy MD, Solomon TM (2016). Temporal relations between methamphetamine use and HIV seroconversion in gay, bisexual, and other men who have sex with men. *J Health Psychol*, 21(1), 93–99.

Halperin JM, Marks DJ (2019). Practitioner review: assessment and treatment of preschool children with attention-deficit/hyperactivity disorder. *J Child Psychol Psychiatry* [Epub ahead of print] doi:10.1111/jcpp.13014.

Harrison AG, Edwards MJ, Parker KCH (2007). Identifying students faking ADHD: preliminary findings and strategies for detection. *Arch Clin Neuropsychol*, 22, 577–588.

Heal DJ, Smith S, Gosden J, Nutt DJ (2013). Amfetamine, past and present: a pharmacological and clinical perspective. *J Psychopharmacol*, 27, 1–18.

Holloway K, Bennett T (2012). Prescription drug misuse among university staff and students: a survey of motives, nature and extent. *Drug Educ Prev Polic*, 19, 137–144.

Hooberman D, Stein TA (1984). Treatment of attention deficit and borderline personality disorders with psychostimulants: case report. *J Clin Psychiatry*, 45, 441–442.

Hornig-Rohan M, Amsterdam JD (2002). Venlafaxine versus stimulant therapy in patients with dual diagnosis ADD and depression. *Prog Neuropsychopharmacol Biol Psychiatry*, 26(3), 585–589.

Humphreys KL, Eng T, Lee SS (2013). Stimulant medication and substance use outcomes: a meta-analysis. *JAMA Psychiatry*, 70, 740–749.

Husain M, Mehta MA (2011). Cognitive enhancement by drugs in health and disease. *Trends Cogn Sci*, 15(1), 28–36.

Huss M, McBurnett K, Cutler AJ, et al. (2019). Distinguishing the efficacy and sedative effects of guanfacine extended release in children and adolescents with attention-deficit/hyperactivity disorder. *Eur Neuropsychopharmacol*, 29, 432–443.

Iaccarino MA, Philpotts LL, Zafonte R, Biederman J (2018). Stimulant use in the management of mild traumatic brain injury: a qualitative literature review. *J Atten Disord* [Epub ahead of print] doi:10.1177/1087054718759752.

Ioannidis K, Chamberlain SR, Müller U (2014a). Ostracizing caffeine from the pharmacological arsenal for ADHD: was this a correct decision? A literature review. *J Psychopharmacol*, 28, 830–836.

Ioannidis K, Serfontein J, Müller U (2014b). Bulimia nervosa patient diagnosed with previously unsuspected adult ADHD: clinical case report, literature review, and diagnostic challenges. *Int J Eat Disord*, 47 (4), 431–436.

Iwanami A, Saito K, Fujiwara M, Okutsu D, Ichikawa H (2019). Randomized, double-blind, placebo-controlled, phase 3 study of guanfacine extended release in adults with attention-deficit/hyperactivity disorder. Presented at 7th World Congress on ADHD, Lisbon, Portugal.

Jackson CO (1971). The amphetamine inhaler: a case study of medical abuse. *J Hist Med*, 26, 187–196.

Kessler RC, Adler L, Barkley R, et al. (2006). The prevalence and correlates of adult ADHD in the United States: results from the National Comorbidity Survey Replication. *Am J Psychiatry*, 163(4), 716–723.

Khan A, Fahl Mar K, Brown WA (2017). Does the increasing placebo response impact outcomes of adult and pediatric ADHD clinical trials? Data from the US Food and Drug Administration 2000–2009. *J Psychiatr Res*, 94, 202–207.

Koblan KS, Hopkins SC, Sarma K, et al. (2016). Assessment of human abuse potential of dasotraline compared to methylphenidate and placebo in recreational stimulant users. *Drug Alcohol Depend*, 159, 26–34.

Konstenius M, Jayaram-Lindström N, Guterstam J, et al. (2014). Methylphenidate for attention deficit hyperactivity disorder and drug relapse in criminal offenders with substance dependence: a 24-week randomized placebo-controlled trial. *Addiction*, 109(3), 440–449.

Kooij JJS (2013). *Adult ADHD: Diagnostic Assessment and Treatment*, 3rd ed. London: Springer.

Kooij JJ, Huss M, Asherson P, et al. (2012). Distinguishing comorbidity and successful management of adult ADHD. *J Atten Disord*, 16(5 Suppl), 3–19.

Kooij JJ, Michielsen M, Kruithof H, Bijlenga D (2016). ADHD in old age: a review of the literature and proposal for assessment and treatment. *Expert Rev Neurother*, 16(12), 1371–1381.

Kooij JJS, Bijlenga D, Salerno L, et al. (2019). Updated European Consensus Statement on diagnosis and treatment of adult ADHD. *Eur Psychiatry*, 56, 14–34.

Kooij SJ, Bejerot S, Blackwell A, et al. (2010). European consensus statement on diagnosis and treatment of adult ADHD: the European Network Adult ADHD. *BMC Psychiatry*, 10, 67.

Kratochvil CJ, Newcorm JH, Arnold LE, et al. (2005). Atomoxetine alone or combined with fluoxetine for treating ADHD with comorbid depressive or anxiety symptoms. *J Am Acad Child Adolesc Psychiatry*, 44(9), 915–924.

Levin FR, Mariani JJ, Specker S, et al. (2015). Extended-release mixed amphetamine salts vs placebo for comorbid adult attention-deficit/hyperactivity disorder and cocaine use disorder. *JAMA Psychiatry*, 72(6), 593–602.

Levin FR, Choi CJ, Pavlicova M, et al. (2018). How treatment improvement in ADHD and cocaine dependence are related to one another: a secondary analysis. *Drug Alcohol Depend*, 188, 135–140.

Lichtenstein P, Halldner L, Zetterqvist J, et al. (2012). Medication for attention deficit-hyperactivity disorder and criminality. *N Engl J Med*, 367, 2006–2014.

Lorvic J, Bourgois P, Wenger LD, et al. (2012). Sexual pleasure and sexual risk among women who use methamphetamine: a mixed methods study. *Int J Drug Policy*, 23(5), 385–392.

Lu Y, Sjölander A, Cederlöf M, et al. (2017). Association between medication use and performance on higher education entrance tests in individuals with attention-deficit/ hyperactivity disorder. *JAMA Psychiatry*, 74(8), 815–822.

Magon RK, Latheesh B, Müller U (2015). Specialist community adult ADHD clinics in East Anglia: service evaluation and audit of NICE guideline recommendations. *BJPsych Bull*, 39, 36–140.

Maier LJ, Liechti ME, Herzig F, Schaub MP (2013). To dope or not to dope: neuroenhancement with prescription drugs and drugs of abuse among Swiss university students. *PLoS One*, 8(11), e77967.

Man KKC, Ip P, Chan EW, et al. (2017). Effectiveness of pharmacological treatment for attention-deficit/hyperactivity disorder on physical injuries: a systematic review and meta-analysis of observational studies. *CNS Drugs*, 31, 1043–1055.

Martins S, Tramontina S, Polanczyk G, et al. (2004). Weekend holidays during methylphenidate use in ADHD children: a randomized clinical trial. *J Child Adolesc Psychopharmacol*, 14(2), 195–206.

Matthies S, Philipsen A (2016). Comorbidity of personality disorders and adult attention deficit hyperactivity disorder (ADHD): review of recent findings. *Curr Psychiatry Rep*, 18(4), 33.

McArdle A (2016). Attention deficit hyperactivity disorder. In A Currie, B Owen, eds., *Sports Psychiatry*. Oxford: Oxford University Press, pp. 87–95.

McIntyre RS, Lee Y, Zhou AJ, et al. (2017). The efficacy of psychostimulants in major depressive episodes: a systematic review and meta-analysis. *J Clin Psychopharmacol*, 37, 412–418.

Melendez-Torres GJ, Bonell C, Hickson F, et al. (2016). Predictors of crystal methamphetamine use in a community-based sample of UK men who have sex with men. *Int J Drug Policy*, 36, 43–46.

Moran LV, Ongur D, Hsu J, et al. (2019). Psychosis with methylphenidate or amphetamine in patients with ADHD. *N Engl J Med*, 380, 1128–1138.

Müller U (2008). Pharmacological treatment. In SF Cappa, J Abutalebi, J-F Démonet, P Fletcher, P Garrard, eds., *Cognitive Neurology: A Clinical Textbook*. Oxford: Oxford University Press, pp. 475–498.

Müller-Sedgwick U, Meisel G, Nasri M, Sedgwick-Müller JA (2018). How fast should we titrate methylphenidate in adults with ADHD? A meta-analysis of dose titration regimes in RCTs. presented at 5th Eunethydis International Conference on ADHD, Edinburgh, Scotland.

National Institute for Health and Care Excellence (NICE) (2008). *Attention deficit hyperactivity disorder: diagnosis and management*. Clinical guideline [CG72]. London: National Institute for Health and Care Excellence.

National Institute for Health and Care Excellence (NICE) (2018). *Attention deficit hyperactivity disorder: diagnosis and management*. NICE guideline [NG87]. London: National Institute for Health and Care Excellence.

Newcorn JH, Stein MA, Childress AC, et al. (2013). Randomized, double-blind trial of guanfacine extended release in children with attention-deficit/hyperactivity disorder: morning or evening administration. *J Am Acad Child Adolesc Psychiatry*, 52, 921–930.

NHS England (2016). *The Five Year Forward View for Mental Health*, Mental Health Taskforce. Available at: www.england.nhs.uk/mentalhealth/taskforce (last accessed 24.10.18).

Nigg JT, Johnstone JM, Musser ED, et al. (2016). Attention-deficit/hyperactivity disorder (ADHD) and being overweight/obesity: new data and meta-analysis. *Clin Psychol Rev*, 43, 67–79.

Nussbaum NL (2012). ADHD and female specific concerns: a review of the literature and clinical implications, *J Atten Disord*, 16, 87–100.

Nutt DJ, Fone K, Asherson P, et al.; British Association for Psychopharmacology (2007). Evidence-based guidelines for management of attention-deficit/hyperactivity disorder in adolescents in transition to adult services and in adults: recommendations from the British Association for Psychopharmacology. *J Psychopharmacol*, 21(1), 10–41.

Ogundele MO, Ayyash HF (2018). Review of the evidence for the management of co-morbid tic disorders in children and adolescents with attention deficit hyperactivity disorder. *World J Clin Pediatr*, 7, 36–42.

Ott R, Biller-Andorno N (2014). Neuroenhancement among Swiss students: a comparison of users and non-users. *Pharmacopsychiatry*, 47, 22–28.

Padala PR, Padala KP, Lensing SY, et al. (2018). Methylphenidate for apathy in community-dwelling older veterans with mild Alzheimer's disease: a double-blind, randomized, placebo-controlled trial. *Am J Psychiatry*, 175, 159–168.

Park J, Choi HW, Yum MS, et al. (2018). Relationship between aggravation of seizures and methylphenidate treatment in subjects with attention-deficit/hyperactivity disorder and epilepsy. *J Child Adolesc Psychopharmacol*, 28, 537–546.

Perera B (2018). Attention deficit hyperactivity disorder in people with intellectual disability. *Ir J Psychol Med*, 35, 213–219.

Philipsen A, Richter H, Peters J, et al. (2007). Structured group psychotherapy in adults with attention deficit hyperactivity disorder: results of an open multicentre study. *J Nerv Ment Disord*, 195(12), 1013–1019.

Philipsen A, Limberger MF, Lieb K, et al. (2008). Attention-deficit hyperactivity disorder as a potentially aggravating factor in borderline personality disorder. *Br J Psychiatry*, 192(2), 118–123.

Philipsen A, Jans T, Graf E, et al.; Comparison of Methylphenidate and Psychotherapy in Adult ADHD Study (COMPAS) Consortium (2015). Effects of group psychotherapy, individual counseling, methylphenidate, and placebo in the treatment of adult attention-deficit/hyperactivity disorder: a randomized clinical trial. *JAMA Psychiatry*, 72, 1199–1210.

POMH-UK (2015). *Topic 13b re-audit report. Prescribing for ADHD in children, adolescents and adults.* Prescribing Observatory for Mental Health (POMH), CCQI218 (data on file).

Quinn PO (2005). Treating adolescent girls and women with ADHD: gender-specific issue. *J Clin Psychol*, 61(5), 579–587.

Rabiner DL, Anastopoulos AD, Costello EJ, et al. (2009). The misuse and diversion of prescribed ADHD medications by college students. *J Atten Disord*, 13, 144–153.

Renoux C, Shin JY, Dell'Aniello S, Fergusson E, Suissa S (2016). Prescribing trends of attention-deficit hyperactivity disorder (ADHD) medications in UK primary care, 1995–2015. *Br J Clin Pharmacol*, 82, 858–868.

Reyniers T, Hoornenborg E, Vuylsteke B, Wouters K, Laga M (2017). Pre-exposure prophylaxis (PrEP) for men who have sex with men in Europe: review of evidence for a much needed prevention tool. *Sex Transm Infect*, 93, 363–367.

Rösler M, Fischer R, Ammer R, Ose C, Retz W (2009). A randomised, placebo-controlled, 24-week, study of low-dose extended-release methylphenidate in adults with attention-deficit/hyperactivity disorder. *Eur Arch Psychiatry Clin Neurosci*, 259(2), 120–129.

Roy A, Hechtman L, Arnold LE, et al.; MTA Cooperative Group (2017). Childhood predictors of adult functional outcomes in the multimodal treatment study of attention-deficit/hyperactivity disorder (MTA). *J Am Acad Child Adolesc Psychiatry*, 56(8), 687–695.

Royal College of Psychiatrists (RCPsych) Psychopharmacology Committee (2017). *Use of Licensed Medicines for Unlicensed Applications in Psychiatric Practice*, 2nd ed. College Report CR210. London: Royal College of Psychiatrists. Available at: www.bap.org.uk/pdfs/CR210-December2017.pdf (last accessed 8.8.19).

Ruggiero S, Clavenna A, Reale L, et al. (2014). Guanfacine for attention deficit and hyperactivity disorder in pediatrics: a systematic review and meta-analysis. *Eur Neuropsychopharmacol*, 24(10), 1578–1590.

Ruthirakuhan MT, Herrmann N, Abraham EH, Chan S, Lanctôt KL (2018). Pharmacological interventions for apathy in Alzheimer's disease. *Cochrane Database Syst Rev*, (5), CD012197.

Sahakian BJ, Morein-Zamir S (2015). Pharmacological cognitive enhancement: treatment of neuropsychiatric disorders and lifestyle use by healthy people. *Lancet Psychiatry*, 2, 357–362.

Scheffer RE (2007). Concurrent ADHD and bipolar disorder. *Curr Psychiatry Rep*, 9, 415–419.

Scheffer RE, Kowatch RA, Carmody T, Rush AJ (2005). Randomized, placebo-controlled trial of mixed amphetamine salts for symptoms of comorbid ADHD in pediatric bipolar disorder after mood stabilization with divalproex sodium. *Am J Psychiatry*, 162(1), 58–64.

Sedgwick JA (2018). University students with attention deficit hyperactivity disorder (ADHD): a literature review. *Ir J Psychol Med*, 35(3), 221–235.

Seixas M, Weiss M, Müller U (2012). Systematic review of national and international guidelines on attention deficit hyperactivity disorder (ADHD). *J Psychopharmacology*, 26(6), 753–765.

Shanmugan S, Epperson CN (2014). Estrogen and the prefrontal cortex: towards a new understanding of estrogen's effects on executive functions in the menopause transition. *Hum Brain Mapp*, 35(3), 847–865.

Singh I, Bard I, Jackson J (2014). Robust resilience and substantial interest: a survey of pharmacological cognitive enhancement among university students in the UK and Ireland. *PLoS One*, 9(20), e105969.

Slade M (2017). Implementing shared decision making in routine mental health care. *World Psychiatry*, 16(2), 146–153.

Solberg BS, Haavik J, Halmøy A (2019). Health care services for adults with ADHD: patient satisfaction and the role of psycho-education. *J Atten Disord*, 23, 99–108.

Solmi M, Fornaro M, Toyoshima K, et al. (2018). Systematic review and exploratory meta-analysis of the efficacy, safety, and biological effects of psychostimulants and atomoxetine in patients with schizophrenia or schizoaffective disorder. *CNS Spectr* [Epub ahead of print] doi:10.1017/S1092852918001050.

Spruyt K, Gozal D (2011). Sleep disturbances in children with attention-deficit/hyperactivity disorder. *Expert Rev Neurother*, 11, 565–577.

Stein M, Thurmond P, Bailey G (2014). Willingness to use HIV pre-exposure prophylaxis among opiate users. *AIDS Behav*, 18(9), 1694–1700.

Stoffers JM, Völlm BA, Rücker G, et al. (2012). Psychological therapies for people with borderline personality disorder. *Cochrane Database Syst Rev*, (8), CD005652.

Sugden C, Housden CR, Aggarwal R, Sahakian BJ, Darzi A (2012). Effect of pharmacological enhancement on the cognitive and clinical psychomotor performance of sleep-deprived doctors: a randomized controlled trial. *Ann Surg*, 255(2), 222–227.

Surman CBH, Fried R, Rhodewalt L, Boland H (2017). Do pharmaceuticals improve driving in individuals with ADHD? A review of the literature and evidence for clinical practice. *CNS Drugs*, 31, 857–866.

Svedlund NE, Norring C, Ginsberg Y, von Hausswolff-Juhlin Y (2018). Are treatment results for eating disorders affected by ADHD symptoms? A one-year follow-up of adult females. *Eur Eat Disord Rev*, 26, 337–345.

Swanson JM, Arnold LE, Molina BSG, et al.; MTA Cooperative Group (2017). Young adult outcomes in the follow-up of the multimodal treatment study of attention-deficit/hyperactivity disorder: symptom persistence, source discrepancy, and height suppression. *J Child Psychol Psychiatry*, 58(6), 663–678.

Tarrant N, Roy M, Deb S, et al. (2018). The effectiveness of methylphenidate in the management of attention deficit hyperactivity disorder (ADHD) in people with intellectual disabilities: a systematic review. *Res Dev Disabil*, 83, 217–232.

Taylor E (2017). Attention deficit hyperactivity disorder: overdiagnosed or diagnoses missed? *Arch Dis Child*, 102, 376–379.

Taylor E (2019). ADHD medication in the longer term. *Z Kinder Jugendpsychiatr Psychother* [Epub ahead of print] doi:10.1024/1422-4917/a000664.

Thorpy MJ (2015). Update on therapy for narcolepsy. *Curr Treat Options Neurol*, 17(5), 347.

Tomlinson D, Robinson PD, Oberoi S, et al. (2018). Pharmacologic interventions for fatigue in cancer and transplantation: a meta-analysis. *Curr Oncol*, 25, e152–e167.

Torgersen T, Gjervan B, Lensing MB, Rasmussen K (2016). Optimal management of ADHD in older adults. *Neuropsychiatr DisTreat*, 12, 79–87.

Tritsch NX, Sabatini BL (2012). Dopaminergic modulation of synaptic transmission in cortex and striatum. *Neuron*, 76(1), 33–50.

UK Medicines Information (2017). Which medicines should be considered for brand-name prescribing in primary care? Available at: www.sps.nhs.uk/wp-content/uploads/2017/12/UKMi_QA_Brand-name_prescribing_Update_Nov2017.pdf (last accessed 9.8.19).

van Reekum R, Links PS (1994). N of 1 study: methylphenidate in a patient with borderline personality disorder and attention deficit hyperactivity disorder. *Can J Psychiatry*, 39(3), 186–187.

Verrotti A, Moavero R, Panzarino G, et al. (2018). The challenge of pharmacotherapy in children and adolescents with epilepsy-ADHD comorbidity. *Clin Drug Investig*, 38(1), 1–8.

Viktorin A, Rydén E, Thase ME, et al. (2017). The risk of treatment-emergent mania with methylphenidate in bipolar disorder. *Am J Psychiatry*, 174(4), 341–348.

Wilens TE, Morrison NR (2011). The intersection of attention-deficit/hyperactivity disorder and substance abuse. *Curr Opin Psychiatry*, 24(4), 280–285.

Wilens TE, Adler LA, Adams J, et al. (2008). Misuse and diversion of stimulants prescribed for ADHD: a systematic review of the literature. *J Am Acad Child Adolesc Psychiatry*, 47, 21–31.

Wilens TE, Adler LA, Weiss MD, et al.; Atomoxetine ADHD/SUD Study Group (2008). Atomoxetine treatment of adults with ADHD and comorbid alcohol use disorders. *Drug Alcohol Depend*, 96(1–2), 145–154.

Williamson D, Johnston C (2015). Gender differences in adults with attention-deficit/ hyperactivity disorder: a narrative review. *Clin Psychol Rev*, 40, 15–27.

Wilson SJ, Nutt DJ, Alford C, et al. (2010). British Association for Psychopharmacology consensus statement on evidence-based treatment of insomnia, parasomnias and circadian rhythm disorders. *J Psychopharmacol*, 24, 1577–1601.

Wolraich M, Brown L, Brown RT, et al. (2011). ADHD: clinical practice guideline for the diagnosis, evaluation and treatment of attention-deficit/hyperactivity disorder in children and adolescents. *Pediatrics*, 128(5), 1007–1022.

Wood DR, Reimherr FW, Wender PH, Johnson GE (1976). Diagnosis and treatment of minimal brain dysfunction in adults: a preliminary report. *Arch Gen Psychiatry*, 33 (12), 1453–1460.

World Health Organization (2011). *Technical Brief 1: Patterns and consequences of the use of amphetamine-type stimulants (ATS)*. Available at: www.wpro.who.int/hiv/documents/docs/Brief1forweb_850A.pdf (last accessed 1.8.18).

Chapter 14

Drugs to Treat Dementia

Ross Dunne and Alistair Burns

14.1 Introduction

Dementia is a clinical syndrome that is estimated to affect 46 million people worldwide. This number is estimated to increase to 131.5 million by 2050 (Prince et al., 2015). Dementia has a huge impact on people with the condition, their families and on health and social services. In the UK alone, it affects some 850 000 people with an estimated annual cost of £26 billion. It is a progressive neuropsychiatric condition leading to a significant strain on individuals, their families and the wider society. The risk increases with age and the burden of disease is set to rise in the coming years (Prince et al., 2015). While symptomatic treatments for the commonest cause of dementia, Alzheimer's disease, are available, no disease-modifying therapy has emerged and the majority of trials in this space have been negative although there is room for optimism (Aisen, 2017). This chapter starts with a review of the neuropathology of dementia. Subsequent sections cover the basic pharmacology of drugs used to treat dementia and the pharmacological treatment of cognitive dysfunction in dementia and behavioural and psychological symptoms of dementia (BPSD). The chapter ends with a short section on disease-modifying medicines in advanced development.

14.2 Neuropathology of Dementia

14.2.1 Alzheimer's Disease

Alzheimer's disease is best considered a disease with a life-long prodromal phase in which clinical features appear only at the latest stages, usually in later life. The two fundamental pathologies associated with Alzheimer's disease are the accumulation of hyperphosphorylated protein tau (Alois Alzheimer's 'tangles') in the cells of non-thalamic nuclei with diffuse ascending projections which are unmyelinated or poorly myelinated (Braak & Del Tredici, 2015) and amyloid plaques. Tau is a microtubule-associated protein which in normal function switches on and off the stabilization of microtubules, and therefore axons, and thus modulates axonal integrity and perhaps neuroplasticity. The biochemical switch involved is phosphorylation at serine and threonine residues. Many neuromodulators (dopamine, serotonin (5-hydroxytryptamine; 5-HT), noradrenaline) originate in brainstem nuclei with long unmyelinated projections with multiple cortical ramifications. These long, many-branched neurons are energetically expensive because of their relatively large surface area and lack of myelin. Braak believes this high metabolic load and oxidative burden to be responsible for these areas' early vulnerability to degeneration (Braak & Del Tredici, 2015). Even early in life, changes in the noradrenergic locus coeruleus and serotonergic median raphé can be found microscopically on AT-8 immunostaining for tau. Effects on these projections might be responsible for prodromal apathy and early non-cognitive symptoms. As well as brainstem nuclei, the cholinergic basal forebrain nucleus (of Meynert) has been found to be profoundly affected at the earliest clinical stages. Amyloid protein fragments form beta-pleated sheets which accumulate outside the cell – Alzheimer's 'plaques'. Amyloid accumulation in the cortex is now used as a relatively sensitive imaging biomarker for sporadic Alzheimer's disease in those with cognitive impairment established via clinical exam. However, we know that some individuals can prosper despite having detectable 'amyloidosis' in their brain and not reach dementia before death, and others, with specific 'tauopathies', get Alzheimer-like dementias without concomitant amyloid accumulation. So, more disease-specific tau-sensitive nuclear imaging modalities are in development (Jang et al., 2018).

14.2.2 Vascular Dementia

Vascular dementia is characterized by a stepwise decline in cognition and functional ability. Plateaus in both can last for months or years and are punctuated by either frank stroke or subcortical vascular events causing a 'step down'. Such events may be detectable clinically or radiologically on diffusion-weighted MRI or be relatively silent. Ischaemia is the common theme and may manifest after an acute stroke large enough to cause clinical signs (post-stroke dementia), or the sequelae of multiple discrete infarcts may be revealed only later on close neurological examination (multi-infarct dementia). In some, the presence of extensive deep white matter hyperintensities on neuroimaging (in the absence of significant hippocampal or generalized cerebral atrophy) may be the only thing except for the stepwise trajectory of decline confirming the diagnosis of subcortical cerebrovascular disease and vascular dementia.

14.2.3 Dementia with Lewy Bodies and Parkinson's Disease Dementia

Sporadic Parkinson's disease (PD) and Parkinson's disease dementia (PDD) and dementia with Lewy bodies (DLB) are different clinical syndromes caused by aberrant accumulation of alpha-synuclein-containing Lewy pathology (neurites, bodies and plaques). Debate continues about whether these illnesses are a single entity, separate illnesses with a common underlying pathology, or form a spectrum. This spectrum may include progressive supranuclear palsy (PSP), a tauopathy also causing dementia and multiple system atrophy, not known to cause cognitive decline. It is highly likely that those in whom dementia is diagnosed early after the onset of Parkinson's movement disorder (i.e. those with PDD), or those with DLB – where dementia comes first – have significant amounts of traditional Alzheimer's pathology in their brains at post-mortem and even potentially at diagnosis (Irwin et al., 2017). While often oversimplified as a movement disorder caused solely by dopaminergic transmission, there is undoubtedly a profound cholinergic deficit in PD/DLB contributing to neuropsychiatric symptoms and sufferers are likely to benefit from cholinergic medications even more than those with Alzheimer's dementia (Liu et al., 2015; Perry et al., 1985). Involvement of the mesencephalic tegmentum and cholinergic basal forebrain nuclei occurs in Braak's PD neuropathological stage three (Braak et al., 2004). Cumulatively, 80% of people with PD will suffer from dementia.

14.2.4 Frontotemporal Dementias

The frontotemporal dementias can be divided anatomically into those with early frontal and early temporal lobe atrophy, respectively. Clinical and neuropsychological classification divides them into language-predominant and behavioural variants. Pathological classification is into different proteinopathies. These classifications often overlap and clinicopathological correlation can be extremely difficult.

14.3 Basic Pharmacology of Drugs Used to Treat Dementia

14.3.1 Donepezil

Hachiro Sugimoto began work on E2020 (later donepezil) at Esai's Tsukuba Research Laboratories in 1983. His mother had suffered from Alzheimer's disease and, because of what was known about cholinergic deficits in the disease at the time, he had dedicated his early career to screening compounds for anticholinesterase activity. E2020 showed much promise at the bench, in that it reversed scopolamine-induced deficits in rat memory tests, without the physical side effects associated with many other pro-cholinergic compounds (Dawson & Iverson, 1993). It was first launched in the USA in 1997. Donepezil is a reversible inhibitor of acetylcholinesterase (AChE), the enzyme responsible for acetylcholine (ACh) catabolism in the cortical synapse.

Donepezil exhibits dose-independent excretion. The total clearance and renal clearance are also dose independent and the mean values after 10 mg dosing are 9.7 L/h and 0.86 L/h, respectively. The cumulative total urinary and faecal excretion of the sum of unchanged donepezil and its metabolites at 264 hours after the administration of the single 10 mg dose was 36.1% and 8.6% of the dose, respectively. The mean serum protein binding was 92.6%. Food intake does not affect its pharmacokinetics. Evaluation of the mean trough levels and $AUC_{(0-24)}$[1] of donepezil indicated that a steady state was achieved after approximately two weeks of daily dosing (Ohnishi et al., 1993).

Older people absorb donepezil more slowly but its clearance from the body is essentially unaffected by age. Age did not significantly affect maximum peak plasma concentration, AUC or oral clearance (9.1 ± 2.4 L/h). However, in the elderly the steady-state volume of distribution is larger by ~40% (Ohnishi et al., 1993).

14.3.2 Rivastigamine

Rivastigmine is a carbamate inhibitor of AChE and butyryl cholinesterase (BChE). Originally developed from physostigmine by Marta Weinstock-Rosin of Hebrew University in Jerusalem, it was sold to Novartis and marketed as liquid and tablet for use in Alzheimer's disease from 1997 and as a patch from 2007.

An amphiphilic molecule, rivastigmine is quickly widely distributed in the body and brain (cerebrospinal fluid (CSF) T_{max} 1.4–3.8 hours) but is less bioavailable than donepezil after oral dosing (40% versus 100%) because although it is rapidly and completely absorbed it undergoes significant first-pass metabolism (T_{max} of 0.8–1.7 hours (Gobburu et al., 2001; Polinsky, 1998)). Rivastigmine is 40% protein bound (mostly to red blood cells) and has a very short elimination half-life, leading to rapid peaks and prominent troughs in blood and brain levels during daily dosing. However, it binds covalently to serine residues in both the AChE and BChE active sites and it inhibits AChE for at least 12 hours, allaying the neurochemical effects of plasma peaks and troughs (Jann et al., 2002).

The peak levels in the CSF are about 40% of peak plasma levels and display a linear relationship between dose and AUC. Rivastigmine is metabolized by both the cholinesterases, but not by hepatic CYP450 enzymes. Cholinesterase metabolism produces a metabolite (NAP-226–90) which may be later renally excreted after hepatic sulphonyl or demethylated conjugation. Its CSF elimination half-life is from half an hour to 3 hours, suggesting it could take a maximum of 15 hours after peak CSF levels (4 hours) before the drug is 97% eliminated from the CSF.

The AUC of rivastigmine in moderate renal impairment was one to two times higher in one preliminary study, but further studies have not shown clinically significant effects,

[1] AUC_{0-24}: area under the curve from time zero to 24 hours after dosing.

and therefore there is no clear need for dose adjustment in renal impairment (Lefèvre et al., 2016). Studies in severe hepatic impairment are lacking.

14.3.3 Galantamine

Originally derived from the snowdrop *Galanthus nivalis,* galantamine was developed in the USSR by Mashkovsky and Kruglikova-Lvova in the 1950s and industrialized by the Bulgarian Paskov in 1959. It is a phenanthrene alkaloid, similar in structure to codeine, which is unique amongst these three dugs in also having allosteric agonist activity at the nicotinic receptor (Bickel et al., 1991). It was originally marketed as Nivalin, and used to treat paralytic and neuropathic conditions. After the cholinergic hypothesis of Alzheimer's disease was proposed and accepted in the early 1980s interest turned to using cholinesterase inhibitors to treat dementia. Patent problems delayed the introduction of galantamine to treat Alzheimer's disease. It was first licensed to treat Alzheimer's disease in Austria in 1994 and then in Europe and the United States in 2000.

Galantamine has high bioavailability (80–100%) (Bickel et al., 1991; Johansson & Nordberg, 1993) after oral administration with a time to peak plasma levels T_{max} of 1–2 hours. Although eating does not decrease the total absorption, it lowers the peak plasma concentration by 25% and delays absorption by 1–2 hours, which may help blunt some of the side effects associated with peak plasma levels of galantamine. While it is rapidly distributed in all compartments it also accumulates extensively and has only approximately 20–30% plasma protein binding, depending on dose (Bickel et al., 1991).

CYP450 3A4 and 2D6 enzymes metabolize 75% of the drug to *N*-demethyl and ketone metabolites. CYP2D6 metabolism produces its *O*-demethyl active metabolite ('sanguinine'), which is three times as potent in inhibiting AChE, 10 times more selective for AChE and may account for 20% of steady-state activity (Bickel et al., 1991). Galantamine is therefore hepatically metabolized and its metabolites 97% renally excreted but expected large differences between limited and 'super' CYP2D6 metabolizers of the drug have not been found, those with low enzyme activity having only 25% reduced clearance. In moderate hepatic impairment, a slower titration regimen may need to be considered to avoid excessive side effects.

Galantamine's elimination half-life is approximately 5–7 hours, and is slightly longer (20%) in women and the aged (10%) but not enough to consider changing the dose. In theory of course, an aged, female, poor metabolizer could then have a 45% reduced clearance rate, which would be something to consider in terms of dosing, but this has not been specifically experimentally examined or modelled (Bickel et al., 1991; Piotrovsky et al., 2003).

Galantamine has been demonstrated not to significantly interact with risperidone (Huang et al., 2002) but CYP450 enzyme inhibitors paroxetine (2D6), ketoconazole (3A4) and erythromycin (3A4) have been shown to increase blood levels of galantamine.

Both dispersible and sustained-release formulations appear to have similar bioavailability (Zhang & Sha, 2007; Zhao et al., 2005). Intranasal dosing methods appear to reduce the prominent gastrointestinal side effects while producing equivalent clinical efficacy but are not widely used in the UK (Vingtdeux et al., 2008).

Clinical uses in development include galantamine as an antidote to organophosphate poisoning (including nerve agents) and as an anti-smoking medication, and as a cognitive enhancer in schizophrenia, stroke and autism (Ghaleiha et al., 2014; Hilmas et al., 2009; Hong et al., 2012; Pereira et al., 2010).

14.3.4 Memantine

First developed by Eli-Lilly in 1968 to treat diabetes, this turned out to be a non-competitive *N*-methyl-D-aspartate (NMDA) receptor antagonist, which makes it the only drug licensed for dementia which does not act on AChE. Memantine inhibits the NMDA receptor, preventing maximal Ca^{++} influx and thus downstream effects of receptor activation. Why this should improve memory is not yet fully understood.

Memantine is mainly (75%) renally excreted as a glucuronide conjugate, with a linear relationship between plasma clearance and creatinine clearance. This means that elimination is decreased in renal impairment. After a single 20 mg dose, mean $AUC_{(0\text{-inf})}$[2] was 60% higher in the moderately impaired group and more than twice as high (115%) in the severely impaired group (CrCl <30 ml/min), with a linear relationship to creatinine clearance. Elimination half-life also doubled in those with severe renal impairment. Non-specific side effects such as dizziness, myalgia and headache were more common (even after a single dose) in those with severe renal impairment than those with normal renal function (Periclou et al., 2006). On the basis of this single-dose study, one would expect plasma concentrations to rise with increasing renal impairment. Maximum doses should therefore be halved in those with renal impairment. The nuclear receptor single nucleotide polymorphism (SNP) rs1523130 has been identified as a contributor to variation in renal clearance, with CT/TT genotypes clearing memantine 16% slower, but this merely demonstrates one potential interindividual difference and emphasizes the need for comprehensive discussion of potential side effects before prescribing (Noetzli et al., 2013). Sedation may be more related to peak concentrations, which can be mitigated by twice-daily dosing.

The most common adverse effects include dizziness, constipation and somnolence at higher doses. Massive doses (or inadvertent overdoses) can cause dissociative anaesthesia (cf. ketamine, which is also an antagonist at the NMDA receptor) (Glasgow et al., 2017). Patients initiated on memantine should be monitored for hypertension, which has sometimes emerged, although a recent meta-analysis suggested this was no more common than in placebo groups (Jiang & Jiang, 2015).

Cognitive improvement, as assessed by mean scores on the Mini–Mental State Examination (MMSE) and Neuropsychiatric Inventory (NPI), is greater in the moderate to severe group of people with dementia but the overall effect sizes are very modest indeed. In the mild-moderately affected Alzheimer's disease patients, memantine did not separate from placebo (Jiang & Jiang, 2015). The most recent meta-analysis of memantine efficacy in Alzheimer's disease demonstrated very modest clinical effects (nine randomized controlled trials (RCTs), n = 2433) but memantine was associated with less agitation compared with placebo (see below) (Matsunaga et al., 2015a).

14.4 Drug Treatment of Cognitive Dysfunction in Dementia

14.4.1 Alzheimer's Disease

In the UK, the acetylcholinesterase inhibitors (AChEIs) are licensed for mild to moderate Alzheimer's dementia, whereas memantine is licensed for moderate to severe disease. Common side effects of the AChEI medicines are directly related to their underlying mechanism of action, specifically, nausea, dizziness, vomiting and diarrhoea. These

[2] The AUC (from zero to infinity) represents total drug exposure across time.

gastrointestinal symptoms are the main reason for non-adherence though they tend to resolve with time (Campbell et al., 2017).

Donepezil is effective in improving cognition versus placebo at the expense of mostly early gastrointestinal side effects. To avoid these, the medication is usually slowly titrated from 5 mg to 10 mg after a period of four to six weeks. National Institute for Health and Care Excellence (NICE) guidance in the UK recommends an ECG before treating with donepezil, due to risks associated with cholinergic cardiac effects, such as bradycardia, heart block and resultant falls. As the risk is low, but the potential consequence serious, an ECG is warranted before initiating AChEI treatment.

A recent network meta-analysis compared three AChEIs (donepezil, galantamine and rivastigmine) in people with mild to moderate Alzheimer's disease. All of the AChEIs were significantly more efficacious than placebo in improving cognition as measured by the cognitive subscale of the Alzheimer's Disease Assessment Scale (ADAS-Cog) and had similar effect sizes (Kobayashi et al., 2016). The only significant difference between the drugs on the ADAS-Cog was that higher doses of galantamine (24 mg) outperformed the rivastigmine patch. The rivastigmine patch caused less nausea than comparator drugs and caused less dizziness than the oral form of rivastigmine, but there was little other difference in tolerability for specific side effects. In general, the rivastigmine patch is the best tolerated formulation, and oral rivastigmine or high-dose galantamine (24 mg) the least well tolerated. There is little difference in efficacy between the AChEIs, suggesting drugs should be chosen on the basis of tolerability and cost.

Managing patient and carer expectations in the use of these medicines is vital. Their effect sizes are very small indeed, with, for example, rivastigamine in Alzheimer's disease exhibiting a mean difference in MMSE scores of 0.74 points and mean ADAS-Cog difference from placebo of −1.79 points during the duration of a clinical trial (Birks et al., 2009). Nevertheless, perceptions persist amongst patients and families that these medicines will 'slow' or 'pause' the progress of cognitive impairment significantly. Because of their low effect size and the likelihood of side effects, the threshold for ceasing prescribing due to personal reluctance or side effects is low. However, they are cost-effective and some people have clear benefits, so all patients should be offered the opportunity for a trial.

Combination therapy (memantine plus any AChEI) is superior to monotherapy alone (Matsunaga et al., 2015b) but additional effects over AChEI monotherapy are very slight. However, memantine is very well tolerated and justifiably often used for BPSD, so it may be added to the treatment regimen at low clinical risk to the patient, even if the number needed to treat (NNT) to achieve a particular measured cognitive benefit might be high.

Schmidt et al. published guidance advising co-treatment in moderate to severe disease based on meta-analytic evidence (Grossberg et al., 2013; Howard et al., 2012; Schmidt et al., 2015; Tariot et al., 2004). They demonstrated benefits for combination of AChEI + memantine in terms of NPI (behaviour and mood) scores on scales measuring activities of daily living, as well as the CIBIC-plus measure of cognition.

One of the included trials, the 2012 DOMINO study, examined four interventions in those stable on donepezil: (1) stopping donepezil; (2) adding memantine; (3) changing to memantine; and (4) continuing donepezil. They found that a combination was better in terms of cognition and preventing admission to care home, one outcome not included in the Schmidt meta-analysis (Howard et al., 2015).

In Alzheimer's disease, there is very little to distinguish the AChEIs from each other except their side-effect profile. Donepezil is first line but up to half of those who do not benefit from the drug will benefit from another AChEI. Therefore, after consultation, switching should be tried in order to maximize benefit and/or minimize side effects (Auriacombe et al., 2002; Bullock & Connolly, 2002; Engedal et al., 2012; Massoud et al., 2011; Ohta et al., 2017; Sasaki et al., 2014).

Dementia may lead to a disruption of the sleep–wake cycle and ACh is active in sleep–wake switching. While night-time dosing of these medications can often lead to nightmares and initial insomnia, morning dosing with a daytime peak more closely mimics physiological circadian rhythms in ACh function.

Some evidence suggests that higher doses of donepezil (23 mg) may be more effective, at the risk of higher rates of side effects. The 23 mg dose is now licensed in the USA (Cummings et al., 2013; Sabbagh et al., 2016).

14.4.2 Vascular Dementia

Vascular dementia is not characterized by the profound cholinergic deficit found in Alzheimer's or Lewy body dementias (Sharp et al., 2009). Thus, it is surprising that the AChEIs have shown benefit in improving cognition in these illnesses, albeit to a minor degree. However, the risk–benefit appears to be against prescribing as there were significant side effects from AChEI drugs in all trials in this subgroup (Chen et al., 2016). Memantine, which in murine models decreased cognitive impact of stroke, by reducing excitotoxicity (López-Valdés et al., 2014; Trotman et al., 2015), has also shown very modest benefits but a better side-effect profile. It may be that neurochemical modulation has greater effects in a subgroup of patients yet to be identified, and certainly if there is an equivocal or clinically mixed picture of overlapping Alzheimer's and vascular disease then a trial of either memantine or an AChEI is warranted.

Those with vascular dementia do have some cognitive improvement overall on memantine, but do not necessarily benefit clinically significantly (in behaviour or function) because effect sizes are small when vascular dementia is narrowly defined according to research criteria (Kavirajan & Schneider, 2007). However, those with an underlying Alzheimer's disease who also have a subcortical vascular component may still benefit, and there are significant effects in terms of reducing agitation.

In many people there is a mixed picture of smooth, slow cognitive decline interspersed with 'steps down'. It is possible that people with such a picture will have clinical features suggestive of both cerebrovascular and Alzheimer's disease pathology. This may be confirmed by clinical history, neuropsychological assessment and perhaps by finding both medial temporal atrophy and deep white matter changes on neuroimaging. On neuropsychological assessment, a more 'subcortical' picture is often present, with more deficits in free recall than recognition, pronounced slow but accurate processing and less distinct early amnesia than 'pure' Alzheimer's disease. While vascular dementia may be significantly over-diagnosed unless strict criteria are used, a trial of AChEIs in these patients is likely worthwhile if there is probable underlying Alzheimer's disease.

14.4.3 Dementia with Lewy Bodies and Parkinson's Disease Dementia

Clinically, the treatment of these illnesses is complicated by the often competing roles of geriatrician, neurologist and psychogeriatrician, and their sometimes competing drugs.

Treatment with anticholinergics such as oxybutinin for bladder dysfunction in PD is likely to cause cognitive deterioration and worsen visual hallucinations. The presence of dementia and the use of dopamine agonists, rather than merely L-dopa dose, may be better predictors of neuropsychiatric conditions such as visual hallucinations in PD (Ecker et al., 2009; Hinkle et al., 2018; Holroyd et al., 2001; Kavirajan & Schneider, 2007). Both rivastigamine (in the UK) and donepezil (in Asia) are licensed for treatment of Lewy body dementia. Memantine has shown promise (Emre et al., 2010; Wesnes et al., 2014) although the size of its effects varied between DLB and PDD groups and between cognitive and non-cognitive benefits within those groups. In both, participants taking memantine demonstrated global improvements. The British Association for Psychopharmacology (BAP) currently recommends rivastigamine and donepezil for DLB and PDD, with more cautious support for memantine.

14.4.4 Frontotemporal Dementias

The frontotemporal dementias are diseases of degeneration in either or both the frontal and temporal lobes. Clinical presentation is often categorized into behavioural variant or language variants (primary progressive aphasia), but in fact presentations occur along a spectrum. The underlying neuropathology is similarly spectral, and while this means that some patients may have cholinergic deficits ameliorable by AChEIs, it is not yet possible to predict a response on the basis of presentation, and the cholinergic compounds are not recommended routinely.

A recent meta-analysis of just two RCTs (n = 130) of memantine's efficacy in frontotemporal dementia did not find a statistically significant difference from placebo on any measures (Kishi et al., 2015).

14.4.5 Dementia in Those with Learning Disabilities

People with trisomy 21 (Down's syndrome) are at increased risk of Alzheimer's dementia. Other neurodevelopmental disorders may also increase the risk of dementia at an earlier age because of decreased cognitive reserve. However, there is little evidence for the efficacy of the cholinergic drugs or memantine in such subgroups. Memantine is relatively contraindicated for those with a history of seizures. However, such medications may be of use for a trial on an individual patient basis for those with severe behavioural disturbance in the context of dementia. It is vitally important to rule out depression or other acute disorders as a confounder and equally important to attend to the list of basic human needs which may not be able to be communicated.

14.4.6 Anticholinergic Burden in Dementia

Since the first use of pro-cholinergic medications in dementia, the contradiction has been that many drugs used to treat physical and psychiatric conditions in the same patients have profound anticholinergic effects. In younger people noticeable side effects are often limited to those on single drugs with very high anticholinergic potency such as tricyclic antidepressants (e.g. nortryptiline). In older people who are often subject to polypharmacy, the cumulative burden of multiple weakly anticholinergic drugs can be just as important. Many different versions of similar scales exist to quantify cumulative anticholinergic 'burden'. Well-replicated epidemiological studies suggest that those with more cumulative 'burden' have lower cognitive scores and progress more quickly to dementia, even after controlling for age and physical co-morbidity. This must be borne in mind, not only when prescribing, but when reviewing and rationalizing the medication regimen, as should be done regularly (Chew et al., 2008; Fox et al., 2011; Green et al., 2016; Risacher et al., 2016). Anticholinergic burden also increases the risk of delirium in the general population, although some findings in general hospital inpatient populations are more equivocal possibly due to the overwhelming effects of infection and surgery which prevail (van Gool et al., 2010). Equally, certain drugs with anticholinergic burden are used to manage BPSD. Olanzapine scores 3 on the commonly used Anticholinergic Burden Scale and trazodone scores 1. These drugs have been found to independently associate with falls and increased mortality. However, in such studies, the risk component contributed by the cholinergic deficit is difficult to isolate (Pasina et al., 2013; Ruxton et al., 2015; Salahudeen et al., 2015).

14.5 Pharmacological Treatment of Behavioural and Psychological Symptoms of Dementia

14.5.1 Introduction

Behavioural and psychological symptoms of dementia (BPSD) refers to any non-cognitive symptom of dementia, but especially: depression, mood lability, anxiety, agitation, apathy, aggression or psychotic symptoms such as paranoia or hallucinations. BPSD used to be considered the preserve of advanced stages of dementing illnesses. This might be the case for some with pure amnestic cognitive impairment in Alzheimer's disease. However, those with Lewy body dementia are often plagued by hallucinations and depression from the earliest stages of the illness (indeed Alois Alzheimer's disease-defining patient was 55 years old and presented with paranoid delusions). Those with vascular dementia can often suffer hallucinations and mood lability, disinhibition or anxiety depending on the anatomical predilection of white matter damage or discrete stroke. So, the incidence and nature of BPSD depends on underlying pathology, stage of illness, concomitant medication (cf. Anticholinergic Burden, above) as well as the caregiver's approach to the person with dementia and their care environment.

The most important statement to make in this context (a chapter in a textbook on psychopharmacology) is that using a medicine for BPSD is not necessarily first-line. Communication with, and education of, caregivers is paramount. Many aspects of BPSD can be addressed through environmental change or caregiver behaviour change. It is very useful to formulate what individual aspects of BPSD are present using the NPI in one of its many guises (Cummings et al., 1994). The scale can be repeated after an interval to examine for change after changing an aspect of the environment or caregiver behaviour. Any acute change in a person with dementia's behaviour or mental state should initiate a search for physical causes including delirium, infection, constipation, hunger, fatigue, pain, medication changes or omissions or environmental changes. A thorough mental or physical checklist including all usual biological, psychological and social needs is a must.

A so-called 'ABC' chart documenting time, date, antecedents (e.g. what was happening before the episode or in the environment?), behaviour (e.g. how did the person with dementia react?) and consequences (e.g. how did the caregiver react?) is also essential for treating BPSD. An iterative cycle of changing one thing only, then reassessing the behaviour in question, will help understand whether the intervention has worked, gradually 'shaping' the environment and caregiver behaviour to accommodate and manage the behavioural problem.

Levels of BPSD/neuropsychiatric symptoms can be captured using the NPI, but it is not a scale per se, merely a combined set of ordinally ranked subscales. For example, benefits in one domain (decreased agitation scale scores) might be mirrored by increased apathy or tiredness scores, perhaps resulting in a clinically significant improvement in behaviour and life-quality, without a change in overall NPI score. Wang et al. (2015) meta-analyzed the efficacy of selective serotonin reuptake inhibitors (SSRIs), memantine, AChEIs and atypical antipsychotics versus placebo in Alzheimer's dementia with total NPI score as an outcome. They found statistically and clinically significant benefits for AChEIs (specifically galantamine) and antipsychotics olanzapine and aripiprazole but again these improvements were of modest size on average. They further examined NPI/BEHAVE-AD score reduction in all-cause dementia and found clinically small, but statistically significant benefits for memantine, atypical antipsychotics and AChEIs over placebo. However, AChEIs and atypical antipsychotics both resulted in increased adverse events and trial dropouts in the Alzheimer's and all-cause dementia groups (Wang et al., 2015). The following sections review the pharmacological treatments of specific aspects of BPSD, namely depression, sleep disturbance, agitation and aggression, disinhibition and hypersexuality, apathy and psychosis.

14.5.2 Depression

Depression occurs in approximately 40% of people with dementia (Zhao et al., 2016). However, given the deterioration of neuromodulatory centres in preclinical phases of neurodegenerative dementias, efficacy of the traditional medications cannot be assumed. One six-week RCT of venlafaxine demonstrated no difference from placebo. A maximum dose of 131.5 mg was used and there was an extended dose-titration period, which may have meant less of an opportunity for response. Mean scores on the Montgomery–Asberg Depression Rating Scale (MADRS) at baseline were 20, improving to 10 in both groups over six weeks (De Vasconcelos Cunha et al., 2007).

A randomized trial conducted in the UK (Health Technology Assessment Study of the Use of Antidepressants for Depression in Dementia (HTA-SADD)) failed to find an effect over placebo for sertraline or mirtazapine over 13 weeks in those with probable or possible Alzheimer's disease and clinically significant depression. It is notable that the baseline cut-off scores for participants' inclusion were >7 on the Cornell Scale for Depression in Dementia (CSDD) and that the mean baseline score was ~13, improving to 8 over the initial 13 weeks of the study in all three groups (Bannerjee et al., 2013). The maximum doses used were sertraline 150 mg and mirtazapine 45 mg. If these findings are disheartening in terms of drug response, they do at least show that these non-suicidal, moderately depressed people with depression do seem to get better with simple supportive care (as received in the placebo arm of a clinical trial). A previous meta-analysis of depression treatment in all-cause dementia analyzed seven RCTs from 1996 onwards and demonstrated no statistically significant effect of SSRI or tricyclic medications versus placebo for response or remission criteria over 6–12 weeks of treatment (Nelson & Devanand, 2011). Overall, psychological measures are likely to be more effective in mild to moderate depression, in those with mild cognitive impairment or an ability to engage in behavioural therapies, while antidepressants are likely to be more effective in those with a known depression prior to dementia onset, or who cannot engage in the low-level psychological therapies often used in moderate dementia. Expert clinical opinion has long held that electroconvulsive therapy (ECT) may be effectively used in those with severe depression in dementia, although RCTs are lacking and evidence is limited to cases series.

14.5.3 Sleep Disturbance

Sleep disturbance has a prevalence of approximately 40% in people with dementia. In Lewy body diseases, there are specific problems with REM sleep behaviour disorder (RSBD) which affects three-quarters of people with DLB/PDD and can often be treated with low-dose clonazepam, if the possible increased risk of falls is borne in mind. Memantine was found in one post-hoc study of a randomized trial to have decreased the broken sleep associated with RSBD (Larsson et al., 2010). Melatonin has been found to be weakly effective in increasing sleep duration and quality, but with better-quality studies showing less effect (Serfaty et al., 2002). It is not currently recommended by NICE. While risperidone has been found to increase sleep in observational studies, this must be balanced against its risks. In care home patients and those with more advanced disease living at home, it is likely that meaningful daytime activity, daylight, exercise and psychosocial interaction are more effective than drugs in improving insomnia (Sullivan & Richards, 2004). A current National Institute for Health research (NIHR)-funded clinical trial (SYMBAD) is measuring the efficacy of mirtazapine versus placebo in agitation and aggression in dementia, but there is currently little evidence that this medication improves sleep in dementia, despite widespread use and intuitive appeal.

14.5.4 Agitation and Aggression

In the past antipsychotics were widely prescribed to treat agitation and aggression in dementia, a practice now seen as inappropriate. Psychological and behavioural methods for dealing with agitation in dementia have been demonstrated to be both clinically and cost-effective (Livingston et al., 2014) and in general should be first-line treatments. However, it is difficult to eliminate the prescribing of antipsychotics completely, especially in care home populations. Where psychosis is the cause of the agitation, such prescribing is justified. Aggression occurs in 40% of people with dementia and can result in serious harm to others or the patient themselves. It is in situations like this where greatest pressure can be applied to clinicians to prescribe. If antipsychotics are used to treat aggression, then prescriptions should start at the very lowest end of the scale and it is not unusual to find experienced clinicians beginning treatment with 0.25 mg of risperidone or 12.5 mg of quetiapine (sometimes chosen because of a broader dose range). All concerned must be appraised of increased risks of falls, stroke and sudden death and there must be close monitoring for oversedation and extrapyramidal side effects (Schneider-Thoma et al., 2018). The need for and purpose of the medication should be regularly reviewed. Benzodiazepines should be used only for brief periods if needed as they can worsen disinhibition and increase falls risk, then people quickly become tolerant and their agitation may worsen in the withdrawal phase. A large clinical trial is currently underway to compare mirtazapine and carbamazepine with placebo for agitation in dementia (ISRCTN 17411897). However, currently neither carbamazepine nor valproate have enough evidence to recommend their prescription to treat agitation and aggression in dementia. Some preliminary evidence suggested that cyproterone, an anti-testoterone drug, may be of benefit in treating aggression associated with dementia (Bolea-Alamanac et al., 2011) but further studies are needed to determine its efficacy and safety when used in this off-label indication.

14.5.5 Disinhibition and Hypersexuality

Both disinhibition and hypersexuality can be an early feature of frontotemporal dementias or occur at later stages of any of the dementias, likely related to the 'release' caused by the atrophy of the dorsolateral prefrontal cortex. The phenomenon is complex and may in some cases be an exaggerated aspect of premorbid personality. In other cases, it comes as a surprise to caregivers, and can be one of the hardest aspects to deal with. People with dementia have a right to privacy and to continue to have a consensual sexual life with partners as well as other aspects of human sexuality (Haddad & Benbow, 1993a, 1993b). In residential care settings this can result in conflict between the needs of the patient and the professional carers' wishes for dignity at work. Education is again key. Normalization of behaviour that does not pose a risk to others, while addressing distress or compulsion, requires a fine balance. After boredom, loneliness, misinterpreted gestures and privacy have been addressed, pharmacological measure may be considered. Strategies that have been tried to reduce distressing hypersexuality include SSRIs, D_2 antagonists and – in men – cimetidine, which causes a mild reduction in testosterone. However, good RCT evidence for any of these approaches is lacking. Benzodiazepines can worsen cognition and impulse control and cause paradoxical disinhibition in the elderly and should probably be avoided.

14.5.6 Apathy

Apathy is a problem in 20–25% of patients with early Alzheimer's disease and its cumulative incidence is approximately 80%. Similar rates of between 55% and 90% in Huntington's disease, 60% and 90% in PSP and 40% and 60% in PDD are reported. Apathy in dementia is a separate entity from depression, but with overlapping features. Notably, there is often an absence of hopelessness and helplessness and the negative cognitive triad of depression (Beck et al., 1979). However, it can of course also be co-morbid with depressive illness which occurs in 40% of those with PD.

Pagonabarraga et al. (2015) divide apathy into four clinical syndromes: reward deficiency syndrome, emotional distress, executive dysfunction and auto-activation deficit. Dopaminergic systems govern both the 'reward deficiency syndrome', characterized by emotional blunting and diminished emotional resonance, and the auto-activation deficit or failure of self-motivation (Pagonabarraga et al., 2015). Acetylcholinergic deficits are felt to underlie the deficits in executive function, in which there is difficulty redirecting attention, abstracting future plans or manipulating information in working memory. Noradrenergic deficits may underlie the negative affect.

This suggests strategies to address individual dimensions of the apathetic syndrome might be more effective than a more general approach. This dimensional approach is supported by animal studies demonstrating that DA depletion in the substantia nigra pars compacta (SNPC) to levels that do not cause motor problems is still sufficient to cause reward deficits (Drui et al., 2014). Apathy is a prominent syndrome after withdrawal of L-dopa after deep brain stimulation to the subthalamic nucleus (STN-DBS). It is best measured with Lille Apathy Rating Scale (LARS). One six-month RCT of rivastigamine for apathy demonstrated small improvements (Devos et al., 2014). One RCT of the dopamine $D_{2/3}$ agonist piribedil in patients after STN-DBS demonstrated a 30% improvement in scores over placebo (Thobois et al., 2013). Antidepressant medication may actually make apathy worse, although the evidence is poor either way and clinical judgement would seem to advocate treating rather than withholding such relatively safe medications.

14.5.7 Psychosis

Hallucinations (16%) and delusions (31%) are prevalent in Alzheimer's dementia (Zhao et al., 2016). Both Lewy body dementia and vascular dementia are known for prominent visual hallucinations, but no form of dementia is exempt, however, and the C9orf72 form of behavioural variant frontotemporal dementia is renowned for early schizophreniform delusions and hallucinations (Collerton et al., 2015).

As in delirium, a good understanding of the visual neural pathway and the nature of top-down as well as bottom-up visual processing is necessary to place visual hallucinations in their environmental context. Often, merely replacing dim lights and ensuring adequate daytime arousal by avoiding sedating medications can significantly improve symptoms (Sullivan & Richards, 2004). However, in those for whom environmental change is not sufficient, a trial of an AChEI is likely to be beneficial. There is reasonable evidence for the use of rivastigamine in DLB/PDD for treating hallucinations and other aspects of 'behavioural disturbance' and in its patch form avoids the need for daily tablet taking which in moderate to severe dementia can be difficult to achieve. Importantly, AChEIs, unlike dopamine receptor antagonists, are not associated with increased mortality in people with dementia making them a safer option to treat psychotic symptoms.

For those who do not respond to environmental change, cholinergic medications and a review of polypharmacy, and where psychotic symptoms are impairing function or associated with risk to self or others, a tentative trial of an antipsychotic is warranted. In these situations, a six-week course of risperidone or olanzapine is recommended by NICE. Full disclosure to patients and families about the risks of such medications is recommended up-front and NICE has produced a decision aid for patients and caregivers. They recommend '*The antipsychotic should be tried alongside other activities to try to help their distress. It should be used at the lowest dose that helps the person, and for the shortest possible time. The person should be assessed at least every 6 weeks and the antipsychotic should be stopped if it is not helping or is no longer needed*' (NICE, 2018a). If there is a suspicion about underlying Lewy body disease, D_2 antagonists should be used only by an expert. If oral intake or other vital measures deteriorate after stopping these medications, then a trial of longer duration is warranted.

Clozapine, the antipsychotic with least propensity for extrapyramidal side effects, has demonstrated some significant success in treating the psychosis of PDD. Its practical use requires good multidisciplinary team work between specialities managing physical and psychiatric care. Evidence and experience suggest that doses in the order of 5–10% of usual adult doses are effective (e.g. 25–50 mg). If clozapine use cannot be contemplated, for example because of physical health concerns, then quetiapine, at a starting dose of 12.5 mg, may be useful for brief periods under close supervision and after a thorough physical exam including ECG. The newer agent pimavanserin, a 5-HT_{2A} receptor antagonist, has had success in clinical trials for psychosis in PD and one in Alzheimer's disease has also been conducted with significant efficacy (Cummings et al., 2018). However, pimavanserin is currently extremely expensive compared with clozapine, and has not yet had a head-to-head comparison (Meltzer et al., 2010).

14.5.8 The Use of Dopamine Antagonists in Dementia

A third of people with dementia live in care homes, and two-thirds of care home residents have dementia. For many years, dopamine antagonists (antipsychotics) were the mainstay of psychopharmacological treatment of those with 'senile dementia' with agitation or sleep disturbance in care homes or at home. These drugs were undoubtedly overused at the expense of sensitive nursing care and therefore played a role in facilitating neglectful and sometimes inhumane practices. Apart from the influence on care practices, dopamine antagonists have been shown to increase the risk of stroke and sudden death by two to three times in those with dementia irrespective of their class or binding affinity at the D_2 or 5-HT_{2A} receptor (Corbett et al., 2014; Herrmann et al., 2004). Dopamine antagonists can be even more lethal in PD, where the hazard ratio for death at six months in one study was two to three times the control group (Weintraub et al., 2016). Clozapine was not included in the study. In addition, dopamine antagonists can worsen symptoms in people with PDD and dementia.

A dopamine receptor antagonist should only be used to treat BPSD after a full assessment has been conducted to determine the cause of the patient's symptoms and distress (e.g. concomitant infection leading to delirium) and psychosocial treatments and environmental interventions have been considered to reduce distress. Alternative pharmacological approaches should be considered, including rationalizing existing medications, especially if recently added. Introducing or optimizing the use of AChEIs or memantine should be considered next. The NICE (2018b) Dementia Guideline recommends that dopamine antagonists are only considered when a patient is at risk of harming themselves or others or experiences agitation, hallucinations or delusions that cause them severe distress. The lowest effective dose of a dopamine antagonist should be used and regular attempts at, or at least consideration of, withdrawal should be the norm. Decisions about starting and stopping antipsychotics need to be made on an individual patient basis, taking account of benefits and harms. Such decision should involve the family members or carers as well as the patient if possible.

Risperidone is licensed in the UK for the short-term treatment (up to six weeks) of persistent aggression in people with moderate to severe Alzheimer's dementia if this has not responded to non-pharmacological approaches and if there is a risk of self-harm or harm to others. In addition, haloperidol is licensed in the UK to treat psychotic symptoms and persistent aggression in people with moderate to severe Alzheimer's dementia and vascular dementia if non-pharmacological treatments have failed and there is a risk of harm to self or others. However, both risperidone and haloperidol have narrow therapeutic indices in the elderly and are prone to causing or exacerbating extrapyramidal symptoms and increasing falls risk. In the UK, the use of antipsychotics in the treatment of BPSD represents off-label use and should immediately prompt referral to specialist psychiatric services.

Guidelines now recommend that regular attempts are made to withdraw antipsychotics in people with dementia. This is based on the risks associated with antipsychotic treatment and because behavioural complications of dementia are usually intermittent and often do not continue beyond three months. Clinicians and the family members may worry that antipsychotic withdrawal may cause a worsening of the symptoms that the drugs were introduced to treat. A Cochrane review analyzed available evidence to help inform decisions about drug continuation/withdrawal (Van Leeuwen et al., 2018). The researchers assessed all trials in which people with dementia, who had been treated with a dopamine receptor antagonist for at least three months, were randomized to continue treatment or be withdrawn from the drug. Ten studies, conducted in various settings, were included (community = 1; nursing home = 8; both settings = 1). Patients were treated with various antipsychotics and doses. Some studies employed an abrupt and others a gradual withdrawal regimen. Overall, antipsychotic withdrawal seemed to make little or no difference to severity of BPSD or whether or not participants completed the study. However, in both cases the quality of evidence was low. Subgroup analysis suggested that withdrawal may reduce agitation for participants with less severe BPSD at baseline. Two studies suggested that those with psychosis, aggression or agitation that had responded to dopamine receptor antagonists, or who had more severe BPSD at baseline, may worsen behaviourally following withdrawal, i.e. they may benefit from continuing treatment with antipsychotics. In summary, current evidence supports the view that it is generally safe to attempt withdrawal of antipsychotics that have been used to treat BPSD. We would generally recommend a gradual withdrawal regimen.

14.6 New Medicines in Development

At the time of writing, Alzheimer's disease is showing weak signs of response to disease-modifying anti-amyloid immunoglobulins. Approaches such as regulation of brain glucose metabolism, inhibitors of the receptor for end products of glycation (RAGE) and other novel compounds are in active trials. Another approach focuses on the use of already licensed molecules such as minocycline (The MADE trial; ISRCTN 16105064), which can be rapidly trialled as side effects are largely understood and safety concerns can be more rationally allayed. This may result in moving agents from animal models to human use more quickly and cheaply.

For the motor component of PD, the replacement of SNPC dopamine-releasing neurons may well be possible due to stem cell therapies in coming years. However, it is not at all clear what effect this would have on the neuropsychiatric components, and other types of dementia are further from effective treatment. For example, the disseminated white matter destruction caused by widespread cerebrovascular disease is more likely to be prevented through lifestyle change and established stroke risk reduction strategies (e.g. antihypertensives and statins) than reversed through specific pharmacological intervention after cognition has already become impaired. This theme of the impossibility of reconstructing diverse tissue damage speaks to the importance of new studies of preventative interventions, including pharmaceuticals.

The neurodegenerative dementias are diseases with decades-long prodromes which are today largely clinically and radiologically undetectable. Earlier intervention will be necessary to initiate neuron-sparing therapies. The recruitment of clinically well people, merely 'at risk' of dementia, to clinical trials of disease-modifying agents presents its own ethical, technological and logistical difficulties, but will be vital in the development of true disease-modifying therapies in the future.

References

Aisen P (2017). Continuing progress in Alzheimer's disease trials. *J Prev Alz Dis*, 4(4), 211–212.

Auriacombe S, Pere J-J, Loria-Kanza Y, Vellas B (2002). Efficacy and safety of rivastigmine in patients with Alzheimer's disease who failed to benefit from treatment with donepezil. *Curr Med Res Opin*, 18, 129–138. doi:10.1185/030079902125000471.

Banerjee S, Hellier J, Romeo R, et al. (2013). Study of the use of antidepressants for depression in dementia: the HTA-SADD trial – a multicentre, randomised, double-blind, placebo-controlled trial of the clinical effectiveness and cost-effectiveness of sertraline and mirtazapine. *Health Technol Assess*, 17, 1–166.

Beck AT, Rush A, Shaw B, Emery G (1979). *Cognitive Therapy of Depression*. New York: Guilford Press.

Bickel U, Thomsen T, Weber W, et al. (1991). Pharmacokinetics of galanthamine in humans and corresponding cholinesterase inhibition. *Clin Pharmacol Ther*, 50, 420–428.

Birks J, Grimley Evans J, Iakovidou V, Tsolaki M (2009). Rivastigmine for Alzheimer's disease. *Cochrane Database Syst Rev*, (2), CD001191. doi:10.1002/14651858.CD001191.pub2.

Bolea-Alamanac BM, Davies SJ, Christmas DM, et al. (2011). Cyproterone to treat aggressivity in dementia: a clinical case and systematic review. *J Psychopharmacol*, 25(1), 141–145.

Braak H, Del Tredici K (2015). Neuroanatomy and pathology of sporadic Alzheimer's disease. *Adv Anat Embryol Cell Biol*, 215, 1–162.

Braak H, Ghebremedhin E, Rüb U, Bratzke H, Del Tredici K (2004). Stages in the development of Parkinson's disease-related pathology. *Cell Tissue Res*, 318, 121–134.

Bullock R, Connolly C (2002). Switching cholinesterase inhibitor therapy in Alzheimer's disease: donepezil to rivastigmine, is it worth it? *Int J Geriatr Psychiatry*, 17, 288–289.

Campbell NL, Perkins AJ, Gao S, et al. (2017). Adherence and tolerability of Alzheimer's disease medications: a pragmatic randomized trial. *J Am Geriatr Soc*, 65, 1497–1504.

Chen YD, Zhang J, Wang Y, Yuan JL, Hu WL (2016). Efficacy of cholinesterase inhibitors in vascular dementia: an updated meta-analysis. *Eur Neurol*, 75, 132–141.

Chew ML, Mulsant BH, Pollock BG, et al. (2008). Anticholinergic activity of 107 medications commonly used by older adults. *J Am Geriatr Soc*, 56, 1333–1341.

Collerton D, Mosimann UP, Perry E (2015). *The Neuroscience of Visual Hallucinations*. Chichester: John Wiley & Sons.

Corbett A, Burns A, Ballard C (2014). Don't use antipsychotics routinely to treat agitation and aggression in people with dementia. *BMJ*, 349, g6420.

Cummings JL, Mega M, Gray K, et al. (1994). The Neuropsychiatric Inventory: comprehensive assessment of psychopathology in dementia. *Neurology*, 44, 2308–2314.

Cummings JL, Geldmacher D, Farlow M, et al. (2013). High-dose donepezil (23 mg/day) for the treatment of moderate and severe Alzheimer's disease: drug profile and clinical guidelines. *CNS Neurosci Ther*, 19, 294–301.

Cummings J, Ballard C, Tariot P, et al. (2018). Pimavanserin: potential treatment for dementia-related psychosis. *J Prev Alzheimers Dis*, 5(1), 253–258.

Dawson GR, Iversen SD (1993). The effects of novel cholinesterase inhibitors and selective muscarinic receptor agonists in tests of reference and working memory. *Behav Brain Res*, 57, 143–153.

de Vasconcelos Cunha UG, Lopes Rocha F, Ávila de Melo R, et al. (2007). A placebo-controlled double-blind randomized study of venlafaxine in the treatment of depression in dementia. *Dement Geriatr Cogn Disord*, 24, 36–41. doi:10.1159/000102570.

Devos D, Moreau C, Maltête D, et al. (2014). Rivastigmine in apathetic but dementia and depression-free patients with Parkinson's disease: a double-blind, placebo-controlled, randomised clinical trial. *J Neurol Neurosurg Psychiatry*, 85, 668–674. doi:10.1136/jnnp-2013-306439.

Drui G, Carnicella S, Carcenac C, et al. (2014). Loss of dopaminergic nigrostriatal neurons accounts for the motivational and affective deficits in Parkinson's disease. *Mol Psychiatry*, 19, 358–367. doi:10.1038/mp.2013.3.

Ecker D, Unrath A, Kassubek J, Sabolek M (2009). Dopamine agonists and their risk to induce psychotic episodes in Parkinson's disease: a case-control study. *BMC Neurol*, 9, 23. doi:10.1186/1471-2377-9-23.

Emre M, Tsolaki M, Bonucelli U, et al. (2010). Memantine for patients with Parkinson's disease dementia or dementia with Lewy bodies: a randomised, double-blind, placebo-controlled trial. *Lancet Neurol*, 9(10), 969–977.

Engedal K, Davis B, Richarz U, et al. (2012). Two galantamine titration regimens in patients switched from donepezil. *Acta Neurol Scand*, 126, 37–44. doi:10.1111/j.1600-0404.2011.01594.x.

Fox C, Livingston G, Maidment ID, et al. (2011). The impact of anticholinergic burden in Alzheimer's dementia – the laser-AD study. *Age Ageing*, 40, 730–735.

Ghaleiha A, Ghyasvand M, Mohammadi MR, et al. (2014). Galantamine efficacy and tolerability as an augmentative therapy in autistic children: a randomized, double-blind, placebo-controlled trial. *J Psychopharmacol*, 28, 677–685.

Glasgow NG, Povysheva NV, Azofeifa AM, Johnson JW (2017). Memantine and ketamine differentially alter NMDA receptor desensitization. *J Neurosci*, 37, 9686–9704.

Gobburu JVS, Tammara V, Lesko L, et al. (2001). Pharmacokinetic-pharmacodynamic modeling of rivastigmine, a cholinesterase inhibitor, in patients with Alzheimer's disease. *J Clin Pharmacol*, 41, 1082–1090.

Green AR, Oh E, Hilson L, Tian J, Boyd CM (2016). Anticholinergic burden in older adults with mild cognitive impairment. *J Am Geriatr Soc*, 64, e313–e314.

Grossberg GT, Manes F, Allegri RF, et al. (2013). The safety, tolerability, and efficacy of once-daily memantine (28 mg): a multinational, randomized, double-blind, placebo-controlled trial in patients with moderate-to-severe Alzheimer's disease taking cholinesterase inhibitors. *CNS Drugs*, 27, 469–478.

Haddad PM, Benbow SM (1993a). Sexual problems associated with dementia: Part 1. Problems and their consequences. *Int J Geriatr Psychiatry*, 8(7), 547–551.

Haddad PM, Benbow SM (1993b). Sexual problems associated with dementia: Part 2. Aetiology, assessment and treatment. *Int J Geriatr Psychiatry*, 8(8), 631–637.

Herrmann N, Mamdani M, Lanctôt KL (2004). Atypical antipsychotics and risk of cerebrovascular accidents. *Am J Psychiatry*, 161, 1113–1115. doi:10.1176/appi.ajp.161.6.1113.

Hilmas CJ, Poole MJ, Finneran K, Clark MG, Williams PT (2009). Galantamine is a novel post-exposure therapeutic against lethal VX challenge. *Toxicol Appl Pharmacol*, 240, 166–173.

Hinkle JT, Perepezko K, Bakker C, et al. (2018). Onset and remission of psychosis in Parkinson's disease: pharmacologic and motoric markers. *Mov Disord Clin Pract*, 5, 31–38. doi:10.1002/mdc3.12550.

Holroyd S, Currie L, Wooten GF (2001). Prospective study of hallucinations and delusions in Parkinson's disease. *J Neurol Neurosurg Psychiatry*, 70, 734–738. doi:10.1136/jnnp.70.6.734.

Hong JM, Shin DH, Lim TS, Lee JS, Huh K (2012). Galantamine administration in chronic post-stroke aphasia. *J Neurol Neurosurg Psychiatry*, 83, 675–680. doi:10.1136/jnnp-2012-302268.

Howard R, McShane R, Lindesay J, et al. (2012). Donepezil and memantine for moderate-to-severe Alzheimer's disease. *N Engl J Med*, 366, 893–903.

Howard R, McShane R, Lindesay J, et al. (2015). Nursing home placement in the Donepezil and Memantine in Moderate to Severe Alzheimer's Disease (DOMINO-AD) trial: secondary and post-hoc analyses. *Lancet Neurol*, 14, 1171–1181.

Huang F, Lasseter AC, Janssens L, et al. (2002). Pharmacokinetic and safety assessments of galantamine and risperidone after the two drugs are administered alone and together. *J Clin Pharmacol*, 42, 1341–1351.

Irwin DJ, Grossman M, Weintraub D, et al. (2017). Neuropathological and genetic correlates of survival and dementia onset in synucleinopathies: a retrospective analysis. *Lancet Neurol*, 16, 55–65.

Jang YK, Lyoo CH, Park S, et al. (2018). Head to head comparison of [^{18}F] AV-1451 and [^{18}F]

THK5351 for tau imaging in Alzheimer's disease and frontotemporal dementia. *Eur J Nucl Med Mol Imaging*, 45, 432–442.

Jann MW, Shirley KL, Small GW (2002). Clinical pharmacokinetics and pharmacodynamics of cholinesterase inhibitors. *Clin Pharmacokinet*, 41, 719–739.

Jiang J, Jiang H (2015). Efficacy and adverse effects of memantine treatment for Alzheimer's disease from randomized controlled trials. *Neurol Sci*, 36, 1633–1641.

Johansson I, Nordberg A (1993). Pharmacokinetic studies of cholinesterase inhibitors. *Acta Neurol Scand Suppl*, 149, 22–25.

Kavirajan H, Schneider LS (2007). Efficacy and adverse effects of cholinesterase inhibitors and memantine in vascular dementia: a meta-analysis of randomised controlled trials. *Lancet Neurol*, 6, 782–792. doi:10.1016/S1474-4422(07)70195-3.

Kishi T, Matsunaga S, Iwata N (2015). Memantine for the treatment of frontotemporal dementia: a meta-analysis. *Neuropsychiatr Dis Treat*, 11, 2883–2885.

Kobayashi H, Ohnishi T, Nakagawa R, Yoshizawa K (2016). The comparative efficacy and safety of cholinesterase inhibitors in patients with mild-to-moderate Alzheimer's disease: a Bayesian network meta analysis. *Int J Geriatr Psychiatry*, 31, 892–904.

Larsson V, Aarsland D, Ballard C, Minthon L, Londos E (2010). The effect of memantine on sleep behaviour in dementia with Lewy bodies and Parkinson's disease dementia. *Int J Geriatr Psychiatry*, 25, 1030–1038. doi:10.1002/gps.2506.

Lefèvre G, Callegari F, Gsteiger S, Xiong Y (2016). Effects of renal impairment on steady-state plasma concentrations of rivastigmine: a population pharmacokinetic analysis of capsule and patch formulations in patients with Alzheimer's disease. *Drugs Aging*, 33, 725–736.

Liu AKL, Chang RCC, Pearce RKB, Gentleman SM (2015). Nucleus basalis of Meynert revisited: anatomy, history and differential involvement in Alzheimer's and Parkinson's disease. *Acta Neuropathol*, 129, 527–540. doi:10.1007/s00401-015-1392-5.

Livingston G, Kelly J, Lewis-Holmes E, et al. (2014). A systematic review of the clinical effectiveness and cost-effectiveness of sensory, psychological and behavioural interventions for managing agitation in older adults with dementia. *Health Technol Assess*, 18, 1–226, v–vi.

López-Valdés HE, Clarkson AN, Ao Y, et al. (2014). Memantine enhances recovery from stroke. *Stroke*, 45, 2093–2100. doi:10.1161/STROKEAHA.113.004476.

Massoud F, Desmarais JE, Gauthier S (2011). Switching cholinesterase inhibitors in older adults with dementia. *Int Psychogeriatr*, 23, 372–378. doi:10.1017/S1041610210001985.

Matsunaga S, Kishi T, Iwata N (2015a). Memantine monotherapy for Alzheimer's disease: a systematic review and meta-analysis. *PLoS One*, 10(4), e0123289. doi:10.1371/journal.pone.0123289.

Matsunaga S, Kishi T, Iwata N (2015b). Combination therapy with cholinesterase inhibitors and memantine for Alzheimer's disease: a systematic review and meta-analysis. *Int J Neuropsychopharmacol*, 18, pyu115. doi:10.1093/ijnp/pyu115.

Meltzer HY, Mills R, Revell S, et al. (2010). Pimavanserin, a serotonin 2A receptor inverse agonist, for the treatment of Parkinson's disease psychosis. *Neuropsychopharmacology*, 35, 881–892.

National Institute for Health and Care Excellence (NICE) (2018a). *Decision aid: antipsychotic medicines for treating agitation, aggression and distress in people living with dementia*. London: National Institute for Health and Care Excellence. Available at: www.nice.org.uk/guidance/ng97/resources/antipsychotic-medicines-for-treating-agitation-aggression-and-distress-in-people-living-with-dementia-patient-decision-aid-pdf-4852697005 (last accessed 26.1.19).

National Institute for Health and Care Excellence (NICE) (2018b). *Dementia: assessment, management and support for people living with dementia and their carers*. NICE guideline [NG97]. London: National Institute for Health and Care Excellence.

Nelson JC, Devanand DP (2011). A systematic review and meta-analysis of placebo-controlled antidepressant studies in people with depression and dementia. *J Am Geriatr Soc*, 59, 577–585. doi:10.1111/j.1532-5415.2011.03355.x.

Noetzli M, Guidi M, Ebbing K, et al. (2013). Population pharmacokinetic study of memantine: effects of clinical and genetic factors. *Clin Pharmacokinet*, 52, 211–223.

Ohnishi A, Mihara M, Kamakura H, et al. (1993). Comparison of the pharmacokinetics of E2020, a new compound for Alzheimer's disease, in healthy young and elderly subjects. *J Clin Pharmacol*, 33, 1086–1091.

Ohta Y, Darwish M, Hishikawa N, et al. (2017). Therapeutic effects of drug switching between acetylcholinesterase inhibitors in patients with Alzheimer's disease. *Geriatr Gerontol Int*, 17, 1843–1848. doi:10.1111/ggi.12971.

Pagonabarraga J, Kulisevsky J, Strafella AP, Krack P (2015). Apathy in Parkinson's disease: clinical features, neural substrates, diagnosis, and treatment. *Lancet Neurology*, 14, 518–531. doi:10.1016/S1474-4422(15)00019-8.

Pasina L, Djade CD, Lucca U, et al. (2013). Association of anticholinergic burden with cognitive and functional status in a cohort of hospitalized elderly: comparison of the anticholinergic cognitive burden scale and anticholinergic risk scale: results from the REPOSI study. *Drugs Aging*, 30, 103–112.

Pereira EFR, Aracava Y, Alkondon M, et al. (2010). Molecular and cellular actions of galantamine: clinical implications for treatment of organophosphorus poisoning. *J Mol Neurosci*, 40, 196–203.

Periclou A, Ventura D, Rao N, Abramowitz W (2006). Pharmacokinetic study of memantine in healthy and renally impaired subjects. *Clin Pharmacol Ther*, 79, 134–143.

Perry EK, Curtis M, Dick DJ, et al. (1985). Cholinergic correlates of cognitive impairment in Parkinson's disease: comparisons with Alzheimer's disease. *J Neurol Neurosurg Psychiatry*, 48, 413–421.

Piotrovsky V, Van Peer A, Van Osselaer N, Armstrong M, Aerssens J (2003). Galantamine population pharmacokinetics in patients with Alzheimer's disease: modeling and simulations. *J Clin Pharmacol*, 43, 514–523.

Polinsky RJ (1998). Clinical pharmacology of rivastigmine: a new-generation acetylcholinesterase inhibitor for the treatment of Alzheimer's disease. *Clin Ther*, 20, 634–647.

Prince M, Wimo A, Guerchet M, et al. (2015). *World Alzheimer Report 2015 – The Global Impact of Dementia: An Analysis of Prevalence, Incidence, Cost and Trends*. London: Alzheimer's Disease International. Available at: www.alz.co.uk/research/WorldAlzheimerReport2015.pdf (last accessed 10.8.19).

Risacher SL, McDonald BC, Tallman EF, et al. (2016). Association between anticholinergic medication use and cognition, brain metabolism, and brain atrophy in cognitively normal older adults. *JAMA Neurol*, 73, 721–732.

Ruxton K, Woodman RJ, Mangoni AA (2015). Drugs with anticholinergic effects and cognitive impairment, falls and all-cause mortality in older adults: a systematic review and meta-analysis. *Br J Clin Pharmacol*, 80, 209–220.

Sabbagh M, Hans S, Kim S, et al. (2016). Clinical recommendations for the use of donepezil 23 mg in moderate-to-severe Alzheimer's disease in the Asia-Pacific region. *Dement Geriatr Cogn Dis Extra*, 6, 382–395.

Salahudeen MS, Duffull SB, Nishtala PS (2015). Anticholinergic burden quantified by anticholinergic risk scales and adverse outcomes in older people: a systematic review. *BMC Geriatr*, 15, 31.

Sasaki S, Horie Y (2014). The effects of an uninterrupted switch from donepezil to galantamine without dose titration on behavioral and psychological symptoms of dementia in Alzheimer's disease. *Dement Geriatr Cogn Dis Extra*, 4, 131–139. doi:10.1159/000362871.

Schmidt R, Hofer E, Bouwman FH, et al. (2015). EFNS-ENS/EAN Guideline on concomitant use of cholinesterase inhibitors and memantine in moderate to severe Alzheimer's disease. *Eur J Neurol*, 22, 889–898.

Schneider-Thoma J, Efthimiou O, Huhn M, et al. (2018). Second-generation antipsychotic drugs and short-term mortality: a systematic review and meta-analysis of placebo-controlled randomised controlled trials. *Lancet Psychiatry*, 5, 653–663.

Serfaty M, Kennell-Webb S, Warner J, Blizard R, Raven P (2002). Double blind randomised placebo controlled trial of low dose melatonin for sleep disorders in dementia. *Int J Geriatr Psychiatry*, 17, 1120–1127.

Sharp SI, Francis PT, Elliot MSJ, et al. (2009). Choline acetyltransferase activity in vascular dementia and stroke. *Dement Geriatr Cogn Disord*, 28, 233–238. doi:10.1159/000239235.

Sullivan SC, Richards KC (2004). Predictors or circadian sleep-wake rhythm maintenance in elders with dementia. *Aging Ment Health*, 8, 143–152. doi:10.1080/13607860410001649608.

Tariot PN, Farlow MR, Grossberg GT, et al. (2004). Memantine treatment in patients with moderate to severe Alzheimer disease already receiving donepezil. *JAMA*, 291, 317–324.

Thobois S, Lhommée E, Klinger H, et al. (2013). Parkinsonian apathy responds to dopaminergic stimulation of D2/D3 receptors with piribedil. *Brain*, 136, 1568–1577.

Trotman M, Vermehren P, Gibson CL, Fern R (2015). The dichotomy of memantine treatment for ischemic stroke: dose-dependent protective and detrimental effects. *J Cereb Blood Flow Metab*, 35, 230–239. doi:10.1038/jcbfm.2014.188.

van Gool WA, van de Beek D, Eikelenboom P (2010). Systemic infection and delirium: when cytokines and acetylcholine collide. *Lancet*, 375(9716), 773–775. doi:10.1016/S0140-6736(09)61158-2.

Van Leeuwen E, Petrovic M, Azermai M, et al. (2018). Withdrawal versus continuation of long-term antipsychotic drug use for behavioural and psychological symptoms in older people with dementia. *Cochrane Database Syst Rev*, (3), CD007726.

Vingtdeux V, Dreses-Werringloer U, Zhao H, Davies P, Marambaud P (2008). Therapeutic potential of resveratrol in Alzheimer's disease. *BMC Neurosci*, 9, S6.

Wang J, Yu JT, Wang HF, et al. (2015). Pharmacological treatment of neuropsychiatric symptoms in Alzheimer's disease: a systematic review and meta-analysis. *J Neurol Neurosurg Psychiatry*, 86, 101–109.

Weintraub D, Chiang C, Kim HM, et al. (2016). Association of antipsychotic use with mortality risk in patients with Parkinson disease. *JAMA Neurol*, 73, 535–541. doi:10.1001/jamaneurol.2016.0031.

Wesnes K, Aarsland D, Ballard C, Londos E (2014). Memantine improves attention and episodic memory in Parkinson's disease dementia and dementia with Lewy bodies. *Int J Geriatr Psychiatry*, 30(1), 46–54.

Zhang L-J, Sha X-Y (2007). Pharmacokinetics and bioequivalence studies of galantamine hydrobromide dispersible tablet in healthy male Chinese volunteers. *Drug Dev Ind Pharm*, 33, 335–340.

Zhao Q, Janssens L, Verhaeghe T, Brashear HR, Truyen L (2005). Pharmacokinetics of extended-release and immediate-release formulations of galantamine at steady state in healthy volunteers. *Curr Med Res Opin*, 21, 1547–1554.

Zhao QF, Tan L, Wang HF, et al. (2016). The prevalence of neuropsychiatric symptoms in Alzheimer's disease: systematic review and meta-analysis. *J Affect Disord*, 190, 264–271.

Chapter

15 Drugs to Treat Substance Use Disorders

Julia Sinclair and Lesley Peters

15.1 Diagnosis

This chapter deals with drugs used to treat substance use disorders (SUDs) due to nicotine, alcohol, opioids and benzodiazepines. A final section briefly considers other common drugs of misuse.

The updated version of the *Diagnostic and Statistical Manual of Mental Disorders* (DSM-5) marks a change in the conceptualization of how SUDs are diagnosed, from the previous dichotomized categorization of 'abuse' and 'dependence' on substances in DSM-IV to a single broader diagnosis of SUD in DSM-5 (American Psychiatric

Association, 2013). The new diagnosis has a severity rating, measured on a continuum from mild to severe, based on how many of 11 criteria are met:

- Mild: the presence of two to three symptoms.
- Moderate: the presence of four to five symptoms.
- Severe: the presence of six or more symptoms.

Between them, the criteria cover four main aspects of substance use (impaired control, social impairment, risky use and pharmacological) (see Table 15.1).

The International Classification of Diseases (ICD-10) continues to keep the dichotomized definitions of 'harmful use' of a substance (F1x.1) and dependence syndrome (F1x.2) (World Health Organization, 1992).

Harmful use is defined as: *A pattern of psychoactive substance use that is causing damage to health. The damage may be physical (as in cases of hepatitis from the self-administration of injected drugs) or mental (e.g. episodes of depressive disorder secondary to heavy consumption of alcohol).*

A dependence syndrome is diagnosed when a person has three or more physiological, behavioural and cognitive phenomena clustering together over the course of a year, in which the use of a substance takes on a much higher priority than other previously valued behaviours. A key phenomenon of the dependence syndrome is the desire, which may be overpowering, to take a specific psychoactive compound (including alcohol, tobacco or medically prescribed drugs).

A criterion common across the diagnostic classifications for dependence (or severe substance use disorder in DSM-5) is the appearance of a withdrawal syndrome in the relative, or absolute, absence of the substance (Table 15.2). The symptoms and potential complications differ depending on the substance, and these will be covered in detail in subsequent sections. The terms dependence and withdrawal are used in this chapter. Both appear in the ICD-10 classification and are disorders/terms that are familiar to clinicians.

The trajectory of substance use from occasional, through habitual, to daily dependent use is a complex interplay between genetic vulnerabilities, environmental factors as well as habitual and learned behaviours. Management of patients presenting with SUD will need to be tailored depending on: the presenting complaint; the substance that is used; level and duration of use; the severity of the disorder; the presence of any co-morbid SUD; physical and/or mental health conditions; as well as motivation to change.

Management always needs to start with engagement of the patient in the process and understanding their initial aims of treatment (which may well change with time). Following this the focus of treatment may be on harm minimization (which may include substitute prescribing), reduction of use, detoxification or relapse prevention. A psychological framework is the basis of most SUD treatment, exclusively so at less severe levels, but the focus of this chapter is on the drugs used for the management of SUDs, and the assumption is that this is delivered within such a framework.

15.2 Nicotine Dependence and Withdrawal

15.2.1 Pharmacological Effects of Nicotine

Nicotine is an alkaloid found in the leaves of the tobacco plant, *Nicotiana tabacum*. It is the main addictive component of tobacco. However, burning tobacco produces other psychoactive substances, particularly monoamine oxidase B-blocking agents, that means

Table 15.1 Questions to diagnose and assess the severity of DSM-5 alcohol use disorder

'In the past year have you . . .'	Category
Had times when you ended up drinking more, or longer, than you intended?	Impaired control
More than once wanted to cut down or stop drinking, or tried to, but couldn't?	Impaired control
Spent a great deal of time in activities necessary to obtain alcohol, use alcohol, or recover from its effects?	Impaired control
Spent a lot of time drinking? Or being sick or getting over other after effects?	Impaired control
Found that drinking – or being sick from drinking – often interfered with taking care of your home or family? Or caused job troubles? Or school problems?	Social impairment
Continued to drink even though it was causing trouble with your family or friends?	Social impairment
Given up or cut back on activities that were important or interesting to you, or gave you pleasure, in order to drink?	Social impairment
More than once got into situations while or after drinking that increased your chances of getting hurt (such as driving, swimming, using machinery, walking in a dangerous area, or having unsafe sex)?	Risky use
Continued to drink even though it was making you feel depressed or anxious or adding to another health problem? Or after having had a memory blackout?	Risky use
Had to drink much more than you once did to get the effect you want? Or found that your usual number of drinks had much less effect than before?	Pharmacological
Found that when the effects of alcohol were wearing off, you had withdrawal symptoms?	Pharmacological

that smoking is more dependence-producing than nicotine used by other methods, e.g. as snus or in vaping.

Nicotine acts both as a stimulant and a relaxant, activating nicotinic acetylcholine receptors located on glutamate terminals in the ventral tegmental area, leading to release of glutamate. The glutamate acts at glutamate (*N*-methyl-D-aspartate (NMDA)) receptors located on ventral tegmental dopamine neurons so enhancing dopamine in the ventral striatum/nucleus accumbens (Montgomery et al., 2007). This is thought to mediate the reinforcing effect of nicotine. It is rapidly absorbed after smoking producing an effect on the brain within 10–20 seconds. Nicotine increases heart rate, blood pressure, concentration, energy and alertness and reduces stress, anxiety and appetite, and activates the chemoreceptor trigger zone causing vomiting (Koob & Le Moal, 2006).

15.2.2 Nicotine Dependence – Cigarette Smoking

15.2.2.1 Prevalence

According to the Global Burden of Disease study, in 2015 the worldwide age-standardized prevalence of daily smoking was 25.0% (95% uncertainty interval 24.2–25.7) in men and 5.4% (5.1–5.7) in women (Reitsma, 2017). Adult smoking prevalence in England in 2016

Table 15.2 ICD-10 definitions of mental and behavioural disorders due to psychoactive substance use

	Definition
F1x.0 Acute intoxication	A condition that follows the administration of a psychoactive substance, resulting in disturbances in level of consciousness, cognition, perception, affect or behaviour, or other psychophysiological functions and responses. Disturbances are directly related to the acute pharmacological effects of the substance and resolve with time with complete recovery except where tissue damage or other complications have arisen.
F1x.2 Dependence	A cluster of behavioural, cognitive and physiological phenomena that develop after repeated substance use and include three or more of the following in 12 months: 1. Strong desire or sense of compulsion to take the substance 2. Impaired capacity to control substance use 3. Physiological withdrawal state 4. Evidence of tolerance to the effects of a substance 5. Preoccupation with substance use to the detriment of other activities 6. Persistent substance use despite clear evidence of harmful consequences.
F1x.3 Withdrawal state	A group of symptoms occurring on absolute or **relative** withdrawal of a psychoactive substance after persistent use. The onset and course of withdrawal state are time limited and are related to the type of psychoactive substance and the dose being used immediately before the cessation or reduction of use. Withdrawal states may be complicated by the presence of additional features, e.g. delirium, seizures.

was 15.5% and smoking remains the leading preventable cause of illness and premature death (McNeill et al., 2018).

15.2.2.2 Co-morbidity and Harms

People with psychiatric co-morbidity are about twice as likely to be smokers as those without such co-morbidity (Lasser et al., 2000). In 2015 the leading causes of smoking-attributable age-standardized disability-adjusted life years in men and women were cardiovascular diseases (41.2%), cancers (27.6%) and chronic respiratory diseases (20.5%). Smoking was the second-leading risk factor for attributable mortality in men and women after high systolic blood pressure (Reitsma, 2017).

15.2.3 Nicotine Withdrawal

Tolerance to nicotine develops rapidly and complex neuroadaptations with chronic use produce withdrawal symptoms. There is nicotinic receptor desensitization followed by receptor up-regulation during withdrawal. Dopaminergic function is reduced in withdrawal. Withdrawal symptoms include craving, irritability, anxiety, dysphoria, poor concentration, restlessness, increased appetite, disturbed sleep and bradycardia. Onset is 6–12 hours after cessation of smoking, peaking in 1 to 3 days but lasting up to 4 weeks, although protracted withdrawal symptoms such as craving can last for several months (Koob & Le Moal, 2006).

15.3 Drugs to Treat Nicotine Dependence

15.3.1 Nicotine Replacement Therapy

Nicotine replacement therapy (NRT) is available as gum, transdermal patch, nasal and oral sprays, inhalers, sublingual tablets and lozenges.

15.3.1.1 Mechanisms of Action and Pharmacokinetics

NRT reduces craving and nicotine withdrawal symptoms associated with stopping smoking. NRT delivers nicotine to the brain more slowly and at lower doses than smoking although the exact rate and dose depends on the NRT delivery system. Transdermal patches deliver nicotine slowly (peak plasma levels after 9 hours), while other forms of NRT deliver nicotine to the brain more quickly, with nasal and mouth sprays producing peak plasma levels within 10 minutes. The elimination half-life of nicotine is about 2 hours. Nicotine is mainly metabolized in the liver by cytochrome P450 enzymes. The active metabolite, cotinine, has a half-life of 18–20 hours. Excretion of metabolites is renal.

15.3.1.2 Clinical Therapeutics

NRT can be used for smokers wishing to quit or those wishing to reduce before quitting. NRT increases the rate of quitting by 50% to 60% (Hartmann-Boyce et al., 2018). All forms of NRT are effective. Comparing any form of NRT with control, for abstinence the risk ratio (RR) was 1.55 (95% confidence interval (CI) 1.49 to 1.61; 133 studies). The effectiveness of NRT does not appear to be dependent on the intensity of psychosocial support provided (Hartmann-Boyce et al., 2018).

Interactions: There are no established interactions between NRT and other medications. However, constituents in tobacco smoke cause increased metabolism of medications metabolized by CYP1A2 and smoking cessation may therefore result in reduced metabolism and increased plasma levels of these medications, e.g. clozapine.

Contraindications and adverse effects: NRT is contraindicated in hypersensitivity to nicotine. Other precautions are relative given the increased risks from continuing to smoke (see Summary of Product Characteristics). Some of the adverse effects of NRT depend on the formulation used. Nicotine sprays and the inhaler can cause nasal, mouth and throat irritation. Patches can cause skin irritation. Gum and tablets can irritate the inside of the mouth. Gum has been associated with hiccoughs and gastrointestinal disturbance. NRT is associated with possible increased risk of chest pains and palpitations. However, NRT does not increase risk of adverse cardiovascular events in those with pre-existing cardiovascular problems (Hartmann-Boyce et al., 2018). NRT products have lower dependence potential than tobacco smoking but still these products are not generally used for more than a year (McNeill et al., 2018). NRT can be used in pregnancy if non-pharmacological methods have failed. Patches should be removed before going to sleep in pregnant women (National Institute for Health and Care Excellence, NICE, 2010b). NRT in pregnancy is not associated with any serious adverse pregnancy or neonatal events (Coleman et al., 2015).

15.3.2 Varenicline

15.3.2.1 Mechanisms of Action

Varenicline is a selective nicotinic acetylcholine receptor partial agonist. It produces less dopamine release than nicotine (Bordia et al., 2012; Di Ciano et al., 2016) but sufficient to counteract craving and withdrawal symptoms as dopamine levels are low when stopping smoking. As it has higher affinity for the nicotine receptor it also blocks access of nicotine to activate the receptor, thereby reducing the reinforcing effects of smoking (Coe et al., 2005).

15.3.2.2 Pharmacokinetics

Peak plasma levels occur after 3–4 hours. Greater than 90% of varenicline is excreted unchanged in the urine. Adverse effects should be monitored in moderate renal impairment reducing dose if needed, and required in severe renal impairment. Varenicline does not affect cytochrome P450 enzymes. Pharmacokinetics are not altered in hepatic impairment.

15.3.2.3 Clinical Therapeutics

Varenicline is used as an aid to smoking cessation. Varenicline should be started 1–2 weeks before the target quit date. The standard dose is 1 mg bd after a 7-day titration period and the standard treatment duration is 12 weeks. A further 12 weeks of treatment can be considered for maintenance of abstinence for those who have stopped smoking at 12 weeks. For those not able to quit immediately a more gradual approach can be considered. Smoking should be reduced and stopped during the first 12 weeks of treatment and varenicline can then be continued for another 12 weeks for a total of 24 weeks treatment (see Summary of Product Characteristics). Varenicline increases the chances of sustained abstinence from smoking at 6 months or longer between two- and threefold compared with placebo, pooled RR 2.24 (95% CI 2.06 to 2.43; 27 studies) (Cahill et al., 2016). Varenicline was more effective than bupropion at maintaining abstinence at 6 months, pooled RR 1.39 (95% CI 1.25 to 1.54; 5 studies) and more effective than NRT, pooled RR 1.25 (95% CI 1.14 to 1.37; 8 studies) (Cahill et al., 2016). Varenicline, as a 24-week treatment course, has also been shown to be effective in achieving abstinence in those reducing smoking prior to quitting (Ebbert et al., 2015).

Interactions: There are no known significant pharmacokinetic interactions with varenicline and other medications. There is an increased incidence of side effects when used in combination with NRT.

Contraindications and adverse effects: The most frequent adverse effects are nausea (most common), headache, insomnia and abnormal dreams (Cahill et al., 2016). In the presence of adverse effects, the dose can be reduced to 0.5 mg bd. Varenicline should be used cautiously in those at increased risk of seizures. Varenicline should be avoided in pregnancy or during breastfeeding.

There have been concerns about an association between varenicline and serious neuropsychiatric and cardiac adverse events. A large cohort study (Kotz et al., 2015) and systematic review and meta-analysis (Sterling et al., 2016) of varenicline and cardiovascular serious adverse events did not find an association with increased risk of cardiovascular events. The EAGLES study assessed varenicline, bupropion and NRT in smokers with and without a history of psychiatric disorders. Those without a psychiatric history had higher quit rates than those in the psychiatric cohort across all treatments. Adverse event rates were higher in the psychiatric cohort (varenicline 6.5%, bupropion 6.7%, NRT 5.2% and placebo 4.9%) than in the non-psychiatric cohort (varenicline 1.3%, bupropion 2.2%, NRT 2.5% and placebo 2.4%). Apart from a significantly lower risk for the varenicline group compared with placebo in the non-psychiatric cohort, all other comparisons of treatments in both groups were not significant. This suggests that none of the smoking cessation treatments compared with placebo are associated with an increased risk of neuropsychiatric adverse events in smokers with or without psychiatric disorders (Anthenelli et al., 2016). However, as the psychiatric cohorts studied were clinically stable, the authors advise the results may not be generalizable to smokers with untreated or unstable psychiatric disorders, and individuals should be monitored.

15.3.3 Bupropion

15.3.3.1 Mechanism of Action

Bupropion is a noradrenaline and dopamine reuptake inhibitor and also acts as an antagonist at the nicotinic acetylcholine receptor. In most countries (though not in the UK) bupropion is also approved as an antidepressant. The exact mechanism by which bupropion supports smoking cessation is unclear but its dopamine-promoting actions may help by relieving withdrawal symptoms or reducing depressed mood which is a feature of withdrawal (Hughes et al., 2014).

15.3.3.2 Pharmacokinetics

Peak plasma levels of bupropion occur about 3 hours after dosing, with active metabolites peaking at about 6 hours. Bupropion is metabolized in the liver to active metabolites. Bupropion should be used cautiously in those with mild to moderate hepatic impairment with dose reduction and close monitoring for adverse effects. Bupropion undergoes renal excretion and the dose should be reduced in renal insufficiency and in underweight people (e.g. those with anorexia nervosa) in whom plasma protein binding is reduced leading to higher plasma concentrations.

15.3.3.3 Clinical Therapeutics

Bupropion is used as an aid to smoking cessation. The standard dose is 150 mg bd after titration. A target quit date should be set for within the first two weeks of treatment. Treatment should be for seven to nine weeks (see Summary of Product Characteristics). The Cochrane review reports that bupropion increases long-term smoking abstinence, RR 1.62 (95% CI 1.49 to 1.76; 44 studies) (Hughes et al., 2014). Bupropion appears similar in effectiveness to NRT (bupropion versus NRT pooled RR 0.96, 95% CI 0.85 to 1.09; 8 studies) and less effective than varenicline (pooled RR 0.68, 95% CI 0.56 to 0.83; 4 studies). Combining bupropion with NRT did not increase effectiveness. Bupropion may be more effective than NRT for smokers with a history of depression (Stapleton et al., 2013).

Interactions: Bupropion has complex interactions with the cytochrome P450 system. It inhibits CYP2D6 causing potential toxicity with medications metabolized by this pathway and drugs which require activation by CYP2D6 will have reduced efficacy. There is increased seizure risk with co-prescribing of other medications which lower the seizure threshold.

Contraindications and adverse effects: Bupropion should not be prescribed in pregnancy, during breastfeeding or in those with seizures or at increased risk of seizures. The incidence of seizures is approximately 1 in 1000. It is contraindicated in severe hepatic impairment.

Other adverse effects include insomnia (most common), dry mouth, nausea and allergic reactions (Hughes et al., 2014). Bupropion may increase blood pressure, which should be monitored during treatment. As with varenicline there have been concerns about increased risk of neuropsychiatric and cardiac adverse events. Hughes et al. (2014) did not find an increase in psychiatric or cardiac serious adverse effects with bupropion compared with placebo. The EAGLES study reported that bupropion was not associated with an increased risk of these events (see under Varenicline), but individuals should be monitored for adverse psychological effects.

15.3.4 E-Cigarettes (Vaping)

E-cigarettes contain a battery powered heating element that vaporizes a nicotine-containing liquid and the resultant vapour is inhaled – 'vaping'. The prevalence of e-cigarette use in the UK is about 6% of the adult population (McNeill et al., 2018).

15.3.4.1 Pharmacokinetics

E-cigarettes produce peak nicotine levels within 2–5 minutes.

15.3.4.2 Clinical Therapeutics

E-cigarettes are the most common aid used to quit smoking with recent data showing just under 40% of people used e-cigarettes in a quit attempt compared with just under 20% using NRT products (McNeill et al., 2018). Evidence suggests e-cigarettes increase smoking cessation rates (Hartmann-Boyce et al., 2016; McNeill et al., 2018).

Adverse effects: The health risks from e-cigarettes are likely to be significantly less than from tobacco smoking with Public Health England stating, 'vaping is at least 95% less harmful than smoking' (McNeill et al., 2018). However, more research is needed about the long-term risks and health effects, although the Cochrane review reports that smokers using e-cigarettes for up to two years did not have increased health risks compared to those not using e-cigarettes (Hartmann-Boyce et al., 2016). The most commonly reported adverse effects are irritation of mouth and throat, gastrointestinal and respiratory problems. There is a risk of poisoning from accidental or intentional ingestion of the liquid used in e-cigarettes. There is also potential injury from fires and explosions caused by malfunctioning lithium-ion batteries.

15.4 Alcohol Use Disorders

15.4.1 Quantifying Alcohol Use

Use of a validated screening tool, such as the three consumption questions of the Alcohol Use Disorder Identification Test (AUDIT) (Saunders et al., 1993) is recommended as a routine part of all psychiatric assessments. The CAGE questions (Do you think you should **Cut** down/Do you get **Annoyed** being asked about your alcohol/Do you feel **Guilty** about the amount you drink/Do you need an '**Eye Opener**') are no longer recommended. CAGE gives no objective assessment of the frequency and quantity of alcohol use; it has low sensitivity for identifying moderate levels of harm (which may still be a significant contributor to the patient's mental state); it goes against all the principles of motivational interviewing and as such is frequently counter-therapeutic. The AUDIT-Consumption (AUDIT-C) has the added advantage of generating a score between 0 and 12, giving information on a spectrum of alcohol use, which itself can be useful as part of a brief intervention, and indicates when a more comprehensive assessment is required. If a more comprehensive assessment is indicated, the full 10 questions of the AUDIT are advised, which includes sections on harms and symptoms of dependence (Table 15.3).

15.4.2 Pharmacological Effects of Alcohol

Alcohol's effect on the brain is mediated through interaction with the inhibitory gamma-aminobutyric acid (GABA) system, as well as antagonism of the excitatory glutamate system, particularly the NMDA receptor.

Table 15.3 Alcohol Use Disorder Identification Test (AUDIT) questions

AUDIT-C

Questions	Scoring system					Score
	0	1	2	3	4	
1. How often do you have a drink containing alcohol?	Never	Monthly or less	2–4 times per month	2–3 times per week	4+ times per week	
2. How many units of alcohol do you drink on a typical day when you are drinking?	1–2	3–4	5–6	7–9	10+	
3. How often have you had 6 or more units on a single occasion in the last year?	Never	Less than monthly	Monthly	Weekly	Daily or almost daily	

0–4 Low-risk drinking level; a total of 5 indicates increasing or higher-risk drinking (AUDIT-C positive). If AUDIT-C positive, consider asking the remaining 7 AUDIT Questions.

Remaining AUDIT questions

Questions	Scoring system					Score
	0	1	2	3	4	
4. How often during the last year have you found that you were not able to stop drinking once you had started?	Never	Less than monthly	Monthly	Weekly	Daily or almost daily	
5. How often during the last year have you failed to do what was normally expected from you because of your drinking?	Never	Less than monthly	Monthly	Weekly	Daily or almost daily	
6. How often during the last year have you needed an alcoholic drink in the morning to get yourself going after a heavy drinking session?	Never	Less than monthly	Monthly	Weekly	Daily or almost daily	
7. How often during the last year have you had a feeling of guilt or remorse after drinking?	Never	Less than monthly	Monthly	Weekly	Daily or almost daily	
8. How often during the last year have you been unable to remember what happened the night before because you had been drinking?	Never	Less than monthly	Monthly	Weekly	Daily or almost daily	
9. Have you or somebody else been injured as a result of your drinking?	No		Yes, but not in the last year		Yes, during the last year	
10. Has a relative or friend, doctor or other health worker been concerned about your drinking or suggested that you cut down?	No		Yes, but not in the last year		Yes, during the last year	

Total score on all 10 questions (/40): 0–7 lower risk, 8–15 increasing risk, 16–19 higher risk, 20+ possible dependence.

The $GABA_A$ receptor includes a subunit with a binding site for alcohol which then increases GABA inhibitory activity, resulting in reduced anxiety and sedation, at lower levels in non-dependent individuals. Higher levels of increased GABA inhibition lead to slurred speech, ataxia and respiratory depression. In individuals who drink regularly at higher levels, down-regulation of the GABA system develops mediated by changes in the $GABA_A$ complex.

At the same time, in response to higher alcohol consumption leading to glutamate receptor blockade, there is an increase in the number of NMDA receptors to overcome this antagonistic effect of alcohol on the glutamatergic system. The brain habituates to this altered state by increasing glutamate receptor number, so individuals subjectively reach a degree of equilibrium. These receptor changes result in the need to drink more alcohol to obtain the same psychotropic effect (tolerance) and is a core feature of physical dependence on alcohol.

15.4.3 Alcohol Dependence

Alcohol use disorders (AUD) are common and disabling conditions, with 3.3 million deaths (5.9% of global deaths) and 5.1% of the global burden of disease and injury in 2012 attributable to them (World Health Organization, 2014). Alcohol dependence (as per ICD-10) or severe alcohol use disorders (DSM-5) is frequently undertreated, with estimates of treatment in less than 25% of affected individuals in the USA (Hasin et al., 2007) and 10% in Europe (Rehm et al., 2013). There is a good evidence base for the effectiveness of pharmacological treatment in managing alcohol withdrawal symptoms (Amato et al., 2011), in relapse prevention and in reduction of alcohol consumption (Lingford-Hughes et al., 2012; NICE, 2011).

AUD are frequently co-morbid with other psychiatric conditions. A Norwegian Patient Registry study found that AUD was the most common co-morbid SUD in every diagnostic group. Five-year prevalence rates of AUD were 4.4% in patients with depression; 4.6% in schizophrenia; and 8.1% in patients with bipolar disorder (Nesvåg et al., 2015). Similarly, a Danish Psychiatric Register found lifetime prevalence of AUD in individuals with psychoses of 27.6%, bipolar disorder of 27.9% and depression of 20.9% (Toftdahl et al., 2016). UK studies of psychiatric inpatients have found rates of co-morbid AUD of between 37% and 51% in men and 13% and 29% of women on admission (Sinclair et al., 2008; Weaver et al., 2003).

15.4.4 Alcohol Withdrawal: Time Course, Symptoms

Due to the altered GABA/glutamate equilibrium which develops over time with chronic heavy drinking, individuals with moderate to severe AUD or alcohol dependence are at risk of a withdrawal syndrome with any abrupt reduction or cessation of alcohol consumption. Seizures, delirium tremens or Wernicke–Korsakoff syndrome (WKS) may further complicate alcohol withdrawal syndromes, and the primary aim of any of the treatment strategies discussed below is to minimize autonomic signs and symptoms and reduce the risk of complications.

Alcohol withdrawal generally develops between 24 and 72 hours after the last drink of alcohol, but this is extremely variable, and in vulnerable individuals at particularly high levels of consumption may occur while alcohol is still at relatively high levels in the bloodstream. The main signs and symptoms of alcohol withdrawal are caused by the relative lack of intrinsic GABA function combined with unopposed glutamatergic activity: namely tremor, sweating, anxiety, irritability, hypertension, and tachycardia, insomnia, transient illusions and hallucinations. In more severe cases, this can be complicated by tonic-clonic seizures, and worsening autonomic instability, confusion and delusions (delirium tremens) and death.

15.5 Drugs to Manage Alcohol Withdrawal Syndrome

15.5.1 Introduction

Patients presenting with signs and symptoms of alcohol withdrawal syndrome (AWS) require a quantified assessment of their alcohol use. This includes the number of units of alcohol per day, duration of daily drinking, history of any previous seizures, and rating of the severity of any alcohol withdrawal symptoms; using a validated scale (e.g. revised Clinical Institute Withdrawal Assessment for Alcohol scale – CIWA-R) (Sullivan et al., 1989).

The severity of alcohol dependence (which can be objectively assessed by using a validated scale, such as the Severity of Alcohol Dependence Questionnaire (SADQ) (Stockwell et al., 1983)) and risk of complications should determine the setting in which withdrawal from alcohol is undertaken. Patients at high risk of WKS or alcohol withdrawal delirium (delirium tremens) will require an inpatient admission to an acute medical setting, as the facilities for intravenous access, and escalation of acute medical care necessary for their safe management, are rarely available in community or psychiatric settings. Patients should not be offered medically assisted withdrawal from alcohol in the community unless there is adequate provision for monitoring, and a clear management plan for the maintenance of abstinence.

The mainstay of pharmacological treatment for AWS is the use of benzodiazepines to offset the reduced GABAergic function and so attenuate the otherwise unopposed glutamate. There is some evidence for the effectiveness of a number of anticonvulsant compounds which are primarily anti-glutamatergic in the management of alcohol withdrawal, including carbamazepine, topiramate and lamotrigine (Lingford-Hughes et al., 2012). In addition to their impact on GABA-glutamate activity, anticonvulsants will also inhibit voltage-activated sodium channels and therefore further excitatory activity (NICE, 2011). However, the most recent Cochrane review found only one outcome which favoured carbamazepine over a benzodiazepine (oxazepam and lorazepam) and concluded there was insufficient evidence for anticonvulsants in the treatment of alcohol withdrawal (Minozzi et al., 2010).

15.5.2 Managing Uncomplicated Alcohol Withdrawal

There is good evidence for the use of long-acting benzodiazepines (most commonly diazepam and chlordiazepoxide) to manage AWS (Amato et al., 2011; Lingford-Hughes et al., 2012; NICE, 2011). However, there is less agreement on the relative risk–benefit profile of whether these are delivered as a ‘symptom-triggered’ or ‘fixed-dose’ reducing regimen.

A 'symptom-triggered' regimen involves regular monitoring of alcohol withdrawal signs and symptoms using a validated symptom scale, e.g. the CIWA-R (Sullivan et al., 1989) and administering medication against symptom severity. Overall, data suggest that it is safe in well-monitored, specialist inpatient settings with trained staff and for well-motivated outpatients (Elholm et al., 2011), and has similar outcomes in terms of days to completion, use of medication and drinking outcomes compared with use of a fixed-dose schedule (NICE, 2010a).

A fixed-dose schedule, most commonly used in community settings and psychiatric inpatient wards, usually follows one of several (mild, moderate or severe) pre-fixed medication schedules, agreed at an organizational level as part of a clinical alcohol management policy and is based on the assessment of severity of alcohol dependence (see example for chlordiazepoxide below) (NICE, 2011).

The decision as to which schedule to use (fixed-dose or symptom-triggered) will be based on the clinical setting, staffing levels and competencies of staff required to undertake the 2-hourly monitoring. Unless a patient can be managed on a well-resourced unit where regular assessment of withdrawal symptoms can be undertaken, a fixed-dose reducing regimen of a benzodiazepine (diazepam or chlordiazepoxide) four times daily over 5–14 days (see Table 15.4) is recommended over 'symptom-triggered' (as required) prescribing (Lingford-Hughes et al., 2012; NICE, 2011).

15.5.3 Managing Complicated Alcohol Withdrawal

In patients with severe liver disease, oxazepam is preferred over chlordiazepoxide as it is short-acting and excreted primarily through the kidneys (NICE, 2010a). If patients are unable to take oral benzodiazepines, parenteral preparations (e.g. intravenous midazolam or lorazepam) should be considered, but the patient will require ongoing monitoring in a high care environment.

For primary and secondary prevention of seizures, diazepam or lorazepam is recommended. For hallucinations, diazepam is first-line treatment; if there is no response, consider olanzapine 5–10 mg orally (Lingford-Hughes et al., 2012). There is no additional advantage in adding anticonvulsants to benzodiazepines for the prevention of alcohol withdrawal seizures (Haber et al., 2009).

15.5.3.1 Wernicke–Korsakoff Syndrome (WKS)

Wernicke–Korsakoff syndrome (WKS) is an under-recognized complication of alcohol withdrawal. It is caused by acute-on-chronic thiamine (vitamin B_1) deficiency, and can present while a patient is still drinking, but most commonly occurs during alcohol withdrawal. Thiamine is an essential co-enzyme in the glycolytic pathway, required for the metabolism of carbohydrates. Patients drinking at dependent levels frequently derive most of their (low nutrient) calories from alcohol and so have a reduced intake of thiamine from food, and inflammation of the gut mucosa reduces absorption. In addition, the high carbohydrate load from excess alcohol increases the need for thiamine, which accentuates this deficit.

The classical symptom triad of WKS is ataxia, opthalmoplegia and confusion; however, all three signs present in only about 10% of patients, whereas over 80%

Table 15.4 Example of chlordiazepoxide fixed-dose reduction (NICE, 2011)

Daily alcohol consumption	15–25 units		30–49 units		50–60 units
Severity of alcohol dependence	**Moderate SADQ score 15–23**		**Severe SADQ score 30–40**		**Very severe SADQ score 40–60**
Day 1 (starting dose)	15 mg four times a day	25 mg four times a day	30 mg four times a day	40 mg four times a day[a]	50 mg four times a day[b]
Day 2	10 mg four times a day	20 mg four times a day	25 mg four times a day	35 mg four times a day[a]	45 mg four times a day[b]
Day 3	10 mg four times a day	15 mg four times a day	20 mg four times a day	30 mg four times a day	40 mg four times a day[a]
Day 4	5 mg four times a day	10 mg four times a day	15 mg four times a day	25 mg four times a day	35 mg four times a day[a]
Day 5	5 mg twice times a day	10 mg three times a day	10 mg four times a day	20 mg four times a day	30 mg four times a day
Day 6	5 mg at night	5 mg three times a day	10 mg three times a day	15 mg four times a day	25 mg four times a day
Day 7		5 mg twice a day	5 mg three times a day	10 mg four times a day	20 mg four times a day
Day 8		5 mg at night	5 mg twice a day	10 mg four times a day	10 mg four times a day
Day 9			5 mg at night	5 mg three times a day	10 mg four times a day
Day 10				5 mg twice a day	10 mg three times a day
Day 11				5 mg at night	5 mg three times a day
Day 12					5 mg twice a day
Day 13					5 mg at night

SADQ, Severity of Alcohol Dependence Questionnaire.

[a] Doses of chlordiazepoxide in excess of 30 mg four times a day should be prescribed only in severe alcohol dependence. The patient's response to treatment should always be regularly and closely monitored.

[b] Doses in excess of 40 mg four times a day should be prescribed only if there is evidence of very severe alcohol dependence. Such doses are rarely necessary in women and children and never in older people or if there is liver impairment.

present with confusion alone (Harper et al., 1986). Consequently, a presumed diagnosis in any alcohol-dependent patient with confusion (or any of the signs of WKS) is advised (Sechi & Serra, 2007) as is ensuring adequate doses of **parenteral** thiamine (due to the low levels of gastric absorption) especially before giving glucose infusions, which can precipitate WKS in susceptible individuals. Current guidelines advise two pairs of ampules (Pabrinex®) three times per day for five days and to continue until cognitive function is optimized (Lingford-Hughes et al., 2012; NICE, 2010a, 2011). Oral thiamine (100 mg three times daily) should be continued for at least six weeks until patients are eating normally.

15.5.3.2 Alcohol Withdrawal Delirium (Delirium Tremens, DTs)

Alcohol withdrawal delirium (delirium tremens, DTs) occurs 48–72 hours after cessation of drinking, and so patients who have stopped by themselves may present to hospital already in an acutely confused state with cognitive and/or perceptual disturbances. The patient also may exhibit other signs of autonomic hyperactivity, such as tachycardia, hypertension, diaphoresis and high temperatures. The syndrome usually lasts two to three days, but in severe cases can persist for several weeks. Prevalence rates are difficult to determine, but in placebo-treated patients with alcohol dependence enrolled into clinical trials it is approximately 5%. The initial goal of management is to control agitation, which has been shown to reduce the incidence of subsequent adverse events. This requires thorough medical evaluation to identify possible electrolyte imbalances and other complications, and good nursing management in a quiet room to monitor vital signs, ensure good hydration and reduce disorientation.

Benzodiazepines are the first-line treatment for DTs, and if given early in alcohol withdrawal completely prevent their emergence (so should be used in anyone with a prior history of DTs going into a planned withdrawal). Once started it is harder to control and the choice of benzodiazepine will depend on the severity of symptoms and treatment setting. The aim is to achieve and maintain light sedation. Antipsychotic medications are second line as an adjuvant to adequate benzodiazepine doses, to control agitation (Haber et al., 2009). Early studies reported mortality of 10–15% (Lishman, 1998) but with improved management mortality is now lower and estimated to be around 1% (Haber et al., 2009).

15.6 Drugs for Relapse Prevention in Alcohol Dependence

15.6.1 Acamprosate

15.6.1.1 Mechanism of Action

The exact mechanism of action of acamprosate (calcium acetylhomotaurinate) is still uncertain. It is thought to act via several mechanisms affecting multiple neurotransmitter systems, including NMDA and GABA function, both of which are altered during alcohol withdrawal and the early stages of abstinence (Kalk & Lingford-Hughes, 2014). Inhibiting neuronal hyperexcitability by antagonism of excitatory amino acid activity, and reduction of calcium ion fluxes has been suggested as its predominant mechanism of action (Wilde & Wagstaff, 1997). A significant decrease in frontal lobe glutamate has been shown on magnetic resonance spectroscopy (MRS) in patients taking acamprosate in the early stages of abstinence compared with placebo (Umhau et al., 2010). This may account for the reduction in arousal, anxiety and insomnia (all negative reinforcers implicated in relapse back to heavy drinking) seen in patients taking acamprosate in the early stages of abstinence.

15.6.1.2 Pharmacokinetics and Interactions

Acamprosate is derived from homotaurine, a non-specific GABA agonist, and calcium. It has low oral bioavailability (approximately 11%), is not protein bound and is not metabolized by the liver, being excreted unchanged in urine, and so has no impact on drugs subject to hepatic metabolism, or which have an impact on the CYP450 system (Kalk & Lingford-Hughes, 2014). It does not interact with alcohol, diazepam, oxazepam or imipramine, and there is no evidence of an interaction with disulfiram, although naltrexone increases its plasma levels in vivo. Due to its predominately renal excretion, it is generally safe in patients with impaired hepatic function, but potential risks and benefits need to be considered on an individual basis in the elderly and patients with renal insufficiency.

15.6.1.3 Clinical Therapeutics

The standard dose of acamprosate is two tablets (666 mg) three times daily. In patients with renal insufficiency, low weight and the elderly, the recommendation is to start at a lower dose (333 mg three times daily) and monitor renal function.

The evidence base for the effectiveness of acamprosate is robust, involving 19 randomized controlled trials (RCTs) with over 4600 patients with a diagnosis of alcohol dependence, drinking at baseline a mean of 145 units of alcohol per week. A systematic review and meta-analysis (NICE, 2011) rate it as 'high-quality' evidence and overall acamprosate demonstrates 'moderate' efficacy (relative risk of relapse 0.86 (95% CI 0.81 to 0.91)) over placebo in the context of a psychosocial framework for management.

Adverse effects: A major concern when treating patients with addictions is the abuse liability of drugs prescribed. There is no evidence of abuse liability in clinical studies with acamprosate, and none has been shown in animal models. Acamprosate appears safe in overdose: there are reports from two studies of three patients taking intentional overdoses of 8–120 tablets with no 'untoward symptoms'. Gastrointestinal side effects, especially diarrhoea, are significantly more common in patients on acamprosate than placebo; however, these tend to settle within the week. Beyond that it is a drug with minimal interactions, and pharmacovigilance data of 1.5 million patients showed no serious adverse events, with anxiety reported significantly more frequently in the placebo than the acamprosate group (Sinclair et al., 2016).

15.6.1.4 Co-morbid Populations

Only a few trials of acamprosate have been undertaken in patients with alcohol dependence and co-morbid mental illness. Two separate underpowered studies in patients with schizophrenia spectrum disorders and bipolar disorder could not demonstrate any significant efficacy outcomes but showed acamprosate was safe and tolerable in terms of common adverse events.

A meta-analysis of the acamprosate trial database estimated the prevalence of depression across all trials (using the Hamilton Depression Rating Scale – HDRS) and explored the differences in outcome between patients with and without depression. Data on 3354 patients from the 11 studies who had values for the HDRS at baseline and follow-up were analyzed. The prevalence of moderate/severe depression at baseline was 34.4% (range 29–53%). There were no specific safety concerns identified in the co-morbidly depressed subgroup, and the effect of acamprosate on mood was found to be mediated by percentage days' abstinence (Lejoyeux & Lehert, 2011).

15.6.2 Opioid Receptor Antagonists (Naltrexone and Nalmefene)

15.6.2.1 Mechanism of Action

Opioid neurotransmitter systems are important mediators of alcohol consumption. Opioid antagonists naltrexone and nalmefene may reduce alcohol consumption by reducing the positive reinforcing, and pleasurable, effects of alcohol as well as enhancing the sedative and dysphoric properties. μ-, κ- and δ-opioid agonists have been demonstrated to affect alcohol consumption. μ-opioid antagonists may reduce craving for alcohol in response to alcohol cues and may act on frontal cortical-limbic circuits to reduce impulsivity that promotes alcohol drinking and other risky behaviours (Swift, 2013). The main difference in mechanism between naltrexone and nalmefene is that naltrexone is a full antagonist across μ, δ and κ receptors, whereas nalmefene is a weak partial agonist at the κ receptor. It is hypothesized that compared with naltrexone it might reduce the dysphoria and anxiety felt during alcohol withdrawal. Preclinical studies with nalmefene suggest that κ-opioid properties of the drug may normalize a chronically dysregulated κ-opioid receptor–dynorphin system (Mann et al., 2016).

15.6.2.2 Pharmacokinetics and Interactions

Naltrexone and nalmefene are closely related compounds, differing only in that naltrexone has a ketone group at the sixth carbon and nalmefene has a methylene group. Pharmacodynamic half-lives at the μ receptor are similar. Nalmefene is rapidly absorbed and attains >80% μ-opioid receptor occupancy at 3 hours, persisting for 26 hours. It is extensively metabolized in the liver, largely by glucuronidation rather than transformation to a different metabolite; unlike naltrexone there is no identified risk of hepatotoxicity, but clearance of nalmefene was found to be significantly reduced in a small study of patients with liver disease, and inversely proportional to the level of hepatic pathology.

Both compounds are rapidly absorbed and reach peak plasma concentrations within one hour. They are subject to significant first-pass metabolism, creating (in naltrexone) the primary active metabolite 6-beta-naltrexol, the levels of which correlate with adverse events. There is limited evidence for a pharmacokinetic effect of naltrexone on other drugs. The cytochrome P450 enzyme system is not involved in metabolism of naltrexone or 6-beta-naltrexol, so interactions with drugs subject to hepatic metabolism are likely to be minimal. Co-administration with acamprosate significantly increases acamprosate levels and side effects from acamprosate. Caution is advised for patients with liver dysfunction and 5- to 10-fold increases in naltrexone plasma concentrations have been reported in patients with cirrhosis.

For both naltrexone and nalmefene, evidence from a single experimental study (Quelch et al., 2017) suggests they work at the level of basal ganglia (i.e. on dopamine systems, not in cortex), and evidence from RCTs suggests the interaction with alcohol is not dangerous, and neither has not been found to produce physical or psychological dependence (Sinclair et al., 2016).

15.6.2.3 Clinical Therapeutics

Naltrexone is recommended for relapse prevention after detoxification from alcohol. There is a substantial evidence base for its efficacy over placebo on relapse rates in heavy drinking (RR 0.83, 95% CI 0.75 to 0.91) (NICE, 2011), and on relapse to any drinking at three months (RR 0.92, 95% CI 0.86 to 1.00) (Donoghue et al., 2015). It has been found to be more effective in the prevention of return to heavy drinking than the maintenance of abstinence, and therefore may be the first-line choice in those who are unlikely to achieve abstinence immediately. Patients should be advised against the concomitant use of opioids. It has a better tolerability profile in men, so it may be preferable to start at a half dose (25 mg daily) in women.

Nalmefene has an indication for reduction of alcohol consumption in patients with mild to moderate alcohol dependence not in immediate need of detoxification. It can be taken on an 'as required' basis, up to once daily (20 mg). It does not need to be started within specialist services and, as with the other medications, should be given alongside psychosocial support.

Adverse effects and contraindications: The most important reaction from a safety consideration for both naltrexone and nalmefene is with other opioid drugs, and patients need to be advised against their concomitant use. A Cochrane review (Rösner et al., 2010) of 47 studies analyzed available data on side effects that were documented in each study and calculated the risk differences (RD) for each of 46 different side effects listed in between 2 and 25 of the study reports. The most significant side effects attributable to naltrexone were nausea, vomiting, dizziness, abdominal pain, reduced appetite and daytime sleepiness. The side effects profile of nalmefene is similar, with insomnia and nausea being reported significantly more by patients on nalmefene than placebo (Rösner et al., 2010), but its action as a partial agonist at the opioid κ receptor may account for the increased reporting of central nervous system (CNS) symptoms (dizziness, insomnia, disorientation) (Sinclair et al., 2016).

15.6.2.4 Co-morbid Populations

There is no evidence for the use of nalmefene in patients who have co-morbid mental illness. Naltrexone has been subject to a number of clinical trials in patients with alcohol dependence and co-morbid post-traumatic stress disorder (PTSD), depression, bipolar disorder and other psychotic disorders. Overall, there are no specific safety concerns for its use, and some evidence for benefit, and it is recommended (above acamprosate) for relapse prevention in patients with bipolar disorder and co-morbid AUD (Goodwin et al., 2016).

15.6.3 Disulfiram

15.6.3.1 Mechanism of Action

Disulfiram acts by irreversible inactivation of hepatic acetaldehyde dehydrogenase (ALDH) enzymes. In the metabolic pathway of alcohol, ALDH catalyzes the conversion of acetaldehyde into acetic acid, and so when ALDH is deactivated and alcohol is consumed, levels of acetaldehyde rise. This gives rise to an unpleasant systemic reaction, called the disulfiram–alcohol reaction (DAR), which starts within 10 minutes of alcohol consumption and last 30–60 minutes, causing a range of symptoms (flushing, headache, tachycardia, nausea and vomiting) that may be mild or life-threatening. Disulfiram also inhibits the conversion of dopamine to noradrenaline, and the depletion of noradrenaline in the cardiovascular system allows acetaldehyde to act directly on myocardial and vascular tissue to cause flushing, tachycardia and hypotension. Other symptoms include hyperthermia, chest pain, and respiratory depression or hyperventilation. There is substantial intra-individual variation in the severity of the DAR, due to variations in polymorphism enzyme expression, or mutations present in different parts of the alcohol oxidative pathway, as well as the complex metabolic pathway of disulfiram itself, which makes it hard to predict the response in any individual.

15.6.3.2 Pharmacokinetics and Interactions

Disulfiram is metabolized in the liver and inhibits the metabolism of drugs such as phenytoin and warfarin, which use the CYP450 and CYP2E1 systems, leading to increased levels. It also inhibits the metabolism of chlordiazepoxide and diazepam (but not oxazepam), increasing their sedative effects. Some case reports have noted the development of a 'confusional psychosis', reversible on discontinuation, when patients prescribed disulfiram have also taken metronidazole. Patients stable on opioid substitution therapy (OST) and then started on disulfiram reported no adverse events attributable to the combination of OST and disulfiram.

15.6.3.3 Clinical Therapeutics

Undertaking an alcohol challenge in patients on disulfiram is not recommended in clinical practice. Rather, patients and carers should be given clear instructions about potential hazards, and sources of alcohol in consumables. Where appropriate a supportive family member or carer 'witnessing' the patient taking their disulfiram can assist with compliance.

Treatment guidelines (NICE, 2011) recommend the use of disulfiram in combination with a psychological intervention for patients who have successfully withdrawn from moderate to severe alcohol dependence and want to achieve abstinence, and for whom acamprosate or naltrexone are not suitable or preferred. Patients should not be started on disulfiram until at least 24 hours after their last drink and be warned that once established it is not safe to drink alcohol for at least five days after the last dose of disulfiram. Disulfiram can be initiated as a loading dose over four days (e.g. 800 mg, 600 mg, 400 mg, 200 mg), before continuing with a daily dose of 200–250 mg.

Adverse effects and contraindications: The DAR is integral to its use, but careful patient selection and monitoring can mitigate safety risks. It is clearly contraindicated in any patient who does not have a clear plan for the maintenance of abstinence from alcohol, or who is unable to engage with the requirement to check for and avoid alcohol-containing products (including food, mouthwash and skin products). A review of adverse effects noted during RCTs found it to be generally well tolerated over 6–12 months, not causing hepatitis, with drowsiness the only reported adverse event occurring significantly more frequently in patients taking disulfiram (Sinclair et al., 2016). Headache, fatigue and skin rashes and an unpleasant aftertaste occurred more commonly with a disulfiram group than placebo, and improved with dose reduction (Chick et al.,

1992; Ulrichsen et al., 2010). Overdose with disulfiram as a sole agent has relatively low toxicity but given the irreversible effect on ALDH patients require observation until ALDH is active again. Early studies of disulfiram used much higher doses (1–3 g daily), causing a higher burden of serious adverse effects and DAR, including death (Chick, 1999).

15.6.3.4 Co-morbid Populations

The main evidence for using disulfiram in patients with alcohol dependence and co-morbid Axis 1 disorders comes from the Veterans Affairs study (Petrakis et al., 2005). No specific safety concerns were identified regarding the use of disulfiram in patients with psychotic spectrum disorders, PTSD or depression. Earlier concerns about the potential for disulfiram to cause psychosis in vulnerable groups were based on higher doses (1–3 g) and have not been reported recently (Sinclair et al., 2016).

15.6.4 Other Medications

15.6.4.1 Baclofen

Baclofen is a $GABA_B$ agonist used in the treatment of spasticity for many years. Its precise mechanism of action is not fully understood in patients with alcohol dependence. It is rapidly absorbed, and excreted primarily by the kidney unchanged, but there appears to be significant inter-subject variation in absorption and elimination. The lack of hepatic metabolism makes it potentially useful in patients with co-morbid liver disease. The main safety considerations relate to co-administration with other CNS depressants (e.g. opioids, benzodiazepines, tricyclic antidepressants) and antihypertensives. The clinical presentation of baclofen overdose is related to its inhibitory neurotransmitter effects, and includes coma, hypotonia, respiratory depression, seizures and cardiac abnormalities, and at higher doses autonomic effects such as hypotension and CNS depression; the increase in prescriptions for baclofen for AUD has resulted in its use in more episodes of self-poisoning, some resulting in death.

There is much interest in baclofen as a new pharmacological agent for the reduction of alcohol use and maintenance of abstinence. The effectiveness of baclofen in alcohol-dependent patients has been shown in a number of small studies in specific groups (e.g. patients with liver cirrhosis), but more recent large multi-centre trial results have been less compelling or unable to demonstrate a clear dose response. However, a recent international consensus on its use (Agabio et al., 2018) and summary of the extensive clinical experience with baclofen (de Beaurepaire et al., 2018) helps give a balanced overview of its risk–benefit profile. To date, there have been no trials of baclofen in co-morbid psychiatric populations, but secondary analysis of data suggests that it may have a role in alcohol-dependent patients with marked anxiety symptoms (Sinclair et al., 2016).

15.6.4.2 Sodium Oxybate

Sodium oxybate is the sodium salt of gamma-hydroxybutyric acid (GHB), a derivative of GABA, and has also attracted interest (Chick & Nutt, 2012; Nutt et al., 2012) as a therapy for managing AWS and maintaining alcohol abstinence. However, the most recent consideration by the European Medicines Agency (2017) concluded that in the absence of demonstration of efficacy the benefit–risk balance of sodium oxybate was not favourable.

15.7 Opioid Dependence and Withdrawal

15.7.1 Pharmacological Effects of Opioids

Opium is derived from the unripe seed capsule of the opium poppy, *Papaver somniferum*. Opium contains many alkaloids but the main active ingredient is morphine. 'Opiate' refers to a drug derived from opium while 'opioid' refers to all drugs, natural and synthetic, with morphine-like properties.

Heroin (diacetyl morphine, diamorphine) was first synthesized from morphine in 1874. Heroin is more lipid soluble than morphine, therefore enters the brain faster. To act it has to be metabolized to morphine. The potency of opioids is judged by comparison with oral morphine. Codeine and tramadol are examples of weak opioids while morphine, fentanyl and oxycodone are classed as strong opioids.

Opioids produce their effects by activating one or more of the three types of opioid receptor in the brain – μ-, κ- and δ-opioid receptors. Opioid receptors are inhibitory G-protein-coupled receptors. There are three groups of endogenous opioid peptides, derived from precursor polypeptides, which act at these receptors – endorphins (all opioid receptors), enkephalins (highest selectivity for δ) and dynorphins (predominantly κ). A fourth related receptor, the nociceptin receptor, has been identified with its endogenous ligand (Pathan & Williams, 2012). These endogenous opioids have widespread roles as neuromodulators of physiological and affective processes, e.g. neural modulation of anxiety (Colasanti et al., 2011).

Activation of μ receptors results in the classic opioid effects including analgesia, euphoria, respiratory depression and pupillary constriction. One theory is that μ receptor activation also mediates positive reinforcement via inhibiting GABA neurons in the ventral tegmental area with resultant disinhibition of dopamine neurons and increased dopamine release in the nucleus accumbens though this has recently been challenged (see Nutt et al., 2015). κ receptor effects include analgesia, sedation, dysphoria and depersonalization. Other opioid effects include nausea and vomiting, constipation (via actions on gastrointestinal tract receptors), cough suppression and immunosuppression.

With chronic opioid use adaptive changes occur in the CNS to reduce the drug effect and produce tolerance. When opioid use is stopped (or the dose reduced) these neuroadaptations which are drug opposite in nature persist but are unopposed and therefore symptoms of withdrawal are produced. Tolerance develops to the respiratory depressant, euphoric, sedative and analgesic effects but tolerance does not fully develop to pupillary constriction or constipation.

An example of the neuroadaptive changes is up-regulation of noradrenergic activity in the locus coeruleus. As μ-opioid receptors are inhibitory, acute opioid use reduces intracellular cAMP production with reduced noradrenergic activity. With chronic opioid use intracellular cAMP production is up-regulated to maintain homeostasis. On withdrawal from opioids this up-regulated system results in excess noradrenergic activity and opioid withdrawal symptoms – particularly the physical symptoms of withdrawal such as sweating, rhinorrhoea and tachycardia.

Neuroadaptation also occurs within dopamine systems, leading to a hypodopaminergic state associated with the dysphoria of withdrawal (Kosten & George, 2002). These physical and affective symptoms of withdrawal may lead to drug-seeking behaviour via negative reinforcement.

15.7.2 Opioid Dependence

15.7.2.1 Prevalence

According to the Global Burden of Disease 2010 study there were 15.5 million people with opioid dependence worldwide (0.22%, 95% uncertainty interval (UI) 0.20% to 0.25%) with the prevalence higher in males and peaking in the 25- to 29-year-old age group. The estimated prevalence for Western Europe was 0.35% (95% UI 0.32% to 0.39%) and the UK was one of the countries with the highest estimated prevalence (0.48%, 95% UI 0.40% to 0.57%). Using disability-adjusted life years (DALYs) as a measure of overall disease burden, opioid dependence accounted for 9.3 million DALYs, an increase of 73% since 1990 (Degenhardt et al., 2014a).

The estimated prevalence of opioid users in England in 2014/15 per 1000 population was 7.33 (95% CI 7.28 to 7.60) with the highest rates in the North West, North East and Yorkshire and the Humber (Hay et al., 2017). In 2017–18 141 189 individuals were in treatment for opioid dependence with 73% males and median age of 40 (Public Health England, 2018).

15.7.2.2 Co-morbidity and Harm

Harms include those from the direct effects of the drug, e.g. respiratory depression, from the route of use, e.g. injecting related harm and from the impact of dependence on psychosocial functioning. Injecting related harm includes transmission of blood-borne viruses, localized bacterial infections (e.g. clostridia), infective endocarditis, anthrax and deep vein thrombosis. Around half of people who inject drugs have been infected with hepatitis C and 1% with HIV (Public Health England, 2016). Opioid dependence is associated with considerable excess mortality. One review found 6.5 times the expected rate of mortality in an opioid-dependent cohort although higher rates have been reported (Degenhardt et al., 2014b). Opioid overdose and viral hepatitis had the greatest excess mortality rates.

Psychiatric co-morbidity is high. At baseline in the Australian Treatment Outcome Study (ATOS) 25% met DSM-IV criteria for current major depression, 41% met PTSD criteria and 13% had attempted suicide in the previous year (Ross et al., 2005). Depression and personality disorder are the most common co-morbid disorders (Weaver et al., 2003). Coexisting alcohol problems are common (Senbanjo et al., 2007).

15.7.3 Opioid Withdrawal

There is a well-recognized opioid withdrawal syndrome. Signs and symptoms start with craving and anxiety, leading onto yawning, sweating, rhinorrhoea, lacrimation, dilated pupils, gooseflesh, hot and cold flushes, abdominal cramps, loss of appetite, general aches and pains especially in muscle and bones, sleep disturbance, and nausea with vomiting and diarrhoea in more severe cases. Pulse and blood pressure are increased. The symptoms increase from the time since last use of opioids – starting 6 to 12 hours after last use of shorter-acting opioids such as heroin and around 24 to 36 hours after last use of longer-acting drugs such as methadone – and peak around 2 to 3 days for withdrawal from heroin and 4 to 6 days after cessation of methadone.

Assessment tools such as the Clinical Opiate Withdrawal Scale (COWS) (Wesson & Ling, 2003) or the Short Opiate Withdrawal Scale (SOWS) (Gossop, 1990) may be used to measure the severity of opioid withdrawal.

The management of opioid withdrawal using methadone/buprenorphine reducing regimens, α_2-adrenergic agonists and symptomatic medication is discussed below under 'Opioid Detoxification Treatments'.

15.8 Opioid Substitution Therapy

15.8.1 General Principles

There is a high degree of cross-tolerance between opioids acting on the same opioid receptors which facilitates opioid substitution therapy (OST). This generally refers to methadone or buprenorphine. Providing a substitute medication with a long half-life prevents the repeated cycle of intoxication and withdrawal that occurs with heroin. The aim of OST is to reduce heroin-related harms and allow an individual to stabilize their lifestyle and promote recovery. There is substantial evidence that OST reduces the harms from heroin dependence. Large RCTs and observational studies have shown that methadone maintenance treatment increases treatment retention, reduces heroin use, reduces offending behaviour, reduces injecting-related risks, reduces blood-borne virus infections, reduces mortality and increases psychosocial well-being and employment (Mattick et al., 2009; Nolan et al., 2014). Before commencing OST, a comprehensive assessment should be undertaken to establish current dependence with usually daily opioid use. This should include history, physical examination, e.g. injection sites, and drug screening.

15.8.2 Methadone

15.8.2.1 Mechanisms of Action and Pharmacokinetics

Methadone is a μ receptor full agonist with high oral bioavailability. The half-life with repeated dosing is around 24 hours so it is suitable for once-daily dosing. However, there is wide inter-individual and intra-individual variation in half-life (13 to 50 hours). Steady-state plasma levels occur five half-lives (about 5 days) after last dose increase. Blood levels will rise even on the same dose during this period and an initially tolerated dose may cause toxicity a few days later. This is especially important during induction onto methadone (Clinical Guidelines on Drug Misuse and Dependence Update 2017 Independent Expert Working Group, 2017). The peak plasma concentration is around 4 hours after an oral dose. It is metabolized in the liver and therefore caution is required in hepatic impairment. Methadone is metabolized by the cytochrome P450 enzymes CYP3A4 and CYP2D6 and inhibits CYP2D6. Excretion is via urine and faeces.

15.8.2.2 Clinical Therapeutics

Methadone as methadone oral solution 1 mg/1 ml is licensed for OST and can be used for maintenance treatment and for detoxification purposes. Higher methadone doses are more effective at keeping individuals in treatment and reducing heroin use. The optimal dose range after induction and titration is 60 mg to 120 mg daily. Advice on initiating methadone is available via the UK clinical guidelines (Clinical Guidelines on Drug Misuse and Dependence Update 2017 Independent Expert Working Group, 2017) and it may take several weeks to reach an optimal dose. Initial doses will usually be 10–30 mg daily and dose increases should not exceed 5–10 mg per day/every few days with close clinical monitoring for signs of opioid toxicity. In the first week, 'a total weekly increase should not usually exceed 30 mg above the starting day's dose' (Clinical Guidelines on Drug Misuse and Dependence Update 2017 Independent Expert Working Group, 2017). After the first week, incremental increases of 5–10 mg every few days may be required with close monitoring (e.g. ongoing heroin use, signs of opioid toxicity) until dose optimization. In the first few weeks of methadone treatment there is an increased overdose risk. Subsequently, the risk of overdose death during maintenance treatment is low compared with the risks of not being in treatment (Sordo et al., 2017).

Interactions: Methadone prolongs the QTc interval in a dose-dependent way and caution should be employed when co-prescribing with other QTc prolonging drugs. ECG monitoring may be advisable. Medications which inhibit CYP3A4 will increase methadone blood levels. Examples include antibiotics, e.g. erythromycin, antifungals, e.g. ketoconazole, and antidepressants, e.g. fluvoxamine. The effect of methadone is reduced by medications which induce CYP3A4 such as rifampicin and carbamazepine. Opioid withdrawal symptoms can appear and careful dose titration can be needed. HIV and hepatitis C medications have complex interactions with methadone and advice may be needed from infectious disease specialists. See Annex 5 in the UK clinical guidelines for interactions with methadone. Sedative drugs and alcohol potentiate the respiratory depressant effect of opioids and are associated with methadone fatalities. Co-prescribing of benzodiazepines and opioids has been associated with increased risk of opioid overdose (Sun et al., 2017).

Contraindications and adverse effects: Certain conditions such as head injury, raised intracranial pressure and severe hepatic impairment require review of prescribing and extreme caution. Effects on those with chronic obstructive pulmonary disease need close monitoring (see Summary of Product Characteristics). Adverse effects of methadone include respiratory depression, nausea and vomiting, constipation and drowsiness although actual effects are moderated by tolerance in opioid-dependent individuals. Increased prolactin, menstrual irregularities and sweating are seen with prolonged use. There is an established neonatal abstinence syndrome with methadone use in pregnancy.

Monitoring: ECG monitoring is recommended for methadone doses over 100 mg daily or at lower doses with other risk factors, e.g. co-prescribing of other QTc prolonging drugs or CYP3A4 inhibitors, cardiac or liver disease, electrolyte abnormalities (MHRA, 2006). Prescribers must balance the need for a pretreatment ECG while considering the risk from delaying entry to OST, or missing an opportunity for entry to OST. When increasing methadone doses in those with risk factors or in those increasing to over 100 mg methadone daily a pre-increase ECG and post-stabilization ECG should be considered (Clinical Guidelines on Drug Misuse and Dependence Update 2017 Independent Expert Working Group, 2017).

NICE recommends that methadone and buprenorphine should be administered daily, under supervision, for at least the first three months. In the UK this is generally via a community pharmacist. Supervision should be relaxed only when the patient's compliance is assured (NICE, 2007a). In reality, a pragmatic approach is taken depending on local resources, commissioning and clinicians' risk management. New patients should generally have their OST supervised on a daily basis. The duration of supervised dispensing will depend on assessment of clinical progress and risk factors. Circumstances where supervised consumption should be continued or its introduction considered include during titration, with polysubstance misuse, with ongoing regular illicit drug use, with excessive alcohol use, where there is an overdose risk including through deliberate self-harm, where there is risk of the medication being diverted and where there are children at home, especially for methadone.

Drug testing can be used to monitor treatment compliance and the impact of OST on illicit drug use. Drug screening tests using urine or oral fluid are routinely used in clinical practice.

15.8.3 Buprenorphine

15.8.3.1 Mechanisms of Action

Buprenorphine is a partial μ agonist meaning it has opioid-like effects but these are milder than a full agonist – less euphoria, sedation, positive reinforcement and respiratory depression. Buprenorphine shows a ceiling effect for respiratory depression as the dose increases and rarely results in death from overdose due to respiratory depression (Office for National Statistics, 2017a). Taking buprenorphine with alcohol and/or other CNS depressant drugs can result in fatal opioid overdose. It has high affinity for μ-opioid receptors and will displace a full agonist such as heroin or methadone and as buprenorphine's effects are milder this can result in 'precipitated' opioid withdrawal. To minimize the risks of precipitated withdrawal buprenorphine should not be started until around 12 hours after last use of a short-acting opioid such as heroin or at least 24 hours after last use of a longer-acting opioid such as methadone (or ideally not until opioid withdrawal symptoms begin). Due to its high affinity for the opioid receptor buprenorphine (at effective doses) should also block the effects of additional opioids. As well as having μ agonist activity buprenorphine is a κ antagonist. Opioid drugs which activate the κ receptor tend to cause dysphoria so buprenorphine may theoretically be beneficial to mood.

15.8.3.2 Pharmacokinetics

The duration of effects is dose related, lasting 24–72 hours at doses of 16 mg and above. Peak plasma levels occur around 2 hours after dosing. Bioavailability is around 50% after sublingual dosing. Buprenorphine is metabolized in the liver and undergoes mainly biliary excretion. Buprenorphine is metabolized by the cytochrome P450 enzymes CYP3A4 and CYP2D6. It also acts as an inhibitor of CYP3A4 and CYP2D6.

15.8.3.3 Clinical Therapeutics

Buprenorphine as a sublingual tablet is licensed for OST and can be used for maintenance treatment and for detoxification purposes. The UK clinical guidelines give advice on dose initiation. For managing heroin dependence, the typical initial dose on day one is 4–8 mg, with the dose on day two 8–16 mg. Dividing the daily dose during induction (especially on day one) may reduce precipitated withdrawal. The optimal dose range is 12–16 mg daily, although some individuals will need more. The maximum daily dose is 32 mg. For individuals transferring from methadone to buprenorphine in the community the methadone dose should generally be 30 mg daily or less to minimize adverse effects during transfer (Clinical Guidelines on Drug Misuse and Dependence Update 2017 Independent Expert Working Group, 2017). After stabilization less than daily dosing may be possible to support engagement with other activities, e.g. work (see Summary of Product Characteristics).

There is a strong evidence base for the effectiveness of buprenorphine in OST. Higher doses of buprenorphine (16 mg and above) are more effective at treatment retention but only high doses suppressed heroin use better than placebo (Mattick et al., 2014). Unlike methadone, buprenorphine is not associated with an increased overdose risk during induction (Sordo et al., 2017).

Other formulations of buprenorphine are available. A rapidly dissolving oral lyophilisate product is licensed in the UK. It should be noted that there is different bioavailability between different buprenorphine products. Buprenorphine implants are not licensed in the UK but are approved in the USA and long-acting injectable buprenorphine is in clinical trials.

Interactions: Buprenorphine's high affinity at the μ receptor means that opioid analgesics may be less effective and buprenorphine may precipitate withdrawal in individuals on regular opioid analgesics. Sedative drugs and alcohol potentiate CNS depression. As with methadone, medications which inhibit or induce CYP3A4 may affect buprenorphine levels. Similarly, HIV and hepatitis C medications have complex interactions with buprenorphine and advice may be needed from infectious disease specialists. See Annex 5 in the UK clinical guidelines for interactions with buprenorphine. In general, buprenorphine is easier to use in people taking antiretroviral medications.

Contraindications and adverse effects: As buprenorphine blocks the additional use of opioids it is not suitable for those with chronic pain issues requiring opioid analgesics. The safer respiratory depressant profile of buprenorphine is adversely affected when it is used with other sedatives or misused, e.g. by injection, and deaths have occurred. The most common adverse effects are insomnia, headache and nausea. Precipitated withdrawal may occur if initiation is incorrect (see above). A neonatal abstinence syndrome may occur with buprenorphine use in pregnancy though less severe than with methadone (Jones et al., 2010). There is potential for liver damage especially if there are pre-existing risk factors and it is contraindicated in severe hepatic impairment.

Monitoring: Baseline liver function tests and regular monitoring are recommended. Urine or oral fluid drug screens can be used to monitor compliance.

15.8.4 Buprenorphine/Naloxone

Buprenorphine is also available as a sublingual tablet combined with the opioid antagonist naloxone in a buprenorphine:naloxone ratio of 4:1. This was developed due to concerns over the misuse of the buprenorphine-only preparation by intravenous injection. Taking the buprenorphine/naloxone tablet as prescribed results in only a buprenorphine effect (as naloxone is not absorbed) but if the tablet is misused by intravenous injection the naloxone is active and will cause opioid withdrawal symptoms in dependent opioid users.

15.8.5 Methadone Versus Buprenorphine

Both methadone and buprenorphine are effective treatments for opioid dependence. The choice of drug should be determined on history of opioid dependence, commitment to a particular treatment strategy and the risk/benefits of each treatment (NICE, 2007a). Key outcomes in OST are retention in treatment and cessation of illicit opioid use. The most recent Cochrane review reports that methadone is superior to buprenorphine in treatment retention and methadone is equally as effective at stopping illicit opioid use (Mattick et al., 2014). A follow-up study of long-term outcomes found that both methadone and buprenorphine (as buprenorphine/naloxone) reduced illicit opioid use but that there was greater opioid use and less treatment retention in the buprenorphine group (Hser et al., 2016). Poorer retention with buprenorphine has been a consistent finding attributed to too low initial dosing and too slow increase to therapeutic dose with resultant patient discomfort during the induction phase and the fact that it may be easier to stop buprenorphine. However, a more recent long-term follow-up study showed improved retention with buprenorphine over time (presumably as clinicians gained experience in more effective and quicker induction procedures and patients became familiar with buprenorphine) although retention was still better with methadone (Burns et al., 2015).

15.8.6 Other Opioid Substitution Treatments

15.8.6.1 Dihydrocodeine and Slow-Release Oral Morphine

Dihydrocodeine and slow-release oral morphine (SROM) are not licensed in the UK for use in OST.

Morphine is a full μ-opioid receptor agonist. SROM preparations are given once daily. Dihydrocodeine has been used for maintenance treatment in opioid dependence but there are concerns about the short half-life with the need for multiple daily doses and large numbers of tablets with risks of diversion (Clinical Guidelines on Drug Misuse and Dependence Update 2017 Independent Expert Working Group, 2017; Robertson et al., 2006). There is a small evidence base for the use of SROM in OST (Beck et al., 2014). The UK clinical guidelines recommend that 'SROM should only be prescribed when first-line OST treatments have been considered and are judged to be inappropriate' (Clinical Guidelines on Drug Misuse and Dependence Update 2017 Independent Expert Working Group, 2017).

15.8.6.2 Injectable Opioid Treatment

Prescribing pharmaceutical heroin, heroin-assisted treatment (HAT), is an option for those who have failed with other optimized OST. HAT increases retention and reduces illicit heroin compared with oral methadone (Strang et al., 2015). However, treatment costs are considerably higher than with oral methadone and supervised HAT may currently be considered a low volume, high-intensity treatment (Strang et al., 2015) to be delivered within specialist services and settings only. Methadone is also available in an injectable formulation but again is a specialist treatment option.

15.9 Opioid Detoxification Treatments

15.9.1 Methadone/Buprenorphine Reducing Regimens

Detoxification should be a readily available treatment option for opioid-dependent people who have expressed an informed choice to become abstinent (NICE, 2007b). Methadone or buprenorphine should be offered as first-line treatment in detoxification taking into account any existing prescribing of OST and patient preference. The medicine on which an individual has been maintained should normally be used to start the detoxification (NICE, 2007b). The detoxification period is usually considered up to 4 weeks for residential detoxification and up to 12 weeks in the community. Some individuals may wish to start gradual reduction of their OST before completing the final detoxification phase. Reducing doses of methadone or buprenorphine are effective. From methadone the reduction rate in the community may be around 5 mg every one or two weeks. With buprenorphine reductions of 2 mg every two weeks can be made until 2 or 4 mg with final reductions being around 400 μg (Clinical Guidelines on Drug Misuse and Dependence Update 2017 Independent Expert Working Group, 2017). Some people may want to reduce at a quicker rate.

There is no difference in completion rates between methadone and buprenorphine although there is some evidence of an earlier and more marked peak of withdrawal symptoms with methadone (Law et al., 2017). Though there is also a suggestion that withdrawal symptoms may resolve quicker with buprenorphine (Gowing et al., 2016).

For methadone a gradual, stepped taper with periods of stabilization on lower doses may increase success rates with Nosyk et al. (2012) reporting greater success with tapering schedules of between 12 and 52 or more weeks compared to less than 12 weeks. In a RCT of buprenorphine taper durations in a community setting in young people aged 16–24 years old, a 56-day taper resulted in more opioid-negative drug screens and greater treatment retention than a 28-day taper (Marsch et al., 2016).

Residential opioid detoxification should be considered for those with unsuccessful previous community detoxification attempts, who are prescribed high-dose opioid substitution treatment, who have significant co-morbid physical or mental health problems, who require concurrent detoxification from other substances in addition to opioids, e.g. alcohol, benzodiazepines, or who lack social support, e.g. homeless (NICE, 2007b).

15.9.2 Alpha$_2$-Adrenergic agonists

Alpha$_2$-adrenergic agonists such as clonidine and lofexidine can also be used for the symptomatic treatment of opioid withdrawal and lofexidine is licensed in the UK for this purpose. Lofexidine may be particularly useful for those who have decided not to use methadone or buprenorphine for detoxification, have decided to detoxify within a short time period or have lower levels of dependence (NICE, 2007b).

15.9.2.1 Mechanisms of Action and Pharmacokinetics

Lofexidine acts presynaptically on α_2-adrenergic receptors to reduce the noradrenergic hyperactivity that occurs in opioid withdrawal. Peak plasma levels occur 3 hours after dosing. It is metabolized in the liver and renally excreted.

15.9.2.2 Clinical Therapeutics

Lofexidine detoxification schedules are between 7 and 10 days with doses starting at 0.8 mg daily (4 × 0.2 mg tablets) and increasing gradually by 2 to 4 tablets daily to a maximum of 2.4 mg (12 tablets) in divided doses. The dose is then reduced over subsequent days. Lofexidine is effective for the management of opioid withdrawal and has similar efficacy to short (around 10 days) methadone reducing regimens (Gowing et al., 2016). Additional symptomatic medication is usually needed to manage opioid withdrawal symptoms. Baseline blood pressure and pulse should be measured. Daily review is needed initially, especially as doses are being increased, to monitor opioid withdrawal symptoms, blood pressure and pulse. Low blood pressure/bradycardia may need dose reduction or in some cases treatment being stopped. Doses should be reduced gradually over 2 to 4 days to reduce the risk of rebound hypertension.

Interactions: Lofexidine enhances the sedative effects of CNS depressants and the effects of antihypertensives.

Contraindications and adverse effects: Caution should be used in those with a history of cardiovascular disease. Lofexidine may prolong the QT interval and pre-treatment ECG should be considered and risk factors reviewed before prescribing. Adverse effects include sedation, dry mouth, dizziness, hypotension and bradycardia.

15.9.3 Symptomatic Medication for Opioid Withdrawal

To manage opioid withdrawal symptoms additional medication, beyond the detoxification agent, may be needed. This is especially likely with lofexidine schedules. Typical symptoms and symptomatic prescribing options are as follows:

- diarrhoea – loperamide
- nausea and vomiting – metoclopramide or prochlorperazine
- abdominal cramps – mebeverine
- agitation and anxiety – diazepam
- insomnia – diazepam or zopiclone
- aches and pains – paracetamol, aspirin, ibuprofen.

When adopting symptomatic prescribing, the prescriber should consult appropriate clinical guidelines and the Summary of Product Characteristics. Caution is needed with the potential for multiple drug interactions and individuals should be monitored closely.

15.10 Naltrexone for Relapse Prevention in Opioid Dependence

15.10.1 Mechanisms of Action and Pharmacokinetics

Naltrexone is a non-selective opioid antagonist with a high affinity for the μ-opioid receptor (see Section 15.6.2.1). It blocks the effect of heroin and other opioids by preventing access to the receptor. It will precipitate withdrawal in currently opioid-dependent individuals by displacing the opioid from the receptor.

15.10.2 Clinical Therapeutics

Oral naltrexone is recommended for relapse prevention by NICE for those highly motivated to remain abstinent (NICE, 2007c). One of the major issues with oral naltrexone is poor compliance but it is an effective treatment if adherence can be assured (Minozzi et al., 2011). To enhance compliance different formulations of naltrexone have been developed. Injectable sustained-release naltrexone is licensed in the USA for use in opioid and alcohol dependence but not in the UK. Naltrexone implants are not licensed and a recent review concluded that better research was required to establish safety and efficacy (Larney et al., 2014).

Due to the risks of precipitating opioid withdrawal as described above, before starting naltrexone a drug screen should be taken and test negative for opioids, just prior to administration of a test dose. For urine on-site tests this may be 5 days after last use of buprenorphine, 7 days after last use of short-acting drugs such as heroin, codeine and dihydrocodeine and up to 14 days after methadone. A 25 mg test dose (half a tablet) should be given and the client observed for 1 hour to ensure no adverse effects particularly any precipitated withdrawal. The standard dose is then 50 mg daily from day 2. It is possible to take naltrexone every 2 or 3 days, e.g. 100 mg Monday and Wednesday and 150 mg on a Friday, and this may be an option if supervised consumption is being used. NICE recommends that naltrexone is continued 'for up to 6 months, or longer for those benefiting from the drug who want to continue with it' (NICE, 2007c).

Interactions, contraindications and adverse effects: Naltrexone is contraindicated in currently opioid-dependent individuals and in those with an opioid-positive drug screen. Naltrexone should not be used with other opioid-containing medications (see also Section 15.6.2.3). Careful management is required if opioids are needed for acute/emergency pain relief. With planned, elective surgery, naltrexone can be stopped 48–72 hours beforehand. Attempts to overcome the blockade by administering larger doses of opioids may result in acute, potentially fatal, opioid overdose. Liver function tests should be taken pre-treatment and monitored during treatment.

15.11 Management of Opioid Overdose and Take-Home Naloxone

15.11.1 Opioid Overdose

In the UK deaths from opioid overdose have been increasing since 2012 and are the highest on record (Office for National Statistics, 2017a). Most are heroin related but there is an increasing number of deaths from synthetic opioid agonists of the fentanyl class. Opioid substitution treatment is associated with considerably reduced overdose deaths in illicit opioid users compared with periods out of treatment (Sordo et al., 2017). Overdose risk increases markedly in the first month following leaving opioid substitution treatment due to loss of tolerance. This increased risk seems irrespective of whether or not discharge was in a successful, planned way (Pierce et al., 2016). High-risk situations associated with loss of opioid tolerance include prison release, discharge from hospital or residential treatment, detoxification and stopping naltrexone.

Naloxone is used in hospital settings and by paramedics for opioid overdose reversal. It is a prescription-only medicine but the Human Medicines (Amendment) (No. 3) Regulations 2015 enables naloxone to be supplied to individuals by drug services without prescription – 'take-home naloxone'. There is a drive to increase access to take-home naloxone for opioid-dependent individuals, their families and carers (Public Health England, 2017a).

15.11.2 Take-Home Naloxone

15.11.2.1 Mechanisms of Action and Pharmacokinetics

Naloxone is a short-acting non-selective opioid receptor antagonist which is active parenterally. It displaces agonist opioids from the μ receptor, thereby reducing opioid effects and, importantly, the respiratory depressant effects. The half-life is about an hour and repeated doses of naloxone may be needed to reverse opioid overdose especially those with opioids of the fentanyl class. It is rapidly metabolized in the liver.

15.11.2.2 Clinical Therapeutics

Take-home naloxone is distributed by drug treatment services to opioid users at risk of opioid overdose and to family members/carers, friends and peers. Take-home naloxone is often packaged as a pre-filled syringe with 5 × 400 μg doses of naloxone. Training in overdose awareness and use of naloxone is given before distribution of take-home naloxone kits. Administration is intramuscular with 400 μg initially, with further 400 μg doses given incrementally every 2–3 minutes until an effect is noted or medical assistance arrives (Clinical Guidelines on Drug Misuse and Dependence 2017) Independent Expert Working Group, 2017. Naloxone (and indeed other opioid antagonists, e.g. naltrexone and nalmefene) can also be administered in the form of a concentrated nasal spray.

Interactions, contraindications, adverse effects and monitoring: Use of naloxone in opioid-dependent patients when not indicated or at too high a dose can lead to acute withdrawal including life-threatening symptoms of pulmonary oedema and cardiac arrhythmias. After use of naloxone individuals must be carefully monitored as the effect of opioids can be longer than the effect of naloxone.

15.12 Benzodiazepine Dependence and Withdrawal

15.12.1 Introduction

The clinical effects and pharmacology of benzodiazepines are described in Chapter 8. This section primarily focuses on benzodiazepine misuse rather than on dependence in prescribed therapeutic dose users. Those misusing benzodiazepines may use with other drugs and alcohol, use once-daily dosing to maximize euphoric or sedative effects, escalate doses with sometimes very high self-reported doses and use in a 'binge' pattern rather than on a daily basis. There is a much stronger evidence base on the management of therapeutic dose use than on the management of benzodiazepine dependence in illicit, high-dose users (Lingford-Hughes et al., 2012).

15.12.2 Benzodiazepine Misuse

15.12.2.1 Prevalence

In England and Wales 0.4% of adults aged 16–59 and 0.6% of those aged 16–24 reported using non-prescribed tranquillisers in the last year (Office for National Statistics, 2017b). Individuals with a history of substance misuse are at increased risk of misusing benzodiazepines. Misuse is common among heroin users. Among individuals in treatment for opioid problems in 2016/17 11% reported problematical benzodiazepine use (Public Health England, 2017b).

15.12.2.2 Harms

Benzodiazepine use has been associated with poorer clinical outcomes in those on opioid substitution treatment and there is increased opioid toxicity including overdose with concurrent benzodiazepine use (Darke et al., 2010; Nielsen et al., 2007; Sun et al., 2017). Drug-related deaths where benzodiazepines are mentioned on the death certificate have continued to rise in England and Wales with 406 such deaths registered in 2016 compared with 284 in 2012 (Office for National Statistics, 2017a). Benzodiazepines are commonly detected in deaths associated with methadone and heroin.

15.12.3 Benzodiazepine Withdrawal

Benzodiazepine withdrawal can manifest with a wide range of symptoms. Their severity will depend on the dose and duration for which benzodiazepines were taken and how abruptly they were stopped. Common symptoms include increased anxiety, insomnia, irritability and perceptual changes. The duration of withdrawal symptoms will partly depend on the half-life of the benzodiazepine in question but symptoms usually last less than four weeks. Further information on benzodiazepine withdrawal symptoms is provided in Chapter 8.

15.13 Pharmacological Management of Benzodiazepine Withdrawal/Dependence

15.13.1 General Principles

Management of benzodiazepine dependence in therapeutic dose use includes minimal interventions (e.g. self-help booklets), gradual dose reduction and gradual dose reduction with additional psychological or pharmacological treatments. Cognitive behavioural therapy plus gradual dose reduction increases cessation rates compared with gradual dose reduction alone at four-week and three-month follow-up but not in the longer term (Darker et al., 2015).

Careful (and often extended) assessment is required with a clear treatment goal before initiating benzodiazepine prescribing in opioid or other illicit drug users. There should be clear evidence of benzodiazepine dependence and withdrawal symptoms usually supported by several positive urine drug screens. A time-limited reduction regimen should be agreed at the outset with the aim of managing withdrawal symptoms and supporting detoxification. Alternative management should be used for problems such as anxiety and insomnia. Opioid substitution treatment should be optimized in opioid-dependent benzodiazepine users and benzodiazepine needs reassessed after this.

15.13.2 Benzodiazepine Reducing Regimens

Benzodiazepines should be converted to diazepam due to its long half-life, dose flexibility and the ability to prescribe daily via instalment prescribing (Clinical Guidelines on Drug Misuse and Dependence Update 2017 Independent Expert Working Group, 2017). Specialist advice about transfer to diazepam should be sought for those with hepatic impairment. Dispensing should be daily especially if there is co-prescribing of OST. The *British National Formulary* (BNF) has a dose equivalence table for diazepam and other sedative-hypnotics. The BNF suggests withdrawal rates of about one-eighth of the daily dose every fortnight. In opioid users a typical regimen would be to reduce the daily dose by 5 mg per fortnight until around 20–30 mg diazepam daily and then by 2 mg per fortnight, although the rate could be increased to weekly reductions or decreased to monthly as clinically indicated. Starting doses above 30 mg diazepam equivalent per day are not generally indicated and there is no need to match the often high self-reported doses to avoid serious adverse effects (Lingford-Hughes et al., 2012). Adverse effects of benzodiazepines and interactions are described in Chapter 8.

15.13.3 Carbamazepine for Managing Withdrawal

Some clinical services have used carbamazepine for inpatient benzodiazepine detoxification. Carbamazepine has been shown to reduce the withdrawal symptoms from benzodiazepines (Garcia-Borreguero et al., 1991; Schweizer et al., 1991).

15.13.4 Maintenance Benzodiazepine Prescribing

There is currently little evidence to support long-term substitute prescribing of benzodiazepines in benzodiazepine misuse (Clinical Guidelines on Drug Misuse and Dependence Update 2017 Independent Expert Working Group, 2017) although the possibility of benzodiazepine substitution treatment for those unable to successfully withdraw has been suggested (Bakker & Streel, 2016; Liebrenz et al., 2010). Rarely longer-term prescribing may be indicated in this population. Examples include verified long-term prescribing (to continue it must be determined that benefits outweigh the harms; and reducing and stabilizing on a lower dose may be an appropriate initial goal, especially if above 30 mg diazepam equivalent daily) and the presence of co-morbid mental health problems (prescribing to be agreed with mental health team).

15.13.5 Z-Drugs: Zaleplon, Zolpidem and Zopiclone

The clinical effects, adverse effects and pharmacology are described in Chapter 8. Dependence does occur with these medications (Hajak et al., 2003; Victorri-Vigneau et al., 2007). Withdrawal symptoms are similar to those of benzodiazepine withdrawal. In cases of dependence, withdrawal should be managed by gradual dose reduction of the Z-drug or by switching to diazepam and subsequent reduction. Additional psychosocial support should be provided.

Table 15.5 Summary of club drugs and novel psychoactive substances (for full details see Novel Psychoactive Treatment UK Network (NEPTUNE), 2015)

Drug/1° Route	Primary (proximal) target/*Main effects*	Common presentation	Management (limited evidence)
GHB –Oral	GHB & $GABA_B$ receptor agonist *Euphoria, relaxation, sociability*	**Withdrawal** (duration 3–21 days) Insomnia, tremor, agitation, delirium, seizures, myoclonic jerks **Toxicity** – CNS depression	Complex, manage in acute care setting Benzodiazepines, symptom triggered Barbiturates in refractory cases Symptom-focused supportive treatment
Dissociatives e.g. Ketamine/PCP/ methoxetamine intranasal/oral/injected	NMDA receptor antagonist *Stimulant at low dose, hallucinogenic and dissociative at higher doses*	Short half-life so rarely presents as toxicity. Main presentation as complication of poly-drug intoxication or withdrawal	Symptom-focused supportive treatment
Amphetamine group Cocaine MDMA	Release DA ± NA and block reuptake Blocks DA reuptake site Blocks serotonin and DA reuptake *Stimulant effects*	**Toxicity** – agitation, anxiety, psychotic symptoms, cardiovascular toxicity, serotonin syndrome, hyperthermia, delirium	Symptom-focused supportive treatment
Mephedrone & synthetic cathinones –nasal/oral	Increase synaptic concentration of DA, NA and serotonin (MA reuptake inhibitor) *Stimulant and sympathomimetic effects*	**Toxicity** – agitation, psychotic symptoms, cardiovascular toxicity, seizures, serotonin syndrome	Symptom-focused supportive treatment
Cannabis	Cannabis CB_1 receptor agonist	Psychological dependence	Rarely presents acutely
Synthetic cannabinoids (e.g. 'spice') – smoked/inhaled	Synthetic cannabinoid receptor agonist (SCRA)	**Toxicity** – confusion, cognitive impairment, paranoia, psychotic symptoms Psychological dependence	Symptom-focused supportive treatment
Psychodelics – swallowed/ injected	Agonists at serotonin $5\text{-}HT_{2A}$ receptors *Hallucinogen*	Generally lower risk profile, but also have stimulant properties so may present with agitation, anxiety, psychotic symptoms, cardiovascular toxicity	

DA, dopamine; MA, monoamine; MDMA, 3,4-methylenedioxymethamphetamine; NA, noradrenaline; PCP, phencyclidine.

15.14 Other Common Drugs of Misuse

The classification systems for SUD allow that drugs whose psychotropic effects fall within broadly defined substance categories may manifest a range of clinical presentations including intoxication, dependence and withdrawal. In reality, there are not describable syndromes for many currently used substances. Consequently, while the evidence base for the treatment of withdrawal, relapse prevention or harm minimization for AUD, opioid dependence, nicotine and benzodiazepine dependence is well established, the situation is different for a wide range of 'club drugs', including novel psychoactive substances (NPS).

The pharmacology of NPS mean that they may have different effects depending on dosage, route of administration and time from ingestion, and often a single substance can have a broad range of psychotropic effects. However, they can broadly be considered as follows: depressant drugs, stimulant drugs, hallucinogenic drugs and synthetic cannabinoids (Novel Psychoactive Treatment UK Network (NEPTUNE), 2015).

The pace of arrival of new substances means that increasingly the clinician will need to rely on accurate observation of presenting signs and symptoms and base the management plan on an understanding of the presumed pharmacology of the ingested drug. Clearly, where the patient is uncertain what they have taken, particularly in cases of polysubstance use, the picture will be further complicated and will need to be kept under constant review. Table 15.5 gives some examples of the main substances currently in use, their presentation and mode of action, but this is subject to significant geographical variations in use, and local up-to-date information from a reliable source should always be sought (e.g. TOXBASE or NEPTUNE) (Novel Psychoactive Treatment UK Network (NEPTUNE), 2015).

References

Agabio R, Sinclair J, Addolorato G, et al. (2018). Baclofen for the treatment of alcohol use disorder: the Cagliari Statement. *Lancet Psychiatry*, 5, 957–960.

Amato L, Minozzi S, Davoli M (2011). Efficacy and safety of pharmacological interventions for the treatment of the Alcohol Withdrawal Syndrome. *Cochrane Database Syst Rev*, (6), CD008537.

American Psychiatric Association (2013). *Diagnostic and Statistical Manual of Mental Disorders*, 5th ed. Arlington, VA: American Psychiatric Association.

Anthenelli RM, Benowitz NL, West R, et al. (2016). Neuropsychiatric safety and efficacy of varenicline, bupropion, and nicotine patch in smokers with and without psychiatric disorders (EAGLES): a double-blind, randomised, placebo-controlled clinical trial. *Lancet*, 387, 2507–2520.

Bakker A, Streel E (2016). Benzodiazepine maintenance in opiate substitution treatment: good or bad? A retrospective primary care case-note review. *J Psychopharmacol*, 31, 62–66.

Beck T, Haasen C, Verthein U, et al. (2014). Maintenance treatment for opioid dependence with slow-release oral morphine: a randomized cross-over, non-inferiority study versus methadone. *Addiction*, 109, 617–626.

Bordia T, Hrachova M, Chin M, McIntosh JM, Quik M (2012). Varenicline is a potent partial agonist at $\alpha6\beta2^*$ nicotinic acetylcholine receptors in rat and monkey striatum. *J Pharmacol Exp Ther*, 342, 327–334.

Burns L, Gisev N, Larney S, et al. (2015). A longitudinal comparison of retention in buprenorphine and methadone treatment for opioid dependence in New South Wales, Australia. *Addiction*, 110, 646–655.

Cahill K, Lindson-Hawley N, Thomas KH, Fanshawe TR, Lancaster T (2016). Nicotine receptor partial agonists for smoking cessation. *Cochrane Database Syst Rev*, (5), CD006103.

Chick J (1999). Safety issues concerning the use of disulfiram in treating alcohol dependence. *Drug Saf*, 20, 427–435.

Chick J, Nutt DJ (2012). Substitution therapy for alcoholism: time for a reappraisal? *J Psychopharmacol*, 26, 205–212.

Chick J, Gough K, Falkowski W, et al. (1992). Disulfiram treatment of alcoholism. *Br J Psychiatry*, 161, 84–89.

Clinical Guidelines on Drug Misuse and Dependence Update 2017 Independent Expert Working Group (2017). *Drug misuse and dependence: UK guidelines on clinical management*. London: Department of Health.

Coe JW, Brooks PR, Vetelino MG, et al. (2005). Varenicline: an α4β2 nicotinic receptor partial agonist for smoking cessation. *J Med Chem*, 48, 3474–3477.

Colasanti A, Rabiner E, Lingford-Hughes A, Nutt D (2011). Opioids and anxiety. *J Psychopharmacol*, 25, 1415–1433.

Coleman T, Chamberlain C, Davey M-A, Cooper SE, Leonardi-Bee J (2015). Pharmacological interventions for promoting smoking cessation during pregnancy. *Cochrane Database Syst Rev*, (12), CD010078.

Darke S, Ross J, Mills K, et al. (2010). Benzodiazepine use among heroin users: baseline use, current use and clinical outcome. *Drug Alcohol Rev*, 29, 250–255.

Darker CD, Sweeney BP, Barry JM, Farrell MF, Donnelly-Swift E (2015). Psychosocial interventions for benzodiazepine harmful use, abuse or dependence. *Cochrane Database Syst Rev*, (5), CD009652.

de Beaurepaire R, Sinclair JMA, Heydtmann M, et al. (2018). The use of baclofen as a treatment for alcohol use disorder: a clinical practice perspective. *Front Psychiatry*, 9, 708.

Degenhardt L, Charlson F, Mathers B, et al. (2014a). The global epidemiology and burden of opioid dependence: results from the global burden of disease 2010 study. *Addiction*, 109, 1320–1333.

Degenhardt L, Larney S, Randall D, Burns L, Hall W (2014b). Causes of death in a cohort treated for opioid dependence between 1985 and 2005. *Addiction*, 109, 90–99.

Di Ciano P, Guranda M, Lagzdins D, et al. (2016). Varenicline-induced elevation of dopamine in smokers: a preliminary [^{11}C]-(+)-PHNO PET study. *Neuropsychopharmacology*, 41, 1513–1520.

Donoghue K, Elzerbi C, Saunders R, et al. (2015). The efficacy of acamprosate and naltrexone in the treatment of alcohol dependence, Europe versus the rest of the world: a meta-analysis. *Addiction*, 110, 920–930.

Ebbert JO, Hughes JR, West RJ, et al. (2015). Effect of varenicline on smoking cessation through smoking reduction: a randomized clinical trial. *JAMA*, 313, 687–694.

Elholm B, Larsen K, Hornnes N, Zierau F, Becker U (2011). Alcohol withdrawal syndrome: symptom-triggered versus fixed-schedule treatment in an outpatient setting. *Alcohol Alcohol*, 46, 318–323.

European Medicines Agency (2017). Alcover (granules in sachet) and associated names. London: European Medicines Agency.

Garcia-Borreguero D, Bronisch T, Apelt S, Yassouridis A, Emrich HM (1991). Treatment of benzodiazepine withdrawal symptoms with carbamazepine. *Eur Arch Psychiatry Clin Neurosci*, 241, 145–150.

Goodwin G, Haddad P, Ferrier I, et al. (2016). Evidence-based guidelines for treating bipolar disorder: revised third edition recommendations from the British Association for Psychopharmacology. *J Psychopharmacol*, 30, 495–553.

Gossop M (1990). The development of a short opiate withdrawal scale (SOWS). *Addict Behav*, 15, 487–490.

Gowing L, Farrell M, Ali R, White JM (2016). Alpha2-adrenergic agonists for the management of opioid withdrawal. *Cochrane Database Syst Rev*, (5), CD002024.

Haber P, Lintzeris N, Proude E, Lopatko O (2009). *Guidelines for the Treatment of Alcohol Problems*. Canberra: Commonwealth of Australia.

Hajak G, Müller WE, Wittchen HU, Pittrow D, Kirch W (2003). Abuse and dependence potential for the non-benzodiazepine hypnotics zolpidem and zopiclone: a review of case reports and epidemiological data. *Addiction*, 98, 1371–1378.

Harper CG, Giles M, Finlay-Jones R (1986). Clinical signs in the Wernicke-Korsakoff complex: a retrospective analysis of 131 cases diagnosed at necropsy. *J Neurol Neurosurg Psychiatry*, 49, 341–345.

Hartmann-Boyce J, McRobbie H, Bullen C, et al. (2016). Electronic cigarettes for smoking cessation. *Cochrane Database Syst Rev*, (9), CD010216.

Hartmann-Boyce J, Chepkin SC, Ye W, Bullen C, Lancaster T (2018). Nicotine replacement therapy versus control for smoking cessation. *Cochrane Database Syst Rev*, (5), CD000146.

Hasin DS, Stinson FS, Ogburn E, Grant BF (2007). Prevalence, correlates, disability, and comorbidity of DSM-IV alcohol abuse and dependence in the United States: results from the National Epidemiologic Survey on Alcohol and Related Conditions. *Arch Gen Psychiatry*, 64, 830–842.

Hay G, Rael dos Santos A, Swithenbank Z (2017). *Estimates of the Prevalence of Opiate Use and/or Crack Cocaine Use, 2014/15: Sweep 11 Report. Public Health England*. Liverpool: Public Health Institute, John Moores University.

Hser Y-I, Evans E, Huang D, et al. (2016). Long-term outcomes after randomization to buprenorphine/naloxone versus methadone in a multi-site trial. *Addiction*, 111, 695–705.

Hughes JR, Stead LF, Hartmann-Boyce J, Cahill K, Lancaster T (2014). Antidepressants for smoking cessation. *Cochrane Database Syst Rev*, (1), CD000031.

Jones HE, Kaltenbach K, Heil SH, et al. (2010). Neonatal abstinence syndrome after methadone or buprenorphine exposure. *New Engl J Med*, 363, 2320–2331.

Kalk NJ, Lingford-Hughes AR (2014). The clinical pharmacology of acamprosate. *Br J Clin Pharmacol*, 77, 315–323.

Koob GF, Le Moal M (2006). Nicotine. In GF Koob, M Le Moal, eds., *Neurobiology of Addiction*. Amsterdam: Elsevier.

Kosten TR, George TP (2002). The neurobiology of opioid dependence: implications for treatment. *Sci Pract Perspect*, 1, 13–20.

Kotz D, Viechtbauer W, Simpson C, et al. (2015). Cardiovascular and neuropsychiatric risks of varenicline: a retrospective cohort study. *Lancet Respir Med*, 3, 761–768.

Larney S, Gowing L, Mattick RP, et al. (2014). A systematic review and meta-analysis of naltrexone implants for the treatment of opioid dependence. *Drug Alcohol Rev*, 33, 115–128.

Lasser K, Boyd J, Woolhandler S, et al. (2000). Smoking and mental illness: a population-based prevalence study. *JAMA*, 284, 2606–2610.

Law FD, Diaper AM, Melichar JK, et al. (2017). Buprenorphine/naloxone versus methadone and lofexidine in community stabilisation and detoxification: a randomised controlled trial of low dose short-term opiate-dependent individuals. *J Psychopharamcol*, 31, 1046–1055.

Lejoyeux M, Lehert P (2011). Alcohol-use disorders and depression: results from individual patient data meta-analysis of the acamprosate controlled studies. *Alcohol Alcohol*, 46, 61–67.

Liebrenz M, Boesch L, Stohler R, Caflisch C (2010). Agonist substitution – a treatment alternative for high-dose benzodiazepine-dependent patients? *Addiction*, 105, 1870–1874.

Lingford-Hughes AR, Welch S, Peters L, Nutt DJ (2012). BAP updated guidelines: evidence-based guidelines for the pharmacological management of substance abuse, harmful use, addiction and comorbidity: recommendations from BAP. *J Psychopharmacol*, 26, 899–952.

Lishman W (1998). *Organic Psychiatry: The Psychological Consequences of Cerebral Disorder*. Oxford: Blackwell Science, pp. 315–323.

Mann K, Torup L, Sørensen P, et al. (2016). Nalmefene for the management of alcohol dependence: review on its pharmacology, mechanism of action and meta-analysis on its clinical efficacy. *Eur Neuropsychopharmacol*, 26, 1941–1949.

Marsch LA, Moore SK, Borodovsky JT, et al. (2016). A randomized controlled trial of buprenorphine taper duration among opioid-dependent adolescents and young adults. *Addiction*, 111, 1406–1415.

Mattick RP, Breen C, Kimber J, Davoli M (2009). Methadone maintenance therapy versus no opioid replacement therapy for opioid dependence. *Cochrane Database Syst Rev*, (3), CD002209.

Mattick RP, Breen C, Kimber J, Davoli M (2014). Buprenorphine maintenance versus placebo or methadone maintenance for opioid dependence. *Cochrane Database of Systematic Reviews*, (2), CD002207.

McNeill A, Brose LS, Calder R, Bauld L, Robson D (2018). *Evidence review of e-cigarettes and heated tobacco products. A report commissioned by Public Health England*. London: Public Health England.

MHRA (2006). *Current Problems in Pharmacovigilance*, Vol. 31. London: Medicines and Healthcare products Regulatory Agency.

Minozzi S, Amato L, Vecchi S, Davoli M (2010). Anticonvulsants for alcohol withdrawal. *Cochrane Database Syst Rev*, (3), CD005064.

Minozzi S, Amato L, Vecchi S, et al. (2011). Oral naltrexone maintenance treatment for opioid dependence. *Cochrane Database Syst Rev*, (4), CD001333.

Montgomery AJ, Lingford-Hughes AR, Egerton A, Nutt DJ, Grasby PM (2007). The effect of nicotine on striatal dopamine release in man: a [11C] raclopride PET study. *Synapse*, 61, 637–645.

National Institute for Health and Care Excellence (NICE) (2007a). *Methadone and buprenorphine for the management of opioid dependence*. Technology appraisal guidance [TA114]. Manchester: National Institute for Health and Care Excellence.

National Institute for Health and Care Excellence (NICE) (2007b). *Drug misuse: opiate detoxification*. Clinical guideline [CG52]. Manchester: National Institute for Health and Care Excellence.

National Institute for Health and Care Excellence (NICE) (2007c). *Naltrexone for the management of opioid dependence*. Technology appraisal guidance [TA115]. Manchester: National Institute for Health and Care Excellence.

National Institute for Health and Care Excellence (NICE) (2010a). *Alcohol-use disorders: diagnosis and management of physical complications*. Clinical guideline [CG100]. Manchester: National Institute for Health and Care Excellence.

National Institute for Health and Care Excellence (NICE) (2010b). *Smoking: stopping in pregnancy and after childbirth*. Public health guideline [PH26]. Manchester: National Institute for Health and Care Excellence.

National Institute for Health and Care Excellence (NICE) (2011). *Alcohol-use disorders: diagnosis, assessment and management of harmful drinking and alcohol dependence*. Clinical guideline [CG115]. Manchester: National Institute for Health and Care Excellence.

Nesvåg R, Knudsen GP, Bakken IJ, et al. (2015). Substance use disorders in schizophrenia, bipolar disorder, and depressive illness: a registry-based study. *Soc Psychiatry Psychiatr Epidemiol*, 50, 1267–1276.

Nielsen S, Dietze P, Lee N, Dunlop A, Taylor D (2007). Concurrent buprenorphine and benzodiazepines use and self-reported opioid toxicity in opioid substitution treatment. *Addiction*, 102, 616–622.

Nolan S, Dias Lima V, Fairbairn N, et al. (2014). The impact of methadone maintenance therapy on hepatitis C incidence among illicit drug users. *Addiction*, 109, 2053–2059.

Nosyk B, Sun H, Evans E, et al. (2012). Defining dosing pattern characteristics of successful tapers following methadone maintenance treatment: results from a population-based retrospective cohort study. *Addiction*, 107, 1621–1629.

Novel Psychoactive Treatment UK Network (NEPTUNE) (2015). *Guidance on the management of acute and chronic harms of club drugs and novel psychoactive substances*. (online). London. (last accessed 19.2.18).

Nutt DJ, Lingford-Hughes A, Chick J (2012). Through a glass darkly: can we improve clarity about mechanism and aims of medications in drug and alcohol treatments? *J Psychopharmacol*, 26, 199–204.

Nutt DJ, Lingford-Hughes A, Erritzoe D, Stokes P (2015). The dopamine theory of addiction: 40 years of highs and lows. *Nat Rev Neurosci*, 16, 305–312.

Office for National Statistics (2017a). *Deaths related to drug poisoning in England and Wales: 2016 registrations. Statistical Bulletin*. London: Office for National Statistics.

Office for National Statistics (2017b). *Drug misuse: findings from the 2016/17 CSEW*. London: Home Office.

Pathan H, Williams J (2012). Basic opioid pharmacology: an update. *Br J Pain*, 6, 11–16.

Petrakis IL, Poling J, Levinson C, et al. (2005). Naltrexone and disulfiram in patients with alcohol dependence and comorbid psychiatric disorders. *Biol Psychiatry*, 57, 1128–1137.

Pierce M, Bird SM, Hickman M, et al. (2016). Impact of treatment for opioid dependence on fatal drug-related poisoning: a national cohort study in England. *Addiction*, 111, 298–308.

Public Health England (2016). *Shooting up: infections among people who injected drugs in the UK, 2015. An update: November 2016*. London: Public Health England.

Public Health England (2017a). *Take-home naloxone for opioid overdose in people who use drugs*. London: Public Health England.

Public Health England (2017b). *Adult substance misuse statistics from the National Drug Treatment Monitoring System (NDTMS)*. London: Public Health England.

Public Health England (2018). *Adult substance misuse statistics from the National Drug Treatment Monitoring System (NDTMS)*. London: Public Health England.

Quelch DR, Mick I, McGonigle J, et al. (2017). Nalmefene reduces reward anticipation in alcohol dependence: an experimental functional magnetic resonance imaging study. *Biol Psychiatry*, 81, 941–948.

Rehm J, Shield K, Gmel G, Rehm M, Frick U (2013). Modeling the impact of alcohol dependence on mortality burden and the effect of available treatment interventions in the European Union. *Eur Neuropsychopharmacol*, 23, 89–97.

Reitsma M (2017). Smoking prevalence and attributable disease burden in 195 countries and territories, 1990–2015: a systematic analysis from the Global Burden of Disease Study 2015. *Lancet*, 389, 1885–1906.

Robertson JR, Raab GM, Bruce M, et al. (2006). Addressing the efficacy of dihydrocodeine versus methadone as an alternative maintenance treatment for opiate dependence: a randomized controlled trial. *Addiction*, 101, 1752–1759.

Rösner S, Hackl-Herrwerth A, Leucht S, et al. (2010). Opioid antagonists for alcohol dependence. *Cochrane Database Syst Rev*, (12), CD001867.

Ross J, Ross J, Teesson M, et al. (2005). The characteristics of heroin users entering treatment: findings from the Australian treatment outcome study (ATOS). *Drug Alcohol Rev*, 24, 411–418.

Saunders JB, Aasland OG, Amundsen A, Grant M (1993). Alcohol consumption and related problems among primary health care patients: WHO collaborative project on early detection of persons with harmful alcohol consumption – I. *Addiction*, 88, 349–362.

Sechi G, Serra A (2007). Wernicke's encephalopathy: new clinical settings and recent advances in diagnosis and management. *Lancet Neurol*, 6, 442–455.

Senbanjo R, Wolff K, Marshall J (2007). Excessive alcohol consumption is associated with reduced quality of life among methadone patients. *Addiction*, 102, 257–263.

Sinclair JMA, Latifi AH, Latifi AW (2008). Co-morbid substance misuse in psychiatric inpatients: prevalence and association with length of inpatient stay. *J Psychopharmacol*, 22, 92–98.

Sinclair JM, Chambers SE, Shiles CJ, Baldwin DS (2016). Safety and tolerability of pharmacological treatment of alcohol dependence: comprehensive review of evidence. *Drug Saf*, 39, 627–645.

Sordo L, Barrio G, Bravo MJ, et al. (2017). Mortality risk during and after opioid substitution treatment: systematic review and meta-analysis of cohort studies. *BMJ*, 357, j1550.

Stapleton J, West R, Hajek P, et al. (2013). Randomized trial of nicotine replacement therapy (NRT), bupropion and NRT plus bupropion for smoking cessation: effectiveness in clinical practice. *Addiction*, 108, 2193–2201.

Sterling LH, Windle SB, Filion KB, Touma L, Eisenberg MJ (2016). Varenicline and adverse cardiovascular events: a systematic review and meta-analysis of randomized controlled trials. *J Am Heart Assoc*, 5, e002849.

Stockwell T, Murphy D, Hodgson R (1983). The severity of alcohol dependence questionnaire: its use, reliability and validity. *Br J Addict*, 78, 145–155.

Strang J, Groshkova T, Uchtenhagen A, et al. (2015). Heroin on trial: systematic review and meta-analysis of randomised trials of diamorphine-prescribing as treatment for refractory heroin addiction. *Br J Psychiatry*, 207, 5–14.

Sullivan JT, Sykora K, Schneiderman J, Naranjo CA, Sellers EM (1989). Assessment of alcohol withdrawal: the revised Clinical Institute Withdrawal Assessment for Alcohol scale (CIWA-Ar). *Br J Addict*, 84, 1353–1357.

Sun EC, Dixit A, Humphreys K, et al. (2017). Association between concurrent use of prescription opioids and benzodiazepines and overdose: retrospective analysis. *BMJ*, 356, j760.

Sweizer E, Rickets K, Case WG, Greenblatt DJ (1991). Carbamazepine treatment in patients discontinuing long-term benzodiazepine therapy. Effects on withdrawal severity and outcome. *Arch Gen Psychiatry*, 48, 448–452.

Swift RM (2013). Naltrexone and nalmefene: any meaningful difference? *Biol Psychiatry*, 73, 700–701.

Toftdahl NG, Nordentoft M, Hjorthøj C (2016). Prevalence of substance use disorders in psychiatric patients: a nationwide Danish population-based study. *Soc Psychiatry Psychiatr Epidemiol*, 51, 129–140.

Ulrichsen J, Nielsen MK, Ulrichsen M (2010). Disulfiram in severe alcoholism – an open controlled study. *Nord J Psychiatry*, 64, 356–362.

Umhau JC, Momenan R, Schwandt ML, et al. (2010). Effect of acamprosate on magnetic resonance spectroscopy measures of central glutamate in detoxified alcohol-dependent individuals: a randomized controlled experimental medicine study. *Arch Gen Psychiatry*, 67, 1069–1077.

Victorri-Vigneau C, Dailly E, Veyrac G, Jolliet P (2007). Evidence of zolpidem abuse and dependence: results of the French Centre for Evaluation and Information on Pharmacodependence (CEIP) network survey. *Br J Clin Pharmacol*, 64, 198–209.

Weaver T, Madden P, Charles V, et al. (2003). Comorbidity of substance misuse and mental illness in community mental health and substance misuse services. *Br J Psychiatry*, 183, 304–313.

Wesson DR, Ling W (2003). The Clinical Opiate Withdrawal Scale (COWS). *J Psychoactive Drugs*, 35, 253–259.

Wilde MI, Wagstaff AJ (1997). Acamprosate. *Drugs*, 53, 1038–1053.

World Health Organization (1992). *ICD-10: International Statistical Classification of Diseases and Related Health Problems*. Geneva: World Health Organization.

World Health Organization (2014). *Global status report on alcohol and health 2014*. Available at: www.who.int/substance_abuse/publications/global_alcohol_report/en/ (last accessed 11.8.19).

Chapter 16

Electroconvulsive Therapy and Neuromodulation Therapies

David Christmas and Keith Matthews

16.1 Introduction

The International Neuromodulation Society (2016) defines therapeutic neuromodulation as *'the alteration of nerve activity through targeted delivery of a stimulus, such as electrical stimulation or chemical agents, to specific neurological sites in the body'*. The term encompasses a wide range of approaches that extend from non-invasive techniques such as transcranial magnetic stimulation (TMS) to the use of implanted devices such as a vagal nerve and deep brain stimulation systems. This chapter reviews the principal neuromodulation therapies relevant to psychiatry. These have been used primarily in treatment-resistant depression, though studies have defined this to differing degrees of stringency. Outside of psychiatry, neuromodulation is widely used. Examples include: spinal cord stimulation for chronic neuropathic pain; deep brain stimulation for Parkinson's disease, essential tremor, dystonia and epilepsy; and carotid artery stimulation for hypertension. This is a rapidly developing field.

Electroconvulsive therapy (ECT) is the oldest and most widely used neuromodulation therapy in medicine. Its effectiveness in treating depression is supported by meta-analysis of randomized controlled trials (RCTs) and it has one of the largest effect sizes of any treatment in psychiatry. The United States Food and Drug Administration (FDA) has approved several neuromodulation therapies: vagus nerve stimulation (VNS) for the treatment of severe recurrent depression that had failed to respond to pharmacotherapy (2005); repetitive transcranial magnetic stimulation (rTMS) for the treatment of major depression that has not responded to one course of antidepressant medication (2008) and the treatment of obsessive-compulsive disorder (OCD) (2018); and deep brain stimulation (DBS) for the treatment of OCD (2018). It should be noted that these approvals relate to specific medical devices. The clinical role of these therapies in psychiatry, outside of these indications, and of other neuromodulation therapies, remains to be established.

16.2 Electroconvulsive Therapy (ECT)

16.2.1 History and Mechanism of Action

In 1938, the Italians Ugo Certletti and Lucio Bini were the first to use electricity applied to the scalp to treat mental disorders; replacing the use of intravenous metrazol that had been introduced by Ladislas Meduna. For around 15 years or more, seizures were 'unmodified' and generated an increased risk of fractures because of strong muscle contractions. In 1953, Adderley and Hamilton described the use of succinylcholine (a depolarizing muscle relaxant) to modify the seizures. They used an inflated blood-pressure cuff to isolate an arm in order to observe the underlying seizure (Adderley & Hamilton, 1953). In the UK this practice has been replaced by EEG monitoring to measure the duration of the seizure.

Today, ECT in most countries is modified, i.e. an anaesthetic and muscle relaxant are administered so that the patient is not conscious during the treatment and the tonic-clonic seizure is controlled with minimal movements occurring. The electrical stimulus is adjusted to ensure a seizure between 20 and 50 seconds long. In Scotland, accreditation of ECT centres is performed by the Scottish ECT Audit Network (SEAN) and all mental health units where ECT is performed take part in audit and outcome monitoring. In

England and Wales, the ECT Accreditation Service (ECTAS) has established standards for ECT centres and approximately 80% of centres are accredited.

The mechanism of action of ECT remains unknown although it is known to affect multiple neurotransmitter systems (Nutt et al., 1989). Increases in cortisol and prolactin (for example) typically return to pretreatment levels within several hours and increases in prolactin are associated with the seizure itself rather than being specific effects of ECT. Electroconvulsive stimulation (ECS), the equivalent of ECT in animal models, has been shown to stimulate neurogenesis in the hippocampus in animal models, with dose-dependent effects (Madsen et al., 2000); and there is convergent evidence that ECT increases both brain volume (particularly the hippocampus) and the integrity of white matter tracts connecting frontal and temporal regions (Gbyl & Videbech, 2018). Additionally, animal models indicate that ECS increases brain-derived neurotrophic factor (BDNF) expression in the ventral hippocampus (Enomoto et al., 2017), and increases in BDNF are also seen in humans (Rocha et al., 2016). However, increases in hippocampal volume do not seem to be associated with clinical response (Oltedal et al., 2018). Ultimately, it is unlikely that there is a single mechanism of action; rather, there are a number of underlying processes that contribute to clinical response.

Reflecting a shift away from neurotransmitter-focused models of psychiatric disorders, interest in recent years has examined changes in both brain structure and function; incorporating models of psychiatric illness that involve dysfunction in neural circuits as better frameworks for understanding illness. Recent functional neuroimaging studies have reported that reductions in 'frontal connectivity' (the extent to which different neural regions and circuits are interconnected functionally) are associated with symptom improvement following ECT (Perrin et al., 2012). These findings are broadly consistent with theories that the 'dorsal nexus' (a region of high connectivity between a cognitive control network, default mode network and an affective network) may play a role in depressive symptomatology (Sheline et al., 2010), and that ECT may affect key pathways directly.

16.2.2 Indications

There are three main contemporary indications for ECT: major depressive disorder; mania that is unresponsive to other treatments; and schizophrenia. There are no comprehensive systematic reviews of ECT for schizophrenia or bipolar disorder.

16.2.2.1 Depression

Major depression is the most common indication for ECT. Differences in the way in which indication is recorded between England and Wales, and Scotland make direct comparisons difficult, but between 67% and 88% of patients receiving ECT in the UK receive it for depression (see Table 16.1).

A number of groups have conducted systematic reviews and meta-analysis of the efficacy of ECT for depression. The UK ECT Review Group reviewed published data regarding ECT and reported outcomes from ECT against sham ECT, inpatient treatment alone and pharmacotherapy (UK ECT Review Group, 2003). Six trials comparing ECT versus sham ECT were included. There were 256 patients in these studies and most patients were inpatients with varying forms of depressive illness. Electrode placement was variable, and both sine-wave and brief-pulse stimulation

Table 16.1 ECT for depression in the UK

Indication	England and Wales (%) (Buley et al., 2017)	Scotland (%) (SEAN, 2017)
Moderate depression that has not responded to drug treatments and psychological treatment/depressive episode without psychosis	43	39
Severe depression that is life-threatening, and where a rapid response is required, or where other treatments have failed/depressive episode with psychosis	45	28

was used. There was a statistically significant benefit of real ECT (standardized mean difference −0.91 95% confidence interval (CI) −1.27 to -0.54) which was equivalent to an improvement of 9.7 on the Hamilton Depression Rating Scale in favour of real ECT. Rates of discontinuation between groups (examined by three trials) were similar.

Only one trial (139 patients) compared ECT versus inpatient treatment alone. The average reduction in Hamilton Depression Rating Scale in favour of ECT was 3.6 points.

The UK ECT Review Group review included 19 trials (1184 patients) comparing ECT with pharmacotherapy. As above, electrode placement and frequency of treatment varied between studies and medication use was heterogeneous. Overall, there was an effect size of −0.80 (95% CI −1.29 to −0.29) in favour of ECT; equivalent to an improvement of 5.2 on the Hamilton Depression Rating Scale in favour of ECT. Patients were slightly more likely to discontinue ECT than pharmacotherapy.

The FDA reviewed the evidence for ECT in order to update their classification of ECT devices (FDA, 2011). Five ECT versus sham ECT for depression studies were included. The FDA concluded that there is a benefit for real ECT of about 7.1 points on the Hamilton Depression Rating Scale. Eight studies were included comparing ECT with pharmacotherapy and the FDA reported that the average improvement in Hamilton Depression Rating Scale was 5.0 points in favour of ECT.

The strong evidence base for using ECT in depression is reflected in current guidelines. The British Association for Psychopharmacology guidelines for treating depression recommend that ECT 'should be considered as a first-line treatment for major depression in urgent and emergency situations' but also that it 'could be considered where: patients express a clear choice; or the patient has relapsed and there has been a previous response to ECT' (Cleare et al., 2015). Similarly, the American Psychiatric Association (APA) and the Canadian Network for Mood and Anxiety Treatments (CANMAT) both give strong recommendations for the use of ECT as first- or second-line treatments for depression (American Psychiatric Association, 2010; Milev et al., 2016). The current National Institute for Health and Care Excellence (NICE) guidelines on ECT also recommend ECT for 'severe depressive illness' (National Institute for Clinical Excellence, 2003).

16.2.2.2 Mania

Rates of ECT use for mania are lower than depression, but approximately 3% of patients undergoing ECT are receiving it on account of a prolonged or severe manic episode (Buley et al., 2017). Clinical guidelines still include a recommendation for ECT for mania, resistant mixed affective states, or mania occurring during pregnancy (American Psychiatric Association, 2002; Goodwin et al., 2016). The current NICE guidelines on ECT identify a 'prolonged or severe manic episode' as an indication (National Institute for Clinical Excellence, 2003).

The UK ECT Review Group identified only one small trial comparing ECT with medication and one study comparing ECT and medication with medication alone (UK ECT Review Group, 2003). ECT combined with medication was more effective than ECT alone, but no meta-analysis was possible.

Comparisons between different stimulus dosing regimens and electrode placements are lacking, and there are very few good quality studies of ECT for mania. Consequently, many clinicians will default to bilateral ECT in cases of mania, but it is not possible to make clear recommendations about electrode placement.

16.2.2.3 Schizophrenia

Rates of ECT use for schizophrenia have declined over time and the proportion of patients receiving ECT for schizophrenia in England and Wales is likely to be less than 2% of all patients receiving ECT (Buley et al., 2017).

There remain significant uncertainties about the use of ECT for schizophrenia but there is systematic review support for the use of ECT for patients with schizophrenia, particularly when a rapid improvement is required and/or when response to other treatment strategies is limited (Tharyan & Adams, 2005). There is no compelling evidence of long-term benefit and effects are likely to be short term.

The UK ECT Review Group analyzed outcome data from six trials containing a total of 140 patients; two of which were excluded because they were small and reported on catatonic schizophrenia only. The authors reported significant heterogeneity among studies. Of the four studies (each containing 20–30 participants) comparing ECT with sham ECT, the pooled effect size was 0.22 in favour of ECT but the 95% confidence interval included zero so it is difficult to draw conclusions (UK ECT Review Group, 2003).

16.2.2.4 Catatonia

A 1995 systematic review of 70 studies of treatment of catatonia (comprising 270 treatment episodes in 178 patients) included ECT in 20% of these (Hawkins et al., 1995). Response rates in this group were 85% (compared with 70% with benzodiazepines) but most studies were case reports and details about previous treatments and clinical histories are lacking. However, the authors concluded that ECT should be used after benzodiazepines have failed.

A more recent review of ECT for catatonia included 564 patients from 28 RCTs and observational studies (Leroy et al., 2018). The quality of studies was low and the authors excluded 18 studies because of missing data. The quantitative analysis included pre- and post-ECT details for 211 patients; mainly from open studies. Overall, there was evidence of a marked treatment benefit, but the authors exercised caution because of the low-quality evidence and lack of RCT data. The current NICE guidelines on ECT include catatonia, along with 'severe depressive illness' and 'prolonged or severe manic episode' as indications (National Institute for Clinical Excellence, 2003).

16.2.3 Contraindications

There are few absolute contraindications that relate to ECT itself; most of the cautions relate predominantly to anaesthetic safety. Medical conditions that would normally exclude a course of ECT include: recent myocardial infarction; significant cardiac dysrhythmia; poorly controlled congestive cardiac failure; or unstable angina (Benbow & White, 2013).

Some other contraindications exist because of the risk of raised intracranial and intravascular pressure; the main one being the presence of a space-occupying lesion of the brain where patients are at an increased risk of deterioration if treated with ECT (Krystal & Coffey, 1997).

The presence of a vagus nerve stimulator or deep brain stimulator is not a contraindication to ECT. The published data would suggest that ECT can be used safely for those with implanted VNS (Burke & Husain, 2006) and there are numerous case reports of ECT being used to treat patients with DBS (for example: Erickson & Carty, 2015; Vila-Rodriguez et al., 2014). For VNS, stimulation is usually stopped just before ECT and restarted shortly afterwards.

There is some limited simulation-based data to suggest that ECT electrode placement should be influenced by the location of burr holes in the case of DBS (Deng et al., 2010). For both VNS and DBS, concomitant ECT should only be given in centres where the treating teams have experience in programming stimulators.

16.2.4 Safety and Adverse Effects

16.2.4.1 Safety Considerations

ECT is generally a safe treatment and it is the anaesthetic component of the treatment that confers many of the associated risks. With regards to mortality, Watts et al. (2011) reported no deaths associated with ECT between 1999 and 2010 and concluded that the mortality rate was less than 1 death per 73 440 treatments. These probably represent the most contemporary estimate of safety. Another US study covering ECT treatments in Texas between 1993 and 1998 reported a mortality rate of less than 2 per 100 000 treatments and no deaths occurred during ECT (Shiwach et al., 2001). In a registry study conducted in Denmark, Munk-Olsen et al. (2007) reported a lower overall mortality rate in those that had received ECT, compared with inpatients that had not; although the suicide rate was slightly higher, possibly reflecting a greater severity of illness in those receiving ECT.

16.2.4.2 Cognitive Adverse Effects

Detailed understanding of the cognitive effects of ECT is limited by several factors: the impact of depression upon cognition, including autobiographical memory; the multiple domains of memory and cognition being tested; a lack of consistency in the tools used to assess memory in studies; and differences between subjective reporting of memory versus objective testing.

With regard to non-autobiographical memory, Semkovska and McLoughlin (2010) systematically reviewed and meta-analyzed 24 cognitive variables reported in 84 studies and including 2981 patients. They did not include any tests of retrograde amnesia. In three-quarters of variables, decreases in cognitive performance were seen in the first three days after ECT. Between 4 and 15 days, only one variable showed impairment, and after 15 days 57% of variables showed improvement compared with baseline testing. These variables included tests of working memory, processing speed and anterograde memory.

A lack of standardized autobiographical memory assessments limits the reliable reporting of the effects of ECT on autobiographical memory. However, there is little doubt that such effects occur. There is some evidence that semantic memory (dates, names of people, places etc.) is unaffected by ECT while episodic memory (recall of details of events) is affected by ECT for up to three months and is unrelated to improvements in mood (Jelovac et al., 2016).

Fraser et al. (2008) identified 15 studies published between 1980 and 2008 that met criteria for inclusion in their systematic review. A range of measures were used. However, there were some consistent findings that can help inform clinicians and patients. Most studies found that reported memory loss occurred in the period of six months prior to ECT; more distant autobiographical memory was generally preserved. Interestingly, objective testing found that any memory deficits generally do not persist beyond six months after ECT, but subjective reports differed and many patients reported autobiographical memory deficits lasting longer than six months. Unilateral ECT appeared less likely to cause autobiographical memory problems than bilateral ECT and the likelihood of memory problems was related to the extent to which the dose was above the patient's seizure threshold. Additionally, brief-pulse ECT was less likely to cause autobiographical memory problems than sine-wave ECT.

Although there is reassuring evidence of only a temporary effect on objective measures of cognition (Semkovska & McLoughlin, 2010), many people receiving ECT report varying degrees of memory impairment. Some of the differences between subjective and objective reporting of memory impairment have been suggested to reflect the effects of underlying depressed mood on subjective memory; which is consistent with the reported correlations between subjective memory impairment and severity of depression which both improve over time (Ng et al., 2000).

A registry-based study from Sweden (including 1212 patients) reported that subjective memory worsening was present in 26% of those receiving ECT. It was reported more commonly by women and more often in those who were between 18 and 39 years than in the over 65s. Subjective memory worsening was less common in those who achieved remission following ECT and brief-pulse ECT was more likely to cause memory problems than ultra-brief pulse (Brus et al., 2017).

16.2.4.3 Non-Cognitive Adverse Effects

Other relatively common adverse effects (and the percentage of courses in which the adverse effect occurs) include: headache (32%); muscle aches (16%); and nausea (8%) (SEAN, 2017). The Scottish audit data report that cardiovascular side effects occurred in 2% of episodes, and prolonged seizures occurred in fewer than 1% of episodes. Most complaints of pain are easily managed with simple analgesia given just after treatment.

16.2.5 Factors Affecting Outcome

16.2.5.1 Patient-Related Factors

Several characteristics in depressed patients have been associated with response to ECT. These are summarized in Table 16.2.

There is a degree of inconsistency in the extent to which different studies have found the same predictors. However, some of the more consistent predictors of ECT response include: older age; presence of psychotic symptoms; presence of melancholic features; and a high level of suicidal behaviour. These features were also identified by a recent review of clinical predictors (Pinna et al., 2018).

A higher level of previous non-response to treatment and the presence of personality disorder both appear to be predictors of a less favourable response; although it should be noted that most people undergoing ECT have already demonstrated non-response to approximately six robust antidepressant and augmentation trials (Hazari et al., 2013) and many still respond.

16.2.5.2 Stimulation-Related Factors

Electrode placement has important effects on tolerability and effectiveness of ECT. In an RCT involving 80 depressed patients, Sackeim et al. (2000) compared high-dose right unilateral (RUL) ECT and bilateral (BL) ECT and examined response rates and adverse effects two months later. Both BL and RUL ECT were comparable with regards to response rates (65%) and there were no group differences between relapse rates (53%). However, they reported that retrograde amnesia was higher with BL ECT, leading them to conclude that RUL ECT is equally effective but less likely to produce cognitive adverse effects.

This was not confirmed by Kellner et al. (2010) who randomized 230 people with unipolar or bipolar depression to one of three electrode placements: bifrontal (1.5× seizure threshold); bilateral (1.5× seizure threshold); and right unilateral (6× seizure threshold). Remission rates were: bifrontal (61%); bilateral (64%); and right unilateral (55%). Cognitive side effects did not differ significantly between groups. There was a finding that bilateral ECT had a slightly quicker effect.

These findings are reflected in recent guidelines with CANMAT suggesting that high-dose RUL ECT or BL ECT are comparable first-line options for ECT but if there is no response to RUL ECT after four to six treatments, then switching to BL ECT should be considered (Milev et al., 2016). Indeed, where a quicker clinical response is required, many clinicians would recommend BL ECT as the preferred treatment.

The waveform and frequency of the electrical stimulus have changed significantly during the development of ECT. A sine-wave electrical stimulus has now been replaced by 'brief-pulse' with 'ultra-brief-pulse' ECT being a more recent development. Brief-pulse ECT requires less energy to produce a generalized seizure than sine-wave stimulation but with no reduction in efficacy; and recovery rates are faster. Modern ECT machines deliver a constant current, square-wave stimulus, with total charge (measured in millicoulombs) being the most commonly used measure of 'dose'. Pulse width (the duration of each pulse) is typically 0.5–2 ms. In most cases, greater doses are delivered by giving a longer stimulus duration.

Table 16.2 Predictors of better outcome following ECT for depression

Variable	de Vreede et al. (2005)	Gupta et al. (2000)	Kindler et al. (1991)	Loo et al. (2011)	Medda et al. (2014)	Nordenskjöld et al. (2012)	Pande et al. (1988)	Prudic et al. (1990)
Number of subjects in analysis	53	22	52	75	208	990	48	53
Older age	+					+		
Greater severity			–	+		+	–	
Longer duration of illness		+	–	+	–			
Psychotic symptoms	–			+	–	+		
Suicidal symptoms		+						
Presence of personality disorder	–					–		
Greater somatic symptoms (e.g. worse appetite)		+					–	
Greater treatment-resistance	–			–				–
Previous ECT course				+				
Preserved insight					+			
Better self-care					+			
Outpatients vs. inpatient						–		

Key: (+) associated with a better response; (–) associated with a worse response.

A systematic review comparing brief-pulse RUL ECT and ultra-brief-pulse RUL ECT was undertaken by Tor et al. (2015). They identified six studies with a total of 689 patients. Although brief-pulse RUL ECT was more effective and required fewer treatment sessions, it caused significantly higher rates of cognitive side effects.

The choice of pulse width is ultimately a decision to be made between the patient and the treating doctor based on clinical priorities. The consensus is that first-line treatment should use brief-pulse ECT. However, where there is previous experience of problematic cognitive side effects or where this is a concern for the patient, ultra-brief-pulse ECT could be considered.

16.2.6 Relapse Prevention

The high likelihood of relapse after treatment with ECT is well recognized. Even with continuation pharmacotherapy, approximately 50% of people will experience a relapse within 12 months of a successful course of ECT, and 37% of people will relapse within 6 months of treatment (Jelovac et al., 2013).

The best evidence for prophylaxis after a successful course of ECT is for nortriptyline ± lithium and for maintenance ECT (discussed below). Sackeim et al. (2001) randomized 84 patients who had remitted with ECT to either: nortriptyline (n = 27); nortriptyline and lithium (n = 28); or placebo (n = 29). Patients were followed up for 24 weeks. The relapse rates for each treatment were: nortriptyline (60%); nortriptyline and lithium (39%); and placebo (84%). Kellner et al. (2006) also found nortriptyline and lithium to be more efficacious than placebo, and equivalent to maintenance ECT; although overall rates of relapse remained high.

There may be some additional benefit from the addition of psychological therapy. Brakemeier et al. (2014) examined response rates following successful RUL ECT with continuation pharmacotherapy plus one of three add-ons: cognitive behavioural therapy (CBT); continuation ECT; or no add-on. Sustained response rates after six months were: CBT (77%); ECT (65%); and medication-only (33%).

16.2.7 Maintenance ECT

In this section, maintenance ECT (M-ECT) is used to describe continuing ECT (at a lower frequency than the index treatment course) that is intended to prevent the relapse or recurrence of the index episode.

There are relatively few prospective studies of M-ECT. Kellner et al. (2006) randomized 201 patients with unipolar depression who had remitted with bilateral ECT to continuation ECT (10 treatments over six months) or continuation pharmacotherapy (six months of nortriptyline augmented with lithium). Relapse rates after six months were 37.1% in the M-ECT group and 31.6% in the pharmacotherapy group. Those receiving M-ECT had a slightly longer (but not statistically significant) time to relapse (9.1 ± 7.0 weeks vs. 6.7 ± 4.6 weeks).

In a small but similar study of older patients (mean age 70 years) treated with ECT for psychotic depression, 17 were randomized to nortriptyline alone and 16 were randomized to ECT in combination with nortriptyline and followed up over two years (Navarro et al., 2008). Those receiving continuation ECT received weekly treatment for one month, then fortnightly for a further month, followed by ECT monthly. At 12-month follow-up, the rate of relapse/recurrence was eight times higher in those who did not receive ECT. Tolerability was similar between groups.

In a systematic review of M-ECT, van Schaik et al. (2012) included RCTs (n = 3); prospective cohort studies (n = 5); retrospective cohort studies with matched comparison group (n = 3); and retrospective cohort studies (n = 11). Participants were over the age of 55 and nine studies reported on M-ECT in elderly patients only. The authors concluded that M-ECT was at least as effective as continuation psychopharmacology and commented that M-ECT is generally well tolerated.

M-ECT continues to be used in clinical practice and data from Scotland indicate that M-ECT represented around 3% of ECT episodes in 2009 and approximately 8% of episodes in 2015 (SEAN, 2016). In England and Wales, around 10% of patients receiving ECT were receiving a maintenance course of treatment (Buley et al., 2017).

A key clinical challenge is that despite the reported benefits of M-ECT for some people, the rates of relapse or recurrence following ECT remain high and treatment pathways for those whose symptoms return after M-ECT and antidepressant prophylaxis are uncertain.

16.3 Repetitive Transcranial Magnetic Stimulation (rTMS)

16.3.1 History and Mechanism of Action

The observation that rapidly switching and alternating magnetic fields can induce a current in a conductor within those magnetic fields was made by Michael Faraday in 1831. The same principle of using electromagnetic stimulation to affect brain functioning was demonstrated in 1985 when an external pulsed magnetic field was used to cause movements of limbs by stimulating the motor cortex (Barker et al., 1985). A system for repetitive transcranial magnetic stimulation (rTMS) was approved by the FDA in 2008 and an approval for its use in OCD was granted in 2018. The mechanism of rTMS is unknown, with competing theories including: changes in neuroplasticity; neuroprotective mechanisms, including neurogenesis; and neurotrophic effects on underlying cerebral tissue (Chervyakov et al., 2015).

Imaging studies have provided support for the suggestion that rTMS has effects on connectivity. It is thought that neurostimulation of external cortical targets such as the dorsolateral prefrontal cortex (DLPFC) can have 'downstream' modulating effects on deeper neuronal targets. In a functional neuroimaging study looking at resting state in 98 patients who were receiving DLPFC rTMS, Fox et al. (2012) reported correlations between changes in resting-state connectivity and clinical response to rTMS. Similar findings have recently been reported by Philip et al. (2018). The dysregulation within neural circuits between the DLPFC, other cortical areas and the limbic system has been well described, and the commonly used target of DLPFC for the treatment of depression is consistent with this model (Baeken & De Raedt, 2011).

16.3.2 Principles of Treatment

Current implementations of TMS involve the placing of an external wand, connected to a field generator, over specific areas of the cortex for periods of 20–30 minutes daily with the intention of causing neuroelectric changes in the underlying cortex. rTMS typically involves the delivery of regularly repeated pulses of TMS. High-frequency (HF) rTMS stimulation refers to frequencies of ≥ 1 Hz (i.e. 1 pulse per second), but 10 Hz is a common setting for rTMS in clinical studies. Low-frequency (LF) rTMS refers to stimulation frequencies of 1 Hz or less.

More recent developments include the use of lower-frequency stimulation (T-PEMF; transcranial pulsed electromagnetic fields) and intermittent theta-burst stimulation (iTBS). The latter differs from conventional rTMS in that pulses are delivered in bursts of three, at a frequency of 50 Hz. Magnetic seizure therapy (MST) involves generating a generalized seizure using a modified rTMS stimulus instead of a directly applied electrical stimulus. It is argued that seizures generated by MST have fewer effects on brain areas such as the hippocampus and can therefore cause fewer neurocognitive side effects (Lisanby et al., 2003). Most clinical trials of rTMS have used once-daily stimulation but twice-daily protocols are emerging. These promise equivalent efficacy with a shorter total duration of treatment, but studies continue to be small and have short periods of follow-up.

The optimum dosing regimen remains unclear, unfortunately. Some recent studies have tested greater stimulation frequency (twice daily) as well as different types of stimulation (T-PEMF) but effectiveness appeared to be related to total duration of treatment rather than frequency of treatment (Straasø et al., 2014).

16.3.3 Indications and Evidence Appraisals

16.3.3.1 Depression

There are at least 20 systematic reviews and meta-analyses of rTMS for depression, covering the period 2001–17. Sixty-five per cent of them have been published after 2010. The summary presented here will focus on two recent and large meta-analyses which provide the largest overview of RCTs of rTMS.

Health Quality Ontario conducted a health technology assessment of TMS for treatment-refractory depression in 2016 (Health Quality Ontario, 2016). They included 23 studies where rTMS had been compared with either ECT or sham treatment. Patients were aged 18 or over, and 80% of patients had failed to respond to at least two previous antidepressant treatment trials.

The total number of patients was 1156. Patients had severe depression (baseline Hamilton Depression Rating Scale score >25) in 11/23 studies (44%), with baseline scores being in the moderate range (19–24) in the remainder of studies.

The degree of treatment resistance varied between studies. In 16/23 (69.6%) studies, patients had failed to respond to two or more antidepressants while 7/23 (30.4%) studies included patients who had failed to respond to only one antidepressant trial. Patients received antidepressants alongside rTMS in 69.6% of studies.

The duration of follow-up was relatively short for most studies. Most studies reported follow-up of two to four weeks and the longest periods of follow-up were three to four months (three studies) and six months (one study).

The weighted mean difference between rTMS and sham TMS was 2.3 points on the Hamilton Depression Rating Scale in favour of rTMS. The equivalent effect size was 0.33 (95% CI 0.17 to 0.50).

When rTMS was compared with ECT, six studies including a total of 266 patients were included. The weighted mean difference between rTMS and ECT was 6.0 points on the Hamilton Depression Rating Scale in favour of ECT. This was equivalent to an effect size of 0.67 (95% CI 0.10 to 1.23). There was a high degree of heterogeneity between studies. The finding of greater efficacy for ECT is consistent with earlier meta-analyses (Berlim et al., 2013; Ren et al., 2014).

The European Network for Health Technology Assessment conducted an update of the Health Quality Ontario review (EUnetHTA, 2017). They identified an additional two studies which were included alongside the 23 studies identified by Health Quality Ontario, although the total number of included patients was similar at 1180. Overall findings were similar to those reported above.

The NICE published guidance on the use of rTMS for depression in 2015 and concluded that: 'The evidence on repetitive transcranial magnetic stimulation for depression shows no major safety concerns. The evidence on its efficacy in the short-term is adequate, although the clinical response is variable. Repetitive transcranial magnetic stimulation for depression may be used with normal arrangements for clinical governance and audit' (NICE, 2015). They acknowledged the uncertainty regarding patient selection, stimulation regimens, and the lack of reliable data about longer-term outcomes from rTMS. A recent position statement from the Royal College of Psychiatrists supported the use of rTMS in the context of robust treatment protocols, sufficient staffing, and prospective outcome monitoring and reporting (RCPsych Committee on ECT and Related Treatments, 2017).

16.3.3.2 Obsessive-Compulsive Disorder

There are at least four systematic reviews and meta-analyses of rTMS for OCD but only the two most recent ones will be considered.

Trevizol et al. (2016) included 15 RCTs (483 patients) comparing active rTMS and sham rTMS. The overall effect (Hedges' *g*) was 0.45 (95% CI 0.2 to 0.7) in favour of active rTMS. Some cautions are advised, however. The median number of patients receiving rTMS in these studies was 15 (range 9–40) and the median follow-up period was 3 weeks (range 1–6 weeks). Most studies are, therefore, short and small. Seven different brain areas were stimulated across the 15 studies: DLPFC (bilateral (n = 3), right (n = 5) and left (n = 3)); orbitofrontal cortex (right (n = 1), left (n = 1)); supplementary motor area (SMA; n = 2) and DLPFC + SMA (n = 1). Baseline severity was not reported in the meta-analysis.

Zhou et al. (2017) identified 20 RCTs (791 patients) comparing real rTMS with sham rTMS for the treatment of OCD. Patients were reported as 'treatment-resistant' in 90% of studies. As with Trevizol et al. (2016), the size of most studies is small (median = 23, range = 10–95) and the duration of follow-up is short (median = 4 weeks, range = 1–12 weeks). Only 20% reported intention-to-treat outcomes. The overall effect size (Hedges' *g*) for rTMS was 0.71 (95% CI 0.55 to 0.87). Greater response was seen in those patients who were not treatment refractory and did not have co-morbid depression. In 2018 the FDA granted marketing approval for a specific deep TMS system for the treatment of OCD.

16.3.3.3 Other Indications

rTMS is currently being explored for a number of other indications. McClelland et al. (2016) conducted an RCT of a single session of rTMS for anorexia nervosa (AN). The study (including 49 patients) was largely negative, with no reported effects on 'core AN symptoms' – a measure that combined a number of anorexia-related experiences. A small RCT of rTMS for bulimia involving 14 female patients found no difference between real and sham rTMS. The role of rTMS in treating eating disorders is, therefore, largely unknown.

A number of small studies (for example: Aleman et al., 2007; Dlabac-de Lange et al., 2015; Goyal et al., 2007) have reported improvements in auditory hallucinations and/or negative symptoms of schizophrenia. However, more recent meta-analysis has suggested that non-specific (i.e. placebo) effects may account for the improvements reported in clinical trials of rTMS for hallucinations (Dollfus et al., 2016).

There has been increasing interest in the role of neuromodulation in the treatment of neurodegenerative disorders such as Alzheimer's disease. Indeed, rTMS has been frequently used as a research tool to explore the cortical excitability of patients with Alzheimer's disease. Currently, there are no large studies reporting sustained clinical and functional benefits from the use of rTMS in Alzheimer's disease (Nardone et al., 2014).

16.3.4 Contraindications

Due to the potential for induced currents in the loop antenna of cochlear implants (which themselves contain a permanent magnet), rTMS is not suitable for patients with cochlear implants; although definitive data on harm and safety are lacking. This is currently the only absolute contraindication to rTMS. Other metallic devices that come into close contact with the rTMS coil (such as syringe drivers or internal pulse generators) will introduce the same risk and rTMS should not be used.

16.3.5 Safety and Adverse Effects

rTMS is generally a safe and well-tolerated treatment. Although it induces electrical currents, this has no meaningful effect on intracranial conductors such as aneurysm clips. Jewellery and other conductors are removed before rTMS treatment, thereby reducing the potential for interference with the electromagnetic field.

Those receiving longer courses of treatment are potentially exposed to cumulative doses of electromagnetic fields, but this is not considered to be a safety risk (Braga & Petrides, 2007).

There are numerous studies of TMS being used in paediatric cases, predominantly for investigation and monitoring rather than treatment. Consequently, most studies have used single-pulse TMS (sTMS) or paired-pulse TMS (ppTMS). Reviews of the use of TMS in children have not identified any serious adverse effects (Frye et al., 2008) but since TMS can influence neuronal plasticity and in the context of greater plasticity in developing brains, more research is needed before use of rTMS in children is likely to be widespread.

There have been many case reports of women undergoing treatment with rTMS while pregnant with no adverse effects and a recent trial of rTMS in 30 depressed pregnant women found good tolerability with no emergent adverse effects (Hızlı Sayar et al., 2014). Since electromagnetic fields diminish exponentially with distance, it is unlikely that rTMS represents a measurable risk to the unborn fetus.

The rest of this section focuses on adverse effects associated with rTMS and iTBS rather than other forms of TMS since these are the most common forms of stimulation used in the treatment of psychiatric disorders. These adverse effects are summarized in Table 16.3.

Table 16.3 Adverse effects from high-frequency rTMS and theta burst stimulation

	HF-rTMS	iTBS
Rare	• Hearing changes • Induction of seizures (less than 1% risk in people without epilepsy) • Burns from scalp electrodes	• Induction of seizures (2%) • Burns from scalp electrodes (possible, but not reported)
Possible	• Development of hypomania (especially with left DLPFC stimulation)	• Dizziness (22%)
Common	• Headache • Local (scalp) pain/ discomfort • Neck pain • Paraesthesia	• Headache • Local (scalp) pain/discomfort • Neck pain • Paraesthesia

Adapted from Rossi et al. (2009).

In general, approximately 40–50% of patients will report a combination of headache, pain or discomfort during stimulation with rTMS or iTBS. In clinical studies, the dropout rate from pain or discomfort is less than 2% (Rossi et al., 2009) and the discomfort rapidly resolves on termination of stimulation. Rates of seizure induction appear broadly similar at 1–2%. Although induction of mania has been reported, the rates between real rTMS and sham rTMS are similar (0.73–0.84%) and not statistically significant (Xia et al., 2008).

16.4 Vagus Nerve Stimulation (VNS)

16.4.1 History and Mechanism of Action

The potential for VNS to have central effects on cortical activity was described in the cat in 1938 (Bailey & Bremer, 1938). The first open case series of VNS for medication-refractory epilepsy was published in 1990 (Penry & Dean, 1990) and controlled trials were published shortly after (Ben-Menachem et al., 1994). Open studies of the effects of VNS in the treatment of depression were conducted shortly after (Rush et al., 2000).

The mechanism of action (in terms of antidepressant effect) is unknown, although plausible hypotheses about central effects of peripheral stimulation have emerged based on our knowledge of the vagus nerve and neuroimaging studies. Eighty per cent of fibres in the vagus nerve are afferent and carry information back to the brain. The vagus nerve terminates in the nucleus tractus solitarius in the brainstem and from there, fibres connect to the locus coeruleus. From the locus coeruleus, most of the outputs are noradrenergic and there are afferents to many brain areas that are involved in mood regulation: hypothalamus; hippocampus; amygdala; orbitofrontal cortex; and cingulate gyrus. There are also afferents to the thalamus.

16.4.2 Principles of Treatment

VNS involves the surgical implantation of a helical electrode that is wrapped around the left cervical vagus nerve in the neck. It is often proposed that cardiac effects are reduced with left-sided placement, but this remains undetermined, and the electrode is positioned below the cardiac branch of the vagus nerve. The electrode is connected to an implanted pulse generator (IPG) by a wire that is tunnelled under the skin. The IPG sits in the left anterior chest wall in a similar position to a cardiac pacemaker. The whole procedure takes approximately 2 hours and is usually performed under a general anaesthetic, although subsequent replacement of the IPG can be done under local anaesthetic.

Two weeks after implantation, the IPG is programmed using a handheld computer that is connected to a programming wand. In the clinic, the patient holds the wand over the IPG which allows the clinician to programme the device and tailor stimulation according to clinical response and adverse effects.

In most clinical studies and in clinical practice, stimulation occurs for 30 seconds every 5 minutes (30/300 seconds) and repeats continuously over a 24-hour period (a 'duty cycle' of 10%). The frequency of the pulse is typically 20 Hz and the pulse width ranges from 130 microseconds to 500 microseconds. Often, shorter pulse widths can be selected to improve tolerability of adverse effects such as discomfort, pain and voice alteration. The stimulating current is commenced low (e.g. 0.25 mA) and is gradually increased, according to tolerability, over multiple clinic visits in the following weeks. Typical current settings range from 0.75 mA to 2.0 mA; although the relationship between stimulating current and response is not fully determined.

16.4.3 The Status of VNS in Current Guidelines

NICE conducted a review of VNS in 2009, concluding that the evidence was of generally low quality and the use of VNS for depression required good patient selection, the involvement of a psychiatrically led multidisciplinary team, and a robust process of clinical audit and follow-up (NICE, 2009).

The current British Association of Psychopharmacology (BAP) antidepressant guidelines state that VNS: ' ... *has limited evidence of efficacy, and no positive double-blind RCTs, but could be considered in patients with chronic and/or recurrent depression who have failed to respond to four or more antidepressant treatments*' and they also express the recommendation that: VNS ' ... *should only be undertaken in specialist centres with prospective outcome evaluation and where provision for long-term follow-up is available*' (Cleare et al., 2015).

The Royal College of Psychiatrists Committee on ECT and Related Treatments, based on the lack of high-quality RCT evidence, considers VNS to be an investigational treatment (RCPsych Committee on ECT and Related Treatments, 2017).

16.4.4 VNS in Depression

The main outcome studies of VNS for depression were numbered D01–D04, and these were followed by a dosing study (D21) and long-term registry-based follow-up study (D23). The key characteristics of these studies are shown in Table 16.4.

It should be noted that there is a degree of duplicate publication in that not all the patients reported are unique. The total number of unique patients with VNS is, therefore, smaller than the total number of patients reported in the various studies; something overlooked by NICE in their 2009 guidance (NICE, 2009).

Overall, the findings from medium- to longer-term open studies are consistent. At 12-month follow-up, the response rate for those receiving VNS is 40–50%, and those who

Study name	Location	Study type	Key references	n	Longest follow-up	Unipolar: bipolar	Chronic	Previous ECT	No. of failed treatment trials (mean ± SD)	Response / remission	Comments
D01	USA	Open study	Marangell et al., 2002; Nahas et al., 2005	59	24 m	73%:27%	–	–	4.8 ± 2.7	42%/22%	–
D02	USA	RCT	Rush et al., 2005a	235	10 wks	90%:10%	68%	53%	3.5 ± 1.3	Response: 15% (active) vs. 10% (sham)	10-week RCT followed by 12-month follow-up (open label)
D02	USA	Open study	Rush et al., 2005b	202	12 m	90%:10%	68%	53%	3.5 ± 1.3	27%/16%	–
D03	Europe	Open study	Bajbouj et al., 2010	49	24 m	73%:27%	53%	50%	3.5 ± 1.3	53%/39%	European replication of D01
D04	USA	VNS vs. TAU	George et al., 2005	205 (VNS) vs. 124 (TAU)	12 m	90%:10%	68%	53%	3.5 ± 1.3	27%/16% (VNS) 13%/4% (TAU)	Included patients from D02
D21	USA	RCT	Aaronson et al., 2012	301	50 wks	79%:21%	–	57%	–	Response: 36% (LOW dose); 48% (MEDIUM dose); 37% (HIGH dose)	Participants were randomized to different 'doses' of VNS
D23	USA	VNS vs. TAU	Aaronson et al., 2017	494 (VNS) vs. 301 (TAU)	5 yrs	73%:27%	–	57%	8.2 ± 3.3	68%/43% (VNS) 41%/26% (TAU)	Included patients from D21

TAU, treatment as usual.

achieve response are likely to maintain response for 2–5 years as long as stimulation persists. Response tends to be cumulative, with response rates at 3 months being around 20% and rising to around 40% at 12 months.

So far, there has only been one RCT of VNS versus sham stimulation (D02) and the blinded phase only lasted 10 weeks (Rush et al., 2005a). The response rate was 15.2% in the active stimulation group versus 10% in the sham stimulation group; a non-statistically significant result. Overall, the study was negative on its primary outcome measure (response on the 24-item Hamilton Depression Rating Scale) but positive on the secondary outcome measure (response on the 30-item Inventory of Depressive Symptomatology Self-Report). Since one might predict a high non-specific response rate from a treatment that is difficult to blind and involves invasive surgery, the absence of longer RCTs with adequate blinding means that there is insufficient evidence currently that would exclude such effects.

The paucity of RCTs of VNS for depression means that meta-analyses are limited. However, Martin and Martín-Sánchez (2012) conducted a meta-analysis of published trials. Although they were cautious in their conclusions, highlighting heterogeneity of the data and study designs, they found a combined effect size of 1.3 (95% CI 1.2 to 1.4) in favour of VNS, with some evidence of greater effects in studies with patients with greater severities of depression.

There are limited data relating to VNS for very chronic and more treatment-refractory populations, although small case series and secondary analyses of larger studies suggest that response rates may be broadly comparable; albeit slightly lower than those in more heterogeneous populations (Christmas et al., 2013).

There is currently little evidence for clear dose–response relationships with VNS in depression (Aaronson et al., 2012). A similar finding has been reported for VNS in epilepsy (DeGiorgio et al., 2005). There is some evidence that different pulse widths can have varying brain effects (Mu et al., 2004), but the clinical relevance is unknown. In practice, clinicians will increase the stimulating current progressively to the best balance between maximized current and tolerability, with a shortening of the pulse width being used to improve tolerability.

16.4.5 Contraindications

There are a small number of situations when VNS is contraindicated. These include: presence of a cardiac pacemaker; previous history of neck surgery that would make implantation difficult; significant cardiac dysrhythmia; and previous left or bilateral cervical vagotomy.

Once the VNS system is implanted, shortwave diathermy is contraindicated because of the risk of induction of current in the VNS electrodes and consequent damage to the vagus nerve. Additionally, the same possibility exists with MRI and although it is possible to perform MRI with a VNS system in situ, it can only be done safely with a separate head coil and where there is expertise in the imaging department. The risk generally reduces after the device is explanted, but since the helical electrode remains in perpetuity, high-intensity MRI scanning (>1.5 Tesla) is cautioned against.

The presence of a VNS device is not a contraindication to ECT (Burke & Husain, 2006), although it usually requires the attendance of a technician to stop and restart VNS before and after each ECT treatment.

16.4.6 Safety and Adverse Effects

Adverse effects are consistent across studies and can typically be separated into stimulation-related effects and non-stimulation-related effects. The most common stimulation-related adverse effect is voice alteration, occurring in around 60% of patients. This is experienced as hoarseness and is present only during periods of active stimulation and generally does not disappear over time. Dysphagia (present in around 13% of patients at 3 months) generally reduces over time. Similarly, around 25% of patients will experience coughing during stimulation at 3 months but this reduces to approximately 6% at 12 months.

Non-stimulation adverse effects relate to surgical and hardware complications. VNS implantation is a relatively safe procedure, but certain risks are involved. Approximately 30% of patients will have post-operative pain around the wounds but this usually responds to analgesia. The risk of post-operative infection is generally small (3–5%) and can be managed with antibiotics. A temporary vocal cord paralysis can occur in approximately 1 in 100 patients. Although this is a post-operative complication, it can sometimes require removal of the device. The most common hardware-related complication is a malfunctioning or fractured lead.

16.5 Deep Brain Stimulation (DBS)

16.5.1 History and Mechanism of Action

DBS in its current form first became established as a treatment when Alim-Louis Benabid and colleagues implanted electrodes in the subthalamic nucleus in order to treat Parkinson's disease (Limousin et al., 1995). Small trials in OCD soon followed (Nuttin et al., 1999), with initial targets mirroring successful ablative targets such as the anterior limb of the internal capsule. Mood changes in individuals with Parkinson's disease were noted and the first case series of DBS for depression was published by Helen Mayberg and colleagues in 2005 (Mayberg et al., 2005). The FDA approved a DBS system for the treatment of OCD (2018). DBS is also approved by the FDA to treat specific movement disorders and as an add-on treatment in refractory epilepsy.

The mechanism of action of DBS is unknown but it has been proposed that suppression of hyperactivity in the subgenual cingulate cortex may be the key feature of response to DBS in this area (Mayberg, 2009). The changes in brain 'circuitry' induced by DBS in other areas are not understood. The pathways involved in the development of tremor in Parkinson's disease, for example, are much better understood than the circuitry of the more complex symptomatology seen in depressive illness or OCD.

It was initially hypothesized that DBS provided a reversible mechanism of inhibition ('inhibition hypothesis'); a theory supported using targets that mirrored traditional lesion surgery, which inevitably created disruption to neuronal circuitry. However, debates regarding whether DBS is excitatory, inhibitory or modulatory have persisted and it is not clear whether a common mode of action explains all the effects of DBS irrespective of site.

The 'disruption hypothesis' argues that information flow in key pathways is abnormal in illness states, and by blocking or stimulating alternative information routes, a more normal mode of action can be introduced (Chiken & Nambu, 2016). Such models have developed out of movement disorders DBS where we have a clearer understanding of the pathways affecting normal and abnormal movements.

16.5.2 Outcome Studies

16.5.2.1 DBS for Depression

There are outcomes from over 230 patients, reported in at least 25 studies of DBS for depression; although only 73% of patients are unique. Most studies are open case series and 50% of studies have seven or fewer participants. One-third of studies had four or fewer participants. The maximum number of participants in a single published study was 30, although the BROADEN RCT of subgenual cingulate DBS included 90 patients: 60 patients receiving active stimulation versus 30 receiving sham stimulation over six months blinded phase. This study failed a futility analysis in late 2014 and was terminated prematurely. The average duration of follow-up was 13 months but 41% of patients had less than one year of follow-up.

The DBS target across all trials was as follows: subgenual cingulate gyrus (SG25; n = 75); ventral capsule/ventral striatum (VC/VS; n = 44); anterior limb of internal capsule (ALIC; n = 25); nucleus accumbens (NAcc; n = 14); medial forebrain bundle (MFB; n = 11); inferior thalamic peduncle (ITP; n = 1); and lateral habenula (n = 2).

The overall response rate (including all targets) is 37% and this ranges from 30% (NAcc) to 41% (MFB). In general, between 30% and 40% of patients in open studies showed a treatment response and there is little clear difference in outcomes between targets.

There have only been two large prospective RCTs of DBS for depression. The RECLAIM study randomized 30 patients to 16 weeks of either active DBS or sham DBS, with the target site being the ventral capsule/ventral striatum. There was then a 24-month open continuation phase. The primary outcome was percentage response on the Montgomery–Asberg Depression Rating Scale (MADRS).

Patients were chronically depressed (mean duration of current episode = 11.4 years) and 97% had previously had ECT. Only one-third of patients were ECT responders. One-third had previously had VNS as well.

At 16 weeks, there was no difference in response rate between active (20%) and sham (14%) groups. Improvement on the MADRS score was not statistically significantly different either: a reduction of 25% in the sham group versus 20% in the active group.

It is possible that the trial was not long enough to demonstrate significant differences between groups but it is equally possible that both groups benefitted from non-specific effects of treatment and that there was no additional benefit from active stimulation. The BROADEN study also found no significant difference between active and sham stimulation during the six-month blinded phase and a further six months after both groups had received active stimulation, there was no further advantage from DBS (Holtzheimer et al., 2017).

There is ongoing discussion about why DBS for depression failed to demonstrate benefit after so much promise was shown in open-label and uncontrolled trials. While people speculate about more precise targeting of specific fibre tracts and better patient selection, it is possible that non-specific (i.e. placebo) effects are not only more significant in these patient populations than previously thought, but also that such effects are long-lasting.

16.5.2.2 DBS for Obsessive-Compulsive Disorder

There have been at least 60 study reports, including outcomes from almost 370 patients. However, only 55% of these studies are reporting unique patients. As with DBS for depression, small case series predominate. The median number of patients in all studies was 3 (range 1–26) and only 1 in 6 studies had more than 10 patients. Only 60% of patients had outcomes reported beyond 12 months.

Seven targets (where four or more patients were included) were reported: VC/VS (n = 60); NAcc (n = 48); bed nucleus of stria terminalis (BNST; n = 25); subthalamic nucleus (STN; n = 17); ALIC (n = 12); ITP (n = 4); and thalamus (n = 4).

Combined response rates are as follows: VC/VS (53%); NAcc (17%); BNST (52%); STN (12%); and ALIC (50%). It should be noted that it was not possible to determine response rate for 88% of patients undergoing STN DBS. It is, therefore, difficult to draw clear conclusions but for most targets the response rate is approximately 50%.

There are at least five trials of DBS for OCD that involve a double-blinded cross-over design. Abelson et al. (2005) followed up four patients who underwent four randomized 'on-off' blocks of three weeks involving stimulation of the ALIC. Patients underwent open stimulation subsequently. Yale-Brown Obsessive Compulsive Scale (Y-BOCS) scores during the OFF phase ranged from 23 to 39, with a mean of 29.3. During the ON phase, Y-BOCS scores had a mean of 26.5 (range 10–37.5). Only one patient showed a reduction of more than 35% during blinded testing with no change being observed in the other three patients.

Mallet et al. (2008) randomly assigned eight patients to either active or sham stimulation of the STN in a cross-over design. Each blinded phase lasted three months. At the end of both blinded phases, the mean Y-BOCS score during active stimulation was 19 compared with 28 during sham stimulation. Scores on the Global Assessment of Functioning (GAF) scale also increased from a mean of 43 to 56 during active stimulation. Differences on both scales were statistically significant. The study group reported 15 serious adverse events (for more on this see below).

Goodman et al. (2010) used a randomized, blinded, staggered-onset design over 3 months (with a 12-month follow-up) to compare active stimulation of the ALIC with sham stimulation. The study was small (n = 6) but at the end of 12 months, 4/6 (67%) patients had responded and there was no evidence of response during the early months when patients were receiving sham stimulation.

Denys and colleagues (2010) employed a two-week double-blind cross-over phase following an eight-month open treatment phase of NAcc DBS in 16 patients with refractory OCD; 14 of whom completed the sham-controlled phase. The difference between active and sham stimulation was 8.3 points on the Y-BOCS scale, a difference of 25%. Following the sham-controlled phase, patients regained their previous trajectory (and response), supporting the argument that the differences were due to stimulation.

In a small blinded, cross-over trial involving six patients Tyagi et al. (2017) randomized patients to DBS of the VC/VS, the STN and a combination of both. Each stimulation period lasted 12 weeks. Improvement in baseline Y-BOCS score was greatest with stimulation of the VC/VS (53%) compared with stimulation of the STN (42%), with only modest benefits from combined stimulation (62%).

16.5.3 Safety and Adverse Effects

The risks of DBS reflect combinations of the target site in terms of operative complexity, and the brain regions being targeted. Saleh and Fontaine (2015) reviewed the published data on adverse effect reporting in studies of DBS for OCD, Tourette syndrome and depression. Overall, they included studies with 272 patients in them. The total proportion of people experiencing an adverse effect, irrespective of severity (by disorder) were: OCD (95%); Tourette syndrome (61%); and depression (45%). Adverse effects can be divided into two broad categories: those that relate to the neurosurgical procedure and the introduction of hardware; and those that relate to the effects of DBS on key brain areas involved in mood, cognition and behaviour.

In the study by Saleh and Fontaine (2015), the most common neurosurgical adverse effects for all disorders were: hardware-related (14%); infection (8%); and intracranial haemorrhage (2%). Overall mortality was 0.4%.

Across all disorders (n = 272), the most common adverse effects were: mood changes (16%); anxiety (9%); suicidality (6%); apathy (5%); sexual dysfunction (5%); psychosis (2%); and completed suicide (0.7%) (Saleh & Fontaine, 2015).

Mood changes were more common in patients with OCD, and were more common in ALIC- (44%) and NAcc-stimulated patients (43%) than STN (33%).

The rates of DBS-induced hypomania and more marked behavioural disturbance (such as novelty-seeking, impulsivity) appear to be much higher with certain stimulation sites. Around 31% of patients with stimulation in the ALIC/VC-VS/NAcc areas experienced mood changes.

16.6 Other Neuromodulation Technologies

16.6.1 Transcranial Direct Current Stimulation (tDCS)

One of the first controlled studies conducted into the effects of applying a constant direct current to the scalp in an attempt to affect underlying neuronal activity and improve depression concluded that: '*Neither positive nor negative polarization is associated with therapeutic change in depressed patients differing from that following placebo treatment. Polarization appears to be therapeutically inert*' (Arfai et al., 1970). A constant current of 250 μA was used for 8 hours per day for six days per week, with a total duration of two weeks or 12 applications. Electrodes were placed on the forehead. All patients were female.

In the ensuring 40–50 years, people have continued to explore the possibility of changing brain activity with the application of an electrical current to the scalp and there are now over 12 controlled trials of tDCS for depression. It has also been used to treat schizophrenia, substance misuse and Alzheimer's disease. tDCS devices are available to buy online, promising improvements in cognitive function and reaction time, and various unsubstantiated claims are made about improving video game performance.

Those purchasing such devices may be disappointed to hear that a systematic review involving 59 studies reporting cognitive changes following tDCS found no evidence of a significant effect on any cognitive domain, leading the authors to conclude that '*Our quantitative review does not support the idea that tDCS generates a reliable effect on cognition in healthy adults*' (Horvath et al., 2015).

While it is possible that weak direct current stimulation may have effects on brain function, we have yet to demonstrate that this has a clinically meaningful effect. A recent study in 15 healthy controls found little difference between tDCS and transcranial random noise stimulation (tRNS) where the oscillating current results in no net current flow (Ho et al., 2015).

The evidence of a meaningful treatment effect remains weak. There are two relatively recent systematic reviews of tDCS for major depression. Brunoni et al. (2016) included patient-level data from six sham-controlled RCTs involving 289 patients. Active tDCS was found to be superior to sham stimulation for both response (odds ratio (OR) 2.44, 95% CI 1.38 to 4.32) and remission (OR 2.38, 95% CI 1.22 to 4.64). The numbers needed to treat (NNT) were 7 for response and 9 for remission. The authors found that treatment resistance (failure to respond to ≥2 antidepressant treatment trials) predicted non-response. The majority of patients in the studies were non-chronic with durations of index depressive episode ranging from means of 6 weeks to 61 weeks.

Palm et al. (2016) reviewed 10 RCTs, 11 open studies and 9 case reports of tDCS for depression. They reported on previous meta-analyses but did not conduct a meta-analysis of their own; highlighting the small sample sizes and unreliable findings from existing clinical trials. They concluded that although tDCS is well tolerated with few side-effects, there remain unanswered questions about the effectiveness of tDCS as a treatment for depression; and they noted that effects seem to diminish with increasing treatment resistance.

At the current time, tDCS is not supported by sufficient data for it to represent a treatment option for depression and there is a possibility that claims for its effect on neurological functioning are exaggerated.

16.6.2 Transcutaneous Vagus Nerve Stimulation (tVNS)

Transcutaneous vagus nerve stimulation (for depression) involves the use of externally applied current to the only place on the body that is innervated by the vagus nerve; namely, a small part of the ear surrounding the external auditory meatus. Stimulation involves 1 mA of current applied for 30 minutes, twice a day, 5 days per week, for up to 12 weeks.

The evidence for tVNS as a treatment for depression is limited and blinding patients receiving tVNS is difficult because of the experience of sensation during stimulation.

In two RCTs of tVNS versus sham stimulation (total participants 37), Hein et al. (2013) reported mean improvements on the Hamilton Depression Rating Scale of 12.6 ± 6.0 in the tVNS group compared with 4.4 ± 9.0 in the sham group over two weeks. Of the 37 patients, only two participants had durations of depressive episode longer than 12 months, and most participants had depressive episodes of only 1–3 months. Again, the observation of effects within such a short period of time (which conflicts with the pattern of response seen in VNS) may reflect non-specific (i.e. placebo) effects.

In a couple of slightly longer non-randomized studies over 12 weeks, Rong et al. (2016) reported outcomes from 91 patients who received 12 weeks of tVNS and also from 69 patients who received 4 weeks of sham stimulation followed by 8 weeks of active stimulation. The treatments were administered by the patients themselves at home and the switch occurred by changing electrodes from a dummy set to an active set. Participants underwent 30 minutes of stimulation (or sham) for 5 days each week. Outcomes were assessed at 4 weeks for the comparison between active and sham and 12 weeks for the whole cohort. It was, therefore, a cross-over study involving twice as long with active stimulation than with sham stimulation. The difference between groups at the end of the 4 weeks active versus sham was 4.6 points on the 24-item Hamilton Depression Rating Scale. However, the success of the blinding is unknown and 15 participants in the sham group withdrew early due to lack of effect. The study outcomes were not intention-to-treat, so the risk of bias is high.

Ultimately, there is insufficient reliable outcome data to support the conclusion that tVNS has a meaningful treatment effect and many better-quality studies are required before it can be considered to represent a realistic treatment option.

References

Aaronson ST, Carpenter LL, Conway CR, et al. (2012). Vagus nerve stimulation therapy randomized to different amounts of electrical charge for treatment-resistant depression: acute and chronic effects. *Brain Stimul*, 6, 631–640.

Aaronson ST, Sears P, Ruvuna F, et al. (2017). A 5-year observational study of patients with treatment-resistant depression treated with vagus nerve stimulation or treatment as usual: comparison of response, remission, and suicidality. *Am J Psychiatry*, 174, 640–648.

Abelson JL, Curtis GC, Sagher O, et al. (2005). Deep brain stimulation for refractory obsessive-compulsive disorder. *Biol Psychiatry*, 57, 510–516.

Adderley DJ, Hamilton M (1953). Use of succinylcholine in ECT. *BMJ*, 1, 195–197.

Aleman A, Sommer IE, Kahn RS (2007). Efficacy of slow repetitive transcranial magnetic stimulation in the treatment of resistant auditory hallucinations in schizophrenia: a meta-analysis. *J Clin Psychiatry*, 68, 416–421.

American Psychiatric Association (2002). *Practice Guideline for the Treatment of Patients with Bipolar Disorder*, 2nd ed. Arlington, VA: American Psychiatric Association.

American Psychiatric Association (2010). *Practice Guideline for the Treatment of Patients with Major Depressive Disorder*, 3rd ed. Washington, DC: American Psychiatric Association. Available at: http://dx.doi.org/10.1176/appi.books.9780890423387.654001 (last accessed 31.8.19).

Arfai E, Theano G, Montagu JD, Robin AA (1970). A controlled study of polarization in depression. *Br J Psychiatry*, 116, 433–434.

Baeken C, De Raedt R (2011). Neurobiological mechanisms of repetitive transcranial magnetic stimulation on the underlying neuro circuitry in unipolar depression. *Dialogues Clin Neurosci*, 13, 139–145.

Bailey P, Bremer F (1938). A sensory cortical representation of the vagus nerve (with a note on the effects of low blood pressure on the cortical electrogram). *J Neurophysiol*, 1, 405–412.

Bajbouj M, Merkl A, Schlaepfer TE, et al. (2010). Two-year outcome of vagus nerve stimulation in treatment-resistant depression. *J Clin Psychopharmacol*, 30, 273–281.

Barker AT, Jalinous R, Freeston IL (1985). Non-invasive magnetic stimulation of human motor cortex. *Lancet*, 325, 1106–1107. http://dx.doi.org/http://dx.doi.org/10.1016/S0140-6736(85)92413-4.

Ben-Menachem E, Manon-Espaillat R, Ristanovic R, et al. (1994). Vagus nerve stimulation for treatment of partial seizures: 1. A controlled study of effect on seizures. *Epilepsia*, 35, 616–626.

Benbow SM, White J (2013). Safe ECT practice in people with a physical illness. In J Waite, A Easton, eds., *The ECT Handbook*, 3rd ed. London: Royal College of Psychiatrists, pp. 184–190.

Berlim MT, Van den Eynde F, Daskalakis ZJ (2013). Efficacy and acceptability of high frequency repetitive transcranial magnetic stimulation (rTMS) versus electroconvulsive therapy (ECT) for major depression: a systematic review and meta-analysis of randomized trials. *Depress Anxiety*, 30, 614–623.

Braga RJ, Petrides G (2007). Somatic therapies for treatment-resistant psychiatric disorders. *Braz J Pschiatry*, 29(Suppl 2), S77–S84.

Brakemeier EL, Merkl A, Wilbertz G, et al. (2014). Cognitive-behavioral therapy as continuation treatment to sustain response after electroconvulsive therapy in depression: a randomized controlled trial. *Biol Psychiatry*, 76, 194–202.

Brunoni AR, Moffa AH, Fregni F, et al. (2016). Transcranial direct current stimulation for acute major depressive episodes: meta-analysis of individual patient data. *Br J Psychiatry*, 208, 522–531.

Brus O, Nordanskog P, Båve U, et al. (2017). Subjective memory immediately following electroconvulsive therapy. *J ECT*, 33, 96–103.

Buley N, Copland E, Hodge S (2017). *ECT Minimum Dataset 2016–17: Activity Data Report – England, Wales, Northern Ireland & Republic of Ireland*. London: Royal College of Psychiatrists.

Burke MJ, Husain MM (2006). Concomitant use of vagus nerve stimulation and electroconvulsive therapy for treatment-resistant depression. *J ECT*, 22, 218–222.

Chervyakov AV, Chernyavsky AY, Sinitsyn DO, Piradov MA (2015). Possible mechanisms underlying the therapeutic effects of transcranial magnetic stimulation. *Front Hum Neurosci*, 9, 303.

Chiken S, Nambu A (2016). Mechanism of deep brain stimulation: inhibition, excitation, or disruption? *Neuroscientist*, 22, 313–322.

Christmas D, Steele JD, Tolomeo S, Eljamel MS, Matthews K (2013). Vagus nerve stimulation for chronic major depressive disorder: 12-month outcomes in highly treatment-refractory patients. *J Affect Disord*, 150, 1221–1225.

Cleare A, Pariante CM, Young AH, et al. (2015). Evidence-based guidelines for treating depressive disorders with antidepressants: a revision of the 2008 British Association for Psychopharmacology guidelines. *J Psychopharmacol*, 29, 459–525.

de Vreede IM, Burger H, van Vliet IM (2005). Prediction of response to ECT with routinely collected data in major depression. *J Affect Disord*, 86, 323–327.

DeGiorgio C, Heck C, Bunch S, et al. (2005). Vagus nerve stimulation for epilepsy: randomized comparison of three stimulation paradigms. *Neurology*, 65, 317–319.

Deng ZD, Hardesty DE, Lisanby SH, Peterchev AV (2010). Electroconvulsive therapy in the presence of deep brain stimulation implants: electric field effects. *Engineering in Medicine and Biology Society (EMBC), 2010 Annual International Conference of the IEEE 2010*, 2049–2052.

Denys D, Mantione M, Figee M, et al. (2010). Deep brain stimulation of the nucleus accumbens for treatment-refractory obsessive-compulsive disorder. *Arch Gen Psychiatry*, 67, 1061–1068.

Dlabac-de Lange JJ, Bais L, van Es FD, et al. (2015). Efficacy of bilateral repetitive transcranial magnetic stimulation for negative symptoms of schizophrenia: results of a multicenter double-blind randomized controlled trial. *Psychol Med*, 45, 1263–1275.

Dollfus S, Lecardeur L, Morello R, Etard O (2016). Placebo response in repetitive transcranial magnetic stimulation trials of treatment of auditory hallucinations in schizophrenia: a meta-analysis. *Schizophr Bull*, 42, 301–308.

Enomoto S, Shimizu K, Nibuya M, et al. (2017). Activated brain-derived neurotrophic factor/TrkB signaling in rat dorsal and ventral hippocampi following 10-day electroconvulsive seizure treatment. *Neurosci Lett*, 660, 45–50.

Erickson JM, Carty J (2015). Safe and effective electroconvulsive therapy using multiple parameters over 5 years in a patient with deep brain stimulator. *J ECT*, 31, 278–279.

EUnetHTA (2017). *Repetitive Transcranial Magnetic Stimulation for Treatment-Resistant Major Depression. Project ID: WP4-ACB-CA-5.* Diemen: European Network for Health Technology Assessment.

FDA (2011). FDA Executive Summary. Prepared for the January 27–28, 2011 meeting of the Neurological Devices Panel: Meeting to Discuss the Classification of Electroconvulsive Therapy Devices (ECT). Silver Spring, MD: US Food and Drug Administration.

Fox MD, Buckner RL, White MP, Greicius MD, Pascual-Leone A (2012). Efficacy of transcranial magnetic stimulation targets for depression is related to intrinsic functional connectivity with the subgenual cingulate. *Biol Psychiatry*, 72, 595–603.

Fraser LM, O'Carroll RE, Ebmeier KP (2008). The effect of electroconvulsive therapy on autobiographical memory: a systematic review. *J ECT*, 24, 10–17.

Frye RE, Rotenberg A, Ousley M, Pascual-Leone A (2008). Transcranial magnetic stimulation in child neurology: current and future directions. *J Child Neurol*, 23, 79–96.

Gbyl K, Videbech P (2018). Electroconvulsive therapy increases brain volume in major depression: a systematic review and meta-analysis. *Acta Psychiatr Scand*, 138, 180–195.

George MS, Rush AJ, Marangell LB, et al. (2005). A one-year comparison of vagus nerve stimulation with treatment as usual for treatment-resistant depression. *Biol Psychiatry*, 58, 364–373.

Goodman WK, Foote KD, Greenberg BD, et al. (2010). Deep brain stimulation for intractable obsessive compulsive disorder: pilot study using a blinded, staggered-onset design. *Biol Psychiatry*, 67, 535–542.

Goodwin GM, Haddad PM, Ferrier IN, et al. (2016). Evidence-based guidelines for treating bipolar disorder: revised third edition recommendations from the British Association for Psychopharmacology. *J Psychopharmacol*, 30, 495–553.

Goyal N, Nizamie SH, Desarkar P (2007). Efficacy of adjuvant high frequency repetitive transcranial magnetic stimulation on negative and positive symptoms of schizophrenia: preliminary results of a double-blind sham-controlled study. *J Neuropsychiatry Clin Neurosci*, 19, 464–467.

Gupta N, Avasthi A, Kulhara P (2000). Clinical variables as predictors of response to electroconvulsive therapy in endogenous depression. *Indian J Psychiatry*, 42, 60–65.

Hawkins JM, Archer KJ, Strakowski SM, Keck PE (1995). Somatic treatment of catatonia. *Int J Psychiatry Med*, 25, 345–369.

Hazari H, Christmas D, Matthews K (2013). The clinical utility of different quantitative methods for measuring treatment resistance in major depression. *J Affect Disord*, 150, 231–236.

Health Quality Ontario (2016). Repetitive transcranial magnetic stimulation for treatment-resistant depression: a systematic review and meta-analysis of randomized controlled trials. *Ont Health Technol Assess Ser*, 16, 1–66.

Hein E, Nowak M, Kiess O, et al. (2013). Auricular transcutaneous electrical nerve stimulation in depressed patients: a randomized controlled pilot study. *J Neural Transm (Vienna)*, 120, 821–827.

Hızlı Sayar G, Ozten E, Tufan E, et al. (2014). Transcranial magnetic stimulation during pregnancy. *Arch Womens Ment Health*, 17, 311–315.

Ho K-A, Taylor JL, Loo CK (2015). Comparison of the effects of transcranial random noise stimulation and transcranial direct current stimulation on motor cortical excitability. *J ECT*, 31, 67–72.

Holtzheimer PE, Husain MM, Lisanby SH, et al. (2017). Subcallosal cingulate deep brain stimulation for treatment-resistant depression: a multisite, randomised, sham-controlled trial. *Lancet Psychiatry*, 4, 839–849. http://dx.doi.org/10.1016/S2215-0366(17)30371-1.

Horvath JC, Forte JD, Carter O (2015). Quantitative review finds no evidence of cognitive effects in healthy populations from single-session transcranial direct current stimulation (tDCS). *Brain Stimul*, 8, 535–550.

International Neuromodulation Society (2016). Welcome to the International Neuromodulation Society. Available at: www.neuromodulation.com (last accessed 21.12.16).

Jelovac A, Kolshus E, McLoughlin DM (2013). Relapse following successful electroconvulsive therapy for major depression: a meta-analysis. *Neuropsychopharmacology*, 38, 2467–2474.

Jelovac A, O'Connor S, McCarron S, McLoughlin DM (2016). Autobiographical memory specificity in major depression treated with electroconvulsive therapy. *J ECT*, 32, 38–43.

Kellner CH, Knapp RG, Petrides G, et al. (2006). Continuation electroconvulsive therapy vs pharmacotherapy for relapse prevention in major depression: a multisite study from the Consortium for Research in Electroconvulsive Therapy (CORE). *Arch Gen Psychiatry*, 63, 1337–1344.

Kellner CH, Knapp R, Husain MM, et al. (2010). Bifrontal, bitemporal and right unilateral electrode placement in ECT: randomised trial. *Br J Psychiatry*, 196, 226–234.

Kindler S, Shapira B, Hadjez J, et al. (1991). Factors influencing response to bilateral electroconvulsive therapy in major depression. *Convuls Ther*, 7, 245–254.

Krystal AD, Coffey CE (1997). Neuropsychiatric considerations in the use of electroconvulsive therapy. *J Neuropsychiatry Clin Neurosci*, 9, 283–292.

Leroy A, Naudet F, Vaiva G, et al. (2018). Is electroconvulsive therapy an evidence-based treatment for catatonia? A systematic review and meta-analysis. *Eur Arch Psychiatry Clin Neurosci*, 268, 675–687.

Limousin P, Pollak P, Benazzouz A, et al. (1995). Effect of parkinsonian signs and symptoms of bilateral subthalamic nucleus stimulation. *Lancet*, 345, 91–95.

Lisanby SH, Luber B, Schlaepfer TE, Sackeim HA (2003). Safety and feasibility of magnetic seizure therapy (MST) in major depression: randomized within-subject comparison with electroconvulsive therapy. *Neuropsychopharmacology*, 28, 1852–1865.

Loo CK, Mahon M, Katalinic N, Lyndon B, Hadzi-Pavlovic D (2011). Predictors of response to ultrabrief right unilateral electroconvulsive therapy. *J Affect Disord*, 130, 192–197.

Madsen TM, Treschow A, Bengzon J, et al. (2000). Increased neurogenesis in a model of electroconvulsive therapy. *Biol Psychiatry*, 47, 1043–1049.

Mallet L, Polosan M, Jaafari N, et al. (2008). Subthalamic nucleus stimulation in severe obsessive-compulsive disorder. *N Engl J Med*, 359, 2121–2134.

Marangell LB, Rush AJ, George MS, et al. (2002). Vagus nerve stimulation (VNS) for major depressive episodes: one year outcomes. *Biol Psychiatry*, 51, 280–287:

Martin JLR, Martín-Sánchez E (2012). Systematic review and meta-analysis of vagus nerve stimulation in the treatment of depression: variable results based on study designs. *Eur Psychiatry*, 27, 147–155.

Mayberg HS (2009). Targeted electrode-based modulation of neural circuits for depression. *J Clin Invest*, 119, 717–725.

Mayberg HS, Lozano AM, Voon V, et al. (2005). Deep brain stimulation for treatment-resistant depression. *Neuron*, 45, 651–660.

McClelland J, Kekic M, Bozhilova N, et al. (2016). A randomised controlled trial of neuronavigated repetitive transcranial magnetic stimulation (rTMS) in anorexia nervosa. *PLoS One*, 11, e0148606.

Medda P, Mauri M, Toni C, et al. (2014). Predictors of remission in 208 drug-resistant depressive patients treated with electroconvulsive therapy. *J ECT*, 30, 292–297.

Milev RV, Giacobbe P, Kennedy SH, et al. (2016). Canadian Network for Mood and Anxiety Treatments (CANMAT) 2016 Clinical Guidelines for the Management of Adults with Major Depressive Disorder: Section 4. Neurostimulation Treatments. *Can J Psychiatry*, 61, 561–575.

Mu Q, Bohning DE, Nahas Z, et al. (2004). Acute vagus nerve stimulation using different pulse widths produces varying brain effects. *Biol Psychiatry*, 55, 816–825.

Munk-Olsen T, Laursen TM, Videbech P, Mortensen PB, Rosenberg R (2007). All-cause mortality among recipients of electroconvulsive therapy: register-based cohort study. *Br J Psychiatry*, 190, 435–459.

Nahas Z, Marangell LB, Husain MM, et al. (2005). Two-year outcome of vagus nerve stimulation (VNS) for treatment of major depressive episodes. *J Clin Psychiatry*, 66, 1097–1104.

Nardone R, Tezzon F, Höller Y, et al. (2014). Transcranial magnetic stimulation (TMS)/repetitive TMS in mild cognitive impairment and Alzheimer's disease. *Acta Neurol Scand*, 129, 351–366.

National Institute for Clinical Excellence (2003). *Guidance on the use of electroconvulsive therapy*. Technical appraisal guidance [TA59]. London: National Collaborating Centre for Mental Health. Available at: www.nice.org.uk/Guidance/TA59 (last accessed 31.8.19).

National Institute for Health and Care Excellence (NICE) (2009). *Vagus nerve stimulation for treatment-resistant depression*. Interventional procedures guidance [IPG330]. London: National Collaborating Centre for Mental Health.

National Institute for Health and Care Excellence (NICE) (2015). *Repetitive transcranial magnetic stimulation for depression.*

Interventional procedures guidance [IPG542]. London: National Collaborating Centre for Mental Health. Available at: http://nice.org.uk/guidance/ipg542 (last accessed 31.8.19).

Navarro V, Gasto C, Torres X, et al. (2008). Continuation/maintenance treatment with nortriptyline versus combined nortriptyline and ECT in late-life psychotic depression: a two-year randomized study. *Am J Geriatr Psychiatry*, 16, 498–505.

Ng C, Schweitzer I, Alexopoulos P, et al. (2000). Efficacy and cognitive effects of right unilateral electroconvulsive therapy. *Journal of ECT*, 16, 370–379.

Nordenskjöld A, von Knorring L, Engström I (2012). Predictors of the short-term responder rate of electroconvulsive therapy in depressive disorders – a population based study. *BMC Psychiatry*, 12, 115.

Nutt DJ, Gleiter CH, Glue P (1989). Neuropharmacological aspects of ECT: in search of the primary mechanism of action. *Convul Ther*, 5, 250–260.

Nuttin B, Cosyns P, Demeulemeester H, Gybels J, Meyerson B (1999). Electrical stimulation in anterior limbs of internal capsules in patients with obsessive-compulsive disorder. *Lancet*, 354, 1526.

Oltedal L, Narr KL, Abbott C, et al. (2018). Volume of the human hippocampus and clinical response following electroconvulsive therapy. *Biol Psychiatry*, 84, 574–581.

Palm U, Hasan A, Strube W, Padberg F (2016). tDCS for the treatment of depression: a comprehensive review. *Eur Arch Psychiatry Clin Neurosci*, 266, 681–694.

Pande AC, Krugler T, Haskett RF, Greden JF, Grunhaus LJ (1988). Predictors of response to electroconvulsive therapy in major depressive disorder. *Biol Psychiatry*, 24, 91–93.

Penry JK, Dean JC (1990). Prevention of intractable partial seizures by intermittent vagal stimulation in humans: preliminary results. *Epilepsia*, 31(Suppl 2), S40–S43.

Perrin JS, Merz S, Bennett DM, et al. (2012). Electroconvulsive therapy reduces frontal cortical connectivity in severe depressive disorder. *Proc Natl Acad Sci U S A*, 109, 5464–5468.

Philip NS, Barredo J, van 't Wout-Frank M, et al. (2018). Network mechanisms of clinical response to transcranial magnetic stimulation in posttraumatic stress disorder and major depressive disorder. *Biol Psychiatry*, 83, 263–272.

Pinna M, Manchia M, Oppo R, et al. (2018). Clinical and biological predictors of response to electroconvulsive therapy (ECT): a review. *Neurosci Lett*, 669, 32–42.

Prudic J, Sackeim HA, Devanand DP (1990). Medication resistance and clinical response to electroconvulsive therapy. *Psychiatry Res*, 31, 287–296.

RCPsych Committee on ECT and Related Treatments (2017). *Statement on Neurosurgery for Mental Disorder (NMD), also known as Psychiatric Neurosurgery (Position statement CERT 05/17).* London: Royal College of Psychiatrists.

Ren J, Li H, Palaniyappan L, et al. (2014). Repetitive transcranial magnetic stimulation versus electroconvulsive therapy for major depression: a systematic review and meta-analysis. *Prog Neuropsychopharmacol Biol Psychiatry*, 51, 181–189.

Rocha RB, Dondossola ER, Grande AJ, et al. (2016). Increased BDNF levels after electroconvulsive therapy in patients with major depressive disorder: a meta-analysis study. *J Psychiatr Res*, 83, 47–53.

Rong P, Liu J, Wang L, et al. (2016). Effect of transcutaneous auricular vagus nerve stimulation on major depressive disorder: a nonrandomized controlled pilot study. *J Affect Disord*, 195, 172–179.

Rossi S, Hallett M, Rossini PM, Pascual-Leone A; Safety of TMS Consensus Group (2009). Safety, ethical considerations, and application guidelines for the use of transcranial magnetic stimulation in clinical practice and research. *Clin Neurophysiology*, 120, 2008–2039.

Rush AJ, George MS, Sackeim HA, et al. (2000). Vagus nerve stimulation (VNS) for treatment-resistant depressions: a multicenter study. *Biol Psychiatry*, 47, 276–286.

Rush AJ, Marangell LB, Sackeim HA, et al. (2005a). Vagus nerve stimulation for treatment-resistant depression: a randomized, controlled acute phase trial. *Biol Psychiatry*, 58, 347–354.

Rush AJ, Sackei HA, Marangell LB, et al. (2005b). Effects of 12 months of vagus nerve stimulation in treatment-resistant depression: a naturalistic study. *Biol Psychiatry*, 58, 355–363.

Sackeim HA, Prudic J, Devanand DP, et al. (2000). A prospective, randomized, double-blind comparison of bilateral and right unilateral electroconvulsive therapy at different stimulus intensities. *Arch Gen Psychiatry*, 57, 425–434.

Sackeim HA, Haskett RF, Mulsant BH, et al. (2001). Continuation pharmacotherapy in the prevention of relapse following electroconvulsive therapy: a randomized controlled trial. *JAMA*, 285, 1299–1307.

Saleh C, Fontaine D (2015). Deep brain stimulation for psychiatric diseases: what are the risks? *Curr Psychiatry Rep*, 17, 1–14.

SEAN (2016). *SEAN Annual Report 2016. A Summary of ECT in Scotland for 2015.* Edinburgh: Scottish ECT Audit Network.

SEAN (2017). *SEAN Annual Report 2017. A Summary of ECT in Scotland for 2016.* Edinburgh: Scottish ECT Audit Network.

Semkovska M, McLoughlin DM (2010). Objective cognitive performance associated with electroconvulsive therapy for depression: a systematic review and meta-analysis. *Biol Psychiatry*, 68, 568–577.

Sheline YI, Price JL, Yan Z, Mintun MA (2010). Resting-state functional MRI in depression unmasks increased connectivity between networks via the dorsal nexus. *Proc Natl Acad Sci U S A*, 107, 11020–11025.

Shiwach RS, Reid WH, Carmody TJ (2001). An analysis of reported deaths following electroconvulsive therapy in Texas, 1993–1998. *Psychiatr Serv*, 52, 1095–1097.

Straasø B, Lauritzen L, Lunde M, et al. (2014). Dose-remission of pulsating electromagnetic fields as augmentation in therapy-resistant depression: a randomized, double-blind controlled study. *Acta Neuropsychiatr*, 26, 272–279.

Tharyan P, Adams CE (2005). Electroconvulsive therapy for schizophrenia. *Cochrane Database Syst Rev*, (2), CD000076. doi:10.1002/14651858.CD000076.pub2.

Tor PC, Bautovich A, Wang MJ, et al. (2015). A systematic review and meta-analysis of brief versus ultrabrief right unilateral electroconvulsive therapy for depression. *J Clin Psychiatry*, 76, e1092–e1098.

TrevizoL AP, Shiozawa P, Cook IA, et al. (2016). Transcranial magnetic stimulation for obsessive-compulsive disorder: an updated systematic review and meta-analysis. *J ECT*, 32, 262–266.

Tyagi H, Zrinzo L, Akram H, et al. (2017). A randomised controlled trial of deep brain stimulation in obsessive compulsive disorder: a comparison of ventral capsule/ventral striatum and subthalamic nucleus targets. *J Neurol Neurosurg Psychiatry*, 88, A8–A9.

UK ECT Review Group (2003). *Systematic Review of the Efficacy and Safety of Electroconvulsive Therapy*. London: Department of Health.

van Schaik AM, Comijs HC, Sonnenberg CM, et al. (2012). Efficacy and safety of continuation and maintenance electroconvulsive therapy in depressed elderly patients: a systematic review. *Am J Geriatr Psychiatry*, 20, 5–17.

Vila-Rodriguez F, McGirr A, Tham J, Hadjipavlou G, Honey CR (2014). Electroconvulsive therapy in patients with deep brain stimulators. *J ECT*, 30, e16–e18.

Watts BV, Groft A, Bagian JP, Mills PD (2011). An examination of mortality and other adverse events related to electroconvulsive therapy using a national adverse event report system. *J ECT*, 27, 105–108.

Xia G, Gajwani P, Muzina DJ, et al. (2008). Treatment-emergent mania in unipolar and bipolar depression: focus on repetitive transcranial magnetic stimulation. *Int J Neuropsychopharmacology*, 11, 119–130.

Zhou D-D, Wang W, Wang G-M, Li D-Q, Kuang L (2017). An updated meta-analysis: short-term therapeutic effects of repeated transcranial magnetic stimulation in treating obsessive-compulsive disorder. *J Affect Disord*, 215, 187–196.

Chapter 17

Psychotropic Drug Treatment in Childhood and Adolescence

David Coghill and Nicoletta Adamo

17.1 Introduction

While the use of medication to treat psychiatric problems is less common in children and adolescents than in adults, rates of prescription are increasing for these groups. Notwithstanding a significant increase in the number and quality of clinical trials of psychotropic medications in children and adolescents there are continuing concerns that increases in rates of prescribing still outstrip the evidence base. For example, the prescribing of antipsychotics for children 7–12 years of age in primary care within the UK almost tripled between 1992 and 2005, with the prescribing of 'atypical antipsychotics' increasing 60-fold from 1994 to 2005 (Rani et al., 2008). It is not clear whether this increase in prescribing of antipsychotics to children should be viewed as an indication of appropriate clinical practice in the management of often very complex and debilitating conditions or raising concerns about safety. The truth is likely to be a combination of the two.

Against this backdrop it is clearly important for mental health professionals managing children and adolescents to have a good understanding of the appropriate use of psychotropic medications including both their potential benefits and adverse effects in these populations. Although many of the issues are similar to those in adults, there are important differences. This chapter will focus on these differences and will not revisit ground covered in the previous chapters on specific medications. In particular, we will not address the pharmacological management of attention deficit hyperactivity disorder

(ADHD) in any detail as this has been comprehensively reviewed in Chapter 13. We therefore strongly suggest that while this chapter could be read in isolation it should be read as a part of the whole book.

17.2 General Principles

For most of the common psychiatric disorders affecting children and adolescents psychological therapies are recommended as first-line treatments. While it is increasingly understood that medication treatment will be first line in many, but not all, cases of ADHD and for those with schizophrenia and bipolar disorder, current guidance suggests psychological approaches as first line for anxiety, depression, post-traumatic stress disorder (PTSD), attachment disorders, obsessive-compulsive disorder, eating disorders, substance use disorders, tic disorders, oppositional defiant and conduct disorders and the irritability and aggression that is common in autism spectrum disorder (ASD) and intellectual disability. Medications can however contribute to the treatment of all of these disorders particularly where psychological therapies have either failed or only partially improved the clinical presentation. It is important that medical and non-medical clinicians working in child and adolescent mental health services or within a paediatric setting do not fall into the trap of adopting a polarized view about medication and psychological approaches to treatment. They can complement each other well if used together thoughtfully and knowledgeably.

When medication is used to treat children and adolescents with psychiatric disorders, it is nearly always deployed alongside psychosocial interventions and integrated into a total treatment package; it is uncommon for it to be the only form of intervention. One benefit of medication, often undervalued by clinicians, is the ability to allow someone to become more able to take full advantage of a psychotherapeutic intervention. On the other hand, there are clear indications that psychotropic medications are being increasingly used in children and adolescents. There is also a growing concern that in some instances medications are being used either to compensate a lack of availability of and access to adequate high-quality psychosocial treatment, or as a 'quick fix' for problems that would more appropriately be managed through a psychological intervention.

Most of the conditions for which medication is useful affect older children and adolescents (see Table 17.1), and it is unusual to prescribe for preschool children. The reaction of very young children to psychotropic medication is often unpredictable with an increased rate of adverse effects compared to older children. Furthermore, some drugs (e.g. fluoxetine) have been demonstrated in animal studies to lead to lasting developmental changes to the immature brain (Shrestha et al., 2014) and the implications of this for humans remain unclear. We therefore suggest clinicians approach the use of any of the medications mentioned in this chapter with great caution in the very young child (≤ 5 years). They should continue to exert a degree of caution for those medications not adequately trialled in children and young people while the brain is still developing (which we now understand extends well into young adulthood – late 20s).

It is also very important always to consider whose benefit a medication is being prescribed for. It is for example becoming more common for the parents or teachers of children with a disruptive behaviour disorder to ask for medication to make their child easier to manage. If this results in improved family relationships, a more settled

Table 17.1 Summary of drug use in child and adolescent psychiatry

Class	Main drugs within class used in children and adolescents	Main indications
Stimulants	Methylphenidate Amphetamines Lisdexamfetamine	ADHD Binge eating disorder
Non-stimulant ADHD medications	Atomoxetine	ADHD
Alpha$_2$ agonists	Guanfacine Clonidine	ADHD Tourette syndrome Sleep disorders
Serotonin reuptake inhibitors Selective	Citalopram Escitalopram Fluoxetine Fluvoxamine Paroxetine Sertraline	Anxiety OCD Depression
Less selective	Clomipramine	
Other antidepressants	Bupropion Venlafaxine	ADHD Treatment-resistant depression
Atypical antipsychotics	Risperidone Aripiprazole Quetiapine Olanzepine	Schizophrenia Mania Tourette syndrome Irritability, aggression (in ASD and ID)
Mood stabilizers	Carbamazepine Valproate Lithium Lamotragine Gabapentin Topiramate	Mania, bipolar disorder Irritability, mood instability, aggression

ID, intellectual disability; OCD, obsessive-compulsive disorder.

household or classroom and a happier child then it can be justified, but enabling an easier life for adult caregivers or educators is insufficient reason to prescribe.

Children are not alone in their ambivalence about taking medication on a regular basis but for many adolescents it is an even more unwelcome imposition. This is particularly true if a decision to start a medication is made simply on the basis of a discussion with parents. Adherence can be improved if the clinician takes time to have an individual discussion with the child/young person about why the medication is being prescribed, what the benefits may be, what adverse effects can be expected, how long before any positive effects will be seen and how long it is anticipated the course will be.

These discussions form the necessary basis for informed consent and are good practice even with children too young to be fully competent to grant or withhold consent. Most people only remember a small proportion of what has been said in clinic so the use of developmentally appropriate handouts describing the drug in question are often helpful and much more likely to be of use than the data sheets supplied by the manufacturers.

Not all children find swallowing tablets and capsules easy, and liquid preparations of medicines are often not available. It may be necessary to teach a child how to swallow a tablet using a graded series of small cake decorations and sweets, ensuring that swallowing a solid item is always followed by a drink. Parents need to be reminded to keep medications safe and secure and should supervise the taking of them. This is particularly important with controlled drugs such as the stimulants.

17.3 Off-Label Prescribing

There continues to be frequent misunderstandings about the use of medications that are not 'licensed' for children and that therefore need to be used 'off-label'. A drug licence is a 'marketing authorization' to promote a drug for a specified indication that has been granted to a pharmaceutical company by a national regulatory body (e.g. the Medicines and Healthcare products Regulatory Agency (MHRA) in the UK; the European Medicines Agency (EMA) in Europe; the Food and Drugs Administration (FDA) in the USA). A licence is only granted when the regulator is convinced that there is enough information about efficacy and safety on this medication for the specified disorder and in the population under consideration (e.g. children, adolescents, adults). Off-label prescribing occurs when medication use falls outside the scope of the marketing authorization with respect to one or more of four key domains (the '4 Ds'): (1) the disorder being treated; (2) the demographics (primarily age) of the patient; (3) the dosage being prescribed and route of administration; and (4) the duration of treatment (Baldwin & Kosky, 2007). Prescribing a medicine in a circumstance that is specified as contraindicated would also constitute off-label use. However, it is important to recognize that prescribing a drug that is contraindicated is not the same as using one outside the '4 Ds', as the latter use may often be very appropriate.

Until recently, most companies did not test new drugs on children and there was no requirement or incentive for them to do so. As a consequence, few new drugs (across the whole of medicine) were licensed for use in children. Conversely, recently the FDA, EMA and MHRA have developed new regulations and guidance. Following an initiative taken by the FDA, the EMA (the advice of which, at least until the terms of Brexit are determined, covers the MHRA in the UK) developed the Paediatric Regulation (European Medicines Agency, 2007), which established a system of obligations, rewards and incentives to ensure that medicines are regularly researched, developed and authorized to meet the therapeutic needs of children. This regulation compels companies to consider the potential paediatric use of medicinal products they develop and conduct a specific programme of research where there is potential for use in this population. The main aims are to improve the availability of evidence on appropriate, and inappropriate, use of medicines for children, to facilitate the development and availability of medicines and to ensure that those medicines for use in children are of high quality, safe, ethically researched and authorized appropriately. At the same time, it is also an attempt to ensure that children are not subjected to unnecessary trials or that the authorization of medicines for use in adults is not delayed while waiting for this evidence. The major consequences of the EU Paediatric Regulation are summarized in Box 17.1 (reproduced from Sharma et al., 2016).

It is important to recognize that prescribing 'on-label' certainly does not guarantee safety or effectiveness for that treatment. It remains the responsibility of the prescriber to understand and appraise the evidence base, and acknowledge any risks associated with prescribing. Paediatricians and child and adolescent psychiatrists are often anxious about recommending the off-label use of psychotropic medications, as are general practitioners

Box 17.1 The Paediatric Regulation (http://bit.ly/1jLqHXM)

The key measures included in the regulation are:

- The setting up of an expert committee within the EMA: the Paediatric Committee (PedCo)
- A requirement for companies to submit data on the use of a edicine in children in accordance with an agreed paediatric investigation plan (PIP) when applying for marketing authorisation for medicines or line-extensions for existing patent-protected medicines
- A system of waivers for medicines unlikely to benefit children
- A system of deferrals to ensure that medicines are tested in children only when it is safe to do so and to prevent a delay the authorisation of medicines for adults
- A reward for complying with the requirement in the form of a six-month extension to the Supplementary Protection Certificate
- For orphan medicines a reward for compliance in the form of an extra two years of market exclusivity added to the existing ten years awarded under the EU's Orphan Regulation
- A new type of marketing authorisation, the Paediatric Use Marketing Authorisation (PUMA), to attract new paediatric indications for off-patent products
- Measures to maximise the impact of existing studies on medicines for children
- An EU inventory of the therapeutic needs of children to focus the research, development and authorisation of medicines
- An EU network of investigators and trial centres to carry out the required R&D (European Network of Paediatric Research at the European Medicines Agency, Enpr-EMA, http://bit.ly/18hvTw8)
- A system of free scientific advice for the industry, provided by the EMA
- A public database of paediatric studies
- A provision on EU funding for research to stimulate the development and authorisation of off-patent medicines for children.

The EMA has also included detailed guidance as to what evidence is required on paediatric populations before MA will be given to new medications for a range of psychiatric disorders. These regulations include a welcome focus on longer-term safety and developmental issues. There is currently advice for:

- ADHD (http://bit.ly/1O2XRPp)
- Schizophrenia (http://bit.ly/1GDBptm)
- Depression (http://bit.ly/1LRvvBN)
- Autism (draft) (http://bit.ly/1P12rMs)

who are often asked to prescribe drugs off-label, under the auspices of a shared-care protocol. This anxiety and reluctance is often a result of a misplaced medico-legal fear of litigation should a practitioner prescribe a medication off-label and the patient develop an adverse reaction. In the UK independent prescribers can prescribe any medication (licensed, unlicensed or off-label) so long as a *reasonable body of medical opinion* would support this prescription (UK Government, 1983). Prescribing unlicensed medicines or medicines outside the recommendations of their licence will however alter (and probably increase) the prescriber's professional responsibility and potential liability. The prescriber should therefore be able to justify and feel competent about using such medicines. It is also important to discuss with the patient and/or their carer that the prescribed medicine is either unlicensed or being used off-label. Where off-label prescribing for children and adolescents is supported by an evidence base and, ideally, published clinical guidelines, then off-label prescribing practice would be easily defensible. In contrast, where the evidence is less clear-cut but the clinician feels that there is a pressing clinical need to consider second- or third-line off-label medication it is sensible to seek a second opinion to support the prescribing decision.

Guidelines on off-label prescribing have been published by the Royal College of Psychiatrists (RCPsych) (Royal College of Psychiatrists, 2007), the Royal College of Paediatrics and Child Health (RCPCH) (Royal College of Paediatrics and Child Health, 2013), *British National Formulary for Children* (Joint Formulary Committee, 2019) and Medicines for Children (Medicines for Children, 2015). The guidance and evidence for off-label prescribing of psychotropic medication to children and adolescents was reviewed recently by an expert group from the British Association of Psychopharmacology who made several helpful recommendations for clinical practice (Sharma et al., 2016):

1. Be familiar with the evidence base for the psychotropic agent, including its pharmacokinetic profile in children, the potential for adverse effects, any drug–drug interactions and differences in bioavailability/stability of the intended formulation.
2. Prescribing an off-label medicine may have advantages over a licensed one. Hence, licensed drugs and formulations should not always be prescribed and supplied in preference to an off-label drug or formulation. A prescribing decision (including a decision not to prescribe) should incorporate knowledge of the overall evidence base and the needs of the individual child.
3. When the evidence base for an off-label medication is lacking or the benefit/risk profile appears potentially unfavourable, obtain a second opinion from another doctor (and perhaps another member of the multidisciplinary team) before prescribing.
4. Explain the potential benefits and side effects to the patient and their parents/carers and document this discussion in the medical record.
5. Provide information leaflets for off-label medications specifying use in children and adolescents, including indications, dosage and route of administration.
6. 'Start low and go slow' and actively monitor response using standardized instruments and whether there are any adverse effects.

17.4 Paediatric Dosing, Titration and Variation in Pharmacokinetics

While children and adolescents may require lower doses of medication than adults, a common error amongst prescribers is to be over cautious and reduce the dose too much. In general, paediatric practice, doses are most often calculated according to a child's body weight or surface area. In a prepubertal child this can help to estimate a starting dose of a psychotropic, but for many medications in psychopharmacological practice the weight/dose relationship is not closely correlated and it is more effective to titrate the dose against the symptom and/or functional response, as well as adverse effects, in order to identify an optimal dose rather than to aim at a particular mg/kg target dose. Drug response does however generally vary with age, weight, sex and disease state as these impact on pharmacokinetics (absorption, distribution, metabolism and excretion). Developmental factors that influence these parameters are important to consider when working out the dose of medication to use. It is also important to note that the processes of development are not linear across the various body systems and children are not, physiologically or pharmacologically, scaled down adults. In recent years dose-finding studies are becoming more common in child and adolescent psychopharmacology but have never been adequately conducted for many of the older more established medications. By their early teens, young people usually need adult doses of psychotropic medications. Although not yet fully grown, their livers are healthy and so for many psychotropics much of the orally administered drug will be broken down by first-pass metabolism before it reaches the brain. As noted below, children and young people may in fact metabolize medications more efficiently than adults. For example, for medications such as stimulants where there is a strong association between pharmacokinetics and pharmacodynamics (Sonuga-Barke et al., 2004), the level and frequency of dosing may need to be greater for children and adolescents than that for adults.

The extent and rate of absorption of a drug after oral administration is determined by gastrointestinal factors. These closely resemble those of the adult after the first year of life. Rates of absorption of some medications may however be slightly faster in children and peak levels reached earlier. Some paediatric medicines are administered as liquids, which are more quickly absorbed than pills. Once absorbed, distribution is influenced by the size of the body water and fat compartments and the binding capacity of plasma and tissue proteins. Fat distribution varies across childhood, rising during the first year, falling towards puberty and increasing again from puberty through to adulthood. Large fat stores slow the elimination of fat-soluble drugs (e.g. fluoxetine) from the body.

Hepatic metabolism develops gradually in the first year of life, peaks in early childhood and by middle childhood (6–12 years) is twice that of adults. It then plateaus down to adult values in the early teens. For some medications a transient decrease in metabolism has been reported in the few months before puberty. This is possibly due to the competition with sex hormones for hepatic enzymes. Thus, for drugs with a primary hepatic metabolism (e.g. most antidepressants, amphetamines, atomoxetine), many children may require higher mg/kg doses than adults. Kidney function also develops at different rates but resembles that of adults by the first year. Of the Caucasian population, 5–10% show slow hepatic metabolism of a number of drugs as a consequence of normal genetic variance (see Chapter 5).

The clinical response to and side-effect profile of a drug can be altered by developmental immaturity. Children may also have differences in drug receptor sensitivity compared to adults. Effective plasma ranges in children may be different to those in adults; for example, children require a slightly lower range for chlorpromazine, haloperidol and phenytoin. Such differences may be due to decreased protein binding and increased free fraction of drug rather than increased receptor sensitivity.

Therapeutic drug monitoring is the measurement of drug levels in body fluids (predominantly blood) and the use of these levels to adjust dose. In child and adolescent psychopharmacology, therapeutic ranges have been suggested for lithium, imipramine and nortriptyline and the anticonvulsants used for mood stabilization, such as valproate and carbamazepine (Rosen, 2017; Ryan, 1990; Rylance & Moreland, 1980). It is hardly ever used for other medications.

As noted above it is common practice to titrate dose, and sometimes frequency of administration, for psychotropic medications in childhood and adolescence. In order to effectively titrate to an optimum response, the goals of treatment need to be clarified and accurately measured at baseline before starting on the first dose of medication. The most convenient way to measure outcomes is through the use of standardized scales. These can be clinician administered (our preference) or filled in by the patient/parent /carer/teacher and administered face to face, over the phone or by email. It is also important to routinely collect information about adverse effects. Again, a standardized approach is preferable. Unfortunately, it is not yet routine for mental health clinicians or paediatricians to routinely collect such standardized information during their routine clinical work; however, evidence is emerging that doing so can result in substantial improvements in clinical outcomes (Coghill & Seth, 2015).

17.5 Adverse Effects

For many medications the patterns of adverse effects in children and adolescents are similar to those seen in adults. However, there is also a general pattern whereby adverse effects occur more frequently in younger patients and in particular those with intellectual disability and other severe neurodevelopmental disorders such as ASD and Tourette syndrome. One particular class of medications for which children and adolescents are at a particularly increased risk is the antipsychotics. This is seen not just for first-generation antipsychotics but also for second-generation drugs. While these more recent medications are associated with less extrapyramidal side effects than some of the older typical antipsychotics, in particular haloperidol, the prevalence of obesity, diabetes mellitus, metabolic and cardiovascular side effects are considerably higher in younger patients than they are in adults (Fraguas et al., 2011). This is particularly important to recognize as the general belief that these second-generation antipsychotics are safer due to lower rates of extrapyramidal symptoms with a lower risk for tardive dyskinesia has almost certainly made a significant contribution to the rapid rise in their use in children and young people, particularly as an attempt to reduce aggressive behaviours in those with intellectual disability or other neurodevelopmental disorders.

A further complicating factor is that, in addition to the increase in prescribing, there has also been an increase in the duration of treatment, often reflecting the lack of an effective exit strategy from prescribing. This further increases the risk of serious adverse effects. Developmental factors also increase the impact of certain adverse events. For example, the hypogonadism that can occur secondary to raised prolactin levels may have a more serious long-term impact on younger people who have not yet reached peak bone density. Despite the fact that clinical guidelines and structured reviews have focused heavily on the monitoring of adverse effects for a range of disorders (Cortese et al., 2013; Kendall et al., 2013) anecdotal evidence suggests that a structured approach to monitoring is still largely absent.

17.6 Drug Treatments for Depression in Children and Adolescents

The National Institute for Health and Care Excellence (NICE) guidelines for depression in children and adolescents are clear that antidepressant medications should not generally be used as an independent initial treatment for depression in children and adolescents (National Collaborating Centre for Mental Health, 2015). They suggest that specific psychological therapy is offered to all patients with moderate to severe depression. In young people (12–18 years), the combination of medication treatment with psychological therapy can be considered for initial treatment of moderate to severe depression instead of psychotherapy on its own. Fluoxetine is currently the only antidepressant recommended as a first-line medication for depression in children and adolescents.

Following an influential Cochrane review (Hazell & Mirzaie, 2013) which demonstrated that tricyclic antidepressants to be of unlikely benefit in the treatment of depression in children and adolescents and likely to have significant adverse events, there was a rapid increase in the use of selective serotonin reuptake inhibitors (SSRIs) in children and adolescents. Initial use significantly outstripped the evidence base. There are now, several randomized controlled trials (RCTs) comparing SSRIs with placebo in children and adolescents although these are not all of high quality. There are consistently positive RCTs for fluoxetine, mixed results for sertraline, citalopram and escitalopram (all reviewed comprehensively in Usala et al., 2008) and negative results for paroxetine, venlafaxine, nefazodone and mirtazapine (all unpublished 'data on file'). A comprehensive network meta-analysis of trials within this age group concluded that only fluoxetine was statistically significantly more effective than placebo (Cipriani et al., 2016). In terms of tolerability the network meta-analysis suggests that fluoxetine is also better than duloxetine and imipramine and that imipramine, venlafaxine and duloxetine are less well tolerated than placebo (Cipriani et al., 2016).

The publicly funded Treatment for Adolescents with Depression Study (TADS) in the USA (March et al., 2004) and the Adolescent Depression Antidepressants and Psychotherapy Trial (ADAPT) in the UK (Goodyer et al., 2007) investigated combination treatment with cognitive behavioural therapy (CBT) and an SSRI (in TADS this was fluoxetine, in ADAPT it was most often fluoxetine) compared with the SSRI alone (in both studies), CBT alone (TADS only) and placebo (TADS only). In the 12-week TADS, both combination treatment and fluoxetine alone were more effective than placebo, with the combination being the most effective treatment. In TADS, CBT alone was less effective than fluoxetine and no more effective than placebo. In the 28-week ADAPT study both the SSRI and SSRI + CBT groups improved, but there was no significant difference between the two groups.

Taken together these data support the conclusions of NICE regarding the acute management of depression in children and adolescents, namely that in young people (12–18 years), the combination of an antidepressant plus a psychological therapy can be considered for initial treatment of moderate to severe depression instead of psychotherapy on its own. It is estimated however that only around 60% of young people with depression will respond adequately to initial treatment with an SSRI so it is important to consider the most appropriate response for those whose response is suboptimal. The National Institute of Mental Health-funded Treatment of Resistant Depression in Adolescents (TORDIA) trial, was designed to investigate alternative treatments for the other 40%. The study included adolescents whose depression had not responded to an 'adequate trial' of an SSRI and they were randomized to one of four treatments (switch to another SSRI; switch to venlafaxine; switch to another SSRI + CBT; switch to venlafaxine + CBT) (Brent et al., 2008; Emslie et al., 2010). Over the first 12 weeks, just under 50% of participants had responded to the switch in treatment. The combination of CBT and a switch to another antidepressant resulted in a higher rate of clinical response than did a medication switch alone. For those who had a simple switch of medication, a switch to another SSRI was just as effective as a switch to venlafaxine and resulted in fewer adverse effects (Brent et al., 2008). At week 12 after randomization, responders continued in their assigned treatment arm while non-responders received open treatment (a switch to another antidepressant, augmentation, or the addition of CBT or other psychotherapy) for a further 12 weeks. At 24 weeks 38.9% of those enrolled in the study had achieved remission with the likelihood of remission much higher (61.6% vs. 18.3%) among those who had already demonstrated clinical response by week 12 (Emslie et al., 2010). All participants were treated naturalistically from week 24 onwards and the remission rate rose to 50% by week 48 and to 61% by week 72. However, 72% of participants still had at least one residual symptom of depression, such as irritability or low self-esteem, at week 72, and 11% met diagnostic criteria for major depression. We agree with the overall conclusions of the study authors that clinicians should pay significant attention to patients who do not respond in the first six weeks of treatment and consider either a combination treatment or switching to another SSRI in such cases.

17.7 Suicidality

Although several non-psychiatric factors are associated with increased risk of suicidal ideations and suicidal behaviour, suicidality and depression are of course closely linked and regular assessment of risk for suicide is a key part of management of depression. In children and adolescents this has been complicated by the suggestion of an association between treatment with antidepressants and suicidality. Regulatory agencies in the United States, the United Kingdom and other countries issued a series of warnings regarding a link between antidepressant use and suicidality in those under 18 years of age starting in 2003 (Leslie et al., 2005). In 2003 the FDA in the United States recommended that paroxetine was not used to treat young people with major depressive disorder because of a possible increased risk of suicidal thoughts and behaviour. Two years later, in 2005, the FDA implemented a black box warning to all antidepressants warning of increased suicidality when these drugs were used in children and adolescents. This was based on a meta-analysis that showed that the rate of suicidal ideation and behaviour in children randomized to antidepressants was double that seen in those randomized to placebo (Hammad et al., 2006). In 2003 the MHRA and the Committee for Safety of Medicines (CSM) in the UK advised against using venlafaxine and SSRI antidepressants, with the exception of fluoxetine, to treat major depressive disorder in under-18-year-olds due to lack of efficacy and increased suicidality (Murray et al., 2005). These warnings have understandably caused a degree of alarm for patients, their families and clinicians.

A more recent Cochrane meta-analysis showed that for 16- to 18-year-old patients with a depressive disorder there was an increased risk of suicidal behaviours and ideations (there were no completed suicides in the included trials) for those on antidepressants compared with those receiving placebo (17 trials; n = 3229; risk ratio 1.58; 95% confidence interval (CI) 1.02 to 2.45) (Hetrick et al., 2012). Those treated with an antidepressant had lower depression severity scores and higher rates of response/remission than those treated with placebo but the size of these effects was small. A meta-analysis of 372 RCTs of antidepressants versus placebo in adults with a range of disorders showed that the effect of antidepressants on suicidal behaviour (completed suicide, attempted suicide or preparatory acts) and ideation varies by age (Stone et al., 2009). Antidepressants, compared with placebo, were associated with an increased risk for suicidality (i.e. thoughts and actions) and suicidal behaviour in adults under 25 years that was similar to that seen in the earlier FDA meta-analysis in children and adolescents (Hammad et al., 2006). In contrast, in adults aged 25–64 years, antidepressants had a neutral effect on suicidal behaviour and possibly a protective effect for suicidal ideation. In adults aged 25–64 years, antidepressants reduced the risk of suicidality and also suicidal behaviour (Stone et al., 2009).

There are various methodological problems in interpreting data on suicidality from RCTs of antidepressants and problems also exist with approaches to post-marketing surveillance (Le Noury et al., 2015). The impact of regulatory warnings about antidepressant use in under 18s has been the subject of intense and ongoing debate. For example, Gibbons et al. (2007) identified an inverse relationship between decreases in SSRI use and increase in suicide in adolescents following the issue of the warnings. In contrast, Sparks and Duncan (2013) suggest that while in the years following such warnings there was a reduction in previous trends for prescription growth, overall paediatric antidepressant prescriptions did not decline significantly and that although rates of youth suicide did rise, this increase has only been seen in more recent years suggesting that they may not be directly related to changes in prescribing. In the adult population things appear to be clearer with ecological data from across 29 European countries suggesting that increased SSRI use is generally linked to lower suicide rates (Gusmao et al., 2013) and direct trial evidence that SSRIs do not increase suicidality and suicidal behaviour when data on adults of all ages are pooled (Stone et al., 2009).

So, where does this leave the clinician? We would recommend that antidepressants should only be prescribed to under 18s and younger adults if the benefits appear likely to outweigh the possible risks. This decision will need to be made on an individual patient basis. The bar to initiate prescribing is higher than in adults. Patients of any age who start antidepressant treatment should be reviewed regularly to detect clinical worsening, suicidality or changes in behaviour but such monitoring is of particular importance in paediatric patients. The patient and, if appropriate, key relatives need to be informed of the potential risk of increased suicidality. In general, fluoxetine is the antidepressant of choice to treat depression in those under 18 years of age.

There are ongoing efforts to test new pharmacological treatments to manage the immediate suicidal risk in children and young people. Clinical trials are being conducted at present on the efficacy, safety and tolerability of ketamine to support the licence for treatment of acute suicidal ideations (e.g. www.clinicaltrialsregister.eu/ctr-search/trial/2016-004422-42/), a new avenue of treatment with promising initial results in both adult and paediatric populations.

17.8 Medication Treatments for Autism Spectrum Disorders

The use of medications in ASD also often includes off-label prescribing. Beyond the core characteristics and symptoms of ASD, individuals with ASD often present with associated troublesome behaviours and co-morbid disorders (Simonoff et al., 2008). Until there are effective drug treatments for the core symptoms of ASD, pharmacological treatments in ASD are focused on the management of the associated challenging behaviours and co-morbid symptoms. The most common targets for treatment are: self-injurious behaviour, aggression to others or objects and property, tantrums, yelling/screaming, stereotypies, hyperactivity, impulsivity and agitation. Even though the evidence for efficacy and safety of pharmacological treatments for these various target symptoms is rather sparse, a working knowledge of what has been studied is helpful in planning clinical work. There are however concerns that the use of these medications has increased considerably over recent years and it is essential that clinicians think about possible non-pharmacological interventions before reaching for the prescription pad. This is particularly so for those working in a solely medical setting or in relative isolation where the temptation to use medication, because of difficulties accessing other services, is even greater.

For many individuals with ASD, irritability and aggression are among the most impairing symptoms. They are also the best studied with respect to pharmacological interventions. Various antipsychotics, mood stabilizers, antidepressants (clomipramine) and other agents (clonidine, amantadine, naltrexone, pentoxifylline) have been investigated for reduction of irritability in the context of ASD. Irritability is in fact the only symptom for which there are medications approved for use in ASD, although only in the USA (risperidone from 2006, and aripiprazole from 2009). Indeed, irritability in ASD was the first case in which the FDA accepted a symptom, rather than a disorder, as an indication for treatment. Risperidone received the indication for prescription to children over five years of age and a body weight of 9.1 kg and aripiprazole to children older than six years. The effect size is around 1.2 for risperidone (0.5–3.5 mg/day) and 0.6–0.9 for aripiprazole (5, 10, 15 mg/day). Extrapyramidal side effects, weight gain, dizziness and somnolence are the most important adverse effects associated with these medications. The positive effects on irritability and aggression do not appear to be secondary to somnolence. Of the drugs prescribed off-label, valproic acid (sodium valproate) in doses resulting in blood valproate levels of 87–110 μg/ml has been shown to reduce irritability scores on the Clinical Global Impression (CGI) irritability subscale in a majority (62.5%) of children and adolescents with ASD and results in statistically significant improvements in scores on the irritability subscale of the Aberrant Behavior Checklist (Hollander et al., 2010). While there is some emerging data to suggest that lurasidone may have some efficacy in reducing irritability the findings are not yet conclusive. It may however be a reasonable alternative, before haloperidol and ziprasidone, for those who experience tolerability issues with risperidone and aripiprazole or whose symptoms are refractory to these drugs (McClellan et al., 2017).

The management of ADHD symptoms in ASD has not been studied extensively (Bratt et al., 2017). This is in part due to the only recent possibility to diagnose ADHD in ASD following the revision of the classification systems (DSM-5). The limited available evidence, however, suggests that (i) treatment should be similar to that for routine cases of ADHD; (ii) the effect sizes are somewhat lower than those seen in children and adolescents with ADHD without ASD (i.e. they are only moderate for stimulant medications); and (iii) adverse effects are more likely in the group with ADHD and ASD. The maxim of 'start low and go slow' should be applied when prescribing any medications for ADHD in children and young people with ASD and medication doses increased with caution. However, too much caution can also be an issue resulting in suboptimal treatment of the ADHD symptoms and missed evidence of effectiveness that may extend beyond ADHD symptom reduction. It is important to also consider that side effects that are peculiar to ASD may emerge with ADHD medications. For example, while stimulant medications reduce attention deficits and hyperactivity-impulsivity symptoms, they may increase stereotypies (Malone et al., 2005). Initial evidence that guanfacine significantly reduces hyperactivity-impulsivity as well as oppositional behaviours (Politte et al., 2018) in children with ASD also suggests that it might be worth switching to guanfacine after unsuccessful trials with stimulants earlier than what would be appropriate in patients without ASD.

On the basis of various neurobiological hypotheses, antipsychotics, antidepressants and mood stabilizers have been studied as potential treatments for the reduction of stereotypies and repetitive behaviours in children and adolescents with ASD. RCTs of aripiprazole (Marcus et al., 2009; Owen et al., 2009) and risperidone (McDougle et al., 2005) both reported significant improvement in more than 50% of study participants. Statistically but not clinically significant response has also been reported for fluoxetine and valproic acid (Hollander et al., 2005, 2010), haloperidol and clomipramine (Remington et al., 2001). Modest although significant improvements of stereotyped behaviours following treatment with guanfacine have been reported (Politte et al., 2018).

The search for new medications to treat ASD is being very actively pursued at present and results from the EU-funded programmes of work are eagerly awaited (www.eu-aims.eu/; www.mind-project.eu).

17.9 Pharmacological Management of Tics and Tourette Syndrome

The decision about whether to focus on managing the tics in patients with tic disorders and Tourette syndrome (from now grouped together as TS) is complicated by several factors. Although TS is defined by the presence of motor and vocal tics, it is often complicated by associated difficulties such as obsessions and compulsions, aggressive and oppositional behaviour, ADHD symptoms, mood instability, anxiety and depression. As a consequence, the quality of life in young people with TS is influenced both by the tics themselves, which can cause social, emotional, functional and subjective discomfort (leading in some cases to severe self-mutilation), and by the presence of these common co-morbid symptoms and conditions. Indeed, several groups have demonstrated that subjective impairment does not necessarily equate with objective tic severity: some individuals with relatively severe tics experience only mild impairment, whereas in other cases mild tics may be associated with significant suffering (Scahill et al., 2006). Eddy et al. (2011) also investigated the clinical correlates of quality of life in TS and again found that the most significant factors affecting quality of life were co-morbid anxiety, ADHD, obsessive-compulsive symptoms, depression and dysthymia. As each of these conditions is a potential treatment target in itself, it is important that the clinician considering pharmacotherapy for TS first identifies whether there are associated target symptoms to be treated and then seeks to match these symptoms to an appropriate medication. Even when the decision is to focus on the treatment of tics, there are several factors that make treatment planning and assessment of response more difficult. These include the high interindividual variability of symptoms, and the waxing and waning of tics over time (Roessner et al., 2011).

Many of those with significant TS do not require pharmacological treatment. Most people with TS do not seek medical advice or support and many of those who seek advice find psychoeducation and a watch-and-wait approach to be adequate. There are also a range of effective non-pharmacological approaches available (Verdellen et al., 2011). The European Society for the Study of Tourette Syndrome (ESSTS) guidelines suggest that medication should be considered when tics cause:

- subjective discomfort (e.g. pain or injury)
- sustained social problems for the patient (e.g. social isolation or bullying)
- social and emotional problems for the patient (e.g. reactive depressive symptoms)
- functional interference (e.g. impairment of academic achievements).

There are a wide range of theories about the pathophysiological imbalances and neurochemical disruptions that underpin the development of tics. While alterations in the dopaminergic system are at the forefront of most people's thinking, other imbalances, such as in the serotonergic, noradrenergic, glutamatergic, GABAergic, cholinergic and opioid systems are also possible targets. It is therefore unsurprising that a broad range of medications have been considered as potentially helpful managing TS. However, the main support thus far is for modulation of the dopaminergic system particularly through blockade of the postsynaptic D_2 receptors. Dopamine receptor antagonists (antipsychotics) and other drugs studied for use in TS have been comprehensively reviewed by the ESSTS guidelines group (Roessner et al., 2011). They note the scarcity of high-quality studies that adequately assess both efficacy and safety. The best evidence for efficacy is for haloperidol and pimozide, both of which are relatively pure dopamine receptor antagonists. There is some indication that pimozide may be more effective and have a more favourable adverse reaction profile than haloperidol, although its potential cardiac effects are concerning. Despite this evidence, and due to the higher risk for adverse events, these medications have been replaced in clinical practice by the atypical antipsychotics which block both dopamine and serotonin receptors. Within this group the best evidence is for risperidone. While risperidone and the other second-generation antipsychotics certainly have a lower risk for extrapyramidal side effects compared with haloperidol, they are still associated with a wide range of adverse reactions, including sedation, weight gain, extrapyramidal symptoms, neuroleptic malignant syndrome and tardive dyskinesia. Of the others the dopamine receptor partial agonist aripiprazole is often favoured by clinicians, given the lower probability of weight gain and promising effects in patients who had not responded to previous treatments (Zheng et al., 2016).

Although, compared with the antipsychotics, the evidence to support the efficacy of clonidine for the management of TS is less robust, clonidine (and possibly guanfacine) among the α-adrenoceptor agonists may also improve ADHD symptoms alongside suppression of mild to moderate tics. In addition, clonidine tends to alleviate initial insomnia and reduce anxiety (Sandor, 1995). While other medications have been studied and are sometimes used in clinical practice the evidence for their efficacy is limited and often contradictory.

A final consideration is the management of coexisting TS and ADHD. Managing these children and young people is often extremely challenging. Clinical judgement is required to balance the relative impairment from ADHD symptoms and tics before deciding the best approach to treatment. There has been a long-standing controversy as to whether the stimulant medications used to treat ADHD also increase tics.

Double-blind placebo-controlled studies have demonstrated that stimulants are highly efficacious in the treatment of core ADHD symptoms in patients with co-morbid TS, and while there is an increase of tics in some patients (around 25%), in the majority of cases, these medications do not increase either tic severity or frequency, nor are they linked to new onset of tics (Cohen et al., 2015). It is therefore generally accepted that, when the aim is to control ADHD symptoms, stimulants remain a first-line treatment choice. Atomoxetine, a non-stimulant treatment for ADHD, does not appear to increase tic frequency or severity, and in clinical trials there is some evidence of a reduction in tic severity as well as a reduction in ADHD symptoms (Allen et al., 2005). Atomoxetine may therefore be considered as a first-line medication for some patients with ADHD, also upon preference of the patient and their family, and co-morbid tics and as the next choice for cases where a stimulant medication leads to either the *de novo* appearance of tics or an exacerbation of pre-existing tics. As noted above clonidine or guanfacine may also be considered in monotherapy or in combination with psychostimulants.

References

Allen AJ, Kurlan RM, Gilbert DL, et al. (2005). Atomoxetine treatment in children and adolescents with ADHD and comorbid tic disorders. *Neurology*, 65, 1941–1949.

Baldwin DS, Kosky N (2007). Off-label prescribing in psychiatric practice. *Adv Psychiatr Treat*, 13, 414–422.

Bratt AM, Masanyero-Bennie B, Kelley SP (2017). A meta-analysis of the efficacy of immediate release methylphenidate to reduce hyperactivity in children with autistic spectrum disorder. *J Pharm Sci Exp Pharmacol*, 2017, 11–20.

Brent D, Emslie G, Clarke G (2008). Switching to another SSRI or to venlafaxine with or without cognitive behavioral therapy for adolescents with SSRI-resistant depression: the TORDIA randomized controlled trial. *JAMA*, 299, 901–913.

Cipriani A, Zhou X, Del Giovane C, et al. (2016). Comparative efficacy and tolerability of antidepressants for major depressive disorder in children and adolescents: a network meta-analysis. *Lancet*, 388, 881–890.

Coghill D, Seth S (2015). Effective management of attention-deficit/hyperactivity disorder (ADHD) through structured re-assessment: the Dundee ADHD Clinical Care Pathway. *Child*

Adolesc Psychiatry Ment Health, 9, 52. doi:10.1186/s13034-015-0083-2.

Cohen SC, Mulqueen JM, Ferracioli-Oda E, et al. (2015). Meta-analysis: risk of tics associated with psychostimulant use in randomized, placebo-controlled trials. *J Am Acad Child Adolesc Psychiatry*, 54, 728–736.

Cortese S, Holtmann M, Banaschewski T, et al. (2013). Practitioner review: current best practice in the management of adverse events during treatment with ADHD medications in children and adolescents. *J Child Psychol Psychiatry*, 54, 227–246.

Eddy CM, Cavanna AE, Gulisano M, et al. (2011). Clinical correlates of quality of life in Tourette syndrome. *Mov Disord*, 26, 735–738.

Emslie GJ, Mayes T, Porta G, et al. (2010). Treatment of resistant depression in adolescents (TORDIA): week 24 outcomes. *Am J Psychiatry*, 167, 782–791.

European Medicines Agency (2007). *Regulation (EC) No 1901/2006 of the European Parliament and of the Council on medicinal products for paediatric use, as amended by Regulation (EC) No 1902/2006* (online). Available at: www.ema.europa.eu/ema/index.jsp?curl=pages/regulation/document_listing/document_listing_000068.jsp (last accessed 12.6.18).

Fraguas D, Correll CU, Merchan-Naranjo J, et al. (2011). Efficacy and safety of second-generation antipsychotics in children and adolescents with psychotic and bipolar spectrum disorders: comprehensive review of prospective head-to-head and placebo-controlled comparisons. *Eur Neuropsychopharmacol*, 21, 621–645.

Gibbons RD, Brown CH, Hur K, et al. (2007). Early evidence on the effects of regulators' suicidality warnings on SSRI prescriptions and suicide in children and adolescents. *Am J Psychiatry*, 164, 1356–1363.

Goodyer I, Dubicka B, Wilkinson P, et al. (2007). Selective serotonin reuptake inhibitors (SSRIs) and routine specialist care with and without cognitive behaviour therapy in adolescents with major depression: randomised controlled trial. *BMJ*, 335, 142.

Gusmao R, Quintao S, McDaid D, et al. (2013). Antidepressant utilization and suicide in Europe: an ecological multi-national study. *PLoS One*, 8, e66455.

Hammad TA, Laughren T, Racoosin J (2006). Suicidality in pediatric patients treated with antidepressant drugs. *Arch Gen Psychiatry*, 63(3), 332–339.

Hazell P, Mirzaie M (2013). Tricyclic drugs for depression in children and adolescents. *Cochrane Database Syst Rev*, (6), CD002317.

Hetrick SE, McKenzie JE, Cox GR, Simmons MB, Merry SN (2012). Newer generation antidepressants for depressive disorders in children and adolescents. *Cochrane Database Syst Rev*, (11), CD004851.

Hollander E, Phillips A, Chaplin W, et al. (2005). A placebo controlled crossover trial of liquid fluoxetine on repetitive behaviors in childhood and adolescent autism. *Neuropsychopharmacology*, 30, 582–589.

Hollander E, Chaplin W, Soorya L, et al. (2010). Divalproex sodium vs placebo for the treatment of irritability in children and adolescents with autism spectrum disorders. *Neuropsychopharmacology*, 35, 990–998.

Joint Formulary Committee (2019). *British National Formulary for Children* (online). London: BMJ Group and Pharmaceutical Press.

Kendall T, Hollis C, Stafford M, Taylor C; Guideline Development Group (2013). Recognition and management of psychosis and schizophrenia in children and young people: summary of NICE guidance. *BMJ*, 346, f150.

Le Noury J, Nardo JM, Healy D, et al. (2015). Restoring Study 329: efficacy and harms of paroxetine and imipramine in treatment of major depression in adolescence. *BMJ*, 351, h4320.

Leslie LK, Newman TB, Chesney PJ, et al. (2005). The Food and Drug Administration's deliberations on antidepressant use in pediatric patients. *Pediatrics*, 116, 195–204.

Malone RP, Gratz SS, Delaney MA, Hyman SB (2005). Advances in drug treatments for children and adolescents with autism and other pervasive developmental disorders. *CNS Drugs*, 19, 923–934.

March J, Silva S, Petrycki S, et al.; Treatment for Adolescents with Depression Study (TADS) Team (2004). Fluoxetine, cognitive-behavioral therapy, and their combination for adolescents with depression: Treatment for Adolescents with Depression Study (TADS) randomized controlled trial. *JAMA*, 292, 807–820.

Marcus RN, Owen R, Kamen L, et al. (2009). A placebo-controlled, fixed-dose study of aripiprazole in children and adolescents with irritability associated with autistic disorder. *J Am Acad Child Adolesc Psychiatry*, 48, 1110–1119.

McClellan L, Dominick KC, Pedapati EV, Wink LK, Erickson CA (2017). Lurasidone for the treatment of irritability and anger in autism spectrum disorders. *Expert Opin Investig Drugs*, 26, 985–989.

McDougle CJ, Scahill L, Aman MG, et al. (2005). Risperidone for the core symptom domains of autism: results from the study by the autism network of the research units on pediatric psychopharmacology. *Am J Psychiatry*, 162, 1142–1148.

Medicines for Children (2015). *Unlicensed Medicines* (online). Available at: www.medicinesforchildren.org.uk/unlicensed-medicines (last accessed 12.6.18).

Murray ML, Thompson M, Santosh PJ, Wong IC (2005). Effects of the Committee on Safety of Medicines advice on antidepressant prescribing to children and adolescents in the UK. *Drug Saf*, 28(12), 1151–1157.

National Collaborating Centre for Mental Health (2015). *Depression in children and young people: identification and management in primary, community and secondary care.* Clinical guideline [CG28]. London: National Institute for Health and Clinical Excellence.

Owen R, Sikich L, Marcus RN, et al. (2009). Aripiprazole in the treatment of irritability in children and adolescents with autistic disorder. *Pediatrics*, 124, 1533–1540.

Politte LC, Scahill L, Figueroa J, et al. (2018). A randomized, placebo-controlled trial of extended-release guanfacine in children with autism spectrum disorder and ADHD symptoms: an analysis of secondary outcome measures. *Neuropsychopharmacology*, 43, 1772–1778.

Rani F, Murray ML, Byrne PJ, Wong IC (2008). Epidemiologic features of antipsychotic prescribing to children and adolescents in primary care in the United Kingdom. *Pediatrics*, 121, 1002–1009.

Remington G, Sloman L, Konstantareas M, Parker K, Gow R (2001). Clomipramine versus haloperidol in the treatment of autistic disorder: a double-blind, placebo-controlled, crossover study. *J Clin Psychopharmacol*, 21, 440–444.

Roessner V, Plessen KJ, Rothenberger A, et al.; ESSTS Guidelines Group (2011). European clinical guidelines for Tourette syndrome and other tic disorders. Part II: pharmacological treatment. *Eur Child Adolesc Psychiatry*, 20, 173–196.

Rosen MS (2017). Lithium in child and adolescent bipolar disorder. *Am J Psychiatry Resid J*, 12, 3–5.

Royal College of Paediatrics and Child Health (2013). *The use of unlicensed medicines or licensed medicines for unlicensed applications in paediatric practice.* London: Royal College of Paediatrics and Child Health.

Royal College of Psychiatrists (2007). *Use of Licensed Medicines for Unlicensed Applications in Psychiatric Practice*, 2nd ed. College Report CR210. London: Royal College of Psychiatrists.

Ryan ND (1990). Heterocyclic antidepressants in children and adolescents. *J Child Adolesc Psychopharmacol*, 1, 21–31.

Rylance GW, Moreland TA (1980). Drug level monitoring in paediatric practice. *Arch Dis Child*, 55, 89–98.

Sandor P (1995). Clinical management of Tourette's syndrome and associated disorders. *Can J Psychiatry*, 40, 577–583.

Scahill L, Erenberg G, Berlin CM Jr, et al.; Tourette Syndrome Association Medical Advisory Board: Practice Committee (2006). Contemporary assessment and pharmacotherapy of Tourette syndrome. *NeuroRx*, 3, 192–206.

Sharma AN, Arango C, Coghill D, et al. (2016). BAP Position Statement: Off-label prescribing of psychotropic medication to children and adolescents. *J Psychopharmacol*, 30, 416–421.

Shrestha SS, Nelson EE, Liow JS, et al. (2014). Fluoxetine administered to juvenile monkeys:

effects on the serotonin transporter and behavior. *Am J Psychiatry*, 171, 323–331.

Simonoff E, Pickles A, Charman T, et al. (2008). Psychiatric disorders in children with autism spectrum disorders: prevalence, comorbidity, and associated factors in a population-derived sample. *J Am Acad Child Adolesc Psychiatry*, 47, 921–929.

Sonuga-Barke EJ, Swanson JM, Coghill D, Decory HH, Hatch SJ (2004). Efficacy of two once-daily methylphenidate formulations compared across dose levels at different times of the day: preliminary indications from a secondary analysis of the COMACS study data. *BMC Psychiatry*, 4, 28.

Sparks JA, Duncan BL (2013). Outside the black box: re-assessing pediatric antidepressant prescription. *J Can Acad Child Adolesc Psychiatry*, 22, 240–246.

Stone M, Laughren T, Jones ML, et al. (2009). Risk of suicidality in clinical trials of antidepressants in adults: analysis of proprietary data submitted to US Food and Drug Administration. *BMJ*, 339, b2880.

UK Government (1983). UK Medical Act 1983 (c54).

Usala T, Clavenna A, Zuddas A, Bonati M (2008). Randomised controlled trials of selective serotonin reuptake inhibitors in treating depression in children and adolescents: a systematic review and meta-analysis. *Eur Neuropsychopharmacol*, 18, 62–73.

Verdellen C, van de Griendt J, Hartmann A, Murphy T; ESSTS Guidelines Group (2011). European clinical guidelines for Tourette syndrome and other tic disorders. Part III: behavioural and psychosocial interventions. *Eur Child Adolesc Psychiatry*, 20, 197–207.

Zheng W, Li XB, Xiang YQ, et al. (2016). Aripiprazole for Tourette's syndrome: a systematic review and meta-analysis. *Hum Psychopharmacol*, 31, 11–18.

Chapter 18

Psychotropic Drug Treatment in Later Life

Simon J. C. Davies

18.1 Introduction

In this chapter, important issues which may be encountered when prescribing medications to older adults will be discussed. It must be remembered that medication is only one of several valuable approaches in treating psychiatric disorders in the elderly and it is often necessary to integrate expertise in drug prescribing with psychotherapy and social interventions, although discussion of these is beyond the scope of this review. The first part of the chapter examines population demographics in relation to older age psychiatry and the fact that the evidence base for using many psychiatric medications in older people is more meagre than in younger adults. This is followed by a review of the pharmacodynamic and pharmacokinetic changes seen in older adults, which can impact on prescribing. The final part of the chapter considers common psychiatric disorders (depression, anxiety disorders, insomnia, psychotic disorders, bipolar disorder, attention deficit hyperactivity disorder (ADHD), substance misuse). For each disorder, the evidence base for pharmacological treatment in the older adults is reviewed together with key interactions and side effects of commonly used medications. This includes considering the impact of physical disorders such as renal and hepatic impairment and cardiovascular morbidity where relevant. Drugs used to treat dementia are not covered in this chapter as this is the subject of Chapter 14.

18.2 Population Demographics

Around 7% of the world's population was aged 65 or more in 2009. However, older adults represent a much greater proportion of the populations in developed countries, for example the proportion aged 65 or over in the United Kingdom is currently 18%. While many western nations, such as the UK, France and Sweden had reached the point where 14% of their populations were aged 65 or more before 1980, heavily populated developing countries such as China and Brazil are expected to reach this mark in the next 10 to 20 years (Kinsella & He, 2009). Psychiatric disorders are common in the elderly. In terms of disability-adjusted life years (DALYs) lost in the global population aged over 60, a World Health Organization study suggested that Alzheimer's disease and other dementias accounted for the greatest number of DALYs lost to psychiatric disorders, followed by depressive disorders, anxiety disorders, schizophrenia, alcohol use disorder, drug use disorders and bipolar disorder (Department of Health Statistics and Informatics of the World Health Organization, 2015).

The number of individuals with dementia has increased markedly in recent decades in line with increases in life expectancy and is expected to continue to increase (Prince et al., 2013). Projections based on a large Canadian longitudinal study suggest that the risk on reaching age 65 of developing dementia at some point before death is around 42% (95% confidence interval (CI) 38–46%) (Carone et al., 2014). However, while the prevalence at age 90 was estimated to be 29%, at age 80 it is around 10% and at age 65 only 1%. It should be noted therefore that the great majority of people aged over 65 do not have dementia or even mild cognitive impairment. Indeed, many continue to work into their eighth and even ninth decades, some in positions of great responsibility, many are very active in the community in retirement and many are essential carers for a spouse, parent, adult child, grandchild or other family member.

The prevalence of affective disorders in older adults appears to be considerably less than that in younger age groups. For instance, the Epidemiologic Catchment Area study (ECA) reported a one-month prevalence of 2.5 % in older adults, compared with 4.6 % in younger age groups (Regier, 1988). A more recent study (Gum et al., 2009), the National Comorbidity Survey Replication, also in the United States, confirmed this observation, but highlighted that the burden of these disorders in older adults may be underestimated through underdiagnosis and lack of representation of high-risk individuals in their sample (such as those with severe medical illnesses). Bipolar disorder appears to be less common than unipolar depression with a prevalence between 0.5% and 1% (Satajovic et al., 2015) which is only around one-third of that observed in younger adults (Depp & Jeste, 2004).

There has been debate in terms of defining when ‘old age’ begins, or from what age should patients be eligible to receive care from a dedicated old age psychiatry service. The boundary is most commonly drawn at 65 years, although 60 is not uncommon. Some ‘old age psychiatry’ services will restrict care at the younger end of the age range (e.g. between 60 and 65) to specific diagnoses or where disorders such as depression, bipolar disorder or psychotic disorders have not occurred earlier in life. Furthermore, some authors draw a distinction between ‘young-old’ (i.e. up to 80 years) and ‘old-old’ (greater than 80 years), while the term ‘oldest-old’ has been used to describe individuals aged over 85.

18.3 Pharmacological Studies in the Elderly

A challenge in making decisions on pharmacological treatments for psychiatric disorders in older adults is that although they exhibit biological and clinical features which may differ from those aged below 65 years, there are few robust randomized trials for psychotropic medications conducted specifically in the elderly. Researchers conducting trials may be reluctant to include older participants due to the likelihood of co-morbid medical disorders and pharmacokinetic or pharmacodynamic differences. This means that prescribers treating older adults will need to give consideration to the full range of psychotropic drugs that are used in younger adults, including drugs that have no successful randomized trial demonstrating safety and efficacy specifically in the elderly. With trials in the elderly in depression, and more so in bipolar disorder, schizophrenia and anxiety disorders being relatively few in number, the old age psychiatrist will by necessity have to extrapolate evidence of efficacy from younger populations into the older adults they need to treat. Where trials in the elderly do exist to support the use of certain medications, they will add weight to the perceived value of the drug studied for use in the elderly – but not to the extent that they would automatically be preferred to drugs with positive trial evidence of effect only in younger populations. A good example would be the choice between selective serotonin reuptake inhibitors (SSRIs) to treat depression when prescribing to the elderly. After sertraline, escitalopram is the SSRI most widely used in younger adults but unlike fluoxetine and paroxetine, it has no successful randomized trials specifically in late-life depression as both of the studies undertaken with escitalopram in older adults reported no significant advantage in efficacy over placebo. Nevertheless, escitalopram remains a more popular choice than fluoxetine or paroxetine when prescribing to older adults for depression and is recommended in recent guidelines (MacQueen et al., 2016). This situation appears to have arisen from the combination of our willingness to extrapolate evidence of escitalopram's efficacy from trials in younger people to the elderly, coupled with concerns relating to the suitability of fluoxetine (e.g. risk of P450 interactions) and paroxetine (e.g. risk of anticholinergic effects) in older populations.

The issue in prescribing psychotropic drugs to older adults is therefore not only 'Is there a trial specific to the elderly?' but also 'When I extrapolate evidence from studies in younger populations, what are the issues I need to be vigilant for in the elderly, and more specifically, what safety issues might I encounter?' The latter question requires consideration of several factors, as follows:

1. What age-associated changes might impact on drug pharmacokinetics or pharmacodynamics, or might reduce capacity to cope with changes that will result from introducing a new drug?
2. What pathological changes/disease states are present that may be exacerbated by introducing a new drug or may prevent the drug from being effective or safe?
3. What co-prescribed medication is my patient taking that could lead to pharmacokinetic or pharmacodynamic interactions?

18.4 Age-Related Pharmacodynamic Changes

Ageing is associated with numerous changes to bodily systems, including many that impact on the central nervous system. Brain volume and weight reduce with age, while ventricles and sulci widen. Neuronal loss occurs throughout life but impacts more on white matter after the age of 50 (Esiri & Morris, 1997). A further consequence of ageing is reduction in neurotransmission for many of the transmitter systems implicated in psychiatric disorders. This is of great relevance to pharmacotherapy, since sensitivity or responsivity may change both in neurotransmitter systems, which psychotropic drugs target for their therapeutic effect, and also in systems on which these drugs exert an impact as side effects.

More specifically, pharmacodynamic changes influence the relationship of circulating drug concentration with observed response (Bowie & Slattum, 2007). Drug pharmacodynamics can be altered through age-related changes in the function of neurotransmitter systems such as the number of available receptors or receptor affinity (Bowie & Slattum, 2007; Singh & Bajorek, 2015) or of allied hormonal systems, or homeostatic mechanisms. These changes impact many neurotransmitter systems such as the monoamine transmitters dopamine, noradrenaline and serotonin, and acetylcholine (Rehman & Masson, 2001). Examples include reduced baroreceptor responsivity or sensitivity with age (making orthostatic hypotension more likely), decreased numbers of dopamine D_2 receptors (leading to increased sensitivity to extrapyramidal symptoms), increased monoamine oxidase availability and decreased acetylcholine availability (causing greater sensitivity to anticholinergic effects).

18.4.1 Changes to Neurotransmitter System Function

18.4.1.1 Monoamines (Dopamine, Noradrenaline and Serotonin)

Many psychotropic drugs have actions on monoamine neurotransmitter systems. These include drugs used in depression and anxiety, in psychosis and in ADHD. The dopaminergic system exhibits pronounced changes with ageing, most notably in the tuberoinfundibular pathway. Age-related decline in dopamine D_2 receptors have been reported in many brain areas (including the caudate, putamen, substantia nigra and globus pallidus (Morgan et al., 1987)) and may explain the increased sensitivity of older adults to extrapyramidal side effects, seen especially with conventional antipsychotic agents. Important age-related changes have also been described in the noradrenaline system, with reduction of neuronal density in the locus coeruleus. For serotonin several imaging studies have reported small reductions with ageing in the binding availability for serotonin receptors implicated in regulation of mood and anxiety, including the 5-HT_{1A} receptor (Møller et al., 2007) and the 5-HT_2 receptor (Adams et al., 2004), although the ramifications of these changes are not clear.

18.4.1.2 Acetylcholine

Numerous drugs have anticholinergic effects (Chew et al., 2008; Rudolph et al., 2008), including many antipsychotic drugs and older antidepressants. Advancing age is associated with decreased acetylcholine availability and receptor numbers (for example in the caudate, putamen, hippocampus and frontal cortex (Rinne, 1987)). The consequence is greater sensitivity to anticholinergic effects in older adults such that drugs with anticholinergic activity are more likely to cause discernible deficits centrally, such as cognitive impairment, and peripherally, such as dry mouth, urinary retention and constipation, as will be described further in the section relating to antipsychotic drugs.

18.4.1.3 Gamma-Aminobutyric Acid (GABA) System

Most anxiolytics and hypnotics (notably benzodiazepines and Z-drugs) act on the GABA system, although some non-benzodiazepine anxiolytics, such as pregabalin, buspirone and hydroxyzine, work through other systems as do some drugs used to promote sedation (e.g. antihistamines and trazodone). Both traditional benzodiazepines (such as the anxiolytics diazepam, alprazolam, lorazepam and clonazepam, and hypnotics such as temazepam and nitrazepam) and the newer class of Z-drugs (including zopiclone, zaleplon and zolpidem), which were introduced in the 1990s, also exert a hypnotic action through their effects on GABA neurotransmission.

Older adults appear to be at risk of increased sensitivity to benzodiazepine effects. Many studies conclude that apparent increased sensitivity to a specific drug dosage can be explained by pharmacokinetics, for example Greenblatt et al. (1991) reported that increased sedation and impairment on psychomotor performance and memory were related to triazolam plasma concentrations, which were greater in elderly subjects. However, a minority of studies have suggested that benzodiazepine sensitivity may be increased independently of pharmacokinetic factors. For example, increased sensitivity to psychomotor, sedative and memory effects were reported in the elderly in a study in which alprazolam was maintained at a similar plateau concentration in both young and older participants to avoid the impact of pharmacokinetic differences (Bertz et al., 1997). This effect does not appear to be attributable to alterations in binding affinity of the GABA/benzodiazepine receptor but might be explained by changes in receptor density.

18.4.1.4 Opioid System

While there is little quantification in the literature relating to humans on age-related changes in the functioning of the opioid system (such as alterations in receptor sensitivity or density), older adults are more vulnerable to side effects when using opioid drugs. While pain relief is mediated through agonism of central μ-opioid receptors, opiate use inevitably activates peripheral μ-opioid receptors such as those in the gastrointestinal system where agonism leads to the commonly observed problem of constipation (Chokhavatia et al., 2016). Older adults, especially those aged over 80, are especially vulnerable to this side effect.

18.4.2 Changes in Homeostatic Mechanisms

Other important pharmacodynamic changes in older adults are linked to the decline of homeostatic systems, relating to control of water balance, posture, circulatory responses and thermoregulation (Bigos et al., 2013), and may interfere with the ability to adapt to physiological effects of medication. For example, ageing is associated with decreased baroreceptor responsivity, which means that orthostatic hypotension is more likely with medications such as prazosin and tricyclic antidepressants (TCAs). Co-prescription of diuretics may exacerbate this problem through their reduction of fluid volume. Further examples of impairments in homeostatic mechanisms include the reduction in peripheral parasympathetic nervous system responses which are dependent on acetylcholine and muscarinic cholinergic receptors, and the increased risk of syndrome of inappropriate antidiuretic hormone secretion (SIADH) when prescribed antidepressants. As a general principle, failure of homeostatic mechanisms creates vulnerabilities which may be exacerbated by drug treatment. For example, the increased risk of falls in older adults is of multifactorial origin, with poor control of posture and orthostatic responses being contributory mechanisms. These problems may be exacerbated by the use of prescribed medications including most psychotropic drugs.

18.5 Age-Related Pharmacokinetic Changes

Pharmacokinetics relates to the impact of bodily systems on ingested drugs, including their absorption, distribution and elimination (see Chapter 4). Ageing can be associated with a wide variety of pharmacokinetic changes. In addition, people are more likely to develop disease as they become older. This has two consequences which add to pharmacokinetic complexity in the elderly. Firstly, organs or body systems already subject to age-related changes may be compromised by dysfunction due to pathological states. Secondly, drugs and other treatments administered to treat diseases or their consequences may themselves cause issues through drug interactions.

Some changes associated with ageing principally affect the absorption process. These include increases in gastric pH, delayed gastric emptying, reduced splanchnic blood flow, decreased gastrointestinal luminal surface and reduction in gastric motility (Klotz, 2009), all of which will tend to reduce absorption (Singh & Bajorek, 2015) leading to the onset of drug actions being delayed.

Changes which affect drug distribution include the relative increase in body fat, which increases the volume of distribution and half-life of most psychotropic drugs since they are lipophilic. Ageing is also associated with reductions in lean body mass and total body water. Serum albumin tends to decrease, which will result in a greater free fraction of any drug that is highly protein bound such as warfarin.

First-pass hepatic metabolism is reduced with age due to reduced hepatic blood flow, so for most drugs there is an increase in bioavailability with ageing. Other changes which impact metabolism and elimination are the increased likelihood that the liver and/or kidneys will function suboptimally with advancing age, thereby slowing down metabolism and/or excretion. Of all pharmacokinetic changes directly associated with ageing, declining renal function is the most consistent finding. A reduction in glomerular filtration rate, amounting to 1 ml/min has been reported for each year over the age of 40 (Wildiers et al., 2003) but around one-third of older adults are reported to have no change in renal function up to the age of 89 years (Lindeman et al., 1985). Reduced renal function is an especially important issue for drugs which are exclusively or predominantly renally excreted such as lithium, amisulpride, sulpiride, gabapentin and pregabalin. Note that a reduction in cardiac output, as occurs in heart failure, will reduce both liver and kidney perfusion, and slow drug elimination through both routes.

The first phase of liver metabolism relies on cytochrome P450 enzymes. While there are many distinct enzymes, it is worth being familiar with a small number of them which together play a prominent role in the metabolism of most psychotropic and non-psychotropic medications. These important enzymes include CYP3A4, CYP2D6, CYP1A2, CYP2C9 and CYP2C19. Among these CYP3A4 is involved in the metabolism of a substantial proportion of psychotropic drugs, the Flockhart table (Flockhart, undated) listing around 80 drugs which are known substrates. There are numerous CYP3A4 inhibitors (Table 18.1), including fluoxetine (through norfluoxetine) and fluvoxamine, while carbamazepine is an inducer of this enzyme. Examples of interactions involving a CYP3A4 inhibitor slowing down the metabolism of a substrate metabolized by this enzyme, and thereby increasing its plasma concentration, include fluoxetine inhibiting zuclopenthixol and erythromycin inhibiting alprazolam. Conversely, adding in the CYP3A4 inducer carbamazepine to the regimen of a person already prescribed haloperidol, a substrate of CYP3A4, would reduce the plasma concentration of the latter and may lead to treatment failure.

After CYP3A4, CYP2D6 (Table 18.2) ranks next in the number of psychotropic and non-psychotropic drugs which are substrates, and its importance in psychiatry is enhanced through paroxetine, fluoxetine and bupropion being strong inhibitors. In the presence of one of these stronger inhibitors any other drug metabolized by CYP2D6 will be broken down more slowly and may have a higher concentration in the blood than

Table 18.1 Psychotropic (and selected other) drugs known to be inhibitors, substrates or inducers of CYP3A4

CYP3A4 inhibitors	
Antidepressants	**Other drugs and substances**
Fluoxetine	Cimetidine
Fluvoxamine	Clarithromycin
	Erythromycin
	Fluconazole
	Ketoconazole
	Verapamil
	HIV antivirals (e.g. indinavir, ritanovir)
	Grapefruit juice

CYP3A4 substrates		
Antidepressants[a]	**Anxiolytics/ hypnotics and antipsychotics**	**Miscellaneous**
Some SSRIs (fluoxetine, escitalopram/citalopram, sertraline)	Alprazolam	Buprenorphine
	Buspirone	Carbamazepine
	Diazepam	Cortisol
Some tricyclics (e.g. amitriptyline, imipramine, nortriptyline)	Midazolam	Dexamethasone
	Suvorexant	Methadone
Mirtazapine		
	Triazolam	Testosterone
Trazodone		
	Zopiclone	Most calcium channel blockers (e.g. amlodipine, diltiazem, nifedipine, verapamil)
Vilazodone	Aripiprazole	
	Haloperidol	
	Lurasidone	Amiodarone
	Quetiapine	
	Risperidone	
	Zuclopenthixol	

[a] Many drugs, including SSRIs and other antidepressants, are metabolized by multiple CYP enzymes.
Adapted from Flockhart (undated).

expected from the dose. CYP2D6 is also important because a proportion of patients (e.g. around 7% of Caucasians) are for genetic reasons 'poor metabolizers' and have little capacity to metabolize drugs by this route.

Table 18.2 Psychotropic (and selected other) drugs known to be inhibitors or substrates of CYP2D6

CYP2D6 inhibitors		
Antidepressants	Other drugs	
Bupropion	Cimetidine	
Duloxetine	Quinidine	
Fluoxetine	Terbinafine	
Paroxetine		
Sertraline (weak)		
CYP2D6 substrates		
Antidepressants[a]	**Antipsychotics**	**Miscellaneous**
All SSRIs	Chlorpromazine	Atomoxetine
Duloxetine	Haloperidol	Codeine
Venlafaxine	Perphenazine	Dexfenfluramine
Many tricylics:	Risperidone	Dextromethorphan
e.g. imipramine,	Zuclopenthixol	Dihydrocodeine
amitriptyline,		Donepezil
clomipramine,		Hydrocodone
nortriptyline		MCPP[b]
Reboxetine		MDMA (ecstasy)
Vortioxetine		Tramadol
		Some β-blockers:
		propranolol
		metoprolol, timolol
		bufaralol, carvedilol

[a] Many drugs, including SSRIs and other antidepressants, are metabolized by multiple CYP enzymes.
[b] MCPP (meta-chlorophenylpiperazine) is a CYP2D6 substrate and is a metabolite of trazodone through a CYP3A4-mediated metabolic step.
Adapted from Flockhart (undated).

CYP1A2 is involved in the metabolism of clozapine (and several other psychotropic drugs) and is responsible for the interaction of clozapine with tobacco smoking (since smoking induces CYP1A2, thereby increasing the rate of clozapine metabolism and decreasing its expected concentration in the blood relative to the dose given). CYP2C9 (inhibited by fluvoxamine) or CYP2C19 (moderately inhibited by fluoxetine) are also potentially important.

With ageing not only is cytochrome P450-based metabolism reduced due to diminished hepatic blood flow, but for certain enzymes there appears to be a further reduction in activity with ageing which cannot be explained by decreased perfusion. However, overall the effect of age-related changes per se on cytochrome P450-mediated metabolism is of lesser importance than the impact of co-prescribed medications which tend to become more prevalent with increasing age (Davies et al., 2004) and are more likely to include drugs known to be inhibitors of specific cytochrome P450 enzymes (Kerr et al., 2014). Similarly, the progressive increase in the number and dose of co-prescribed medications with age is probably the most important factor in accentuating the impact of known genetic polymorphisms, such as being a poor metabolizer with respect to CYP2D6 (Kirchheiner & Seeringer, 2007). Individuals with a poor metabolizer genotype for CYP2D6 may have elevated plasma concentrations of drugs metabolized by this enzyme unless alternative metabolic pathways are available. For example, there is some evidence that CYP2D6 poor metabolizers may be especially susceptible to high drug concentrations when they are elderly (Waade et al., 2014) – which has led to suggestions that a small proportion of elderly patients starting venlafaxine may experience unexpectedly high drug exposure, a risk which could be mitigated by genotyping. A recent pilot study (Finkelstein et al., 2016) has identified that elderly people who experience repeated hospitalizations due to polypharmacy and medication side-effects have a significantly higher frequency of genotypes associated with poor or ultrarapid metabolizer status with respect to pharmacogenetics than do individuals of a similar age who are rarely hospitalized.

Other changes not directly related to the ageing process, or to the increased burden of disease and increased use of prescribed medications, include alterations in diet (e.g. reduced overall intake, or increasing intake of a specific item which can impact on drug metabolism such as grapefruit juice, which is an inhibitor of CYP3A4), changes in smoking status and alcohol use.

18.6 Increased Prevalence of Medical Disorders and Drugs Administered with Advancing Age

Advancing age sees an increased prevalence of medical disorders and drugs administered and both can impact on the pharmacokinetics and pharmacodynamics of antipsychotic drugs that are prescribed. In addition, physical co-morbidity can make older people more vulnerable to adverse drug effects. There are several reasons why elderly patients who require treatment for psychiatric disorders are at greater risk of having medical disorders than the general population. Firstly, the prevalence of many physical disorders increases markedly with age. Hypertension is rare in the third and fourth decades but for individuals aged over 60 is common and increasingly prevalent in each further decade of life. Many other disorders affecting the cardiovascular, respiratory, gastrointestinal and musculoskeletal systems are associated with similar patterns of increased prevalence with ageing. At the same time, certain common psychiatric disorders are associated causally with medical problems. For example, depression has been reported to be an independent risk factor for diabetes and myocardial infarction (Evans et al., 2005). Associations between psychiatric disorders and subsequent medical disorders may be underpinned by biological mechanisms (e.g. increased platelet reactivity in depression increasing the risk of stroke) (Musselman et al., 1996), be attributable to psychotropic drug treatment representing a risk factor for specific physical problems (e.g. clozapine, olanzapine and quetiapine contributing to risk of hypertension, diabetes or hyperlipidaemia), or occur for behavioural reasons (e.g. severe depression or psychotic illness leading to disengagement with medical treatment and supporting services essential to recovery). In addition, sensory problems or cognitive impairment may impair an individual's ability to take medication as prescribed or engage in other health-promoting activities.

With the increased prevalence of medical co-morbidity with advancing age, there is an increased likelihood of older patients who require treatment for psychiatric disorders receiving more drugs, and thereby greater potential for both pharmacokinetic and pharmacodynamic interactions. For example, when prescribing patterns on general adult and 'functional' elderly psychiatric inpatient units (i.e. excluding wards specifically for patients with dementia) were compared (Davies et al., 2004), patients on the functional elderly wards were administered over 70% more drugs per day and were significantly more likely to be taking combinations judged to be potentially clinically important pharmacokinetic interactions through CYP3A4. Examples of pharmacodynamic interactions involving psychotropic drugs include (i) cholinesterase inhibitors with drugs used in overactive bladder (due to opposing actions on the cholinergic system); (ii) L-dopa + a dopamine receptor antagonist used to treat psychosis (due to opposing actions on the dopamine system); (iii) serotonin reuptake inhibitors to treat depression + pro-serotonergic drugs (e.g. L-tryptophan; sumatriptan for migraine – due to additive actions on the serotonergic system); (iv) serotonin reuptake inhibitors + monoamine oxidase inhibitors (MAOIs) (due to potential for the inhibition of monoamine oxidase to leave the patient vulnerable to excessive monoamine actions); and (v) serotonin reuptake inhibitor + antiplatelet drugs (due to the possibility of antiplatelet drugs exacerbating the tendency of serotonin reuptake inhibitors to inhibit platelet activity, thereby increasing the risk of bleeding). Various approaches have been examined to reduce the likelihood of adverse reactions occurring in older adults including those led by pharmacists or other professionals, physician education and technology-based interventions (Gray et al., 2018). When all studies were pooled these interventions had a statistically significant effect and reduced the incidence of adverse drug reactions by 21%.

In summary, the consequence of the increased burden of disease in older people experiencing psychiatric disorders is the potential for increased complexity in every aspect of psychotropic drug treatment. The presence of greater numbers of existing medications and the interactions they may produce when new drugs are added, the disruption of systems involved in drug absorption, distribution, metabolism and excretion, and the impact of medical disorders on neurotransmitter functions and homeostatic mechanisms all contribute to the need for heightened vigilance on the part of the prescriber.

18.7 Pharmacological Treatment of Depression

After dementia, depressive disorders carry the greatest disease burden among the psychiatric disorders in terms of DALYs lost in older adults. Prognosis in treatment of depression is poorer with advancing age as well as in males (Calati et al., 2013). The question of whether increasing age is associated with risk of relapse after remission of depression with drug treatment is a complex one. There is evidence to suggest that age, per se, does not confer increased risk, but the presence and burden of co-morbid medical illnesses is a more clear-cut risk factor, and elderly people are more likely to have these characteristics. As in younger populations, there is evidence that continued treatment with antidepressants after remission reduces likelihood of relapse. A meta-analysis reported a protective effect of continuing antidepressants in studies which followed patients for between 6 and 36 months after remission, both overall and in seven of the eight trials included (Kok et al., 2011). The decision of how long to continue and indeed whether to stop antidepressants is down to patient preference although a pattern of recurrent relapse after antidepressant discontinuation should point towards the need for sustained treatment.

Each of the many antidepressant drugs available for use in younger adults can be used in elderly patients. These include monoamine reuptake inhibitors (e.g. SSRIs, serotonin and noradrenaline reuptake inhibitors (SNRIs), TCAs, bupropion, reboxetine), receptor blockers (e.g. trazodone, mirtazapine, agomelatine), enzyme inhibitors (reversible and irreversible MAOIs) and multimodal drugs (e.g. vortioxetine). Treatment trials specifically in the elderly are fewer in number than those for younger adults, which means that treatment recommendations employ extrapolation of evidence from trials in younger adults. However, there are a reasonable number of randomized trials for depression which have been conducted specifically in the elderly which will be mentioned below. There has been some controversy about whether antidepressants are sufficiently effective in older adults to merit use. A meta-analysis published in 2011 (Tedeschini et al., 2011) suggested that across eight trials identified in individuals aged over 65 antidepressants did not outperform placebo significantly in terms of response rate; however, when trials which included individuals aged over 55 were added, bringing the total to 15, there was a statistically significant benefit in favour of antidepressants. Subsequent studies appear to have offered greater reassurance to prescribers – for instance a meta-analysis which included a larger number of randomized trials by additionally examining unpublished data (Kok et al., 2012) reported that all three antidepressant types examined (SSRIs, TCAs and others) were significantly more likely to be associated with response than was placebo, and when the three groups were combined there was also an association with remission.

For each subtype of antidepressants, there are specific considerations relating to side-effect profile and interactions which must be borne in mind when prescribing in elderly patients, especially those who are frail, have medical co-morbidities or are co-prescribed potentially interacting drugs.

18.7.1 Selective Serotonin Reuptake Inhibitors[1] and Serotonin and Noradrenaline Reuptake Inhibitors

These drug classes are the most widely used in depression in the elderly, and there are several trials in older adults which supplement the well-demonstrated evidence of their efficacy in younger people. In a network meta-analysis of 15 trials in the elderly, the drugs which demonstrated the clearest evidence of efficacy were sertraline, paroxetine and duloxetine (Thorlund et al., 2015). There is some evidence that the elderly take longer to respond and may therefore require longer trials than younger adults.

Selective serotonin reuptake inhibitors (SSRIs) are associated with an increased risk of bleeding, which may be of particular importance in elderly patients taking anticoagulants such as warfarin, or who have a previous history of bleeding incidents. Risk of gastrointestinal bleeding can be mitigated by use of proton pump inhibitors. Both SSRIs and Serotonin and Noradrenaline Reuptake Inhibitors (SNRIs) are associated with reduction in sodium concentration, which means that it is wise to check electrolytes prior to initiation and periodically afterwards. Hyponatraemia most commonly manifests in the first two weeks of treatment, and may lead to symptom such as tiredness, urinary incontinence, low blood pressure, and in more severe cases, vomiting, delirium and hallucinations. Most SSRIs and SNRIs carry limited risk of anticholinergic effects, but an exception is paroxetine, which has some affinity

[1] SSRIs fall within the category of serotonin reuptake inhibitors in NbN.

for muscarinic receptors and therefore a more substantial risk of anticholinergic effects. The consequences of 'anticholinergic burden' are discussed below in the section on drugs used for psychosis.

Many SSRIs and SNRIs inhibit important cytochrome P450 enzymes. In the elderly this is especially important since many patients who require these drugs may already be taking other medications metabolized by these enzymes, and introducing an inhibitor may increase the plasma concentration of co-prescribed drugs unless they can be metabolized by an alternative route. Fluoxetine, which inhibits both CYP3A4 (through norfluoxetine) and CYP2D6, and paroxetine, a strong CYP2D6 inhibitor, can be particularly problematic whereas sertraline, which exerts weaker inhibition, or escitalopram is often easier to use when faced with a patient on multiple medications. Duloxetine is another CYP2D6 inhibitor.

In general, SSRIs should be started at lower doses when treating depression in the elderly. This is due both to increased sensitivity to side effects and also to the likelihood that pharmacokinetic changes (e.g. reduced hepatic enzyme activity and renal function) will result in higher circulating plasma concentrations for a given dose. For SNRIs these effects appear to be less prominent and it is therefore reasonable to use similar starting doses in the elderly as are used in younger adults. However, venlafaxine has an exception in the minority of older adults who are genetically CYP2D6 poor metabolizers; as it is metabolized by CYP2D6 it is very susceptible to having markedly reduced clearance and therefore increased circulating concentrations in this group. One study reported concentrations in elderly CYP2D6 poor metabolizers being eight times greater than in those aged 40 (Waade et al., 2014). If an elderly person starting venlafaxine is known to be a poor metabolizer with respect to CYP2D6 (where genotyping is available) or has a history of poor tolerance to previously used antidepressants or other drugs metabolized by this enzyme it would be wise to start with low doses of 37.5 mg/day or less.

A 2016 Canadian guideline (MacQueen et al., 2016) describes there being a 'dissonance' in the fact that escitalopram is preferred over paroxetine and fluoxetine in both this and earlier guidelines, and in the current practice of most old age psychiatrists since paroxetine and fluoxetine have greater numbers of successful placebo-controlled trials in the elderly, but escitalopram has none – in fact both of the trials undertaken with escitalopram were negative. Even sertraline has only one randomized placebo-controlled trial specifically in the elderly which reported a modest, but significant effect (Schneider et al., 2003). However, old age psychiatrists' tendency to prioritize sertraline and escitalopram illustrates the point that the existence of successful trials specifically in the elderly is merely one of several factors which must be considered when weighing the advantages and disadvantages of competing drugs for use in the elderly. The preference for sertraline and escitalopram is most likely due to (i) the extrapolation of trial evidence and clinical experience from younger patients (although sertraline has performed well in the above-mentioned network meta-analysis for trials in the elderly (Thorlund et al., 2015)); (ii) the lower risk of P450 interactions with sertraline and escitalopram; and (iii) absence of other undesirable features such as paroxetine's association with difficult withdrawal and anticholinergic side effects. However, in recent years evidence has emerged suggesting that citalopram may cause dose-dependent QTc prolongation, a risk factor for ventricular arrhythmia. The evidence linking escitalopram to this problem is less robust (Qirjazi et al., 2016) but guidance in several countries, including the United Kingdom, advises that in people aged over 65, 20 mg/

day should be the maximum dose of citalopram used and 10 mg/day for escitalopram. Although any possible association of escitalopram with QTc prolongation appears to be weaker and less robust than that for citalopram, it may nevertheless make this drug a less attractive choice than it was before this issue emerged.

Among SNRIs, venlafaxine, which has some randomized trial evidence of efficacy specifically in late-life depression (Hewett et al., 2010), appears to be associated with a variety of side effects in the elderly including nausea, dry mouth, dizziness, hyperhidrosis, insomnia, constipation, tremor, anorexia and male sexual dysfunction. Blood pressure monitoring is essential at doses of 150 mg/day or more. Duloxetine has randomized controlled trial (RCT) evidence in older adults including two trials for depression in the elderly in which it was significantly more efficacious than placebo (Katona et al., 2012; Raskin et al., 2007). Of other SNRI drugs available in certain countries, the venlafaxine metabolite desvenlafaxine lacks trials evidence specific to the elderly. However, levomilnacipran, an isomer of milnacipran introduced in the USA in 2013, has an intriguing pharmacological property in addition to its noradrenaline and serotonin reuptake inhibition in that it inhibits an amyloid precursor protein-cleaving enzyme, and so offers the theoretical possibility of reducing amyloid plaque formation in Alzheimer's. Lower doses may be necessary in patients with hepatic or renal disease.

Evidence exists to suggest that SSRIs may be effective in specific subpopulations of older adults. For example, there are trials reporting efficacy in individuals who have had acute myocardial infarction or unstable angina (Glassman et al., 2002). For people with Alzheimer's and co-morbid depression the picture is mixed, with a recent meta-analysis (Ortega et al., 2017) finding no significant benefit of antidepressants over placebo overall across seven trials. Both of the two individual trials that did show a significant treatment effect employed SSRIs as opposed to other antidepressants, but a large multi-centre trial involving sertraline was negative (Rosenberg et al., 2010).

18.7.2 Bupropion

Bupropion may be associated with reduced clearance and the possibility of accumulation in elderly individuals who have poor hepatic function. It is a strong inhibitor of CYP2D6 and is associated with a falls risk through provocation of orthostatic hypotension. The risk of seizures requires consideration. Its use in the elderly is supported by RCT evidence (Weihs et al., 2000) although, like many other antidepressants, not all placebo-controlled trials have demonstrated efficacy in this age group (Hewett et al., 2010).

18.7.3 Tricyclic Antidepressants

The problems inherent in using terms such as tricyclic antidepressants (TCAs) have been discussed in the Editor's Note on Nomenclature that deals with Neuroscience-based Nomenclature (NbN). However, given that the term TCA has been used for approximately 70 years it is unlikely to be abandoned by clinicians in the near future, so it is retained in this chapter. Most of the TCAs exert their therapeutic effect through noradrenaline reuptake inhibition accompanied by varying degrees of serotonin reuptake inhibition, but all impact a range of other pharmacological systems. As a result, TCAs can generally cause a wider range of side effects than subsequently introduced SNRIs (for example venlafaxine and duloxetine) which were more specific in their range of actions. TCAs are no longer considered first-line agents in depression for the elderly. Anticholinergic symptoms may be prominent, although nortriptyline and desipramine may present fewer problems in this area than other tricyclic agents. Clomipramine continues to have a role in treating both depression and obsessive-compulsive disorder (OCD) in the elderly if its anticholinergic side effects can be tolerated (Stage et al., 2002). While nortriptyline's kinetics do not appear to be influenced by advancing age, age has much more profound effects with imipramine which means that standard adult doses will result in appreciably higher circulating concentrations, necessitating dose reduction. Some anticholinergic symptoms are especially problematic in older adults due to pharmacokinetic considerations, for example constipation is more likely as gut motility declines. Another anticholinergic effect which may be problematic in the elderly is impaired cognition. Similarly, other TCA side effects such as α_1-adrenoceptor antagonism leading to orthostatic hypotension can have greater implications in the elderly as baroreceptor reflexes are less able to buffer the blood pressure, which leads to an increased risk of falls. Finally, as elderly individuals may be at greater risk of accidental overdose, a further issue with most TCAs (with the exception of lofepramine) is the association with increased risk of death in overdose relative to SSRIs and SNRIs.

18.7.4 Mirtazapine

Mirtazapine has been compared with paroxetine in a study specific to the elderly and was superior for some efficacy measures and in having fewer discontinuation symptoms (Schatzberg et al., 2002). Mirtazapine may be cleared more slowly in the elderly so it is wise to start at a 7.5 mg dose and increase in 7.5 mg increments. Mirtazapine is often given preference when poor sleep is a feature of depression because it can cause sedation due to high affinity for histamine H_1 receptors, but in the frail elderly the risk of oversedation should be monitored. Note that mirtazapine is sometimes combined with SSRIs/SNRIs based on a small evidence base in younger adults that the combination is more effective than monotherapy (Blier et al., 2010), although this was not replicated in a recent primary care-based trial (Kessler et al., 2018). It should be noted that some combinations, such as fluoxetine-mirtazapine may result in inhibition of mirtazapine metabolism which may require use of lower mirtazapine doses than would be employed if mirtazapine were to be prescribed alone. As in younger adults, mirtazapine has the advantage of carrying little risk of sexual side effects, but the disadvantage of being associated with weight gain.

18.7.5 Trazodone

Trazodone is another drug used for depression which is often selected when sleep problems are present. It is often prescribed off-label for insomnia in the absence of depression due to its α-adrenergic and histamine blockade. Trazodone should be titrated slowly from low starting doses (e.g. 25 mg/day). While for insomnia a typical dose range is 25–100 mg/day, in depression higher doses are often required in the range of 100–200 mg/day or more, and longer trials may be required than would be the standard for younger patients. While the risk of anticholinergic effects is low there is a risk of falls through orthostatic hypotension and of priapism in males. Both CYP2D6 and CYP3A4 are involved in its metabolism so vigilance for interactions is required.

18.7.6 Monoamine Oxidase Inhibitors

Both reversible (moclobemide) and irreversible inhibitors of monoamine oxidase (phenelzine, tranylcypromine) may be used in the elderly, but moclobemide presents fewer issues in terms of dietary restrictions and potential for dangerous drug interactions, although it can be associated with orthostatic hypotension. Moclobemide can be prescribed at similar doses to those used in younger adults. There have been suggestions that as monoamine oxidase becomes more abundant with ageing these drugs have the potential to be more effective in older patients. Moclobemide was also effective in a randomized placebo-controlled trial of elderly patients with depression and dementia or cognitive decline (Roth et al., 1996), with some evidence of improved cognitive function in moclobemide-treated patients. Irreversible monoamine oxidase inhibitors (MAOIs) are reserved only for treatment-resistant depression as well as the occasional patient who had responded well to phenelzine or tranylcypromine at an earlier stage in life (possibly several decades ago when antidepressant choices were far more limited and irreversible MAOIs were therefore used more readily) and chooses to use the same drug again. If recommending irreversible MAOIs to an elderly patient it would be essential to discuss the potential for interactions with foods and other drugs and for the prescriber to be confident that the intended recipient and/or their carers understand the importance of following the restrictions so that the drug can be taken safely.

18.7.7 Vilazodone

This drug has both SSRI-like properties and is a partial agonist of the 5-HT_{1A} receptor. It is a substrate of CYP3A4. It has the useful property of the starting dose of 10 mg/day not needing adjustment in people with declining renal or hepatic function. There are no trials specifically in the elderly, although one successful trial included patients up to the age of 70 years.

18.7.8 Vortioxetine

Vortioxetine is a multimodal antidepressant with agonist, antagonist and partial agonist actions across several serotonin receptors as well as SSRI activity. It is metabolized by CYP2D6. The standard dose of 10 mg/day, which can be increased to 20 mg/day, does not require adjustment in renal or mild to moderate hepatic impairment, although a lower starting dose of 5 mg/day is advised in the case of frailty. It has one RCT specifically for depression in the elderly (Katona et al., 2012) and in this the efficacy of the 5 mg dose was similar to that of 60 mg/day of duloxetine and significantly better than placebo. For vortioxetine only nausea was significantly more common than with placebo but for duloxetine several side effects were observed more frequently. There is some suggestion from this trial that vortioxetine may improve cognitive performance in depression compared with placebo, with improved performance for vortioxetine on both a test of executive function (the Digit Symbol Substitution test) and a test of attention (the Rey Auditory Verbal Learning test); duloxetine only improved the latter.

18.7.9 Agomelatine

This melatonin receptor agonist and serotonin 5-HT_2 receptor antagonist is known for having few sexual side effects and beneficial effects on sleep regulation. A randomized trial for recurrent depressive disorder in the elderly suggested that response rates, if not remission rates, were superior to placebo (Heun et al., 2013).

18.7.10 Reboxetine

The noradrenaline reuptake inhibitor reboxetine has comparative randomized trial data in the elderly in which doses of 4–6 mg/day had similar efficacy to imipramine (50–100 mg/day) but with less incidence of hypotension and serious adverse events (Katona et al., 1999). Caution is advised in frail individuals.

18.7.11 Other Biological Treatments Used in Depression

In younger adults, evidence exists for using several other drugs in the treatment of depression, either as monotherapy or as augmentation of traditional antidepressants. These drugs include lithium, risperidone, olanzapine, quetiapine and aripiprazole, the stimulant methylphenidate, tri-iodothyronine and the anaesthetic agent ketamine. Some of these drugs have evidence for depression specifically in the elderly while others rely on evidence from younger populations, but all are options which may be employed when standard antidepressants have not provided adequate response. For example, there are successful placebo-controlled randomized trials for depression in older adults with quetiapine as monotherapy (Katila et al., 2013) and with aripiprazole added to venlafaxine (Lenze et al., 2015). Methylphenidate has been employed in an RCT in older out-patients in which the combination of methylphenidate with citalopram was compared with methylphenidate + placebo and citalopram + placebo (Lavretsky et al., 2015). The group assigned to the two active drugs was observed to have greater and more rapid response than either of the two groups assigned to monotherapy, although these benefits came at the cost of a sustained increase in heart rate.

Other drugs which may be used in treatment-resistant depression in combination include lithium, which will be discussed more fully later in this chapter in the context of bipolar disorder. There is open randomized trial evidence in that lithium augmentation is more effective in augmenting antidepressants for depression in older adults than is switching to an MAOI (Kok et al., 2007). Tri-iodothyronine augmentation has largely fallen out of use in all ages and its use in the elderly requires caution due to risks associated with cardiovascular function.

Although there have been no trials specific to the elderly, case reports indicate that older patients may benefit from ketamine (intravenously or via intranasal inhalation) in the treatment of depression. Since aspects of cognitive impairment, including poor memory and poor concentration, have been reported in RCTs in younger patients a caveat exists when extrapolating evidence to the elderly in that it remains possible that ketamine may pose some risks in individuals with limited cognitive reserve.

Electroconvulsive therapy (ECT) may be used safely in the elderly to treat depression and other psychiatric disorders (see Chapter 16). Overall, its efficacy is similar to that in younger patients. Advancing age in the absence of medical co-morbidities presents no additional risks. ECT remains an option for depressed patients in the context of early dementia.

The use of rTMS (repetitive transcranial magnetic stimulation) for depression in the elderly is becoming increasingly widespread (see Chapter 16). This non-invasive treatment is typically administered daily, or several times a week and involves the application of a magnetic field to the surface of the scalp. While some initial meta-analyses suggested limited efficacy in the elderly, the evidence base has now advanced to the point where we can be confident that rTMS is as effective in older adults as it is in those aged under 65, provided treatment of sufficient duration and intensity is given. Previous trials which reported reduced efficacy in the elderly appear to have delivered fewer pulses than those in which efficacy was comparable to younger patients (Sabesan et al., 2015). While rTMS is not associated with the rapid response typically seen with ECT, it has the advantages of not requiring anaesthesia and having no association with cognitive deficits, even in subjects having pre-existing cerebrovascular disease.

18.8 Pharmacological Treatment of Anxiety Disorders

Anxiety symptoms are common in the elderly, either as primary disorders, or secondary to depression or other diagnoses. Anxiety disorders amenable to drug treatment include generalized anxiety disorder (GAD), panic disorder, social anxiety disorder and post-traumatic stress disorder. Although anxiety disorders can occur in previously unaffected patients late in life, the majority occur in people who have had previous episodes. In some elderly people who have had a long-standing tendency to worry, anxiety about their health may be a prominent feature, and it is common for such individuals to extend their worries and ruminations to the possible side effects and interactions of their medications. It is therefore especially important when prescribing drugs to treat anxiety disorders that older patients are allowed to discuss their concerns and that the prescriber is able to offer reassurance about the balance of risk and benefits.

18.8.1 SSRIs and SNRIs

As in younger adults, across the various anxiety disorders SSRIs and the SNRI venlafaxine are considered first-line drug treatments in the elderly. For GAD the SNRI duloxetine can also be considered first line. SSRIs are also first line in OCD. There is some randomized trial data to support a number of these agents in elderly populations. There are successful placebo-controlled randomized trials for duloxetine (Alaka et al., 2014) in GAD and citalopram (Lenze et al., 2005) in people with anxiety disorders aged over 65. Escitalopram has one trial in GAD in older adults (Lenze et al., 2009) which showed some advantages over placebo but the difference on the main intention-to-treat analysis was not significant. Venlafaxine is supported in older adults with GAD by a pooled analysis (Katz et al., 2002).

18.8.2 Pregabalin/Gabapentin

Use of pregabalin, described as an 'alternative first-line treatment' for GAD in recent UK guidelines (Baldwin et al., 2014) on the basis of several trials in younger adults, is supported in the elderly by there being one successful randomized placebo-controlled trial which was undertaken exclusively in patients aged over 65 (Montgomery et al., 2008). Both pregabalin and its sister drug gabapentin are renally excreted and therefore dose adjustment is required in cases of renal impairment – where this is suspected it is wise to obtain a blood test for estimated glomerular filtration rate (eGFR) and follow guidelines from a source such as the *British National Formulary*, which advises on regimens and maximum doses for specific ranges of eGFR (Joint Formulary Committee, 2017). Pregabalin and gabapentin can cause dizziness and motor incoordination and can therefore be associated with falls, thus a lower starting dose would be preferred in any elderly person who is frail or has a history of falling. Both drugs can be associated with daytime sedation. If this is problematic, instead of dividing up doses equally, the majority of the daily dose should be given at bedtime.

18.8.3 Benzodiazepines

Several studies report a reduction in benzodiazepine prescription rates in the elderly in recent years (Davies et al., 2018b), although this is offset in part by increases in the use of Z-drugs such as zopiclone for insomnia. There are several successful trials of benzodiazepines for anxiety disorders in the elderly but all were conducted more than 20 years ago. Despite this evidence base, specialist prescribers are often reluctant to offer benzodiazepines to older patients given that they have several pitfalls in this age group, and when they are prescribed will aim to keep the duration of regular use short or else restrict them to use as 'rescue medication' – i.e. for PRN use in emergencies only. However, it remains common for psychiatrists and other prescribers to inherit patients who are already established on benzodiazepines and here the risks of continued use must be balanced against the clinical benefits they have delivered and with the difficulty and discomfort that might result from stopping or reducing them. Due to the potential for declining liver function or hepatic disease in elderly populations, benzodiazepines subject to Phase I metabolism (e.g. nitrazepam) present a risk of accumulation. There is also a risk of pharmacodynamic interactions with other drugs that produce sedation. The association with tolerance and difficult withdrawal observed in younger populations is also relevant in the elderly. Although many patients can stop benzodiazepines successfully if they reduce the dose gradually in small increments, there may be subgroups of elderly patients who are highly sensitive to withdrawal symptoms especially those who have been taking benzodiazepines consistently for many years. The elderly are also at greater risk of falls and fractures from benzodiazepines than younger patients due to effects on coordination, balance and gait (Cumming & Le Couteur, 2003). These risks are dose dependent. The elderly are susceptible to an increased risk of car accidents while taking benzodiazepines and long-acting benzodiazepines, such as diazepam and nitrazepam, are especially implicated (Thomas, 1998). Benzodiazepines are associated with several measurable impairments in cognitive performance, especially in longer-term use (Crowe & Stranks, 2017). However, while benzodiazepines were previously thought to increase risk of dementia, a recent prospective population-based cohort study (Gray et al., 2016) did not support a causal association. Interestingly, in another study (Chung et al., 2016) which employed brain imaging, benzodiazepine use was associated with lesser amyloid aggregation.

18.8.4 Dopamine Receptor Antagonists in Anxiety Disorders

The use of dopamine receptor antagonists (i.e. drugs traditionally referred to as 'antipsychotics') to treat anxiety disorders in any age group represents off-label use. However, there is supportive evidence from trials for using specific drugs in specific anxiety disorders in younger adults. By inference antipsychotics may be prescribed in the elderly for some anxiety disorders. Examples include the use of quetiapine monotherapy in GAD (Maneeton et al., 2016) and aripiprazole, risperidone and haloperidol to augment antidepressants in OCD (Dold et al., 2015). In every case, dopamine receptor antagonists are recommended for use in anxiety disorders only where drug treatments with a more established evidence base such as serotonin reuptake inhibitors, venlafaxine and, in the case of GAD, pregabalin or duloxetine have already been considered.

A further alternative drug in GAD is buspirone, which is not associated with sedation or falls in the elderly, although lower doses are required in the presence of either renal or hepatic impairment.

18.9 Pharmacological Treatment of Insomnia

Guidelines suggest that the first steps in treating insomnia are not pharmacological but involve exclusion of physical, psychiatric and drug-related causes and promotion of good sleep hygiene, such as going to bed at a regular time, avoiding caffeine in the afternoon and evening and ensuring the bedroom is quiet and otherwise appropriate for restful sleep. When medications are required there are a wide range of possibilities to consider in older adults (for review see Shroeck et al., 2016).

Benzodiazepines are still used to counter insomnia, but Z-drugs such as zopiclone, zolpidem and zaleplon (and in some countries the zopiclone isomer eszopiclone) have been progressively replacing them over the past two decades. Zopiclone has the longest half-life of the three, around 4–5 hours but this is typically increased to 8 hours in the elderly. Zaleplon has the shortest half-life of around one hour (Terzano et al., 2003) and may reduce the time to onset of sleep as well as subjectively related sleep quality. For all three of these drugs, lower starting doses are recommended for elderly patients, which are 50% of the adult starting dose.

However, Z-drugs share many of the benzodiazepines' properties, including the possibility of tolerance and risks of falls and fractures. All three Z-drugs have been noted to increase the risk of hip fracture (Berry et al., 2013; Lin et al., 2014) with the risk being increased in individuals with cognitive or functional impairment. Meta-analysis has revealed that zopiclone and zolpidem may be associated with impairments in verbal memory and other measures of cognitive performance (Stranks & Crowe, 2014).

There are various alternative pharmacological approaches for insomnia. In the United Kingdom, melatonin is licensed specifically for insomnia in people aged over 55. It should be noted that to use melatonin within the terms of its licence it should be used for no longer than 13 weeks. Alternative drugs which may be used to promote sleep in older patients, provided the risks and benefits are considered, include trazodone and agomelatine, histamine H_1 receptor antagonists (e.g. chlorpheniramine) and a sub-dopamine receptor-blocking dose of quetiapine. However, when any of the drugs mentioned in this section are used in older patients to encourage sleep, it is essential to consider not only the sleep-promoting drug's side effects, but also the possibility of any existing co-prescribed drugs having sedative or other central nervous system effects which might lead to oversedation or even to confusion. It should be noted that trazodone, which is increasingly used in older adults to promote sleep irrespective of the presence or absence of depression, is, like benzodiazepines, associated with increased risk of falls in this age group (Coupland et al., 2011).

The novel melatonin agonist ramelteon should be used with caution in the elderly as its half-life is typically increased compared with that in younger adults. It may also be subject to interactions with CYP1A2 inhibitors such as fluvoxamine. Another novel agent, the orexin antagonist suvorexant has two trials which have included elderly patients and has shown efficacy at the 30 mg dose (Michelson et al., 2014) in terms of reducing time to onset of sleep and maintaining sleep. Suvorexant is a CYP3A4 substrate necessitating caution with fluoxetine, verapamil, diltiazem and other inhibitors of this enzyme.

18.10 Pharmacological Treatment of Psychotic Disorders

There is a wide range of potential indications for use of dopamine receptor antagonists (i.e. antipsychotics) in the elderly. The majority relate to clinical situations in which such drugs are similarly indicated in younger adults (see Chapter 9). These include the treatment of schizophrenia and related psychotic disorders, mania, the prophylaxis of bipolar affective disorder, as adjuncts to antidepressant drugs in the treatment of depression and OCD, and occasionally as monotherapy in depression and GAD. In older people, dopamine receptor antagonists are sometimes used to treat behavioural and psychological symptoms of dementia (BPSD), including aggression and agitation as well as psychosis. Non-pharmacological approaches are normally used first, but when they are unsuccessful in controlling these symptoms pharmacological treatments may be needed. Leaving aside acetylcholinesterase inhibitors and memantine, which should be optimized where appropriate in patients with BPSD to provide cognitive-enhancing treatment for the underlying dementia, dopamine receptor antagonists have the strongest evidence base for treating agitation and aggression in BPSD in Alzheimer's disease. Risperidone is approved or licensed for short-term use for management of persistent aggression in Alzheimer's unresponsive to non-pharmacological interventions, in both the United Kingdom and Canada. However, use of antipsychotic drugs requires careful consideration and discussion with caregivers due to their association with an increased risk of mortality (Maust et al., 2015) which has to be balanced against the potential benefits of mitigating the wide-ranging consequences of recurrent episodes of agitation and aggressive behaviour. Readers are referred to a recent paper (Davies et al., 2018a) which discusses this balance and describes a sequential drug treatment algorithm for agitation and aggression in Alzheimer's or mixed Alzheimer's/vascular dementia initially developed for hospital inpatient settings where it is now widely used, and to Chapter 14 where use of antipsychotic drugs in BPSD is discussed in detail. Here only the use of dopamine receptor antagonists for functional psychiatric disorders will be reviewed.

When considering the treatment of schizophrenia and related psychotic disorders in the elderly two distinct groups can be identified. The majority of elderly individuals with schizophrenia will have received the diagnosis much earlier in life. While schizophrenia is associated with shorter life expectancy, in the modern era many people who have received this diagnosis will live into their 60s or beyond and will require ongoing treatment. However, a small proportion of elderly people have their first onset of psychosis after 60 and may be considered to have late-onset schizophrenia. Unfortunately, there are few adequate drug trials to guide treatment of the latter group, a Cochrane review (Esali & Ali, 2012) identifying only one trial of sufficiently robust design to meet criteria for inclusion which recruited 44 patients with late-onset schizophrenia, so it is difficult to make evidence-based judgements for this population.

In general, elderly patients who have had a diagnosis of schizophrenia made earlier in life will be offered dopamine antagonists based on any history of previous response or intolerance, consideration of medical problems and potential interactions, and application of the evidence base from younger adults. There are only a small number of RCTs undertaken specifically in the elderly. These trials include a randomized trial comparing risperidone and olanzapine in older patients who had had schizophrenia or schizoaffective disorder for a mean duration of 36 years. Both groups improved over eight weeks but with no statistically significant difference in efficacy between the two, and similar drop-out rates (Jeste et al., 2003). Another trial compared extended-release paliperidone with placebo in patients with schizophrenia aged over 65 (Tzimos et al., 2008). Although the benefits of the active drug over placebo were limited and non-significant the dopamine antagonist was well tolerated. An older trial reported that clozapine and chlorpromazine were equally effective, but clozapine was associated with excess weight gain and tachycardia while chlorpromazine was associated with sedation. Other trials provide some further evidence for using risperidone and olanzapine in elderly patients, although with less robust study design. Outside of these relatively limited examples of trials conducted specifically in the elderly, psychiatrists treating geriatric populations will consider evidence of efficacy in younger populations with schizophrenia but will be especially mindful of the potential for side effects, toxicity and interactions.

All dopamine antagonist drugs present the prescriber with concerns relating to their side-effect profiles. As we have discussed earlier, these concerns carry greater weight than in younger populations due to pharmacokinetic and pharmacodynamic changes associated with ageing (due for example to changes in liver function, renal clearance and cardiac output) and the possibility that elder people will have less reserve to maintain homeostasis in the face of changes associated with drug effects. Examples of dose adjustments required due to pharmacological considerations include the need to reduce risperidone doses where liver function is impaired (as the first metabolic step is mediated mainly by CYP2D6 and partly by CYP3A4). In the case of renal impairment, dose reduction is required both for paliperidone, an active metabolite of risperidone which is mainly renally excreted (Madhusoodanan & Zaveri, 2010), and for risperidone itself since poor renal function will increase the longevity and availability of paliperidone. The increased incidence of medical co-morbidity and the increased potential for drug interactions are, as always, further considerations in elderly patients.

Elderly patients should generally be started on lower initial doses and have the dose titrated more slowly than in younger adults. For example, when using quetiapine, age is a good predictor of reduced clearance so that a low starting dose (25 mg/day) is recommended along with smaller dose increments than would be used in younger adults. The presence of 'frailty' signals the need for further caution and starting doses which may need to be lower still (e.g. 12.5 mg/day in the case of quetiapine). Although frailty has no operationalized definition, it can be inferred by taking account of body mass index/weight, vital signs, mobility and co-morbid medical conditions. Antipsychotic drug side-effects which may be especially problematic in the elderly include anticholinergic effects, neurological effects due to dopamine receptor blockade, as well as sedation, orthostatic hypertension, metabolic side effects and other cardiovascular and haematological problems. All elderly patients taking dopamine receptor antagonists should be monitored carefully for the incidence of these side effects and have metabolic parameters (weight, blood pressure, fasting glucose and lipid profiles) assessed regularly.

Anticholinergic actions, which result from blockade of muscarinic acetylcholine receptors, include deleterious effects on concentration and cognition, as well as impact on peripheral systems leading to urinary retention, constipation, dry mouth (due to reduced salivation), blurred vision, increased pupil size and increased heart rate (Liberman, 2004). In vulnerable populations, these problems can be associated with further complications, including gum ulceration, bowel obstruction, precipitation of acute narrow-angle glaucoma, as well as angina and cardiac events. There are marked differences between dopamine receptor antagonists in their propensity to cause anticholinergic side effects. For example, the Anticholinergic Cognitive Burden Scale (Boustani et al., 2008) rates drugs according to anticholinergic activity based on review of evidence relating to 88 medications thought to have an impact on cognition in older adults, and rates clozapine, olanzapine, quetiapine, promethazine and chlorpromazine as having 'severe anticholinergic activity' while risperidone and haloperidol are rated as mild in this domain.

The elderly are more likely to experience extrapyramidal side effects such as akathisia, dystonias, muscular rigidity and tardive dyskinesia. Extrapyramidal symptoms are most common with high potency dopamine receptor antagonists at higher doses, for example haloperidol. In the elderly these side effects may also increase the risk of falls. Since some of these drugs, e.g. risperidone and quetiapine, may also cause orthostatic hypertension, which itself is associated with falls, and falls risk may be exacerbated by pre-existing medical disorders (e.g. arthritis) or by other co-prescribed medications (e.g. benzodiazepines and TCAs) the danger of increased propensity to falls should always be considered.

Metabolic side effects, impacting on the ability to control blood pressure and manage circulating glucose and lipid concentrations, are especially pertinent in the elderly, in part because individuals are already at increasing risk of hypertension, diabetes and hyperlipidaemia with increasing age. Overall, metabolic symptoms are more problematic with serotonin/dopamine-blocking antipsychotics such as olanzapine but diabetes may be provoked by any antipsychotic (Lipscombe et al., 2009). All of these metabolic disorders can contribute to increased risk of cardiac events. Independently of the increased cardiovascular risk through worsening control of metabolic systems, it should also be noted that many antipsychotics increase the risk of cardiac arrhythmia through QTc prolongation, with quetiapine, olanzapine and ziprasidone thought to carry the highest risk among the newer antipsychotics, while haloperidol is thought to markedly elevate the risk in the presence of low potassium concentrations. Further, there is an association between antipsychotic use and stroke in the elderly which has been identified as being especially worthy of attention when antipsychotics are required to control BPSD of dementia, where the benefits of these drugs must be contrasted with their association with moderate increases in risk of mortality (Maust et al., 2015).

Many dopamine receptor antagonists are associated with sedation. In some cases, this property may be used to good effect, for example when quetiapine is prescribed for a psychiatric disorder and improves sleep as a secondary consequence. However, sedation can also be problematic in the elderly. Sedative effects may be more pronounced and longer-lasting, and in some cases can provoke confusion and disorientation. While prescription of dopamine receptor antagonist drugs is a necessity in many cases when treating elderly patients with functional psychiatric disorders, including first-line treatment in schizophrenia and bipolar disorder and as alternative treatments in depression and anxiety disorders, their many possible side effects and potential to exacerbate pre-existing medical problems and interact with other prescribed drugs mean that vigilance is always required.

Haematological side effects to consider when prescribing in the elderly include the association of clozapine with increased risk of agranulocytosis (Bishara & Taylor, 2014) and leucopenia (O'Connor et al., 2010). Clozapine has also been implicated in cases of myocarditis and life-threatening constipation. However, as in younger age groups, clozapine retains its important role for treatment-resistant schizophrenia (Barak et al., 1999) although slower dose titration is advisable. Although there are no prospective trials of clozapine specifically in the elderly diagnosed with schizophrenia, a recently published retrospective study (Pridan et al., 2015) suggests that mortality rates with clozapine were similar to those in older adults prescribed other antipsychotic drugs, whereas rehospitalization rates were significantly lower.

As discussed earlier in this chapter, older adults are especially sensitive to drugs with anticholinergic properties. In addition to certain dopamine receptor antagonist drugs, TCAs, paroxetine and carbamazepine, it should be recalled that drugs such as procyclidine and benztropine, which may be co-prescribed with dopamine receptor antagonist antipsychotic drugs in order to reduce the impact of extrapyramidal side effects, have strong anticholinergic activity. When these drugs are used in the elderly, especially if they are prescribed alongside other drugs with anticholinergic effects, it is essential to be aware of the possibility of symptoms such as dry mouth and constipation and the risks of urinary retention and of confusion or disorientation.

18.11 Pharmacological Treatment of Bipolar Disorder

18.11.1 Lithium

The relative merits of lithium in relation to anticonvulsants and to dopamine receptor-blocking drugs in the elderly are the subject of much debate in old age psychiatry. Some prescribers are hesitant to use lithium, given that it requires regular assessment of plasma concentration, and other parameters including renal function, electrolytes and thyroid status. It is also necessary to ensure there is a good intake of fluids and salt. Risk of renal toxicity appears to be slightly higher in older people (Close et al., 2014). Neurotoxicity (i.e. neurological sequelae such as tremor or discoordination proceeding to more gross manifestations such as slurred speech, muscular fasciculation, seizures and nystagmus) appears to have a similar risk in the elderly at any specific plasma concentration as for younger people. However, the complexity in the elderly lies in the potential for kidney function to decline and lithium concentrations to increase, provoking toxic neurological effects before the change in renal parameters is detected, which underlines the need for regular monitoring in older patients (every three to six months, and within five to seven days of dose changes or co-prescription/adjustment of antihypertensives or anti-inflammatory drugs (Chen et al., 2017)).

As described earlier, since body fat increases and total body water decreases with age, as a water-soluble drug, the volume of distribution for lithium (i.e. the apparent volume into which lithium would be expected to distribute into based on its concentration in the plasma), which is high in younger people relative to most psychotropic drugs, will tend to decline with age. In general, lower doses of lithium should be used than in younger adults, and the target therapeutic range is lower (typically 0.4–0.8 mmol/L). This is because of increased risk of toxicity at the upper end of the adult therapeutic range –

including risk of peripheral symptoms such as tremor, polyuria and gastrointestinal disturbance and also of cognitive impairment.

However, despite these issues, lithium is effective both as a treatment (for episodes of depression, hypomania and mania) and as a prophylaxis for bipolar affective disorder. A recently published multi-centre randomized trial comparing lithium with valproate in treatment of hypomania and mania (Young et al., 2017) illustrates that it can be used safely in the elderly and is slightly more effective than valproate. Although there are no large trials specifically in the elderly to compare lithium with antipsychotics in bipolar disorder, it has performed well in trials in younger people and has the advantage of avoiding metabolic side effects as well as its known protective effect against suicidality. There is also the suggestion that it might promote synaptic spine growth.

Note that there is a specific concern of giving ECT in patients on lithium treatment, in that ECT can increase permeability of the blood–brain barrier and therefore lead to the brain being exposed to toxic lithium levels and complications such as delirium (Zolezzi, 2016). Prolonged seizures may also occur. There is debate as to whether this combination should be contraindicated entirely in the elderly, but if the lithium must be continued it is advisable to reduce the dose to have its concentration at the lower end of the therapeutic range or withhold the lithium on the day prior to administering ECT.

18.11.2 Anticonvulsants in Bipolar Disorder

Certain anticonvulsants are widely used for the acute treatment and prophylaxis of bipolar disorder in the elderly. The main such drugs are carbamazepine/oxcarbazepine, valproate and lamotrigine. It is important to highlight that efficacy in bipolar disorder is not a class effect of all anticonvulsants. Anticonvulsants can cause a wide range of side effects that can be especially undesirable in older patients. Some side effects are shared between anticonvulsants used in bipolar disorder, for example a study using veterans' data in the United States (Mezuk et al., 2010) reported that while older people with bipolar disorder experience more fractures than those with no psychiatric illness, the risk of fractures is more than doubled in people prescribed any of these drugs, with risk linked to duration of use. Hip fracture was significantly more common in individuals taking 'liver enzyme inducing' anticonvulsants such as carbamazepine, oxcarbazepine and topiramate.

There are placebo-controlled randomized trial data that support the efficacy of valproate in treating acute mania in younger adults (Bowden et al., 1994). However, there are no such data for the use of valproate, or other anticonvulsants, to treat manic episodes in bipolar disorder in the elderly. Randomized trial evidence for valproate in old age bipolar disorder is limited to the comparative study discussed earlier of valproate and lithium, in which valproate was slightly less effective in treating hypomania and mania (Young et al., 2017). The remaining studies are uncontrolled. Nevertheless, valproate and associated preparations are frequently used for treatment and prophylaxis of bipolar disorder in elderly populations. Valproate clearance is reduced in the elderly, and a further complication is that as protein binding of valproate may be reduced in the elderly, plasma levels reported as being in the therapeutic range may be less reliable being confounded by albumin concentration (Lampon & Tutor, 2012). side effects which may occur with increased frequency in the elderly include thrombocytopaenia, neurological symptoms, weight gain and diabetes.

There are no high-quality trials for other anticonvulsant drugs in bipolar disorder specific to the elderly (Chen et al., 2017) and their use relies on evidence inferred from randomized trials in younger age groups. While carbamazepine does not require dose adjustment in healthy older individuals (Punyawudho et al., 2012), it should always be used with caution. Dose titration should be more gradual in patients with hepatic impairment. It has marked anticholinergic activity and may be associated with nausea and ataxia as well as carrying a small risk of leucopenia. It is a strong inducer of CYP3A4, an enzyme which metabolizes numerous psychotropic and non-psychotropic drugs, so dose of co-prescribed medications may need to be increased as carbamazepine is increased to achieve the same therapeutic effect. Carbamazepine, and the related drug oxcarbazepine, is capable of causing hyponatraemia.

Lamotrigine clearance is reduced in the elderly (Wegner et al., 2013), necessitating some dose adjustment, but it remains a treatment option in bipolar disorder especially where depressive episodes predominate, although evidence is inferred from studies in younger adults. Given the small risk of dangerous skin reactions, including Stevens–Johnson syndrome and toxic epidermal necrolysis, dose titration should be slow and gradual and patients must be warned to seek advice if they experience a rash. Although these reactions may not be more common in the elderly than in younger adults, the ramifications, should they occur, may be more serious.

Many guidelines (Goodwin et al., 2016) advise against the use of topiramate in bipolar disorder due to lack of supporting evidence. A further issue in the elderly is that topiramate is associated with cognitive impairment which may be clinically significant in up to half of older adults treated with this drug for its original indication of epilepsy (Sommer & Fenn, 2010). Topiramate may also be employed as a treatment for antipsychotic-induced weight gain (Mizuno et al., 2014) and has a licensed indication for migraine prophylaxis, but the association with cognitive impairment means that it should be used with caution in the elderly whatever the rationale for its introduction.

18.11.3 Dopamine Receptor Antagonists (Antipsychotics) in Treatment of Bipolar Disorder

While many newer antipsychotics have evidence of efficacy for manic episodes in bipolar disorder from randomized trials in adult patients which guides prescription choices in the elderly, evidence from trials conducted specifically in older patients is limited. Quetiapine has positive evidence from a pooled analysis of randomized trials in older adults, asenapine and aripiprazole (Sajatovic et al., 2008) have evidence from open-label trials and risperidone and clozapine have evidence from case series only. Recent work relating to people aged 60 and over (Chen et al., 2017) advises that lithium and valproate are considered first-line treatments for manic episodes, with these antipsychotics used as alternatives if these first-line drugs are ineffective or poorly tolerated, or added in the case of partial response. Nevertheless, dopamine receptor antagonists are used increasingly in bipolar disorder in older adults, both in the treatment of acute manic episodes and in prophylaxis, and in a recent study of individuals with late-life bipolar disorder their prevalence in the post-discharge period greatly eclipsed that of lithium and anticonvulsants (Rej et al., 2016). This may be due to their relative ease of use including lower propensity for drug interactions and toxic effects, albeit at the cost of exposure to the range of metabolic and other side effects described earlier. Quetiapine and lurasidone have evidence of efficacy in bipolar depression in adults aged 55 to 65, although these are based on post-hoc analyses, the lurasidone study being a pooled analysis of patients in this age group from two randomized trials (Sajatovic et al., 2016).

18.12 Psychostimulants and Other Drugs for Attention Deficit Hyperactivity Disorder

In adolescents and adults, methylphenidate and amphetamines have been increasingly used to treat ADHD, with good randomized trial evidence of efficacy. While no trials exist specifically for ADHD in the elderly, a recent paper from Denmark using national prescribing data registers (Ormhøj et al., 2018) illustrates that use of methylphenidate and other drugs for ADHD (atomoxetine and amphetamines) has increased more than twofold in all age groups over 65 in the period 2000–15. However, these data come with the caveat that these drugs may have been used for other indications – for example as palliative care in patients with a cancer, narcolepsy or indeed as an adjunctive treatment for depression as discussed earlier. As with younger patients, stimulant use requires cardiovascular monitoring necessitating regular checking of cardiovascular parameters. Atomoxetine, a noradrenergic reuptake blocker which is not a stimulant, also requires cardiovascular monitoring. It is metabolized by CYP2D6 and may require reduced doses in patients with poor hepatic function or in the presence of CYP2D6 inhibitors.

18.13 Pharmacological Treatments for Substance Misuse

Substance misuse in the elderly includes harmful use of alcohol and other legal drugs (e.g. nicotine), prescribed medications (e.g. benzodiazepines, opioids) and illicit drugs. As has been discussed extensively in this chapter, older adults may be excessively susceptible to the effects of substances due to pre-existing medical issues, pharmacodynamics changes associated with ageing, lack of reserve to cope with the physiological effects associated with substance use, and increased potential for interactions with other prescribed medications. These risks apply whether drugs are being used as prescribed or in the context of abuse – for instance, both benzodiazepines (Nurmi-Lüthje et al., 2006) and opioids (Vestergaard et al., 2006) carry risks of falls and fractures in the elderly, especially those in residential homes and institutional settings, which may be enhanced when they are abused. Similarly, the risk of alcohol-related dementia increases both with intake and with advancing age.

Some medications are indicated specifically for use in substance misuse disorders and may be used in the elderly subject to cautions relating to co-morbid medical disorders. As regards drugs used in alcohol use disorders, there is little data on the use of the anti-craving agent acamprosate in the elderly seeking to maintain abstinence from alcohol, and it should be avoided in individuals with renal impairment. Naltrexone may be problematic due to hepatotoxicity, although nalmefene, which has a similar structure, has not been associated with this problem. If considering disulfiram, which is taken to promote abstinence as it causes an unpleasant physical reaction in the event that alcohol is consumed, dose adjustments are not required but the issue of reduced tolerance to its cardiovascular effects may preclude its use in some older people.

While there is extensive literature on the appropriate use of opioid-based drugs in elderly patients for pain, among drugs employed specifically for opioid misuse, methadone has the best developed evidence base in older adults (Doukas, 2011). One study estimated that around 5% of the 160 000 people receiving methadone maintenance treatment in the United States were aged over 55 and this group tended to have better outcomes than their younger counterparts (Firoz & Carlson, 2004), a finding replicated in other studies (Carew & Comiskey, 2017). Reduced methadone doses are required in renal impairment. Buprenorphine has little data pertaining specifically to the elderly.

18.14 Summary

In this chapter the changes associated with ageing which impact pharmacodynamics and pharmacokinetics have been reviewed. These include not only direct changes in pharmacodynamics and pharmacokinetic parameters, but also the impacts of medical disorders and co-prescribed medications which can reduce tolerance to change, increase propensity for interactions and lower thresholds for toxic effects. While the formulary of available psychotropic drugs for prescribing to older adults is essentially the same as that for those aged under 65, some drugs require evidence to be extrapolated from younger populations. Vigilance for side effects and interactions is paramount.

References

Adams KH, Pinborg LH, Svarer C, et al. (2004). A database of [(18)F]-altanserin binding to 5-HT(2A) receptors in normal volunteers: normative data and relationship to physiological and demographic variables. *Neuroimage*, 21, 1105–1113.

Alaka KJ, Noble W, Montejo A, et al. (2014). Efficacy and safety of duloxetine in the treatment of older adult patients with generalized anxiety disorder: a randomized, double-blind, placebo-controlled trial. *Int J Geriatr Psychiatry*, 29, 978–986.

Baldwin DS, Anderson IM, Nutt DJ, et al. (2014). Evidence-based pharmacological treatment of anxiety disorders, post-traumatic stress disorder and obsessive-compulsive disorder: a revision of the 2005 guidelines from the British Association for Psychopharmacology. *J Psychopharmacol*, 28, 403–439.

Barak Y, Wittenberg N, Naor S, Kutzuk D, Weizman A (1999). Clozapine in elderly psychiatric patients: tolerability, safety, and efficacy. *Compr Psychiatry*, 40, 320–325.

Berry SD, Lee Y, Cai S, Dore DD (2013). Nonbenzodiazepine sleep medication use and hip fractures in nursing home residents. *JAMA Intern Med*, 173, 754–761.

Bertz RJ, Kroboth PD, Kroboth FJ, et al. (1997). Alprazolam in young and elderly men: sensitivity and tolerance to psychomotor, sedative and memory effects. *J Pharmacol Exp Ther*, 281, 1317–1329.

Bigos KL, Bies RR, Pollock BG (2013). Pharmacokinetics and pharmacodynamics in late life. In H Lavretsky, M Sajatovic, C Reynolds, eds., *Late-Life Mood Disorders*. New York: Oxford University Press, pp. 655–674.

Bishara D, Taylor D (2014). Adverse effects of clozapine in older patients: epidemiology, prevention and management. *Drugs Aging*, 31, 11–20.

Blier P, Ward HE, Tremblay P, et al. (2010). Combination of antidepressant medications from treatment initiation for major depressive disorder: a double-blind randomized study. *Am J Psychiatry*, 167, 281–288.

Boustani M, Campbell N, Munger S, Maidment I, Fox C (2008). Impact of anticholinergics on the aging brain: a review and practical application. *Aging Health*, 4, 311–320.

Bowden CL, Brugger AM, Swann AC, et al. (1994). Efficacy of divalproex vs lithium and placebo in the treatment of mania. The Depakote Mania Study Group. *JAMA*, 271(12), 918–924.

Bowie MW, Slattum PW (2007). Pharmacodynamics in older adults: a review. *Am J Geriatr Pharmacother*, 5, 263–303.

Calati R, Salvina Signorelli M, Balestri M, et al. (2013). Antidepressants in elderly: metaregression of double-blind, randomized clinical trials. *J Affect Disord*, 147, 1–8.

Carew AM, Comiskey C (2017). Treatment for opioid use and outcomes in older adults: a systematic literature review. *Drug Alcohol Depend*, 182, 48–57.

Carone M, Asgharian M, Jewell NP (2014). Estimating the lifetime risk of dementia in the Canadian elderly population using cross-sectional cohort survival data. *J Am Stat Assoc*, 109, 24–35.

Chen P, Dols A, Rej S, Sajatovic M (2017). Update on the epidemiology, diagnosis, and treatment of mania in older-age bipolar disorder. *Curr Psychiatry Rep*, 19, 46. https://doi.org/10.1007/s11920-017-0804-8.

Chew ML, Mulsant BH, Pollock BG, et al. (2008). Anticholinergic activity of 107 medications commonly used by older adults. *J Am Geriatr Soc*, 56, 1333–1341.

Chokhavatia S, John ES, Bridgeman MB, Dixit D (2016). Constipation in elderly patients with noncancer pain: focus on opioid-induced constipation. *Drugs Aging*, 33, 557–574.

Chung JK, Nakajima S, Shinagawa S, et al.; Alzheimer's Disease Neuroimaging Initiative (2016). Benzodiazepine use attenuates cortical β-amyloid and is not associated with progressive cognitive decline in nondemented elderly adults: a pilot study using F18-florbetapir positron emission tomography. *Am J Geriatr Psychiatry*, 24, 1028–1039.

Close H, Reilly J, Mason JM, et al. (2014). Renal failure in lithium-treated bipolar disorder: a retrospective cohort study. *PLoS One*, 9(3), e90169. doi:10.1371/journal.pone.0090169. eCollection 2014.

Coupland C, Dhiman P, Morriss R, et al. (2011). Antidepressant use and risk of adverse outcomes in older people: population based cohort study. *BMJ*, 343, d4551.

Crowe SF, Stranks EK (2018). The residual medium and long-term cognitive effects of benzodiazepine use: an updated meta-analysis. *Arch Clin Neuropsychol*, 33, 901–911. doi:10.1093/arclin/acx120.

Cumming RG, Le Couteur DG (2003). Benzodiazepines and risk of hip fractures in older people: a review of the evidence. *CNS Drugs*, 17, 825–837.

Davies SJC, Eayrs S, Pratt P, Lennard MS (2004). Potential for drug interactions involving cytochromes P450 2D6 and 3A4 on general adult psychiatric and functional elderly psychiatric wards. *Br J Clin Pharmacol*, 57, 464–472.

Davies SJ, Burhan AM, Kim D, et al. (2018a). Sequential drug treatment algorithm for agitation and aggression in Alzheimer's and mixed dementia. *J Psychopharmacol*, 32(5), 509–523.

Davies SJC, Jacob B, Rudoler D, et al. (2018b). Benzodiazepine prescription in Ontario residents aged 65 and over: a population-based study from 1998 to 2013. *Ther Adv Psychopharmacol*, 8, 99–114.

Department of Health Statistics and Informatics of the World Health Organization (2015). *Disease burden and mortality estimates. Global Health Estimates 2015: DALYs by age, sex and cause.* Available at: www.who.int/healthinfo/global_burden_disease/estimates/en/index2.html (last accessed 14.8.18).

Depp CA, Jeste DV (2004). Bipolar disorder in older adults: a critical review. *Bipolar Disord*, 6, 343–367.

Dold M, Aigner M, Lanzenberger R, Kasper S (2015). Antipsychotic augmentation of serotonin reuptake inhibitors in treatment-resistant obsessive-compulsive disorder: an update meta-analysis of double-blind, randomized, placebo-controlled trials. *Int J Neuropsychopharmacol*, 18(9), pyv047.

Doukas N (2011). Older adults in methadone maintenance treatment: a literature review. *J Soc Work Pract Addict*, 11, 230–244.

Esiri MM, Morris JH (1997). Practical approach to pathological diagnosis. In MM Esiri, JH Morris, eds., *The Neuropathology of Dementia*. Cambridge: Cambridge University Press, pp. 36–69.

Essali A, Ali G (2012). Antipsychotic drug treatment for elderly people with late-onset schizophrenia. *Cochrane Database Syst Rev*, (2), CD004162.

Evans DL, Charney DS, Lewis L, et al. (2005). Mood disorders in the medically ill: scientific review and recommendations. *Biol Psychiatry*, 58, 175–189.

Finkelstein J, Friedman C, Hripcsak G, Cabrera M (2016). Pharmacogenetic polymorphism as an independent risk factor for frequent hospitalizations in older adults with polypharmacy: a pilot study. *Pharmgenomics Pers Med*, 14, 107–116.

Firoz S, Carlson G (2004). Characteristics and treatment outcome of older methadone-maintenance patients. *Am J Geriatr Psychiatry*, 12, 539–541.

Flockhart D (undated). Flockhart Table P450 Drug Interaction Table. Available at: http://medicine.iupui.edu/clinpharm/ddis/main-table (last accessed 25.3.17).

Glassman AH, O'Connor CM, Califf RM, et al. (2002). Sertraline treatment of major depression in patients with acute MI or unstable angina. Sertraline Antidepressant Heart Attack Randomized Trial (SADHEART) Group. *JAMA*, 288, 701–709.

Goodwin GM, Haddad PM, Ferrier IN, et al. (2016). Evidence-based guidelines for treating bipolar disorder: revised third edition recommendations from the British Association for Psychopharmacology. *J Psychopharmacol*, 30, 495–553.

Gray SL, Dublin S, Yu O, et al. (2016). Benzodiazepine use and risk of incident dementia or cognitive decline: prospective population based study. *BMJ*, 352, i90.

Gray SL, Hart LA, Perera S, et al. (2018). Meta-analysis of interventions to reduce adverse drug reactions in older adults. *J Am Geriatr Soc*, 66, 282–288.

Greenblatt DJ, Harmatz JS, Shapiro L, et al. (1991). Sensitivity to triazolam in the elderly. *N Engl J Med*, 324, 1691–1698.

Gum AM, King-Kallimanis B, Kohn R (2009). Prevalence of mood, anxiety, and substance-abuse disorders for older Americans in the National Comorbidity Survey-Replication. *Am J Geriatr Psychiatry*, 17, 769–781.

Heun R, Ahokas A, Boyer P, et al. (2013). The efficacy of agomelatine in elderly patients with recurrent major depressive disorder: a placebo-controlled study. *J Clin Psychiatry*, 74, 587–594.

Hewett K, Gee MD, Krishen A, et al. (2010). Double-blind, placebo-controlled comparison of the antidepressant efficacy and tolerability of bupropion XR and venlafaxine XR. *J Psychopharmacol*, 24, 1209–1216.

Jeste DV, Barak Y, Madhusoodanan S, Grossman F, Gharabawi G (2003). International multisite double-blind trial of the atypical antipsychotics risperidone and olanzapine in 175 elderly patients with chronic schizophrenia. *Am J Geriatr Psychiatry*, 11, 638–647.

Joint Formulary Committee (2017). *British National Formulary*, No. 73. London: BMJ Group and Pharmaceutical Press, p. 296 and p. 304.

Katila H, Mezhebovsky I, Mulroy A, et al. (2013). Randomized, double-blind study of the efficacy and tolerability of extended release quetiapine fumarate (quetiapine XR) monotherapy in elderly patients with major depressive disorder. *Am J Geriatr Psychiatry*, 21, 769–784.

Katona C, Bercoff E, Chiu E, et al. (1999). Reboxetine versus imipramine in the treatment of elderly patients with depressive disorders: a double-blind randomised trial. *J Affect Disord*, 55, 203–213.

Katona C, Hansen T, Olsen CK (2012). A randomized, double-blind, placebo-controlled, duloxetine-referenced, fixed-dose study comparing the efficacy and safety of LU AA21004 in elderly patients with major depressive disorder. *Int Clin Psychopharmacol*, 27, 215–223.

Katz IR, Reynolds CF, III Alexopoulos GS, Hackett D (2002). Venlafaxine ER as a treatment for generalized anxiety disorder in older adults: pooled analysis of five randomized placebo-controlled clinical trials. *J Am Geriatr Soc*, 50, 18–25.

Kerr KP, Mate KE, Magin PJ, et al. (2014). The prevalence of co-prescription of clinically relevant CYP enzyme inhibitor and substrate drugs in community-dwelling elderly Australians. *J Clin Pharm Ther*, 39, 383–389.

Kessler D, MacNeill SJ, Tallon D, et al. (2018). Mirtazapine added to SSRIs or SNRIs for treatment resistant depression in primary care: phase III randomised controlled trial (MIR). *BMJ*, 363, k4218.

Kinsella K, He W (2009). *An Aging World*. Washington, DC: National Institute on Aging and US Census Bureau.

Kirchheiner J, Seeringer A (2007). Clinical implications of pharmacogenetics of cytochrome P450 drug metabolizing enzymes. *Biochim Biophys Acta*, 1770, 489–494.

Klotz U (2009). Pharmacokinetics and drug metabolism in the elderly. *Drug Metab Rev*, 41, 67–76.

Kok RM, Vink D, Heeren TJ, Nolen WA (2007). Lithium augmentation compared with phenelzine in treatment-resistant depression in the elderly: an open, randomized, controlled trial. *J Clin Psychiatry*, 68, 1177–1185.

Kok RM, Heeren TJ, Nolen WA (2011). Continuing treatment of depression in the elderly: a systematic review and meta-analysis of double-blinded randomized controlled trials with antidepressants. *Am J Geriatr Psychiatry*, 19, 249–255.

Kok RM, Nolen WA, Heeren TJ (2012). Efficacy of treatment in older depressed patients: a systematic review and meta-analysis of double-blind randomized controlled trials with antidepressants *J Affect Disord*, 141, 103–115.

Lampon N, Tutor JC (2012). Apparent clearance of valproic acid in elderly epileptic patients: estimation of the confounding effect of albumin concentration. *Ups J Med Sci*, 117, 41–46.

Lavretsky H, Reinlieb M, St Cyr N, et al. (2015). Citalopram, methylphenidate, or their combination in geriatric depression: a randomized, double-blind, placebo-controlled trial. *Am J Psychiatry*, 172, 561–569.

Lenze EJ, Mulsant BH, Shear MK, et al. (2005). Efficacy and tolerability of citalopram in the treatment of late-life anxiety disorders: results from an 8-week randomized, placebo-controlled trial. *Am J Psychiatry*, 162, 146–150.

Lenze EJ, Rollman BL, Shear MK, et al. (2009). Escitalopram for older adults with generalized anxiety disorder: a randomized controlled trial. *JAMA*, 301, 295–303.

Lenze EJ, Mulsant BH, Blumberger DM, et al. (2015). Efficacy, safety, and tolerability of augmentation pharmacotherapy with aripiprazole for treatment-resistant depression in late life: a randomised, double-blind, placebo-controlled trial. *Lancet*, 386(10011), 2404–2412.

Lieberman, JA, III (2004). Managing anticholinergic side effects. *Prim Care Companion J Clin Psychiatry*, 6(Suppl 2), 20–23.

Lin FY, Chen PC, Liao CH, Hsieh YW, Sung FC (2014). Retrospective population cohort study on hip fracture risk associated with zolpidem medication. *Sleep*, 37, 673–679.

Lindeman R, Tobin J, Shock N (1985). Longitudinal studies on the rate of decline in renal function with age. *J Am Geriatr Soc*, 33, 278–285.

Lipscombe LL, Lévesque L, Gruneir A, et al. (2009). Antipsychotic drugs and hyperglycemia in older patients with diabetes. *Arch Intern Med*, 169, 1282–1289.

MacQueen GM, Frey BN, Ismail Z, et al.; CANMAT Depression Work Group (2016). Canadian Network for Mood and Anxiety Treatments (CANMAT) 2016 Clinical Guidelines for the Management of Adults with Major Depressive Disorder: Section 6. Special Populations: Youth, Women, and the Elderly. *Can J Psychiatry*, 61, 588–603.

Madhusoodanan S, Zaveri D (2010). Paliperidone use in the elderly. *Curr Drug Saf*, 5, 149–152.

Maneeton N, Maneeton B, Woottiluk P, et al. (2016). Quetiapine monotherapy in acute treatment of generalized anxiety disorder: a systematic review and meta-analysis of randomized controlled trials. *Drug Des Devel Ther*, 10, 259–276.

Maust DT, Kim HM, Seyfried LS (2015). Antipsychotics, other psychotropics, and the risk of death in patients with dementia: number needed to harm. *JAMA Psychiatry*, 72, 438–445.

Mezuk B, Morden NE, Ganoczy D, Post EP, Kilbourne AM (2010). Anticonvulsant use, bipolar disorder, and risk of fracture among older adults in the Veterans Health Administration. *Am J Geriatr Psychiatry*, 18, 245–255.

Michelson D, Snyder E, Paradis E, et al. (2014). Safety and efficacy of suvorexant during 1-year treatment of insomnia with subsequent abrupt treatment discontinuation: a phase 3 randomised, double-blind, placebo-controlled trial. *Lancet Neurol*, 13, 461–471.

Mizuno Y, Suzuki T, Nakagawa A, et al. (2014). Pharmacological strategies to counteract antipsychotic-induced weight gain and metabolic adverse effects in schizophrenia: a systematic review and meta-analysis. *Schizophr Bull*, 40, 1385–1403.

Møller M, Jakobsen S, Gjedde A (2007). Parametric and regional maps of free serotonin 5HT1A receptor sites in human brain as function of age in healthy humans. *Neuropsychopharmacology*, 32, 1707–1714.

Montgomery S, Chatamra K, Pauer L, Whalen E, Baldinetti F (2008). Efficacy and safety of pregabalin in elderly people with generalised anxiety disorder. *Br J Psychiatry*, 193, 389–394.

Morgan DG, May PC, Finch CE (1987). Dopamine and serotonin systems in human and rodent brain: effects of age and neurodegenerative disease. *J Am Geriatr Soc*, 35, 334–345.

Musselman DL, Tomer A, Manatunga AK, et al. (1996). Exaggerated platelet reactivity in major depression. *Am J Psychiatry*, 153, 1313–1317.

Nurmi-Lüthje I, Kaukonen JP, Lüthje P, et al. (2006). Use of benzodiazepines and benzodiazepine-related drugs among 223 patients with an acute hip fracture in Finland: comparison of benzodiazepine findings in medical records and laboratory assays. *Drugs Aging*, 23, 27–37.

O'Connor DW, Sierakowski C, Chin LF, Singh D (2010). The safety and tolerability of clozapine in aged patients: a retrospective clinical file review. *World J Biol Psychiatry*, 11, 788–791.

Ormhøj SS, Pottegård A, Gasse C, Rasmussen L (2018). Use of attention-deficit/hyperactivity disorder medication among older adults in Denmark. *Br J Clin Pharmacol*, 84, 1505–1513. doi:10.1111/bcp.13569.

Ortega V, Tabet N, Nilforooshan R, Howard R (2017). Efficacy of antidepressants for depression in Alzheimer's disease: systematic review and meta-analysis. *J Alzheimers Dis*, 58, 725–733.

Pridan S, Swartz M, Baruch Y, et al. (2015). Effectiveness and safety of clozapine in elderly patients with chronic resistant schizophrenia. *Int Psychogeriatr*, 27, 131–134.

Prince, M, Bryce, R, Albanese, E (2013). The global prevalence of dementia: a systematic review and meta-analysis. *Alzheimers Dement (N Y)*, 9, 63–75.

Punyawudho B, Ramsay ER, Brundage RC, et al. (2012). Population pharmacokinetics of carbamazepine in elderly patients. *Ther Drug Monit*, 34, 176–181.

Qirjazi E, McArthur E, Nash DM, et al. (2016). Risk of ventricular arrhythmia with citalopram and escitalopram: a population-based study. *PLoS One*, 11(8), e0160768.

Raskin J, Wiltse CG, Siegal A, et al. (2007). Efficacy of duloxetine on cognition, depression, and pain in elderly patients with major depressive disorder: an 8-week, double-blind, placebo-controlled trial. *Am J Psychiatry*, 164, 900–909.

Regier DA, Boyd JH, Burke JD Jr, et al. (1988). One-month prevalence of mental disorders in the United States. Based on five epidemiologic catchment area sites. *Arch Gen Psychiatry*, 45, 977–986.

Rehman HU, Masson EA (2001). Neuroendocrinology of ageing. *Age Ageing*, 30, 279–287.

Rej S, Herrmann N, Shulman K, et al. (2016). Farewell mood stabilizers? Current psychotropic medication prescribing patterns in late-life bipolar disorder. *Am J Geriatr Psychiatry*, 24(3 Suppl), S86–S87.

Rinne JO (1987). Muscarinic and dopaminergic receptors in ageing human brain. *Brain Res*, 404, 161–168.

Rosenberg PB, Drye LT, Martin BK, et al.; DIADS-2 Research Group (2010). Sertraline for the treatment of depression in Alzheimer disease. *Am J Geriatr Psychiatry*, 18, 136–145.

Roth M, Mountjoy CQ, Amrein R (1996). Moclobemide in elderly patients with cognitive decline and depression: an international double-blind, placebo-controlled trial. *Br J Psychiatry*, 168, 149–157.

Rudolph JL, Salow MJ, Angelini MC, McGlinchey RE (2008). The anticholinergic risk scale and anticholinergic adverse effects in older persons. *Arch Intern Med*, 168, 508–513.

Sabesan P, Lankappa S, Khalifa N, et al. (2015). Transcranial magnetic stimulation for geriatric depression: promises and pitfalls. *World J Psychiatry*, 5(2), 170–181.

Sajatovic M, Coconcea N, Ignacio RV, et al. (2008). Aripiprazole therapy in 20 older adults with bipolar disorder: a 12-week, open-label trial. *J Clin Psychiatry*, 69, 41–46.

Sajatovic M, Strejilevich SA, Gildengers AG, et al. (2015). A report on older-age bipolar disorder from the International Society for Bipolar Disorders Task Force. *Bipolar Disord*, 17, 689–704.

Sajatovic M, Forester BP, Tsai J, et al. (2016). Efficacy of lurasidone in adults aged 55 years and older with bipolar depression: post hoc analysis of 2 double-blind, placebo-controlled studies. *J Clin Psychiatry*, 77(10), e1324–e1331.

Schatzberg AF, Kremer C, Rodrigues HE, Murphy GM Jr (2002). Mirtazapine vs. Paroxetine Study Group. Double-blind, randomized comparison of mirtazapine and paroxetine in elderly depressed patients. *Am J Geriatr Psychiatry*, 10, 541–550.

Schneider LS, Nelson JC, Clary CM, et al.; Sertraline Elderly Depression Study Group (2003). An 8-week multicenter, parallel-group, double-blind, placebo-controlled study of sertraline in elderly outpatients with major depression. *Am J Psychiatry*, 160, 1277–1285.

Shroeck J, Ford J, Conway EL, et al. (2016). Review of safety and efficacy of sleep medicines in older adults. *Clin Ther*, 38, 2340–2372.

Singh S, Bajorek B (2015). Pharmacotherapy in the ageing patient: the impact of age per se (a review). *Ageing Res Rev*, 24(Pt B), 99–110.

Sommer BR, Fenn HH (2010). Review of topiramate for the treatment of epilepsy in elderly patients. *Clin Interv Aging*, 5, 89–99.

Stage KB, Kragh-Sørensen PB; Danish University Antidepressant Group (2002). Age-related adverse drug reactions to clomipramine. *Acta Psychiatr Scand*, 105, 55–59.

Stranks EK, Crowe SF (2014). The acute cognitive effects of zopiclone, zolpidem, zaleplon, and eszopiclone: a systematic review and meta-analysis. *J Clin Exp Neuropsychol*, 36, 691–700.

Tedeschini E, Levkovitz Y, Iovieno N, et al. (2011). Efficacy of antidepressants for late-life depression: a meta-analysis and meta-regression of placebo-controlled randomized trials. *J Clin Psychiatry*, 72, 1660–1668.

Terzano MG, Rossi M, Palomba V, Smerieri A, Parrino L (2003). New drugs for insomnia: comparative tolerability of zopiclone, zolpidem and zaleplon. *Drug Saf*, 26, 261–282.

Thomas RE (1998). Benzodiazepine use and motor vehicle accidents. Systematic review of reported association. *Can Fam Physician*, 44, 799–808.

Thorlund K, Druyts E, Wu P, et al. (2015). Comparative efficacy and safety of selective serotonin reuptake inhibitors and serotonin-norepinephrine reuptake inhibitors in older adults: a network meta-analysis. *J Am Geriatr Soc*, 63, 1002–1009.

Tzimos A, Samokhvalov V, Kramer M, et al. (2008). Safety and tolerability of oral paliperidone extended-release tablets in elderly patients with schizophrenia: a double-blind, placebo-controlled study with six-month open-label extension. *Am J Geriatr Psychiatry*, 16, 31–43.

Vestergaard P, Rejnmark L, Mosekilde L (2006). Fracture risk associated with the use of morphine and opiates. *J Intern Med*, 260, 76–87.

Waade RB, Hermann M, Moe HL, Molden E (2014). Impact of age on serum concentrations of venlafaxine and escitalopram in different CYP2D6 and CYP2C19 genotype subgroups. *Eur J Clin Pharmacol*, 70, 933–940.

Wegner I, Wilhelm AJ, Sander JW, Lindhout D (2013). The impact of age on lamotrigine and oxcarbazepine kinetics: a historical cohort study. *Epilepsy Behav*, 29, 217–221.

Weihs KL, Settle EC Jr, Batey SR, et al. (2000). Bupropion sustained release versus paroxetine for the treatment of depression in the elderly. *J Clin Psychiatry*, 61, 196–202.

Wildiers H, Highley MS, de Bruijn EA, van Oosterom AT (2003). Pharmacology of anticancer drugs in the elderly population. *Clin Pharmacokinet*, 42, 1213–1242.

Young RC, Mulsant BH, Sajatovic M, et al.; GERI-BD Study Group (2017). GERI-BD: a randomized double-blind controlled trial of lithium and divalproex in the treatment of mania in older patients with bipolar disorder. *Am J Psychiatry*, 174, 1086–1093.

Zolezzi M (2016). Medication management during electroconvulsant therapy. *Neuropsychiatr Dis Treat*, 12, 931–939.

Chapter

19

Psychotropic Prescribing in Pregnancy and Lactation

Angelika Wieck and Ian Jones

19.1 Introduction

The decision to prescribe psychotropic medication is always a matter of weighing up potential risks and benefits but at no time is this more difficult than in pregnancy and the post-partum period. This is because the risks do not only relate to the side effects for the mother but also potential adverse outcomes for the pregnancy and the child who may be particularly vulnerable during fetal development and breastfeeding. In addition, there is often a degree of uncertainty about what added risks medication may bring compared with no treatment.

In this chapter we will consider the issues around prescribing in the perinatal period. It is a rapidly changing area with new data constantly emerging. We will therefore focus on general principles that can guide clinicians in working with women at this time, rather than a detailed consideration of the reproductive safety literature itself. The chapter starts by considering the perinatal context and the ways in which a drug can harm the fetus. We then consider the important issues in interpreting the literature in this area before going on to consider the general principles of prescribing. To illustrate these points, we will then consider data on the use of a number of medications in pregnancy – namely, antidepressants, antipsychotics, anticonvulsants and lithium. This section is not intended to be an extensive and exhaustive systematic review, rather we will pick out some studies to discuss in more detail in order to explore the limitations of the data and issues in interpreting the findings as they emerge. This is followed by a brief review of psychotropic prescribing in relation to breastfeeding. The chapter finishes with a brief summary and conclusions.

19.2 The Perinatal Context

Before considering the evidence base around prescribing in pregnancy and the post-partum period, it is important to briefly acknowledge the context in which these difficult decisions are made. Pregnancy and the post-partum period are associated with high levels of psychiatric morbidity with depression the most common medical complication of pregnancy and childbirth. Mental health problems are common during pregnancy or within the first year of giving birth, affecting more than 1 in 10 women (Casanova Dias & Jones, 2016). Conditions include antenatal and post-natal depression, obsessive-compulsive disorder, post-traumatic stress disorder and other anxiety disorders, and post-partum psychosis. These problems can develop suddenly and range from mild to moderate, to extremely severe (Meltzer-Brody et al., 2018). While it is not clear that psychiatric morbidity in general is increased at this time, for severe episodes of illness such as post-partum psychosis affecting around 1 in 1000 women, there is very strong evidence that the post-partum period is high risk (Jones et al., 2014). Women with bipolar disorder in particular are at very high risk of a significant recurrence following childbirth (Di Florio et al., 2013). For women with bipolar disorder, 4 to 5 in every 10 are at risk of having an episode of illness in pregnancy or following childbirth and women are 23 times more likely to be admitted to a psychiatric hospital with an episode of bipolar disorder in the month following childbirth than at any other time in their life (Jones et al., 2014).

In summary, psychiatric disorders are very common in the perinatal period and for some conditions such as bipolar disorder, the post-partum period is a period of very high risk. In addition, these episodes have the potential to cause significant suffering to women and their baby. Suicide remains a leading cause of maternal death and these episodes can impact on the lives of women and their families, disrupting the relationship with the new baby. Perinatal mental illnesses are therefore a major public health issue. As well as having an adverse impact on the mother, they can impact on the emotional, cognitive and physical development of the child, and in some cases, the consequences can be life-long and experienced by the whole family (Stein et al., 2014). The estimated health and social care costs in the UK for perinatal mental health problems is £8.1 billion for each one-year cohort of births and mainly relates to impact that the maternal illness has on the child (Bauer et al., 2014). Decisions about prescribing, or indeed not prescribing, medication must be made, therefore, cognisant of the significant impact that perinatal mental illness can have on women and their families.

19.3 How a Drug Can Affect a Fetus

Since they are relatively small molecules and lipophilic, all psychotropic drugs can pass through the placenta. The amount reaching the fetus varies between drugs but whether this has a bearing on the fetal toxicity of a psychotropic drug is largely unknown.

In the first two weeks after fertilization, maternal medication has an 'all or nothing' effect, it can either kill the embryo or not affect it at all. The most severe consequences of maternal medication occur in the following weeks when organ structures are formed. Drugs reaching the embryo during this stage of development may result in pregnancy loss or a gross anatomical defect. Organ systems differ in the precise timing of the onset and end of the sensitive period for major congenital anomalies with the central nervous system being vulnerable the earliest and longest, from gestational week 3 to 16.

In the second and third trimester a medication used in pregnancy may result in minor congenital anomalies, functional defects and abnormal growth of the fetus or fetal organs that may have important short- and long-term consequences for the child, such as, for example, cognitive and behavioural development. There are a number of other ways in which maternal medication can affect outcome, including gestational diabetes, premature delivery, respiratory problems after birth and neonatal toxicity or withdrawal. In this chapter we will summarize the main findings from research in these areas.

19.4 Problems in Interpreting the Literature on the Safety of Psychotropic Drugs in Pregnancy

There are a number of important considerations when evaluating the reproductive safety literature. Historically, the main limitation has been the lack of available data with the literature consisting of case reports or small case series that are problematic due to the inevitable reporting bias in retrospective studies. For many psychotropic medications we still lack data but for some medications over the past decade the situation has dramatically changed. For example, there have been a large number of population studies reporting the outcome of thousands or even tens of thousands of exposures to selective serotonin reuptake inhibitor (SSRI) antidepressants in pregnancy with the largest study to date reporting the outcome of over 128 000 exposures (Huybrechts, 2015). These very large studies can bring problems of their own, having the power to pick up associations with very small effects that may be statistically significt but of doubtful clinical significance.

Perhaps the most fundamental confounding problem is that women who have a significant mental illness are more likely to have characteristics that are linked to a range of poor pregnancy and infant outcomes, including congenital anomalies. These factors include increased body mass index, physical illnesses, substance misuse, chronic psychosocial stress and low socio-economic status. In most studies information on these confounders is incomplete or patchy. This has hindered comparison with unexposed controls and the combining of data in meta-analyses. Several examples highlighting this important issue will be discussed in this chapter.

A further difficulty in making decisions about psychotropic medications is that for some medications, antiepileptic medication used in the treatment of bipolar disorder for example, the data we have on reproductive safety come from their use in non-psychiatric disorders. Although it may be reasonable to extrapolate the evidence to psychiatric indications, there are possible differences, in dosage for example, that may need to be taken into account.

Many studies reporting reproductive safety do not give any information on the severity of malformations reported, which can vary from minor issues that need no intervention to life-threatening problems requiring major surgery. With regard to minor problems, the fact that women are taking medication may lead to an increased vigilance for malformations with evidence, for example, that women taking drugs are subject to an increased number of ultrasound scans in pregnancy. On the other hand, in the case of more serious malformations, clinicians are more likely to record potential causes, such as the use of medication in early pregnancy, or report this outcome. One example for the latter is an early study linking the Ebstein anomaly with lithium exposure as discussed below.

A further difficulty in weighing up the risks and benefits of medication in pregnancy is that the evidence available tends to focus on the risks, with little data available on the benefits to the woman and the child of effective treatment of the mental illness. This is an area where further research is clearly needed.

Interpretation of studies must always take account of a further methodological issue, namely that of multiple testing. Studies often compare a number of drugs with a large number of malformations racking up a very large number of statistical comparisons which of course are likely then to result in type I errors. In addition, when considering the risks of medication, we always must remember that there is a surprisingly high background malformation rate of around 2–4% of pregnancies. Finally, it is important that the issues of the reproductive safety of medication should not only be considered in women who are pregnant or planning a pregnancy. In the general population around 40% of pregnancies are unintended and there is evidence that the rates in women with mental health conditions will be higher. We must therefore treat all women in their reproductive years with the possibility of pregnancy in mind and discuss pregnancy and contraception with all the women we treat under our care.

19.5 Pharmacokinetics of Psychotropic Drugs in Pregnant and Post-Natal Women

The changes in maternal physiology during pregnancy alter all major pharmacokinetic processes, including absorption, distribution, metabolism and elimination of drugs (Koren & Pariente, 2018). Intestinal motility is reduced resulting in longer gastric and intestinal emptying time which may have implications for the onset of drug action. Gastric acidity is reduced and mucus secretion increased with a potential to alter absorption. There is a 50% increase in plasma volume and a mean increase of body water by eight litres which results in lower peak serum concentrations. Elevated female sex steroid levels lead to an increased metabolizing activity of some cytochrome P450 and other enzymes in the liver and this, together with increased hepatic blood flow, leads to faster elimination of some psychotropic drugs. The reduced availability of albumin for drug binding in pregnancy is not thought to ultimately affect the amount of drugs that circulates in plasma unbound (Koren & Pariente, 2018). Renal plasma flow and glomerular filtration rate increase by up to 50% so that drugs which are primarily excreted unchanged in urine, such as lithium, show lower steady-state concentrations and a higher elimination rate (Koren & Pariente, 2018). Because of this, tight monitoring of lithium levels is recommended in pregnancy and the early post-natal period as described below.

Although there is considerable interindividual variation, clearance of lamotrigine increases gradually from early pregnancy, with over threefold drops in plasma levels being reported. This is caused by oestrogen-induced increases in the hepatic activity of glucuronosyltransferases and increased renal function. Levels increase again within a few days of delivery and return to non-pregnant baselines within the first month post-partum.

The plasma concentrations of several SSRIs and several tricyclic antidepressants have also been reported to decrease in pregnancy (Deligiannidis et al., 2014). Westin et al. (2018) measured antipsychotic drug levels in pregnancy and found a gradual decrease for aripiprazole and quetiapine, but not olanzapine. In the third trimester quetiapine levels were 76% and aripiprazole levels 52% lower than preconception and post-natally. Little data is available for other antipsychotic agents.

Because of uncertainties about therapeutic windows and clinical effectiveness, plasma levels are not routinely measured in the UK for psychotropic drugs other than lithium. However, indications for measurements include a lack of response despite a therapeutic dose, investigation of significant side effects and assessing adherence. In our opinion, measuring plasma levels should be considered more frequently in pregnancy than they currently are. For example, if women with a history of severe mental illness are planning a pregnancy and are currently stable on medication that has the potential to have accelerated metabolism in pregnancy, a plasma level should be considered and the woman's mental state closely monitored once she conceives. If the mental state deteriorates in pregnancy, the baseline drug level, in combination with a repeat measurement, will be helpful in evaluating the potential cause of the deterioration, the adequacy of the dosage and the need for dose adjustment. Therapeutic drug monitoring should also be considered, for example, in patients with psychosis or mania in advanced pregnancy who are initiated on antipsychotic medication, such as aripiprazole or quetiapine, and do not respond.

In the post-partum period, the pharmacokinetic processes normalize but little is known about how rapidly they return to pre-pregnancy states. If a higher medication dosage was used in pregnancy, it should be down-titrated to preconception values after delivery and plasma levels should be repeated from the early post-natal period until they have returned to baseline.

Prospective studies correlating declining psychotropic drug levels with clinical symptoms and developments of mental state after dose adjustments have not been done but are clearly needed in order to test whether this pragmatic approach is effective. Plasma level monitoring is only available in few centres and incurs costs to the service.

19.6 Principles of Prescribing in Preconception or Pregnant Patients

At no other time is it more important to exploit non-pharmacological interventions to the full than during childbearing. Current guidelines in the UK state that 75% of people referred to the 'Improving Access to Psychological Therapy' programme should begin treatment within 6 weeks of referral, and 95% within 18 weeks of referral. In respect of complex psychological interventions for severe disorders, many localities in the UK include childbearing women as one of the priority groups to ensure that treatment can begin within an even shorter time frame. If required, the woman should be offered a referral for dietary advice, and to weight management, smoking cessation and substance misuse clinics. For many childbearing women with moderate to severe mental illness, however, psychotropic medication is the mainstay of management.

19.6.1 Women Who Have Childbearing Potential

Women with psychotic illnesses and depression become pregnant more often unintentionally than other women. This results in a number of risks to pregnancy and infant outcome. Women with unplanned pregnancies, for example, receive antenatal care later, may be less likely to take the universally recommended peri-conceptual folic acid supplements and be more likely to smoke and use illicit drugs and alcohol. Women with affective disorders and unplanned pregnancies are more likely to abruptly stop their psychotropic medication. While they might fear that the drug will harm their child, there is evidence that pregnant women overestimate the risks. In their study of risk perception, Bonari et al. (2005) included callers to a teratology information service who were taking antidepressant, antibiotic or gastric drugs. The reproductive risks were grossly overestimated for all three groups of medications, but particularly so for antidepressants. Interestingly, evidence-based counselling improved the risk estimations (Bonari et al., 2005).

For all of these reasons, it is essential that general adult psychiatrists offer any woman with a severe mental illness who could get pregnant advice on childbearing on a regular basis. In addition to the reproductive safety of medication, the discussion should cover her current pregnancy status, contraception, and the effects of childbearing on her illness and the effects of her illness on childbearing. Discussions about the reproductive safety of prescribed medications need to be carefully recorded in patient's case notes, a practice which is not commonly adhered to (Royal College of Psychiatrists, 2016).

19.6.2 Preconception and Pregnant Women

All women with a history of mental illness who are planning a pregnancy or have recently conceived require advice and support. For common mental disorders this may be from the primary care team but women with more severe conditions, particularly those with bipolar or psychotic disorders, will need specialist psychiatric advice. Ideally this would be through a specialist perinatal community mental health team, if available. In the UK these services are currently being expanded but do not cover all areas. Where specialist perinatal services are not available, expertise will need to come from within general adult psychiatric services.

In the UK, there is a range of helpful websites for health professionals and patients available on the effects of childbearing on mental illness and vice versa (for example the Royal College of Psychiatrists) and the reproductive safety of psychotropic drugs (for example the UK Teratology Information Centre). Comparable information, in different languages, is available in some other countries.

When a woman with a severe mental disorder presents for preconception consultation or in early pregnancy, a detailed review of the psychiatric history, diagnosis and formulation and an estimate of the likely course of her illness in the antenatal and postnatal period is required. This, together with the difficult task of making decisions about medication, requires often more than one appointment, ideally with the patient's partner or significant other.

In the consultation, the advantages and risks of continuing, stopping and restarting medication in pregnancy should be discussed. Other than the reproductive safety, the decision should be based on the woman's illness and treatment history, her social and personal circumstances and her attitude to risks.

When selecting a drug, those with higher teratogenic potential and other risks to offspring should be avoided, as well as agents with little reproductive safety data or where there are other current contentious issues. With few exceptions, differences in the safety between newer antidepressants and individual antipsychotics are small, however, and it is often more important to choose or continue with an agent the woman is known to have responded to.

In the attempt to reduce harm to the fetus, clinicians often substantially reduce the dose of a prescribed medication when women present pregnant or plan to conceive. However, it is important that the dose does not drop below the known therapeutic range or what is effective for the individual patient. This is particularly important for women who are taking medication whose metabolism accelerates in pregnancy.

Sometimes clinicians lower the dose of ongoing psychotropic medication, and in particular antidepressants and lithium, in the last few weeks before the expected delivery date with the intent to avoid intoxication or withdrawal effects for the neonate. There is currently no evidence that this improves neonatal outcome significantly, while it may increase the risks of recurrence for the mother at the most critical time.

Because women may give birth prematurely, it is essential to prepare a written medication plan for the immediate perinatal period several weeks ahead of the expected delivery date, ideally at 32 weeks of pregnancy. It should be distributed, as part of the overall care plan, to the patient and all involved health professionals, including the obstetrician, community midwife, obstetric pharmacist, neonatologist, health visitor and primary care physician. In our experience, this is the time when breakdowns in communication between the many health professionals involved around the delivery occur most frequently and medication errors are being made. This is particularly of concern in women who are at risk of a post-partum relapse of affective psychosis. It is important that the medication plan is detailed, clear and placed in the woman's handheld maternity notes. It should include details about the timing of any planned medication changes, the timetable for any required blood sampling and whom to discuss results and dose adjustments with. Any questions regarding the medication plan should be discussed with the responsible consultant psychiatrist, and if she or he is not available, with another community mental health team (CMHT) member or the mental health liaison team. The patient should also be instructed to bring the medication with her when going into the maternity service for delivery because psychotropic medication will not be readily available there.

19.7 Antidepressant Medication

It is clear that prescriptions of antidepressants in pregnancy have markedly increased in recent decades. For example, in a study of the Danish registries that identified 19 740 pregnancies exposed to an antidepressant at some point during pregnancy, the rate increased from 0.2% in 1997 to 3.2% in 2010 (Jimenez-Solem et al., 2013). The use of antidepressant medication in pregnancy has been associated with changes on a number of pregnancy outcomes with small effects on gestational age, birth weight and APGAR scores (Ross et al., 2013). In addition, there is consistent evidence that exposure to antidepressants in late pregnancy is associated with complications in the neonate following delivery, with a fivefold increased risk of the usually mild and transient post-natal adaptation syndrome (Grigoriadis et al., 2013).

19.7.1 Are Antidepressants Associated with an Increased Risk of Congenital Malformations?

Before 2005 no increased risk of teratogenicity had been demonstrated for antidepressants, either tricyclic antidepressants or SSRIs, but the studies consisted of small cohorts with insufficient power to detect anything other than very large effects. In 2006 two studies reported an increased risk of cardiac defects with exposure to a particular SSRI, paroxetine (an unpublished study from the manufacturer GSK, and Källén and Otterblad, 2007). These studies reported a modest increased risk of cardiac defects, a rate of around 1.5/100 deliveries compared with a risk of 1/100 deliveries in all women. Over the last decade there have been many further studies, examining increasingly large numbers of antidepressant exposures. To summarize this increasingly large evidence base, there have been a number of associations reported between a range of individual antidepressants and various malformations. Two meta-analyses have been conducted, with the first finding fluoxetine (odds ratio (OR) 1.14, 95% confidence interval (CI) 1.01

to 1.30) and paroxetine (OR 1.29, 95% CI 1.11 to 1.49) associated with an increased risk of major anomalies and paroxetine also with cardiac malformations (OR 1.44, 95% CI 1.12 to 1.86) (Myles et al., 2013). The second meta-analysis, however, found antidepressants not to be associated with an increased risk of congenital malformations in general, but did find a statistically significant, but modest, increased risk for cardiovascular malformations that was not clearly of clinical significance (Grigoriadis et al., 2013).

In addition to the issue of large studies finding effects that while statistically significant are of marginal clinical significance, it is not even clear whether the small signal that emerges from the studies is a true effect of the medication or results from confounding. The impact of confounding can be seen by a close examination of the studies. For example, a Finnish registry study found an association with SSRI use in pregnancy and major congenital abnormalities with a modest effect size (OR 1.24, 95% CI 1.1 to 1.39) (Malm et al., 2011). However, when the attempt was made to control for confounders the effect size reduced and became non-significant (OR 1.08, 95% CI 0.96 to 1.22). Women taking antidepressants in pregnancy were less likely to be married, twice as likely to smoke and 20 times more likely to take other psychiatric medication.

Further evidence of the impact of confounding comes from a study of over 2.3 million pregnancies that generated 36 772 SSRI exposures (Furu et al., 2015). The adjusted analysis found a small association with cardiac defects (adjusted OR 1.15) but in further analysis using sibling controls the association disappeared (OR 0.92). As the authors conclude, although the prevalence of cardiac defects was higher in the exposed infants, the lack of an association in the sibling-controlled analyses points against a true teratogenic effect of these drugs.

19.7.2 Do SSRIs Increase Risk of PPHN?

Persistent pulmonary hypertension of the newborn (PPHN) is a rare but severe congenital abnormality with a high morbidity and mortality. An initial report in 2006 found a very strong association with 1% of babies exposed to an SSRI in the second and third trimesters of pregnancy affected (Chambers et al., 2006). As the condition is very rare in the general population this equated to an odds ratio of 6 and caused considerable concern in both women and clinicians. Since then, however, a number of further studies have been published, many with a much larger number of exposures. Some studies have failed to replicate the finding or have found the effect size to be much lower than the initial report. The largest study included data from 128 950 women who filled a prescription for antidepressants in late pregnancy (3.4% of all pregnancies) (Huybrechts et al., 2015). It found the absolute risk of PPHN to be much smaller than the initial study, with an odds ratio of 1.51 (95% CI 1.35 to 1.69). When adjusted for confounders, the odds ratio was even lower and no longer significant (adjusted OR 1.10, 95% CI 0.94 to 1.29).

19.7.3 Are There Long-Term Implications of Taking Antidepressants?

When considering the risks of taking antidepressants in pregnancy, congenital malformations are not the only consideration, longer-term impacts on the development of the exposed child must also be examined. In recent years a particular concern has been the association of SSRI exposure in pregnancy and the subsequent development of autism spectrum disorders (ASDs) in the offspring. An initial study (Croen et al., 2011) of 298 children with ASDs and 1507 controls found a more than twofold increased rate of SSRI exposure in the ASD group (OR 2.2, 95% CI 1.2 to 4.3) and an attributable risk of 2.1%. Questions have been asked about the adequacy of controlling for confounders and a number of further papers have emerged which have addressed this association. Although not all have replicated the original findings a meta-analysis has found further evidence to support this concerning association (pooled crude OR 2.13, adjusted OR 1.81) (Man et al., 2015). Residual confounding also remains a concern in these studies, but a recent paper made a valiant attempt to address this in four sets of analysis (control group of women with psychiatric illness; propensity score analysis; sibling analysis; control group of fathers who took antidepressants). Three of the four methods provided significant support, although attenuated, for the association. The sibling analysis was not significant but had a similar effect size to the unadjusted analysis.

In contrast, a further study also employing Swedish data came to very different conclusions. The authors assessed autism risk and prenatal antidepressant exposure in 179 007 children from the Swedish National Registers followed to age eight and adjusting for potential confounders, in particular the presence of maternal psychiatric disorder (Viktorin et al., 2017). The study concluded that antidepressants during pregnancy were not causally associated with an increased risk of ASD in offspring, rather the results suggesting the association is explained by factors related to the underlying susceptibility to psychiatric disorders.

If antidepressant use in pregnancy is associated with risks, it is also important to address the other side of the risk–benefit equation and look at the outcomes in treated women compared to unmedicated mothers with episodes of illness and their children. Although there are few studies that address this question, there are some data emerging which point to the potential benefits of medication in pregnancy compared with not receiving treatment. In a Danish study, there were non-significant trends for children exposed to antidepressants in pregnancy to do better, when examined at the age of seven, on a range of measures (e.g. hyperactivity/inattention, conduct and emotional problems) than children of mothers whose depression in pregnancy was not treated (Grzeskowiak et al., 2015).

19.7.4 What Are the Implications of Stopping Antidepressants in Relation to Pregnancy?

Finally, an important consideration in making decisions about stopping or continuing antidepressant medication in women who are, or wish to be pregnant, is the impact of stopping medication. In this area the literature is somewhat conflicting. In a study of 201 women with a history of major depression referred to a tertiary mood disorder centre in the USA, 68% of those who discontinued medication experienced a significant recurrence of depression in pregnancy compared with a 26% recurrence in those who remained on antidepressants (Cohen et al., 2006). However, the women in this study predominantly were suffering from a severe unipolar mood disorder with a mean duration of over 15 years and almost half had experienced five or more episodes.

Contrasting results were found by a second study from the USA. In 778 pregnant women with a history of major depression recruited in community settings there was no effect of continuing or stopping antidepressant treatment (hazard ratio 0.88, 95% CI 0.51

to 1.50) (Yonkers et al., 2011). These very different results probably reflect the fact that depression is a heterogeneous condition and emphasizes the need to individualize the risk assessment and options for each woman.

19.8 Dopamine Receptor Antagonists (Antipsychotic Medications)

As in other psychiatric patient groups, there has been an increase in the prescribing of atypical antipsychotics to pregnant women while the use of typical antipsychotics has remained the same or decreased. Prescriptions for dopamine receptor antagonist medications are often discontinued or no longer claimed by pregnant patients. Only 38% of atypical and 19% of typical antipsychotics are still prescribed in the third trimester (Petersen et al., 2014).

19.8.1 Infant and Pregnancy Outcomes

In a meta-analysis of available case-control or cohort studies that included controls and investigated major congenital malformations, Coughlin et al. (2015) examined 13 publications with data on more than 6000 exposed and 1.6 million unexposed children. They found a twofold increase in the rate of major congenital anomalies with heart defects most commonly represented. These malformations were frequently septal defects. There was also a raised incidence of preterm birth (twofold) and small size of the newborn for gestational age (2.5-fold) but no association with miscarriage and stillbirth. The analysis was difficult to interpret because of the small number of included studies and the limited adjustment for confounding factors: only five took into account smoking, one substance misuse and two obesity. One in five patients were taking concomitant antiepileptic medication and antidepressant use was frequent. Low socio-economic status and confounding by indication could not be considered.

Significant progress was made in the landmark study by Huybrechts et al. (2016). The study cohort consisted of the largest sample to date with 9258 women who had filled a prescription of a 'second-generation' antipsychotic in the first trimester and 733 women who had filled a prescription for a 'first-generation' antipsychotic. This large cohort number allowed the assessment of individual second-generation antipsychotics. Unadjusted analyses suggested a small increase in the overall malformation rate and the incidence of cardiac anomalies in particular for second-generation antipsychotics. That increase was also seen for individual second-generation antipsychotics. However, after a broad range of confounding factors were taken into account, the only association that remained significant was an increased risk of general malformations in children exposed to risperidone. When the relationship with dose was explored, the difference to controls was only significant for a daily dose of 2 mg or more. A specific effect of risperidone is difficult to explain with a known biological mechanism and the finding may have arisen by chance. Further studies are required to clarify this finding.

Since the endocrine and metabolic changes in pregnancy enhance vulnerability to diabetes the question arises whether antipsychotic therapy increases the risk of gestational diabetes. There is some evidence that this is the case but the relationship may be explained by a greater body mass index at the beginning of pregnancy in women taking antipsychotics (Bodén et al., 2012).

19.8.2 Neonatal Symptoms

The only study of neonatal health after intrauterine exposure to antipsychotics that included controls and accounted for confounders found that monotherapy with first- and second-generation antipsychotics were not associated with withdrawal symptoms (Habermann et al., 2013).

19.8.3 Neurodevelopment

Current evidence from studies that followed children up to different ages suggests that there are no major long-term neurodevelopmental adverse effects of intrauterine antipsychotic exposure. In one prospective study covering the first 12 months of life after exposure to atypical antipsychotics in utero, an initial worse performance on most scores of the Bayley scales resolved by the end of the first post-natal year (Peng et al., 2013).

19.9 Anticonvulsants Used in Psychiatry

Evidence on the reproductive safety of anticonvulsant drugs is largely based on research of children born to mothers with epilepsy, probably because these drugs were introduced into the treatment of bipolar disorder later. However, there is no known reason why reproductive safety findings would be different if the indication is a mental disorder.

19.9.1 Teratogenic Potential

There is now consistent and compelling evidence that valproate is linked with an excess of major structural defects in the developing fetus. In their systematic review and meta-analysis of cohort and pregnancy register studies, Meador et al. (2008) found an anomaly rate for monotherapy with valproate in the first trimester of 10.7% compared with 3.3% in offspring of healthy control mothers. The most recent meta-analysis including 4455 cases of exposure to valproate monotherapy confirmed an approximately threefold increase compared with control groups (Veroniki et al., 2017a). In regard to specific anomalies, significant differences have not only been reported for spina bifida (OR 12.7) but also for atrial septal defects, cleft palate, hypospadias, polydactyly and craniosynostosis (Jentink et al., 2010) as well as club foot (Veroniki et al., 2017a).

Estimates for a teratogenic risk of carbamazepine have consistently been lower and in the most recent meta-analysis (n = 8437, Veroniki et al., 2017a) the odds ratio was only slightly raised at 1.37 (95% credible interval (CrI) 1.10 to 1.71). Carbamazepine has been implicated in causing spina bifida but the reported risk is much smaller than for valproate. Current evidence suggests that exposure to lamotrigine monotherapy does not alter the overall rate of major congenital malformations (n = 6290 cases, Veroniki et al., 2017a). An initial finding of an increased risk of oral clefts following pregnancy exposure to lamotrigine has not been substantiated by subsequent studies (Tomson & Battino, 2012).

19.9.2 Neurodevelopmental Effects

Earlier concerns about the cognitive development of children exposed to valproate in pregnancy have recently been confirmed (Bromley et al., 2014). Current evidence suggests that, compared with offspring of mothers without epilepsy or with untreated epilepsy, exposed children perform less well on various tests of intellectual development by 8–9 IQ or developmental points (Bromley et al., 2014). In a recent population study, exposed children were also five and three times more likely to have ASD or autism, respectively (Christensen et al., 2013), and the rate was higher than for children whose mothers had discontinued valproate before pregnancy. Taking into account other developmental problems, it has been estimated that 30–40% of exposed young children may be affected by neurodevelopmental problems (European Medicines Agency, 2014).

Lamotrigine has not been suggested to be detrimental to the cognitive development of children, but a recent meta-analysis found a high odds ratio (8.8) for autism (Veroniki et al., 2017b). However, the total sample of exposed children was small (n = 254) and the confidence interval was very large (1.28 to 112.00) so this potentially worrying finding clearly requires further study. Carbamazepine has not been associated with poorer cognitive development in early childhood in the majority of studies (Bromley & Baker, 2017).

19.9.3 Can Valproate-Induced Harm Be Prevented?

A relationship of the teratogenic effect with daily dose of valproate has been widely described although critical thresholds have varied between 600 mg and 1500 mg per day (Tomson & Battino, 2012). It is still too early yet to draw conclusions about the dose dependence of neurocognitive problems. Overall, a safe valproate dose for pregnant women cannot be defined.

The general population incidence of neural tube defects and several other congenital anomalies can be markedly reduced by folic acid use (400 μg daily) from preconception to early pregnancy. Prescription of a high dose of folic acid (4–5 mg daily) to women taking antiepileptic drugs is sometimes recommended because low folate levels have been associated with an increased malformation risk in women taking antiepileptic drugs. However, current evidence suggests that dietary folic acid supplementation at high or low doses does not, or may only partially, prevent teratogenicity in women (Wlodarczyk et al., 2012).

19.9.4 Prescribing Anticonvulsant Medication to Women with Mental Disorders Who Are or Could Get Pregnant

Because of the mounting evidence for widespread harm to offspring, and evidence that there has not been a consistent large decline in valproate prescribing across European countries and indications, the European Medicines Agency (2018) has recently recommended that valproate is not used to treat epilepsy, bipolar disorder or migraine in girls and women who are pregnant. The only group exempted are pregnant women with idiopathic epilepsy whose seizures have been poorly controlled by other antiepileptic medications. Girls or women who are not pregnant but have childbearing potential should only be prescribed valproate if there is no alternative treatment and if a pregnancy prevention programme is followed. These recommendations are now legally binding across European countries. The guidelines by the National Institute for Health and Care Excellence for Antenatal and Postnatal Mental Health in England and Wales (National Institute for Health and Care Excellence, NICE, 2014) go even further and state that valproate should not be offered at all to any woman who is pregnant or could get pregnant, regardless of whether she is using effective contraception.

The pregnancy prevention programme suggested by the European Medicines Agency (2018) and supported by the Medicines and Healthcare products Regulatory Agency (MHRA) in the UK includes an assessment of a woman's potential to become pregnant, pregnancy tests before and during treatment, and counselling about the risks of valproate to unborn children and the importance of effective contraception throughout treatment. Patients are required to have specialist reviews and complete a risk acknowledgement form every year. Valproate packaging are now carrying a visual warning of the pregnancy risks and patients will receive a warning card with each prescription. Pharmacists will be required to discuss the risks every time they dispense valproate to women of childbearing age. The MHRA published a toolkit on their website (Medicines and Healthcare Products Agency, 2019) with educational information and helpful advice for patients and clinicians which we would recommend to use. As a result of the new regulations clinicians can encounter challenging issues in the pharmacological management of patients with complex bipolar disorder and other conditions currently taking valproate. The Royal College of Psychiatrists and the British Association of Psychopharmacology have recently published a position statement discussing the evidence for alternatives to valproate and providing advice on how women can be withdrawn or switched to alternative treatments (Baldwin & Wieck, 2018).

NICE (2014) in the UK also recommends that carbamazepine should not be offered to women who are pregnant or are planning a pregnancy but do not restrict its use in women with childbearing potential. If this drug is considered for a woman with childbearing potential who does not plan a pregnancy, she should be informed about the teratogenic risk and advised to use effective contraception.

19.10 Lithium

In the UK, the use of lithium in pregnancy has been low and prescriptions are discontinued in two-thirds of women in early gestation, reflecting concerns about its reproductive safety. Only 1 in 10 000 pregnant women are prescribed lithium beyond the sixth week of pregnancy (McCrea et al., 2015).

19.10.1 How Teratogenic is Lithium?

A finding of a large increase of the severe cardiovascular anomaly of the Ebstein type, from a general population rate of only 1:20 000 to 2.7% in children exposed to lithium in utero, was reported almost four decades ago. This study, which included only a small number of cases and was based on selective retrospective reporting, nevertheless influenced clinical practice in subsequent decades. The methodological flaws of the study and the low number of Ebstein cases in subsequent reports led the authors of a meta-analysis (McKnight et al., 2012) to conclude that the risk was overestimated. More recently, a European registry-based study covering 5.6 million deliveries reported the largest sample of unexplained Ebstein cases and found that none of the 173 babies had been exposed to lithium in utero (Boyle et al., 2017). Interestingly, there was an association of Ebstein's anomaly with maternal mental illness although this was based on only a small number of cases.

In the largest study of first trimester lithium exposure to date, involving a retrospective cohort of more than 1.3 million pregnant women, Patorno et al. (2017) reported on 663 infants. After adjustment for several important confounders, the rate of cardiac congenital anomalies was slightly increased (OR 1.65, 95% CI 1.02 to 2.68) but much lower than in the historical study. The likelihood of confounding by indication was low because a similar difference was found compared with children who had been exposed to lamotrigine in the first trimester. The teratogenic effect was dose related and only significant when a daily lithium dose of more than 900 mg was prescribed. However, at this dose level, the risk was increased threefold.

There have been few studies of other pregnancy outcomes and no systematic studies of the physical health in newborns who were exposed to lithium in pregnancy but a variety of problems have been described in case reports (for example cardiac arrhythmias, hypoglycaemia, diabetes insipidus, polyhydramnios, thyroid dysfunction, goitre, floppiness, lethargy, hepatic anomalies and respiratory difficulties) (American College of Obstetricians and Gynecologists, 2008). There is one five-year prospective study of 60 children who showed no excess of physical or mental anomalies compared with their unexposed siblings (Schou et al., 1976).

19.10.2 Lithium Use in Pregnancy

Lithium is now recommended as a first-line therapy for the prevention of bipolar episodes in general (Goodwin et al., 2016; see also Chapter 11). In a woman who is planning a pregnancy or who is pregnant in the first trimester and is already taking lithium, a need to switch to an antipsychotic is now less compelling (Wieck, 2017). A patient can stay on lithium if it is clear that she needs maintenance treatment, there is evidence that she has responded to lithium and that the risk of relapse would be high if it was discontinued and replaced by an antipsychotic. If the woman requires a second drug for maintenance treatment in addition to a dopamine receptor antagonist this should be lithium and not valproate or carbamazepine.

19.10.3 Lithium Dosing and Monitoring in the Perinatal Period

Since lithium readily equilibrates across the placenta it is important to avoid blood levels higher than necessary to maintain mood stability. On the other hand, subtherapeutic levels should equally be avoided. Renal function increases until mid-pregnancy and decreases again in the third trimester. Using standardized lithium levels in 1001 clinical samples before, during and after pregnancy, Wesseloo et al. (2017) found that the blood-level-to-dose ratio significantly dropped in the first trimester and was one-third less than before conception in the second trimester with the lowest values occurring at week 17 of pregnancy. There was a gradual return towards preconception levels in the third trimester and the early post-partum period. The creatinine levels showed a similar longitudinal pattern as for lithium.

Although the mean daily dose increased in pregnancy, the proportion of subtherapeutic lithium levels rose from 15% preconception to 62% in the first and second trimester, dropped to 39% in the third trimester and fell below the preconception value after delivery. Only a small number of women relapsed (n = 5) but it is interesting to note that three had evidence of low levels and one had discontinued her medication.

Because of the dynamic changes, the guidelines by NICE (2014) recommend to measure lithium levels more frequently in pregnancy and suggest once a month until week 36 of pregnancy and then weekly. Psychiatrists need to warn obstetricians about the risks of toxic lithium levels in women who develop pre-eclampsia or other conditions with renal impairment. Should this occur, the woman should be managed proactively with a joint care plan by obstetrician and psychiatrist.

During delivery, we would recommend to monitor levels 12 hours after every lithium dose and to repeat this on the first post-natal day. If the result is outside the therapeutic range measurements should be continued in intervals as appropriate. We would also recommend to follow the recommendation by Wesseloo et al. (2017) to continue with at least two measurements in the first two weeks post-natal since renal function only gradually normalizes after delivery.

19.11 Psychotropics and Breastfeeding

19.11.1 Interpreting the Literature

The amount of a maternal drug that reaches the blood circulation of a breastfed infant is the result of perhaps the most complex series of processes in psychopharmacology. It is dependent on the mother's pharmacokinetics, the size, lipophilicity and albumin binding of the drug, the frequency of feeding, the volume and fat content of the milk the baby ingests, the fate of the drug in the infant's gut and its absorption rate, the maturity of the infant liver, and the child's metabolizer status and volume of distribution.

Research on drug levels in infants' circulation is limited but existing data suggest that concentrations are often either low or below assay detection limits. If levels are measurable, they tend to vary widely. Likewise, studies of potential adverse medication effects in breastfed infants are scarce. They consist of uncontrolled observations made on single cases or case series, usually without standardized assessments, and long-term effects remain largely unstudied.

Most research has been conducted on the proportions of psychotropic drugs transferred from the maternal circulation to breast milk. Overall, infants are exposed to much smaller amounts when breastfeeding than during pregnancy, but there are exceptions. A measure of exposure that is frequently used in paediatric practice is the relative infant dose (RID). This is defined as the daily amount of drug ingested by an infant, who is fully breastfed, per kg body weight divided by the maternal daily dose per kg body weight. The infant is assumed to ingest 150 ml/kg milk per day. A value of more than 10% is regarded as generally indicating a higher probability of side effects in the infant (Bennett, 1996).

19.11.2 Principles of Prescribing During Breastfeeding

Although methodological inadequacies in studies measuring RIDs have been noted (Hummels et al., 2016), the measure is in our opinion still useful for clinical purposes as a rough guide for the likelihood of side effects in the child. For example, if a woman has recently given birth and requires an antidepressant or antipsychotic drug for the first time, an agent with a low RID would be the first choice. If a woman with a psychiatric history has, however, responded to an antidepressant or antipsychotic medication with a moderately high RID, for example, then it is reasonable to continue this medication because otherwise the therapeutic effect might be lost for a relatively uncertain gain for the individual child. Drugs with very high RIDs and mood stabilizers need to be considered with caution, as outlined below.

There are limited data on the time course of concentrations of some psychotropic drugs in breast milk which indicate that they follow those in the maternal serum with some delay. However, there is little evidence to support discarding breast milk and delaying breastfeeding after a mother has taken a dose of medication. In addition, this practice would make it even more challenging for the mother to establish or maintain breastfeeding.

Medication that causes excessive sedation should be avoided in post-natal women, if possible, since it can hinder nursing and baby care. If the sedative effect of a medication does not resolve after a short time, switching to a less sedative agent should be considered.

When nursing mothers of premature or unwell infants are prescribed particular caution needs to be exercised. The ability of premature infants to metabolize drugs is less developed than those of term infants and this can lead to drug accumulation. Discussion with a neonatologist is advised.

In terms of general advice, breastfed infants should be monitored for adverse effects such as excessive sedation and poor feeding and other side effects that are seen in adults. Mothers should be advised to seek advice from the health visitor or primary care physician if in doubt.

An excellent resource for prescribers that provides free access to up-to-date evaluations of research on frequently prescribed medications is the Toxnet – LactMed (2019) that is accessible on the World Wide Web.

19.11.3 Antidepressants, Antipsychotics and Breastfeeding

Most antidepressants are transferred in very low concentrations to breast milk whereas venlafaxine, fluoxetine and citalopram are reported to result occasionally in moderately high RIDs (less than 20%, Toxnet – LactMed, 2019).

In respect of dopamine receptor antagonists, small case numbers to date suggest very low transfer of drugs into breast milk except for amisulpride, sulpiride, risperidone and haloperidol where estimated RIDs can approach or exceed 10% (Hale, 2012; Toxnet – Lact Med, 2019). Nevertheless, in published clinical observations of breastfed infants, relatively few adverse effects have been reported (Dayan et al., 2011; Gentile, 2008). One breastfed infant whose mother took clozapine developed agranulocytosis but it is not known whether this was related to pregnancy exposure. We would advise against breastfeeding during clozapine therapy.

19.11.4 Anticonvulsants and Breastfeeding

Breastfed infants whose mothers are taking lamotrigine have relatively high plasma lamotrigine levels which can sometimes reach half of the maternal value. This is thought to be related to the post-partum rise of lamotrigine levels, if the dose is not reduced after delivery, and the limited ability of the neonatal liver to metabolize drugs by glucuronidation.

Occasional adverse effects in breastfed infants have been reported. These include withdrawal symptoms after abrupt weaning, and mild and asymptomatic thrombocytosis (Toxnet – LactMed, 2019). One infant, who had a high plasma level in the context of a high maternal dose of lamotrigine (850 mg daily), was reported to have experienced a severe apnoeic episode (Toxnet – LactMed, 2019).

During maternal therapy with lamotrigine, breastfed infants should be carefully monitored for side effects such as apnoea, skin rash, excessive drowsiness and poor sucking. The infant's plasma level should be measured if there is any concern about its health. Monitoring of the platelet count and liver function may also be advisable (Toxnet – LactMed, 2019). If the child develops a skin rash, breastfeeding should be discontinued until the cause is established.

Lithium easily enters breast milk and in several case reports breastfed infants had serum levels between 10% and 58% of the maternal value (Toxnet – LactMed, 2019). Several instances of infant health problems were described, including suspected lithium intoxication, abnormal thyroid function tests, slow weight gain and delay in motor development (Toxnet – LactMed, 2019). In some cases, it was difficult to establish whether these problems were the result of lithium exposure via breast milk. It has been highlighted that numerous reports also exist of infants without any signs of lithium toxicity or developmental problems and that maternal lithium therapy should not be an absolute contraindication to breastfeeding of full-term infants (Toxnet – LactMed, 2019). We would recommend to exercise great caution when making decisions about breastfeeding in a mother who is medicated with lithium. Some authors recommend monitoring infant serum lithium, serum creatinine, urea and thyroid stimulating hormone in intervals ranging from unspecified to every 4 to 12 weeks. Breastfeeding should be discontinued immediately and the infant evaluated if she or he appears restless or lethargic or has feeding problems.

19.12 Summary and Conclusions

As we hope we have demonstrated, women and the clinicians face very difficult decisions with regard to medication in pregnancy and breastfeeding and until relatively recently there was very little data to guide them. Over the last decade there has been a considerable improvement in the amount and quality of research. For example, much larger studies have been published for antidepressant and antipsychotic use in pregnancy that take better account of confounding factors. However, it is clear that residual confounding is still a big issue in determining the safety of these medications in pregnancy.

What is clear is that there are a number of examples of initial reports over-estimating the magnitude of risk, the association of lithium with heart malformations for example, or SSRIs and persistent pulmonary hypertension of the newborn. Caution is always advisable in responding to the latest reproductive safety scare that is so often exaggerated in the media. It is also a recurring pattern that the better the studies and the more they control for confounders, the less is the apparent impact of medication on negative outcomes. A number of factors related to the prescription of the medication, not least the illness itself, may therefore account for at least some of the increased risk.

In this area, as in so many others in medicine, more research is required. We need better systems to establish the safety or identify risks for currently used drugs in pregnancy and breastfeeding, conducting large naturalistic monitoring studies of routinely collected clinical and other data. In addition to studies highlighting risk, we need to address the benefit side of the risk–benefit equation. Pregnancy and breastfeeding are usual exclusion criteria for drug trials meaning there are little data on the efficacy of medication specifically in the perinatal period. In addition, there has been very little progress in developing interventions specifically for perinatal mental illness. The recent very encouraging, if preliminary, evidence suggesting a 60-hour infusion of the neuro-steroid allopregnanolone may be an effective new treatment for post-partum depression is particularly to be welcomed (Kanes et al., 2017). In addition to studies of medication, we also need well-conducted investigations of non-pharmacological treatments in the perinatal period, such as electroconvulsive therapy, repetitive transcranial magnetic stimulation and light therapy.

While it is right to call for more and better research, studies with ever larger exposure numbers may bring issues of their own. As we have seen when considering the very large studies of antidepressant exposure, it is possible that they may pick up statistically significant associations of very small and doubtful clinical significance. It is therefore vital that clinicians consider the magnitude of the risks, not just their statistical significance.

When weighing up treatment options in the perinatal context, there are often no right or wrong answers and each decision should be made based on the specific history of an individual woman at that particular time. It also means that however helpful and authoritative clinical guidelines are, and whatever decision aids may be developed in this area, there will be no substitute for detailed clinical review and discussion with the patient. Thoughtful and compassionate clinicians working with women and their partners to make difficult decisions will still be central to good management.

References

American College of Obstetricians and Gynecologists (2008). ACOG Practice Bulletin: clinical management guidelines for obstetrician-gynecologists number 92, April 2008. Use of psychiatric medications during pregnancy and lactation. *Obstet Gynecol*, 111, 1001–1020.

Baldwin D, Wieck A (2018). *Withdrawal of, and alternatives to, valproate-containing medicines in girls and women of childbearing potential who have a psychiatric illness*. Royal College of Psychiatrists, PS 04/18. Available at: www.bap.org.uk/pdfs/PS04-18-December2018.pdf (last accessed 15.8.19).

Bauer A, Paronage M, Knapp M, et al. (2014). *The Costs of Perinatal Mental Health Problems*. The London School of Economics, Personal Social Services Research Unit. Available at: http://eprints.lse.ac.uk/59885/1/__lse.ac.uk_storage_LIBRARY_Secondary_libfile_shared_repository_Content_Bauer%2C%20M_Bauer_Costs_perinatal_%20mental_2014_Bauer_Costs_perinatal_mental_2014_author.pdf (last accessed 8.9.19).

Bennett PN (1996). Use of monographs in drugs. In PN Bennett, ed., *Drugs and Human Lactation*. Amsterdam: Elsevier Science Publishers, pp. 67–74.

Bodén R, Lundgren M, Brandt L, et al. (2012). Antipsychotics during pregnancy: relation to fetal and maternal metabolic effects. *Arch Gen Psychiatry*, 69, 715–721.

Bonari L, Koren G, Einarson TR, et al. (2005). Use of antidepressants by pregnant women: evaluation of perception of risk, efficacy of evidence based counseling and determinants of decision making. *Arch Womens Ment Health*, 8(4), 214–220.

Boyle B, Garne E, Loane M, et al. (2017). The changing epidemiology of Ebstein's anomaly and its relationship with maternal mental health conditions: a European registry-based study. *Cardiol Young*, 27(4), 677–685. doi:10.1017/S1047951116001025.

Bromley R, Baker GA (2017). Fetal antiepileptic drug exposure and cognitive outcomes. *Seizure*, 44, 225–231.

Bromley R, Weston J, Adab N, et al. (2014). Treatment for epilepsy in pregnancy: neurodevelopmental outcomes in the child. *Cochrane Database Syst Rev*, (10), CD010236. doi:10.1002/14651858.CD010236.pub2.

Casanova Dias M, Jones I (2016). Perinatal psychiatry. *Medicine*, 44(12), 720–723. doi:http://dx.doi.org/10.1016/j.mpmed.2016.09.006.

Chambers CD, Hernandez-Diaz S, Van Marter LJ, et al. (2006). Selective serotonin-reuptake inhibitors and risk of persistent pulmonary hypertension of the newborn. *N Engl J Med*, 354, 579–587.

Christensen J, Grønborg TK, Sørensen MJ, et al. (2013). Prenatal valproate exposure and risk of autism spectrum disorders and childhood autism. *JAMA*, 309(16), 1696–1703.

Cohen LS, Altshuler LL, Harlow BL, et al. (2006). Relapse of major depression during pregnancy in women who maintain or discontinue antidepressant treatment. *JAMA*, 295, 499–507.

Coughlin CG, Blackwell KA, Bartley C, et al. (2015). Obstetric and neonatal outcomes after antipsychotic medication exposure in pregnancy. *Obstet Gynecol*, 125(5), 1224–1235. doi:10.1097/AOG.0000000000000759.

Croen LA, Grether JK, Yoshida CK, et al. (2011). Antidepressant use during pregnancy and childhood autism spectrum disorders. *Arch Gen Psychiatry*, 68, 1104–1112.

Dayan J, Gaignic-Philippe R, Seligmann C, et al. (2011). Use of antipsychotics and breastfeeding. *Curr Wom Health Rev*, 7, 37–45.

Deligiannidis KM, Byatt N, Freeman MP (2014). Pharmacotherapy for mood disorders in pregnancy: a review of pharmacokinetic changes and clinical recommendations for therapeutic drug monitoring. *J Clin Psychopharmacol*, 34(2), 244–255. doi:10.1097/JCP.0000000000000087.

Di Florio A, Forty L, Gordon-Smith K, et al. (2013). Perinatal episodes across the mood disorder spectrum. *JAMA Psychiatry*, 70(2), 168–175.

European Medicines Agency (2014). CMDh agrees to strengthen warnings on the use of valproate medicines in women and girls. Press release, 21 November 2014. Available at: www.ema.europa.eu/docs/en_GB/document_library/Referrals_document/Valproate_and_related_substances_31/Position_provided_by_CMDh/WC500177637.pdf (last accessed 15.8.19).

European Medicines Agency (2018). New measures to avoid valproate exposure in pregnancy endorsed. Press release, 23 March 2018. Available at: www.ema.europa.eu/docs/en_GB/document_library/Press_release/2018/03/WC500246391.pdf (last accessed 15.8.19).

Furu K, Kieler H, Haglund B, et al. (2015). Selective serotonin reuptake inhibitors and venlafaxine in early pregnancy and risk of birth defects: population based cohort study and sibling design. *BMJ*, 350, h1798. doi:10.1136/bmj.h1798.

Gentile S (2008). Infant safety with antipsychotic therapy in breast-feeding: a systematic review. *J Clin Psychiatry*, 69(4), 666–673.

Goodwin GM, Haddad PM, Ferrier IN, et al. (2016). Evidence-based guidelines for treating bipolar disorder: revised third edition recommendations from the British Association for Psychopharmacology. *J Psychopharmacol*, 30(6), 495–553. doi:10.1177/0269881116636545.

Grigoriadis S, VonderPorten EH, Mamisashvili L, et al. (2013). The effect of prenatal antidepressant exposure on neonatal adaptation: a systematic review and meta-analysis. *J Clin Psychiatry*, 74, e309–e320.

Grzeskowiak LE, Morrison JL, Henriksen TB, et al. (2015). Prenatal antidepressant exposure and child behavioural outcomes at 7 years of age: a study within the Danish National Birth Cohort. *BJOG*, 123, 1919–1928.

Habermann F, Fritzsche J, Fuhlbrück F, et al. (2013). Atypical antipsychotic drugs and pregnancy outcome: a prospective, cohort study. *J Clin Psychopharmacol*, 33(4), 453–462. doi:10.1097/JCP.0b013e318295fe12.

Hale T (2012). *Medications and Mother's Milk*. Amarillo: Hale Publishing.

Huybrechts KF, Bateman BT, Palmsten K, et al. (2015). Antidepressant use late in pregnancy and risk of persistent pulmonary hypertension of the newborn. *JAMA*, 313, 2142–2151.

Huybrechts KF, Hernández-Díaz S, Patorno E, et al. (2016). Antipsychotic use in pregnancy and the risk for congenital malformations. *JAMA Psychiatry*, 73(9), 938–946. doi:10.1001/jamapsychiatry.2016.1520.

Hummels H, Bertholee D, van der Meer D, et al. (2016). The quality of lactation studies including antipsychotics. *Eur J Clin Pharmacol*, 72(12), 1417–1425.

Jentink J, Loane MA, Dolk H, et al.; EUROCAT Antiepileptic Study Working Group (2010). Valproic acid monotherapy in pregnancy and major congenital malformations. *N Engl J Med*, 362(23), 2185–2193.

Jimenez-Solem E, Andersen JT, Petersen M, et al. (2013). Prevalence of antidepressant use during pregnancy in Denmark, a nation-wide cohort study. *PLoS One*, 8(4), e63034. doi:10.1371/journal.pone.0063034.

Jones I, Chandra PS, Dazzan P, Howard LM (2014). Bipolar disorder, affective psychosis, and schizophrenia in pregnancy and the post-partum period. *Lancet*, 384(9956), 1789–1799.

Källén BA, Otterblad OP (2007). Maternal use of selective serotonin re-uptake inhibitors in early pregnancy and infant congenital malformations. *Birth Defects Res A Clin Mol Teratol*, 79, 301–308.

Kanes S, Colquhoun H, Gunduz-Bruce H, et al. (2017). Brexanolone (SAGE-547 injection) in post-partum depression: a randomised controlled trial. *Lancet*, 390(10093), 480–489.

Koren G, Pariente G (2018). Pregnancy-associated changes in pharmacokinetics and their clinical implications. *Pharm Res*, 35(3), 61. doi:10.1007/s11095-018-2352-2.

Malm H, Artama M, Gissler M, et al. (2011). Selective serotonin reuptake inhibitors and risk for major congenital anomalies. *Obstet Gynecol*, 118, 111–120.

Man KK, Tong HH, Wong LY, et al. (2015). Exposure to selective serotonin reuptake inhibitors during pregnancy and risk of autism spectrum disorder in children: a systematic review and meta-analysis of observational studies. *Neurosci Biobehav Rev*, 49, 82–89.

McCrea RL, Nazareth I, Evans SJ, et al. (2015). Lithium prescribing during pregnancy: a UK primary care database study. *PLoS One*, 10(3), e0121024. doi:10.1371/journal.pone.0121024.

McKnight RF, Adida M, Budge K, et al. (2012). Lithium toxicity profile: a systematic review and meta-analysis. *Lancet*, 379(9817), 721–728. doi:10.1016/S0140-6736(11)61516-X.

Meador K, Reynolds MW, Crean S, et al. (2008). Pregnancy outcomes in women with epilepsy: a systematic review and meta-analysis of published pregnancy registries and cohorts. *Epilepsy Res*, 81(1), 1–13. doi:10.1016/j.eplepsyres.2008.04.022.

Meltzer-Brody S, Howard LM, Bergink V, et al. (2018). Postpartum psychiatric disorders. *Nat Rev Dis Primers*, 4, 18022. doi:10.1038/nrdp.2018.22.

Myles N, Newall H, Ward H, et al. (2013). Systematic meta-analysis of individual selective serotonin reuptake inhibitor medications and congenital malformations. *Aust N Z J Psychiatry*, 47(11), 1002–1012. doi:10.1177/0004867413492219.

National Institute for Health and Care Excellence (NICE) (2014). *Antenatal and postnatal mental health – clinical management and service guidance*. Clinical guideline [CG192]. London: National Institute for Health and Care Excellence.

Patorno E, Huybrechts KF, Bateman BT, et al. (2017). Lithium use in pregnancy and the risk of cardiac malformations. *N Engl J Med*, 376(23), 2245–2254. doi:10.1056/NEJMoa1612222.

Peng M, Gao K, Ding Y, et al. (2013). Effects of prenatal exposure to atypical antipsychotics on postnatal development and growth of infants: a case-controlled, prospective study. *Psychopharmacology (Berl)*, 228(4), 577–584. doi:10.1007/s00213-013-3060-6.

Petersen I, McCrea RL, Osborn DJ, et al. (2014). Discontinuation of antipsychotic medication in pregnancy: a cohort study. *Schizophr Res*, 159(1), 218–225. doi:10.1016/j.schres.2014.07.034.

Ross LE, Grigoriadis S, Mamisashvili L, et al. (2013). Selected pregnancy and delivery outcomes after exposure to antidepressant medication: a systematic review and meta-analysis. *JAMA Psychiatry*, 70, 436–443.

Royal College of Psychiatrists, Centre for Care Quality Improvement (2016). *Topic 15a baseline audit report. Prescribing valproate for bipolar disorder*. Available at: www.covwarkpt.nhs.uk/download.cfm?doc=docm93jijm4n2406.pdf&ver=3039 (last accessed 15.8.19).

Schou M (1976). What happened later to the lithium babies? A follow-up study of children born without malformations. *Acta Psychiatr Scand*, 54(3), 193–197.

Stein A, Pearson RM, Goodman SH, et al. (2014). Effects of perinatal mental disorders on the fetus and child. *Lancet*, 384(9956), 1800–1819. http://dx.doi.org/10.1016/S0140-6736(14)61277-0.

Tomson T, Battino D (2012). Teratogenic effects of antiepileptic drugs. *Lancet Neurol*, 11(9), 803–813. doi:10.1016/S1474-4422(12)70103-5.

Toxnet – LactMed (2019). Drugs and Lactation Database – LactMed. Available at: https://toxnet.nlm.nih.gov/newtoxnet/lactmed.htm (last accessed 8.9.19).

Veroniki AA, Cogo E, Rios P, et al. (2017a). Comparative safety of anti-epileptic drugs during pregnancy: a systematic review and network meta-analysis of congenital malformations and prenatal outcomes. *BMC Med*, 15(1), 95. doi:10.1186/s12916-017-0845-1.

Veroniki AA, Rios P, Cogo E, et al. (2017b). Comparative safety of antiepileptic drugs for neurological development in children exposed during pregnancy and breast feeding: a systematic review and network meta-analysis. *BMJ Open*, 7(7), e017248. doi:10.1136/bmjopen-2017-017248.

Viktorin A, Uher R, Reichenberg A, et al. (2017). Autism risk following antidepressant medication during pregnancy. *Psychol Med*, 47, 2787–2796. doi:10.1017/S0033291717001301.

Wesseloo R, Wierdsma AI, van Kamp IL, et al. (2017). Lithium dosing strategies during pregnancy and the postpartum period. *Br J Psychiatry*, 211(1), 31–36. doi:10.1192/bjp.bp.116.192799.

Westin AA, Brekke M, Molden E, et al. (2018). Treatment with antipsychotics in pregnancy: changes in drug disposition. *Clin Pharmacol Ther*, 103(3), 477–484. doi:10.1002/cpt.770.

Wieck A (2017). Prevention of bipolar episodes with lithium in the perinatal period. *Br J Psychiatry*, 211, 3–4.

Wlodarczyk BJ, Palacios AM, George TM, et al. (2012). Antiepileptic drugs and pregnancy outcomes. *Am J Med Genet A*, 158A(8), 2071–2090. doi:10.1002/ajmg.a.35438.

Yonkers KA, Gotman N, Smith MV, et al. (2011). Does antidepressant use attenuate the risk of a major depressive episode in pregnancy? *Epidemiology*, 22, 848–854.

The Clinical Management of Acute Disturbance Including Rapid Tranquillisation

Faisil Sethi, Caroline Parker, Aileen O'Brien and Maxine X. Patel

20.1 Introduction

In psychiatric and emergency healthcare settings, episodes of agitation and violence are relatively common. One meta-analysis reported that 32.4% of patients behaved violently during admission to a psychiatric ward; this was the mean rate of violence based on 122 studies from 11 countries (Bowers et al., 2011). The comparable rate in the UK studies was 41.7%. A study of general adult wards of a UK inner-city mental health trust found violence rates for 49% of men and 39% of women in the 6-month period studied (Hodgins et al., 2007).

Definitions for the terms 'violence' and 'agitation' vary. The World Health Organization defines violence as 'the intentional use of physical force or power, threatened or actual, against oneself, another person, or against a group or community, that either results in or has a high likelihood of resulting in injury, death, psychological harm, maldevelopment, or deprivation' (Krug et al., 2002). The UK National Institute for Health and Care Excellence (NICE) defines violence and aggression as '*a range of behaviours or actions that can result in harm, hurt or injury to another person, regardless of whether the violence or aggression is physically or verbally expressed, physical harm is sustained or the intention is clear*' (NICE, 2015). As far as possible, both on an individual and at a service level, therapeutic interventions should aim to reduce the frequency of incidents of agitation, aggression and violence. When such interventions are unsuccessful, rapid tranquillisation (RT) may be necessary to reduce harm to the patient or to others.

It is important to be specific regarding the definition for RT. The most recent definition by NICE in the UK is '*the use of medication by the parenteral route (usually intramuscular or, exceptionally, intravenous) if oral medication is not possible or appropriate and urgent sedation with medication is needed*' (NICE, 2015). Other guidelines have varied according to whether medication needs to be administered parenterally to meet the definition for RT. When oral emergency medication is included within the definition of RT, there can be confusion regarding whether medication is being given as required (*pro re nata*; PRN), being used as a measure to reduce the need for RT, or whether it can be considered in its own right as RT. For clarity, we refer to RT as only including parenteral options, which is in keeping with recent guidelines (NICE, 2015; Patel et al., 2018).

The goal of RT is to '*calm/lightly sedate the patient, reduce the risk to self and/or others and achieve an optimal reduction in agitation and aggression, thereby allowing a thorough psychiatric evaluation to take place allowing comprehension and response to spoken messages throughout the intervention*' (NICE, 2005). Accepting the definition of RT as referring to medication given in an emergency situation via the parenteral route has the potential advantage that RT incidents may be more clearly defined and recorded. It is important to emphasize that RT should generally be used as a last resort and only if non-pharmacological and oral pharmacological options have been exhausted. A core tenet of pharmacological management is that regular treatment should be optimized both as a primary measure with the aim of reducing the requirement for RT, and to try to avoid further episodes.

20.2 Evidence and Guidelines

Robust evidence regarding RT is sparse due to the ethical and practical difficulties involved in conducting trials. The lack of internationally accepted definitions of the terms 'violence', 'aggression' and indeed 'rapid tranquillisation' can lead to confusion in the literature. Nevertheless, there is a range of guidelines available, based on the evidence that exists and on clinical consensus. Outside of the UK, the American College of Emergency Physicians' guidelines (Lukens, 2006) focused on management in the emergency department and the issue of determining that a patient does not have physical health problems. In October 2010, the American Association for Emergency Psychiatry embarked on Project BETA (Wilson et al., 2012). Over 35 emergency psychiatrists, emergency medicine physicians, mental health clinicians, nurses and patient advocates participated in the project. A range of recommendations from de-escalation to pharmacological recommendations were produced. With a more European perspective, the World Federation of Societies of Biological Psychiatry (WFSBP) created a consensus statement with guidelines for the assessment and management of agitation in psychiatry (Garriga et al., 2016). The data used were extracted from various national treatment guidelines and panels for schizophrenia, as well as from meta-analyses, reviews and randomized controlled trials (RCTs).

The NICE guidelines in the UK include both general recommendations regarding management of violence and aggression and more specific recommendations regarding agents used in RT. The NG10 guideline (NICE, 2015) on the short-term management of violence and aggression in mental health and community settings includes principles for: managing violence and aggression; anticipating and reducing the risk of violence and aggression; preventing violence and aggression; using restrictive interventions in inpatient psychiatric settings; managing violence and aggression in emergency departments, and community and primary care settings; managing violence and aggression in children and young people. This was followed up in 2017 by the NICE Quality Standard [QS154] on violent and aggressive behaviour in people with mental health problems, based on the 2015 guidance (NICE, 2017) (see Table 20.1). Quality Standards identify priority areas for quality improvement in care, and usually cover areas where there is variation in care. Although they are not mandatory, they can help plan and deliver services and serve as audit standards to measure the quality of care.

Table 20.1 NICE Quality Statements for the management of violent and aggressive behaviours in people with mental health problems. Quality Standard [QS154] Published date: June 2017 (NICE, 2017)

Quality Statement 1	People in contact with mental health services who have been violent or aggressive are supported to identify triggers and early warning signs for these behaviours.
Quality Statement 2	People in contact with mental health services who have been violent or aggressive are supported to identify successful de-escalation techniques and make advance statements about the use of restrictive interventions.
Quality Statement 3	People with a mental health problem who are manually restrained have their physical health monitored during and after restraint.
Quality Statement 4	People with a mental health problem who are given rapid tranquillisation have side effects, vital signs, hydration level and consciousness monitored after the intervention.
Quality Statement 5	People with a mental health problem who experience restraint, rapid tranquillisation or seclusion are involved in an immediate post-incident debrief.

In addition to the NICE guidelines, in the UK, the *Maudsley Prescribing Guidelines* form an influential guide including treatment algorithms (Taylor et al., 2018). Guidelines notwithstanding, virtually all mental health organizations have protocols in this clinical area. Innes and Sethi (2012) reviewed recommendations set out in the adult RT documents of UK mental health organizations. A total of 45 RT documents met the inclusion criteria and were examined. There was little consensus as to which drugs should be used for RT in adults. In these documents, 11 clinical decision-making parameters were identified that influenced the selection of drugs for intramuscular (IM) administration (Innes & Sethi, 2012). Most recently, the British Association for Psychopharmacology together with the National Association of Psychiatric Intensive Care and Low Secure Units developed joint evidence-based consensus guidelines on the management of acute disturbance which included recommendations for clinical practice and an algorithm to guide treatment (Patel et al., 2018).

20.3 Non-Pharmacological Alternatives to Rapid Tranquillisation

RT cannot be considered in isolation without considering the practices of restraint and seclusion. Ineffective management of agitation can result in an unnecessary use of these coercive measures, but it may not be possible to safely avoid them altogether.

The NICE definition of manual restraint is a '*skilled, hands-on method of physical restraint used by trained healthcare professionals to prevent service users from harming themselves, endangering others or compromising the therapeutic environment. Its purpose is to safely immobilise the service user*' (NICE, 2015). Manual restraint should be distinguished from mechanical restraint in which straps, belts or other equipment are used to restrict movement; this is very rarely used in the UK.

Seclusion is defined in the Mental Health Act 1983 Code of Practice as '*the supervised confinement and isolation of a patient in a room, away from other patients, in an area from which the patient is prevented from leaving, where it is of immediate necessity for the purpose of the containment of severe behavioural disturbance which is likely to cause harm to others*' (Department of Health, 2015). This is to be differentiated from 'time out', when a patient agrees to spend time in a quiet area away from others, with no restrictions on returning to contact with other patients. This may effectively reduce the requirement for more restrictive interventions, but it is important to ensure that it happens with the full consent of the patient.

Restraint can occur without RT and vice versa. A patient may, once manually restrained, agree to 'time out' or to take oral medication. Generally, however, for a patient to receive RT safely, some form of manual restraint is required. Seclusion may be necessary in cases of risk to others and in this situation if the patient is refusing oral medication, RT would normally be required. However, this can be especially challenging when considering safe post-RT monitoring.

Many countries have introduced strategies to reduce seclusion and restraint; the 'six core strategies' developed in the United States by the National Association of State Mental Health Program Directors have been influential (NASMHPD, 2008) (see Figure 20.1). Some studies have indicated a decrease in seclusion and restraint rates following the introduction of these core strategies (Azeem et al., 2011; Huckshorn, 2006). The strategies include: articulating a philosophy of care that embraces seclusion and restraint

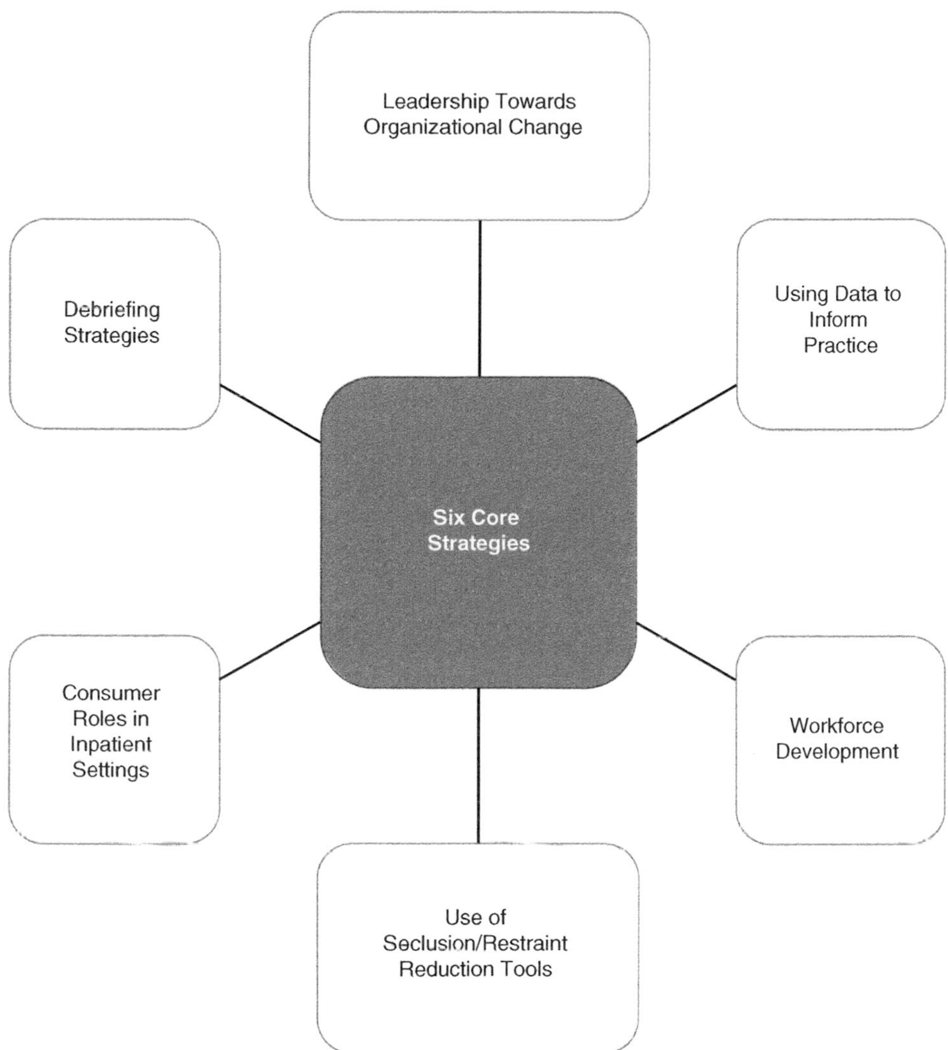

Figure 20.1 Six core strategies to reduce seclusion and restraint use (adapted from NASMHPD, 2008).

reduction; using data in an empirical, 'non-punitive' way to examine and monitor patterns of seclusion and restraint use; developing procedures, practices and training that are based on knowledge and principles of mental health recovery; using assessments and resources to individualize aggression prevention; including consumers, carers and advocates in seclusion and restraint reduction initiatives; conducting an analysis (debrief) of why seclusion and restraint occurred and evaluating the impacts of these practices on individuals with lived experience.

In the UK, the Department of Health published *Positive and Proactive Care* (Department of Health, 2014). This work aimed to reduce all forms of restrictive practices and ensure that they were only used as a last resort in emergency situations; a particular focus was placed on ending prone (face-down) restraint. All providers were asked to publish an annual report on the use of restrictive interventions, with Board oversight of an organizational plan to reduce restrictive practices.

Recognizing the early signs of agitation, with the aim of reducing the need for further restrictive interventions, is important and staff should be trained in the use of techniques aimed at defusing anger and averting aggression. NICE recommends that all staff receive training in de-escalation. De-escalation is defined by NICE as the '*use of techniques (including verbal and non-verbal communication skills) aimed at defusing anger and averting aggression. PRN medication can be used as part of a de-escalation strategy but PRN medication used alone is not de-escalation*' (NICE, 2015). NICE also recommends that people in contact with mental health services who have been violent or aggressive should be supported to (i) identify triggers and early warning signs for these behaviours; (ii) identify successful de-escalation techniques; and (iii) make advance statements about the use of restrictive interventions (NICE, 2017). Price et al. (2015) described seven themes from the literature on de-escalation. The first three related broadly to staff skills, including: characteristics of effective de-escalators; maintaining personal control; and verbal and non-verbal skills. The last four relate to the process of intervening and include: engaging with the patient; when to intervene; ensuring safe conditions for de-escalation; and strategies for de-escalation. Recent guidelines review the evidence on the various components of de-escalation (Patel et al., 2018).

In England, the Safewards model has identified aspects of working in wards that are considered to create potential 'flashpoints' and described strategies to manage these (Bowers, 2014). Bowers et al. (2015) identified many factors that can be originating factors of problems including the culture and environment of the ward, policies and procedures. Modifiers include positive appreciation and support, role modelling and education. The model was subject to a cluster RCT which indicated that staff can successfully intervene to manage flashpoints to reduce conflict and the use of seclusion (Bowers et al., 2015).

Gaskin et al. (2007) described ways that seclusion can be reduced; their review of the literature highlighted the complexity in this area, with no one solution or 'magic bullet'. Interventions described included: increased monitoring and regulation; leadership changes; staff training; introducing new staff; improved staff-to-patient ratios; treatment plan improvement; and even aromatherapy. Recently, one study found that the introduction of body cameras for inpatient staff led to a reduction in untoward incidents (Hardy et al., 2017).

Interventions to reduce restrictive practice including restraint and RT are as complex and multifactorial as the causes of aggression. Caution should be taken when comparing different service models which may differ greatly in terms of both culture and the type of patients. The Prescribing Observatory for Mental Health found the highest rates of RT nationally to be in forensic Child and Adolescent Mental Health Services (CAMHS) and acute learning disabilities (LD) inpatient settings, with high rates in psychiatric intensive care units (PICU) but lower rates in forensic settings, reflecting acuity of situations (POMH-UK, 2017).

20.4 Oral Medication

When non-pharmacological methods fail to diminish acute disturbance, oral medication should be considered before IM options (NICE, 2015). Usually these include promethazine and/or benzodiazepines as tablets, but liquid preparations and orodispersible options can be helpful to ensure compliance. Other options include buccal midazolam or sometimes antipsychotics including inhaled loxapine (see Neuroscience-based Nomenclature Glossary).

20.4.1 Benzodiazepines

Lorazepam is the most commonly used oral benzodiazepine in the management of acute disturbance due to its short half-life (dose of 1–2 mg; time to peak plasma concentration 2 hours; onset of effect 20–30 minutes; time to peak effect 2 hours). Oral diazepam may sometimes be considered but its active metabolites contribute to its long half-life in terms of accumulation and associated risks of side effects (time to peak plasma concentration 30–90 minutes).

Clonazepam can be a useful drug as it also has a liquid oral formulation in addition to tablets but the time to peak effect is long and there is a risk of accumulation (time to peak plasma concentration 1–4 hours; onset of effect 20–60 minutes; time to peak effect 12 hours) (Gillies et al., 2013). Significant side effects of benzodiazepines primarily include respiratory depression and hypotension with its associated increased risk of falls.

Midazolam has an oro-mucosal/buccal formulation (dose of 10–20 mg; time to peak plasma concentration 24 minutes; onset of effect 5–20 minutes; time to peak effect 5–20 minutes). This has a very short half-life of 2–3 hours and its effect is likely to be only for a few hours. In a small observational study, it was found to be effective and well tolerated with target levels of sedation being achieved in over two-thirds of patients within 30 minutes (Taylor et al., 2008).

20.4.2 Antipsychotics (Dopamine Receptor Antagonists and Partial Agonists)

Antipsychotic use for acute disturbance will often involve patients with mania, schizophrenia or another psychotic disorder. As such, any PRN use is likely to be in addition to regularly prescribed antipsychotics and this commonly leads to high-dose prescribing with associated heightened risk of side effects (Patel et al., 2018; RCPsych, 2014). It is important to note that there is no current evidence from RCTs to support the common practice of PRN antipsychotic use and thus current practice appears to be based on clinical experience and prescribing habit rather than high-quality evidence (Douglas-Hall & Whicher, 2015). In addition to sedation, side effects of antipsychotics include QT prolongation, hypotension and extrapyramidal symptoms (see a later section in this chapter and also Chapter 9 for a discussion of these side effects).

Oral haloperidol is the most commonly used antipsychotic in the management of acute disturbance but the Summary of Product Characteristics recommends that an ECG should be available before this drug is prescribed (eMC, 2017), which may not be feasible, and that concomitant antipsychotics should be avoided. The suggested dose is haloperidol 5 mg (time to peak plasma concentration 2–6 hours). Other commonly used oral options include quetiapine 50–100 mg, olanzapine 10 mg (time to peak plasma concentration 5–8 hours), risperidone 1–2 mg (time to peak plasma concentration 1–2 hours) and less commonly aripiprazole 5–10 mg (time to peak plasma concentration 3 hours). A good review of the evidence base for oral antipsychotics was provided by Garriga et al. (2016) who highlighted that second-generation antipsychotics (with high serotonin and histamine receptor antagonist properties) have more recently been recommended over haloperidol for the control of agitation due to a psychiatric illness.

Loxapine is a first-generation antipsychotic (dibenzoxazepine class) that is a potent H_1 receptor antagonist and it has an orally inhaled preparation, with absorption in the lungs, which requires some cooperation from the patient. The recommended dose for acute agitation is 10 mg via a single-use inhaler (time to peak plasma concentration is less than 5 minutes; onset of action is less than 10 minutes). It is contraindicated in respiratory diseases including asthma and chronic obstructive pulmonary disease due to the risk of wheezing and bronchospasm. A bronchodilator such as salbutamol must also be readily available in healthcare facilities which use loxapine for those who do not have a respiratory disease history. Other side effects include a metallic taste and throat irritation (Citrome, 2012). There is RCT evidence to support the use of loxapine, versus placebo, for the management of acute agitation in schizophrenia and bipolar disorder (Kwentus et al., 2012; Lesem et al., 2011). Comparison of loxapine with other medications commonly used in RT is yet to be reported on (Garriga et al., 2016).

20.4.3 Promethazine

This is an antihistamine (phenothiazine derivative with strong H_1 antagonism) with sedative properties. In its oral form it is licensed as an anti-emetic, for the treatment of insomnia in adults, as a sedative in children and for the symptomatic treatment of allergic conditions. Its use for treating acute disturbance is thus off-label. The common dose of promethazine for managing acute disturbance is 25–50 mg (time to peak plasma concentration 1.5–3 hours; onset of effect 20–30 minutes). Side effects include confusion, dry mouth, extrapyramidal symptoms and reduction of seizure threshold. It is sometimes used in combination with an oral benzodiazepine or an oral antipsychotic; and such use is often in the domain PRN or regular medication.

20.5 Parenteral Medication in Rapid Tranquillisation

When patients present with acutely disturbed and violent behaviour that does not respond to de-escalation and other non-drug options, then the use of medication needs to be considered. Oral medication should be offered first. Only if oral medication is actively refused and medication is still considered necessary should parenteral medication be considered (Khwaja & Beer, 2013; NICE, 2015). In such circumstances, the administration of medication parenterally is not without risks, and therefore should not be undertaken lightly.

If patients are not willing to accept oral medication in their agitated and violent state, then parenteral medication needs to be administered by force. For this to occur, the patient will need to be restrained. There are two main parenteral routes of administration: intramuscular (IM) and intravenous (IV). IM administration is usually into the gluteal muscle. This has the advantage of being a large muscle which is readily accessible during restraint but has the disadvantage that the removal of clothing is required for access to the muscle and this is perceived as undignified.

When administering an IM injection to obese patients, care needs to be taken to ensure that the needle goes deep enough to actually enter the muscle and not deposit the medication in the adipose tissue, as this would adversely affect the drug absorption. Following IM administration, the time to maximum plasma concentration (a very crude proxy for time to effect) can range between 15 and 60 minutes (depending on the medication). Arguably, this is not that much faster than some of the oral medications which have a time to maximum plasma concentration around the hour mark (the range is 1–8 hours for the group of oral medications).

IV RT is rarely used in the UK (POMH-UK, 2017) and is generally not recommended (Gillies et al., 2013; Innes & Sethi, 2012; Khwaja & Beer, 2013; NICE, 2015) as although the patient is restrained it still carries the inherent risks of inadvertent arterial administration. Also, registered mental health nurses (RMNs) are not trained to administer IV injections and therefore a doctor (or someone else trained in IV administration techniques) is required. It has the advantage of an extremely rapid onset of action (within 5 minutes).

There are three groups of medication that are generally recommended for parenteral RT: benzodiazepines, antipsychotics and the antihistamine promethazine, and combinations of these groups (Patel et al., 2018). The exact medications used vary between countries and are partly related to availability. The evidence for the efficacy of these agents is relatively small and weak (CADTH, 2015; Gillies, 2013). Trials vary considerably in design and most are small. There have been no large, well-designed RT trials conducted in the UK; all trials used to inform our practice were conducted in other healthcare settings. Depending on the continent or country in which they were conducted, trials vary from asking the patient for informed written consent prior to participation (Breier et al., 2002; Wright et al., 2001) to having endpoints of complete sedation, where consent would have been a challenge (Alexander et al., 2004; Huf et al., 2007; Raveendran et al., 2007; TREC Collaborative Group, 2003).

20.5.1 Benzodiazepines

A benzodiazepine alone is the most common form of parenteral RT administered in the UK (POMH-UK, 2017) and the most widely recommended (Innes & Sethi, 2012; NICE, 2015). Most benzodiazepines are fat soluble, so there can be a risk of accumulation. The following benzodiazepines can be administered IM and are commonly referred to in RT protocols and guidelines:

- Lorazepam IM: In the UK this is the most commonly used (POMH-UK, 2017) and recommended benzodiazepine for IM use (Innes & Sethi, 2012; NICE, 2015); with peak plasma levels at 1–1.5 hours, this is one of the fastest acting agents, which is a key criterion for this intervention. The duration of effect is 6–8 hours; the half-life is 12–16 hours; it does not have any active metabolites so there is no risk of active accumulation. Although this is the benzodiazepine of choice there have been intermittent supply problems over the past decade leading to services looking for alternatives.
- Midazolam IM: Peak plasma levels are achieved within 30 minutes, with a rapid onset of action at 5–20 minutes (Martel, 2005; TREC Collaborative Group, 2003); like lorazepam it has the advantage of no active metabolites; unlike most benzodiazepines, midazolam is water soluble and has a short half-life (1–3 hours) although this can be so short that its duration of effect is insufficient, leading to the need for repeated doses (TREC Collaborative Group, 2003); it has a notably increased risk of respiratory depression compared with other benzodiazepines (Gillies, 2013; TREC Collaborative Group, 2003). For these reasons it is not recommended for use in RT (Patel et al., 2018).

- Diazepam IM: A very erratic absorption pattern, peaking at 1–5 hours; a very long half-life followed by an active metabolite (desmethyldiazepam) with a much longer half-life (20–40 hours) leading to the risk of accumulation; effects last for 24–48 hours. It is not recommended for use in RT (Patel et al., 2018).

IV administration is rarely used in the UK, Diazepam IV has a very quick onset of action (5–10 seconds) and peak concentration (< 1 minute); if the IV route is used it is important to use the correct formulation of diazepam (Diazemuls®). Midazolam IV also exists as does clonazepam IV but there is no licensed version of the latter available in the UK.

For a detailed review of the international evidence and practice of using benzodiazepines for RT refer to Gillies et al. (2013) and also Patel et al. (2018).

20.5.2 Antipsychotics (Dopamine Receptor Antagonists and Partial Agonists)

The following IM antipsychotics are commonly used in RT:

- Haloperidol IM: A first-generation antipsychotic; this is widely available internationally and the most commonly used antipsychotic in RT in the UK (POMH-UK, 2017) with the most RCT data supporting its use (Huf et al., 2016). It has a time to maximum plasma concentration of around 20–40 minutes. However, a baseline ECG is required and it should not be used as monotherapy in RT as measures are required to offset its adverse effects including the risk of acute dystonia (Patel et al., 2018).
- Olanzapine IM: A second-generation antipsychotic; similar efficacy to the combination of haloperidol plus promethazine, but causes fewer extrapyramidal side effects (EPSE) than haloperidol (Breier et al., 2002; Raveendran et al., 2007; Wright et al., 2001). It has a time to maximum plasma concentration of around 15–45 minutes. This should not be administered concurrently with IM benzodiazepines due to the risk of hypotension.
- Aripiprazole IM: A second-generation antipsychotic; in trials this demonstrated greater efficacy compared with placebo at 45 minutes (Tran-Johnson et al., 2007; Zimbroff et al., 2007) but its onset of action was slower than haloperidol IM; of note it has a time to maximum plasma concentration of around an hour. It has lower rates of EPSE compared with IM haloperidol (Andrezina et al., 2006).

20.5.3 Promethazine

Promethazine IM is a potent, long-acting, central sedative antihistamine that is a phenothiazine derivative. It is licensed for sedation and the treatment of insomnia in adults but not for use in RT. Its efficacy has been demonstrated both as monotherapy and, more frequently, in combination with other agents (see below). It has a slower onset of action than other options, such as IM lorazepam. The peak plasma level is reached at 1.5–3 hours, with an onset of action at 20–30 minutes and a half-life of 9.8 ± 4 hours; effects last 4–6 hours but may persist longer.

20.6 Combinations of Medications in Rapid Tranquillisation

It is common practice to administer combinations of two medicines from different groups in RT (POMH-UK, 2017). These would be administered concurrently, but not mixed in the same syringe. Combinations are recommended when single agents are not

Table 20.2 Summary of TREC trials

Sample size	Country	Medicines investigated	Primary outcome	Results	Serious adverse effects
TREC Rio-I (TREC Collaborative Group, 2003)					
301	Brazil	IM midazolam 7.5–15 mg vs. IM haloperidol 5–10 mg + IM promethazine 25–50 mg	Tranquil or sedated at 20 min	IM midazolam (89%) vs. IM haloperidol + IM promethazine (67%) RR: 1.32 (CI: 1.16–1.49)	2
TREC Vellore-I (Alexander et al., 2004)					
200	India	IM lorazepam 4 mg vs IM haloperidol 5–10 mg + IM promethazine 25–50 mg	Tranquil or asleep by 4 hr	IM lorazepam (96%) vs. IM haloperidol + IM promethazine (96%) RR: 1.0 (CI: 0.9–1.06), NS	2
TREC Rio-II (Huf et al., 2007)					
316	Brazil	IM haloperidol 5–10 mg vs. IM haloperidol 5–10 mg + IM promethazine 25–50 mg	Tranquil or asleep at 20 min	IM haloperidol (55%) vs. IM haloperidol + IM promethazine (72%) RR: 1.30 (CI 1.10–1.55) (trial was stopped early)	12
TREC Vellore-II (Raveendran et al., 2007)					
300	India	IM olanzapine 10 mg vs. IM haloperidol 5–10mg + IM promethazine 25–50 mg	Tranquil or asleep at 15 mins	IM olanzapine (87%) vs. IM haloperidol + IM promethazine (91%) RR: 0.96 (CI: 0.34–1.47), NS	4

CI, 95% confidence interval; NS, non-significant; RR, relative risk.

sufficient (NICE, 2015; Patel et al., 2018). There have been four significant randomized RT trials (the TREC trials, see Table 20.2), the details of which are described below, and which were summarized in a Cochrane review (Huf et al., 2016) and also in recent guidelines (Patel et al., 2018).

The NICE (2015) guidelines recommend the use of lorazepam alone, or the combination of haloperidol + promethazine. In general, haloperidol is not recommended as monotherapy due to the greater side-effect burden, which can be reduced by using a lower dose of haloperidol in combination with another agents. The two most common combinations are (i) haloperidol with lorazepam and (ii) haloperidol with promethazine. There are no trial data to compare the efficacy of the two combinations.

- Haloperidol plus lorazepam is the most widely used combination for RT in the UK (POMH-UK, 2017) and has been for many decades. There is some RCT evidence to recommend this combination over IM lorazepam alone in the short term of up to an hour but not thereafter (Zaman et al., 2017).
- The four robust TREC RCTs demonstrated the efficacy and relative safety of haloperidol plus promethazine combination in non-UK settings, and therefore this combination is now recommended in guidelines (NICE, 2015; Patel et al., 2018). However, this combination is not widely used in the UK (POMH-UK, 2017).

20.7 Other Treatments

20.7.1 Ketamine

Ketamine is an *N*-methyl-D-aspartate (NMDA) receptor antagonist and is used as an anaesthetic agent especially in emergency situations. In a psychiatric context, it is usually recommended for use administered by an anaesthetist with full resuscitation equipment availability. In a prospective open-label study for 146 patients, the median time to 'adequate sedation' was significantly shorter at 5 minutes for IM ketamine (5 mg/kg) than for IM haloperidol (10 mg) at 17 minutes (Cole et al., 2016). However, 49% of patients in the IM ketamine group experienced side effects including hypersalivation, vomiting and laryngospasm and 39% required intubation. Use of ketamine is supported by the Royal College of Emergency Medicine, but without comment on the strength of evidence (Gillings et al., 2016). Hence, other guidelines note that ketamine has some evidence for effectiveness but do not recommend it due to the risk of respiratory depression and lack of reversing agent (Patel et al., 2018).

20.7.2 Zuclopenthixol Acetate

This is a first-generation antipsychotic which may be considered for disturbed behaviour but not during RT as its onset is not rapid. Peak serum concentrations are reached 24–36 hours after injection and decline slowly thereafter, reaching about one-third after 3 days. Some studies have shown that sedation usually starts approximately 2 hours after injection and peaks around 12 hours, with some effect for up to 72 hours. Doses are 50–150 mg per injection, up to a maximum of 400 mg over 2 weeks (Taylor et al., 2015). Injections should be given at least 24 hours apart and the patient should be medically and psychiatrically assessed before each injection.

Generally, zuclopenthixol acetate should only be considered for use: (i) after a patient with acute psychosis has required repeated short-acting injections of olanzapine, haloperidol and/or lorazepam; or (ii) in patients who have previously had a good treatment response to zuclopenthixol acetate. Due to the risk of oversedation, this drug should preferably not be used in combination with other parenteral antipsychotics or benzodiazepines. It should not be used in patients who: are accepting oral medication; are antipsychotic naive; are sensitive to extrapyramidal symptoms; are unconscious; have significant hepatic or renal impairment; or have cardiac disease (Taylor et al., 2015).

Jayakody et al. (2012) highlighted that the evidence base for zuclopenthixol acetate is based on small trials with methodological flaws. In comparison with IM haloperidol, there is no evidence to support the superiority of zuclopenthixol acetate (Chin et al., 1998). They concluded that perhaps the only true advantage of using zuclopenthixol acetate is that following its administration, patients generally need fewer injections in the following seven days. There is no evidence to suggest that higher doses offer additional benefit over lower doses (Jayakody et al., 2012).

20.7.3 Barbiturates

IM preparations of amylobarbitone and paraldehyde have been historically used, but current use is extremely rare. In reference to the 1999 *Maudsley Prescribing Guidelines*, after parenteral benzodiazepines and/or antipsychotics failed to have a desired clinical effect, amylobarbitone sodium was given as 500 mg IM or IV following consultant advice. If a response occurred, then oral amylobarbitone sodium 200 mg PRN could be considered. If no response was found after 30 minutes for IM or 60 minutes for IV, then a second dose IM or IV was advised (Kerr & Taylor, 1997; Taylor et al., 1999). In subsequent editions of the *Maudsley Prescribing Guidelines*, the suggested dose of amylobarbitone sodium was reduced to 200 mg IM and subsequent oral doses were not recommended. Further notes were added to highlight that amylobarbitone is a strong respiratory depressant with no pharmacological antagonist. Therefore, facilities for mechanical ventilation should be available (Taylor et al., 2001).

If no response is elicited from use of amylobarbitone, then paraldehyde 5–10 ml IM gluteal (5 ml each side) could be considered, if still available, but only if all other options have failed (Kerr & Taylor, 1997; Taylor et al., 1999, 2001).

20.7.4 Electroconvulsive Therapy (ECT)

This should only be considered when all pharmacological and other methods have failed to contain the disturbed behaviour especially mania that may be life threatening through exhaustion (Khwaja & Beer, 2013). Provision exists in the Mental Health Act 1983 for the emergency use of ECT to prevent a patient from behaving violently or being a danger to themselves or others. ECT is not included in the most recent version of the NICE guidelines for the management of violence (NICE, 2015) but is considered by more recent guidelines (Patel et al., 2018). If using ECT for this purpose, beware that benzodiazepines raise the seizure threshold and they will need to be stopped, at least temporarily, before ECT is administered.

20.8 Special Clinical Settings

20.8.1 Pregnancy

Clinical guidelines from the British Association for Psychopharmacology on the use of psychotropic medication preconception, in pregnancy and post-partum provide guidance on managing acute disturbance in pregnancy (McAllister-Williams et al., 2017). They recommend that a woman should have a clear plan in her records for a relapse of a mental illness and how the associated acute disturbance will be managed, including what medication might be used, and that this plan should be shared. Further, any restraint procedures need to be adapted to avoid possible harm to either fetus or mother. Thus, a pregnant woman must not be laid supine or prone, the former due to risk of obstruction to major blood vessels and the latter due to risk to the fetus. Use of a bean bag is advised so that a woman can be lowered onto it and thereby is in a semi-seated position where she is supported (McAllister-Williams et al., 2017). Where RT is used, this should be according to guidelines (McAllister-Williams et al., 2017; NICE, 2015; Patel et al., 2018). Specifically, a pregnant woman should never be left alone after the use of RT.

For choice of medication, a benzodiazepine or antipsychotic with a short half-life should be considered. The minimal effective dose necessary to reduce agitation or aggression should be used (Galbally et al., 2014). When using regular benzodiazepines, the risk of floppy baby syndrome should be taken into account. For antipsychotics, a minimum effective dose should be considered due to the risk of neonatal extrapyramidal symptoms with repeated and higher doses. If IM formulations are required, these should be administered into the gluteal muscle or lateral thigh (McAllister-Williams et al., 2017).

20.8.2 Intoxication by Drugs and Alcohol

Drug- and alcohol-related acute disturbance can be more severe and longer in duration than that associated with psychiatric illness alone. Commonly used substances that can cause acute disturbance include alcohol, synthetic cannabinoids, stimulants and also gamma-hydroxybutyrate (GHB or G), which is a solvent with a street use for pro-sexual side effects. Identification of substance misuse is predominantly based on clinical assessment as there are no rapid urine or field tests available for club drugs and novel psychoactive substances. Time and supportive management may be safer than adding sedative drugs. In the presence of alcohol or illicit substances, more intensive and frequent monitoring (every 15 minutes) is likely to be required, with particular attention to breathing, airway and level of consciousness (NICE, 2015). For patients with GHB intoxication, admission to a medical intensive care unit for anaesthetic sedation and ventilation may be required.

In general, for RT, the underlying condition also needs to be considered: for alcohol withdrawal in someone with dependency, benzodiazepines are efficacious in reducing the associated signs and symptoms (Lingford-Hughes et al., 2012). For management of patients under the influence of club drugs, information should be sought from the National Poisons Information Service via its telephone services and TOXBASE® database (www.toxbase.org). Intoxication of synthetic cannabinoids can resolve spontaneously but as the clinical presentation can include seizures, hypokalaemia, tachycardia, hypertonia, dyspnoea, syncope, ECG changes, observation and monitoring with supportive measures is advised. Agitation and aggression may be treated with benzodiazepines as these can be reversed if necessary by flumazenil. For example, in one TREC study it was reported that one man with alcohol-induced, and possibly also cocaine-induced, aggression was randomized to IM midazolam and suffered from respiratory depression, becoming cyanotic. After IV flumazenil he made a full recovery (TREC Collaborative Group, 2003).

Occasionally antipsychotics may be used, particularly so if there is a psychotic disorder history and when the psychotic symptoms do not spontaneously resolve (Abdulrahim & Bowden-Jones, 2015). However, it should be remembered that antipsychotics can lower the seizure threshold and also impact on cardiovascular rhythm.

20.9 Adverse Effects and Monitoring

There are a number of considerable non-pharmacological risks associated with the administration of IM RT, including: (i) inherent risk of violence of the situation, to both the patient and others; (ii) risks to both the patient and staff involved in the physical restraint; (iii) risk related to administration technique while under restraint (accuracy, obesity related); (iv) risks to the staff's therapeutic relationship with the patient. These are beyond the remit of this chapter. Here, we will consider some medication specific risks.

20.9.1 Respiratory Depression with Benzodiazepines

All sedative benzodiazepines can cause respiratory depression. When used IM for RT, at doses that will cause sedation, even greater care must be taken. Respiratory depression is more likely with increasing doses, and with benzodiazepines that accumulate on repeated administration, for example, diazepam, which is very long-acting. In the TREC Collaborative Group (2003) trial, IM midazolam was more likely than other benzodiazepines to cause respiratory depression, with very abrupt onset, making this option more risky than IM lorazepam. Wherever parenteral benzodiazepines are prescribed there should be access to flumazenil (the reversal agent) and suitable arrangements for administration which is IV only. That being said, the availability of a reversal agent confers a putative advantage of IM lorazepam over other agents such as IM antipsychotics or indeed ketamine.

20.9.2 Prolongation of QTc Interval with Antipsychotics

Some antipsychotics, particularly haloperidol and olanzapine, are known to increase the corrected QT interval (QTc) on the ECG, even at therapeutic doses. The QT interval is a poor guide to cardiac conductance disturbance because it varies with heart rate, hence the QTc is used. Values vary between genders and are influenced by a number of other factors. There is an approximate relationship between QT prolongation and the risk of sudden death. A QTc of greater than 500 ms puts the patient at increased risk of serious arrhythmias such as ventricular tachycardia and torsade de pointes. Ideally, as the licence for haloperidol recommends, a baseline ECG should be referred to before administering IM haloperidol. However, it is often not possible in the scenario of acute violence to carry out an ECG, and if one has not been done recently, haloperidol should be avoided. The prescriber should consider the risks and benefits of using this treatment and be able to justify their prescribing decision.

20.9.3 Extrapyramidal Side Effects (EPSE) with Antipsychotics

All first-generation antipsychotics (e.g. haloperidol) and some second-generation antipsychotics can cause EPSE. Some EPSE develop over time with repeated doses, but others can develop acutely, including acute dystonic reactions and oculogyric crises. These may be extremely frightening for those experiencing them. Those prescribed parenteral haloperidol should also be prescribed an anticholinergic such as procyclidine.

20.9.4 Monitoring

Antipsychotics can cause other adverse effects, some of which are predictable but others are not (e.g. seizures, neuroleptic malignant syndrome). Parenteral administration generally results in higher peak drug concentrations than oral administration, and usually within an hour of administration. Often IM medication options for RT are administered as an emergency, sometimes to patients who are not well known, and are not able to engage verbally in assessment, making observational assessment of their physical health even more important.

People with mental health problems are at increased risk of coronary heart disease, cerebrovascular disease, diabetes, epilepsy and respiratory disease, all of which can be exacerbated by the effects of RT. To ensure that patients' physical health and safety are given priority, the NICE Quality Standards highlight that all patients given RT should have side effects, vital signs, hydration level and consciousness monitored after the intervention. People given RT need to be monitored *at least* every hour until there are no further concerns about their physical status (NICE, 2017). It is not unusual for more intensive monitoring to be employed (e.g. two to four times per hour or constant monitoring) for periods of time in more complex and high-risk clinical scenarios.

20.10 A Systematic Approach

The aims of RT are to reduce the imminent risk of harm to self or others (through self-harm or violence) in the context of severe agitation. The underlying aetiology of the agitated state may stem from a psychiatric, physical or psychological condition; or of course a combination of these.

A number of guidelines exist which attempt to outline a systematic approach to RT. In general, they are linear in their approach to step-wise decision making as the supposed clinical scenario advances through a spectrum of increasing risk and

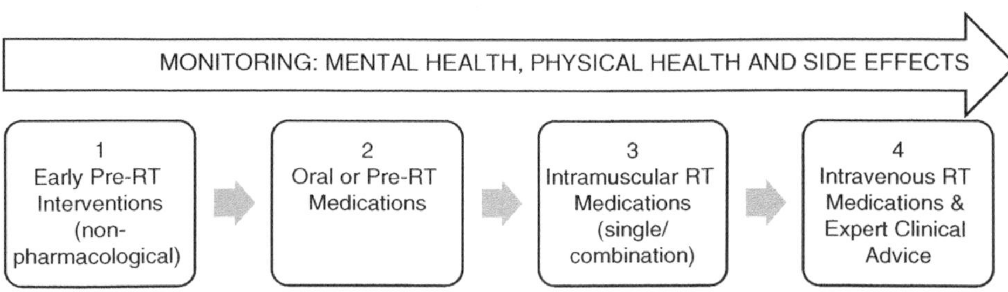

Figure 20.2 Building blocks of RT decision-making tools.

complexity. One such example exists in the *Maudsley Prescribing Guidelines* which tabulates a five-step interventional strategy (Taylor et al., 2018). Other guidelines, such as the American Association for Emergency Psychiatry's Project BETA, stratified their RT algorithm along the lines of different aetiologies of agitation (Wilson et al., 2012).

The clinical reality is complex, and clinical scenarios leading to RT are often not amenable to a linear algorithmic treatment plan. The basic building blocks of most RT decision-making tools incorporate a version of the four steps in Figure 20.2.

The flow from left to right is a pragmatic oversimplification of a multidimensional process sitting in an array of contextual factors which can affect RT decision making at the individual patient level. Arguably steps 1 and 2 could and should occur at any stage in the management of agitation. All four steps sit within a dynamic clinical system and regular (if not constant) monitoring is required to assess benefit versus harm. More recent guidelines are consistent with this approach (Patel et al., 2018).

A range of modifying factors or special circumstances is referred to in guidelines (Patel et al., 2018) and in mental health organizational protocols for RT in the UK (Innes & Sethi, 2012). Modifications, and in some cases separate guidelines, exist for different patient types (for example pregnancy, children, older adults and learning disability), for co-morbid medical disorders and other health states (for example delirium, intoxication, withdrawal). Guidelines seem not to fully capture the nuances of when to use individual RT medications and how to manage the potential medication risks, in a one-size-fits-all type of algorithm. This is most probably due to the paucity of evidence in this risky area of clinical practice and a testament to the clinical complexity.

In a general sense, RT should not be about medication alone; a multidisciplinary approach to managing agitation is more likely to ensure that pre-RT interventions are utilized. Patient engagement can be a significant challenge, but as far as is practicable, and as soon as the clinical and risk picture allows, patient choice and treatment individualization should direct RT planning. The choice of RT or pre-RT intervention will be driven by the nature of the risk associated with the agitated state. What must not get lost in the management of the agitated state is the optimization of the assessment and management of the underlying health disorder.

References

Abdulrahim D, Bowden-Jones O, on behalf of the NEPTUNE Expert Group (2015). *Guidance on the Management of Acute and Chronic Harms of Club Drugs and Novel Psychoactive Substances*. London: Novel Psychoactive Treatment UK Network (NEPTUNE).

Alexander J, Tharyan P, Adams C, et al. (2004). Rapid tranquillisation of violent or agitated patients in a psychiatric emergency setting. Pragmatic randomised trial of intramuscular lorazepam v. haloperidol plus promethazine. *Br J Psychiatry*, 185, 63–69.

Andrezina R, Josiassen RC, Marcus RN, et al. (2006). Intramuscular aripiprazole for the treatment of acute agitation in patients with schizophrenia or schizoaffective disorder: a double blind, placebo-controlled comparison with intramuscular haloperidol. *Psychopharmacology*, 188, 281–292.

Azeem MW, Aujla A, Rammerth M, Binsfeld G, Jones RB (2011). Effectiveness of six core strategies based on trauma informed care in reducing seclusions and restraints at a child and adolescent psychiatric hospital. *J Child Adolesc Psychiatr Nurs*, 24, 11–15. https://doi.org/10.1111/j.1744-6171.2010.00262.x.

Bowers L (2014). Safewards: a new model of conflict and containment on psychiatric wards. *J Psychiatr Ment Health Nurs*, 21, 499–508.

Bowers L, Stewart D, Papadopoulos C, et al. (2011). *Inpatient Violence and Aggression: A Literature Review*. London: Institute of Psychiatry, King's College London.

Bowers L, James K, Quirk A, et al. (2015). Reducing conflict and containment rates on acute psychiatric wards: the Safewards cluster randomised controlled trial. *Int J Nurs Stud*, 52, 1412–1422. https://doi.org/10.1016/j.ijnurstu.2015.05.001.

Breier A, Meehan K, Birkett M, et al. (2002). A double-blind, placebo-controlled dose response comparison of intramuscular olanzapine and haloperidol in the treatment of acute agitation in schizophrenia. *Arch Gen Psychiatry*, 59, 441–448.

Canadian Agency for Drugs and Technologies in Health (CADTH) (2015). *Use of Antipsychotics and/or Benzodiazepines as Rapid Tranquilization in In-Patients of Mental Facilities and Emergency Departments: A Review of the Clinical Effectiveness and Guidelines*. CADTH Rapid Response Reports.

Chin CN, Hamid ARA, Philip G, et al. (1998). A double-blind comparison of zuclopenthixol acetate with haloperidol in the management of acutely disturbed schizophrenics. *Med J Malaysia*, 53(4), 365–371.

Citrome L (2012). Inhaled loxapine for agitation revisited: focus on effect sizes 2 from Phase III randomised controlled trials in persons with schizophrenia or bipolar disorder. *Int J Clin Pract*, 66, 318–325. https://doi.org/10.1111/j.1742-1241.2011.02890.x.

Cole JB, Moore JC, Nystrom PC, et al. (2016). A prospective study of ketamine versus haloperidol for severe prehospital agitation. *Clin Toxicol (Phila)*, 54, 556–562.

Department of Health (DH) (2014). *Positive and Proactive Care: Reducing the Need for Restrictive Interventions*. London: Department of Health. Available at: www.gov.uk/government/publications/positive-and-proactive-care-reducing-restrictive-interventions (last accessed 15.8.19).

Department of Health (DH) (2015). *Mental Health Act 1983: Code of Practice*. London: The Stationery Office. Available at: www.gov.uk/government/uploads/system/uploads/attachment_data/file/435512/MHA_Code_of_Practice.PDF (last accessed 15.8.19).

Douglas-Hall P, Whicher EV (2015). 'As required' medication regimens for seriously mentally ill people in hospital. *Cochrane Database Syst Rev*, (12), CD003441. https://doi.org/10.1002/14651858.CD003441.pub3.

eMC (2017). Summary of Product Characteristics (updated January 2017): Clopixol Acuphase Injection. Available at: www.medicines.org.uk/emc/medicine/1071 (last accessed 15.8.19).

Galbally M, Snellen M, Lewis A (2014). *Psychopharmacology and Pregnancy*. New York: Springer. https://doi.org/10.1007/978-3-642-54562-7.

Garriga M, Pacchiarotti I, Kasper S, et al. (2016). Assessment and management of agitation in psychiatry: expert consensus. *World Biol Psychiatry*, 17(2), 86–128. https://doi.org/10.3109/15622975.2015.1132007.

Gaskin CJ, Elsom SJ, Happell B (2007). Interventions for reducing the use of seclusion in psychiatric facilities. *Br J Psychiatry*, 191, 298–303. https://doi.org/10.1192/bjp.bp.106.034538.

Gillies D, Sampson S, Beck A, Rathbone J (2013). Benzodiazepines for psychosis-induced aggression or agitation. *Cochrane Database Syst Rev*, (4), CD003079. https://doi.org/10.1002/14651858.CD003079.pub3.

Gillings M, Grundlingh J, Aw-Yong M (2016). *Guidelines for the Management of Excited Delirium/Acute Behavioural Disturbance (ABD)*. London: The Royal College of Emergency Medicine, Best Practice Guidance.

Hardy S, Bennett L, Rosen P, et al. (2017). The feasibility of using body worn cameras in an inpatient mental health setting. *Ment Health Fam Med*, 357, 393–400.

Hodgins S, Alderton J, Cree A, Aboud A, Mak T (2007). Aggressive behaviour, victimisation and crime among severely mentally ill patients requiring hospitalisation. *Br J Psychiatry*, 191, 343–350. https://doi.org/10.1192/bjp.bp.106.06.029587.

Huckshorn KA (2006). *Six Core Strategies for Reducing Seclusion and Restraint Use: A Snapshot of Six Core Strategies for the Reduction of S/R*. National Association of State Mental Health Program Directors (NASMHPD). Available at: www.nasmhpd.org/sites/default/files/ConsolidatedSixCoreStrategiesDocument.pdf (last accessed 15.8.19).

Huf G, Countinho ESF, Adams CE; TREC Collaborative Group (2007). Rapid tranquillisation in psychiatric emergency settings in Brazil: pragmatic randomised controlled trial of intramuscular haloperidol versus intramuscular haloperidol plus promethazine. *BMJ*, 335, 869. https://doi.org/10.1136/bmj.39339.448819.AE.

Huf G, Alexander J, Gandhi P, Allen MH (2016). Haloperidol plus promethazine for psychosis-induced aggression. *Cochrane Database of Syst Rev*, (11), CD005146. https://doi.org/10.1002/14651858.CD005146.pub3.

Innes J, Sethi F (2012). Current rapid tranquillisation documents in the UK: a review of the drugs recommended, their routes of administration and clinical parameters influencing their use. *J Psychiatr Intensive Care*, 9, 110–118. https://doi.org/10.1017/S174264641200026X.

Jayakody K, Gibson RC, Kumar A, Gunadasa S (2012). Zuclopenthixol acetate for acute schizophrenia and similar serious mental illnesses. *Cochrane Database Syst Rev*, (4), CD000525. https://doi.org/10.1002/14651858.CD000525.pub3.

Kerr I, Taylor D (1997). Acute disturbed or violent behaviour: principals of treatment. *J Psychopharmacology*, 11, 271–277.

Khwaja M, Beer D (eds.) (2013). *Prevention and Management of Violence: Guidance for Mental Healthcare Professionals*. College Report CR177. London: Royal College of Psychiatrists.

Krug EG, Dahlberg LL, Mercy JA, Zwi, AB, Lozano R (eds.) (2002). *World report on violence and health*. Geneva: World Health Organization.

Kwentus J, Riesenberg RA, Marandi M, et al. (2012). Rapid acute treatment of agitation in patients with bipolar I disorder: a multicentre, randomized, placebo-controlled trial with inhaled loxapine. *Bipolar Disord*, 14, 31–40. https://doi.org/10.1111/j.1399-5618.2011.00975.x.

Lesem MD, Tran-Johnson TK, Riesenberg RA, et al. (2011). Rapid acute treatment of agitation in individuals with schizophrenia: multicentre, randomised, placebo-controlled trial of inhaled loxapine. *Br J Psychiatry*, 198, 51–58. https://doi.org/10.1192/bjp.bp.110.081513.

Lingford-Hughes L, Welch W, Peters L, Nutt D; British Association for Psychopharmacology Expert Reviewers Group (2012). BAP updated guidelines: evidence-based guidelines for the pharmacological management of substance abuse, harmful use, addiction and comorbidity: recommendations from BAP. *J Psychopharmacol*, 26(7), 899–952. https://doi.org/10.1177/0269881112444324.

Lukens TW, Wolf SJ, Edlow JA, et al. (2006). Clinical policy: critical issues in the diagnosis and management of the adult psychiatric patient in the emergency department. *Ann Emerg Med*, 47, 79–99.

Martel M, Sterzinger A, Miner J, Clinton J, Biros M (2005). Management of acute undifferentiated agitation in the emergency department: a randomized double-blind trial of droperidol, ziprasidone, and midazolam. *Acad Emerg Med*, 12(12), 1167–1172.

McAllister-Williams RH, Baldwin DS, Cantwell R, et al. (2017). British Association for Psychopharmacology consensus guidance on the use of psychotropic medication preconception, in pregnancy and postpartum 2017. *J Psychopharmacol*, 31(5), 519–552. https://doi.org/10.1177/0269881117699361.

NASMHPD (2008). *Six Core Strategies to Reduce Seclusion and Restraint Use*. Alexandria, VA: National Association of State Mental Health Program Directors. Available at: www.nasmhpd.org/sites/default/files/Consolidated%20Six%20Core%20Strategies%20Document.pdf (last accessed 15.8.19).

National Institute of Health and Clinical Excellence (NICE) (2005). *Violence: the short-term management of disturbed and violent behaviour in inpatient psychiatric settings and emergency departments*. Clinical guideline [CG25]. London: National Institute for Health and Care Excellence.

National Institute for Health and Care Excellence (NICE) (2015). *Violence and aggression: short-term management in mental health, health and community settings.* NICE guideline [NG10]. London: National Institute for Health and Care Excellence. Available at: http://nice.org.uk/guidance/ng10 (last accessed 15.8.19).

National Institute for Health and Care Excellence (NICE) (2017). *Violent and Aggressive Behaviours in People with Mental Health Problems.* Quality Standard [QS154]. London: National Institute for Health and Care Excellence. Available at: www.nice.org.uk/guidance/qs154 (last accessed 15.8.19).

Patel MX, Sethi FN, Barnes TRE, et al. (2018). Joint BAP NAPICU evidence based consensus guidelines for the clinical management of acute disturbance: de-escalation and rapid tranquillisation. *J Psychopharmacol*, 32(6), 601–640. [This article was also co-published in the *Journal of Psychiatric Intensive Care*]

POMH-UK (2017). *Topic 16a. Rapid tranquillisation in the context of the pharmacological management of acutely-disturbed behaviour.* London: Royal College of Psychiatrists, CCQI263.

Price O, Baker J, Bee P, Lovell K (2015). Learning and performance outcomes of mental health staff training in de-escalation techniques for the management of violence and aggression. *Br J Psychiatry*, 206, 447–455. https://doi.org/10.1192/bjp.bp.114.144576.

Raveendran N, Tharyan P, Alexander J, Adams CE; TREC-India II Collaborative Group (2007). Rapid tranquillisation in psychiatric emergency settings in India: pragmatic randomised controlled trial of intramuscular olanzapine versus intramuscular haloperidol plus promethazine. *BMJ*, 335, 865. https://doi.org/10.1136/bmj.39341.608519.BE.

Royal College of Psychiatrists (RCPsych) (2014). *Consensus Statement on High-Dose Antipsychotic Medication.* College Report CR190. London: Royal College of Psychiatrists.

Taylor D, McConnell D, McConnell H, Abel K, Kerwin R (1999). *The Bethlem and Maudsley NHS Trust Prescribing Guidelines 1999*, 5th ed. London: Martin Dunitz.

Taylor D, McConnell DH, McConnell D, Kerwin R (2001). *Maudsley 2001 Prescribing Guidelines*, 6th ed. London: Martin Dunitz.

Taylor D, Okocha C, Paton C, Smith S, Connolly A (2008). Buccal midazolam for agitation on psychiatric intensive care wards. *Int J Psychiatry Clin Pract*, 12(4), 309–311. https://doi.org/10.1080/13651500802233886.

Taylor D, Paton C, Kapur S (2015). *The Maudsley Prescribing Guidelines in Psychiatry*, 12th ed. West Sussex: Wiley Blackwell.

Taylor D, Barnes TRE, Young AH (2018). *The Maudsley Prescribing Guidelines in Psychiatry*, 13th ed. Hoboken: Wiley Blackwell.

Tran-Johnson TK, Sack DA, Marcus RN, et al. (2007). Efficacy and safety of intramuscular aripiprazole in patients with acute agitation: a randomized, double-blind, placebo-controlled trial. *J Clin Psychiatry*, 68, 111–119.

TREC Collaborative Group (2003). Rapid tranquillisation for agitated patients in psychiatric rooms: a randomised trial of midazolam versus haloperidol plus promethazine. *BMJ*, 327, 708–711. https://doi.org/10.1136/bmj.327.7417.708.

Wilson MP, Pepper D, Currier GW, Holloman, GH Jr, Feifel D (2012). The psychopharmacology of agitation: consensus statement of the American Association for Emergency Psychiatry Project Beta Psychopharmacology Workgroup. *West J Emerg Med*, 13, 26–34. https://doi.org/10.5811/westjem.2011.9.6866.

Wright P, Birkett M, David SR, et al. (2001). Double-blind, placebo-controlled comparison of intramuscular olanzapine and intramuscular haloperidol in the treatment of acute agitation in schizophrenia. *Am J Psychiatry*, 158(7), 1149–1151.

Zaman H, Sampson SJ, Beck ALS, et al. (2017). Benzodiazepines for psychosis-induced aggression or agitation. *Cochrane Database Syst Rev*, (12), CD003079.

Zimbroff DL, Marcus RN, Manos G, et al. (2007). Management of acute agitation in patients with bipolar disorder: efficacy and safety of intramuscular aripiprazole. *J Clin Psychopharmacology*, 27, 171–176.

Antipsychotics, Weight Gain and Metabolic Risk

Stephen J. Cooper and Gavin P. Reynolds

21.1 Introduction

During the last 20 years there has been increased focus on the problem of premature mortality among people with schizophrenia. This has resulted in a focus on weight gain, the development of metabolic problems, the need to understand the mechanisms behind these and the need to identify strategies to manage these problems. Audit programmes have highlighted the poor quality of monitoring for, and management of, physical health problems in people with all types of mental health disorder but particularly for those with psychotic illnesses. Further, weight gain also reinforces service users' negative views of themselves and may lead to poor adherence with treatment (Faulkner et al., 2007; Lester et al., 2011; Weiden et al., 2004). This chapter reviews the effect of antipsychotic drugs (dopamine receptor antagonists and partial agonists) on weight and metabolic risk factors (blood glucose and lipid levels) as well as non-pharmacological risk factors that contribute to reduced life expectancy in those with serious mental illness. The assessment of cardiovascular risk and management of relevant cardiovascular risk factors are reviewed.

21.1.1 Reduced Life Expectancy

The life expectancy of people with schizophrenia is reduced by over 20 years compared with the general population (Tiihonen et al., 2009). A meta-analysis of 18 international studies indicated that 60% of this excess mortality was caused by physical illness (Brown, 1997). Recent large cohort studies in Australia and the USA have confirmed this increased risk of premature mortality and suggest the gap between people with schizophrenia and the general population may be widening (Lawrence et al., 2013; Olfson et al., 2015). Excess deaths from cardiovascular disease (CVD) are the major contributor to this and those with schizophrenia are twice as likely to die from CVD compared to those in the general population (Osborn et al., 2007a, 2015). An increased prevalence of important cardiovascular risk factors is well documented in people with schizophrenia (De Hert et al., 2011).

Observational studies have found that, compared with the general population, the risk of diabetes is higher among people receiving antipsychotic medication (Vancampfort et al., 2013) and higher in people with schizophrenia who have experienced multiple episodes, compared with first-episode and untreated individuals (Mitchell et al., 2013a). Meta-analysis shows that, compared with placebo, most antipsychotic medications are associated with weight gain which in turn increases the likelihood of developing a range of physical illnesses, including diabetes, with its own associated risk of premature mortality, CVD and cancer.

Meta-analysis of 78 publications, which included 24 892 patients, found that 32.5% of people taking antipsychotic medications manifest metabolic syndrome (Mitchell et al., 2013b). Metabolic syndrome refers to the presence of three abnormal findings from the following five risk factors: a measure of central obesity, hypertension, raised fasting glucose, low high-density lipoprotein (HDL) cholesterol and raised triglyceride levels (Alberti et al., 2009).

21.1.2 Risk Factors and Prevention

It is important to recognize the risk factors for development of diabetes and CVD and offer appropriate interventions for these. For people with psychotic illness, cigarette smoking, misuse of alcohol and being overweight are important risk factors for diabetes and CVD (e.g. De Hert et al., 2009a). Significant weight gain and increases in other metabolic indices can be identified within six to eight weeks of commencing antipsychotic treatment (Correll et al., 2014; Foley & Morley, 2011). Early weight gain appears to be a strong predictor of longer-term weight gain (Kinon et al., 2005; Vandenberghe et al., 2015). In the EUFEST study, of individuals experiencing their first episode of schizophrenia, weight gain of ≥7% of initial body weight was found in 65% of the follow-up population at one year (Kahn et al., 2008). A meta-analysis of studies in the general population (Kodama et al., 2014) suggests that, in young adults, for a weight gain corresponding to a 5 kg/m^2 increase in body mass index (BMI) the pooled relative risk of development of type 2 diabetes mellitus is 3.07 (95% confidence interval (CI) 2.49 to 3.79). There was a trend for this effect to be greater for males compared to females.

The ideal is to prevent the development of such risk factors. The National Institute for Health and Care Excellence (NICE) guideline CG178 *Psychosis and schizophrenia in adults: treatment and management* (NICE, 2014a, paragraph 1.1.3.1) recommends that all people with psychosis, and particularly those receiving antipsychotic medications, should be offered a healthy eating and physical activity programme from the outset. It is also important to assess weight and other physical health parameters before starting treatment and then at regular intervals (NICE CG178, paragraphs 1.3.6.1 & 1.3.6.4; Box 21.1 of this chapter).

Choice of initial antipsychotic medication is important. Antipsychotics vary in their liability to induce weight gain (see Table 21.1) and this should be taken into consideration in the discussion regarding choice of initial antipsychotic. However, there is considerable variation between patients in liability to antipsychotic-induced weight gain and there are no tests that will predict the development of any specific adverse effect. A recent meta-analysis of the effects of antipsychotic drugs in the treatment of patients in their first episode of psychosis (Zhu et al., 2017) found limited evidence of clinical superiority of any one drug over another during the first 13 weeks of treatment and recommended that the choice of treatment should be guided primarily by side effects. However, in relation to weight gain, the authors found only superiority of molindone (not available in the UK) over olanzapine, haloperidol and risperidone and superiority of haloperidol over olanzapine.

21.2 Non-Pharmacological Factors Contributing to Reduced Life Expectancy

21.2.1 Excessive Weight Gain and Metabolic Changes

De Hert et al. (2009b) report the prevalence of metabolic syndrome to be elevated by two to three times in people with schizophrenia compared with the general population. Obesity and diabetes are substantially increased in schizophrenia with estimates of relative risk of 1.5–2 (De Hert et al., 2009a) and 2 (Holt & Mitchell, 2015). A Northern Ireland study of people with schizophrenia found a high prevalence of obesity (40%) and metabolic syndrome (38%) (Yevtushenko et al., 2008). These metabolic disturbances are multifactorial in origin (Holt & Mitchell, 2015; Manu et al., 2015).

The impact of psychiatric drugs, especially antipsychotics, on weight gain and metabolic disturbance will be discussed in detail in a later section. In this section we deal with lifestyle factors, often partly related to aspects of schizophrenia, that contribute to weight gain and some of the metabolic pathology. Poor self-care is associated with a poor diet. People with psychosis consume more saturated fat (Ryan et al., 2003), more refined sugar (Stokes & Peet, 2004), less fibre (Osborn et al., 2007b) and less fruit and vegetables (McCreadie et al., 2003) than the general population. Many people with psychotic illness have a rather sedentary lifestyle (Daumit et al., 2005) and take less exercise than the general population (Osborne et al., 2007b). The higher prevalence of smoking in people with schizophrenia, even in the early stages of the illness (Barnes et al., 2006), appears to have no protective effect on body weight and may be associated with increased prevalence of metabolic syndrome (Yevtushenko et al., 2008).

People with schizophrenia are disproportionately represented within inner-city areas where health inequalities are greatest (World Health Organization, 2010). Deprivation is recognized as an important risk factor for diabetes (Connolly et al., 2000) and CVD in the general population and is included in the QRISK2 and QRISK3 algorithms (Hippisley-Cox et al., 2017). People with mental illness are also likely to experience inferior medical care compared with the general population (Mitchell et al., 2009).

Another disease-related factor that may contribute to changes in insulin sensitivity is stress. Psychotic symptoms are usually stressful and anxiety provoking and in addition many patients find some emotional interactions stressful. Stress is an established risk factor for metabolic disease, acting via stimulation of the hypothalamic–pituitary–adrenal (HPA) axis and elevated cortisol secretion. There is evidence that this occurs in many patients who demonstrate dysfunction of the normal cortisol response (reviewed by Toalson et al., 2004).

21.2.2 Genetic Factors

Is there an inherent metabolic pathology in schizophrenia apparent at, or prior to, the onset of psychosis? Could there be a genetic relationship between diabetes and schizophrenia as suggested by the higher prevalence of diabetes in relatives of those with psychotic illness (Mothi et al., 2015)?

The evidence is somewhat equivocal. Studies of young drug-naive first-episode patients have found no significant differences in a range of metabolic parameters including blood glucose, lipids, insulin and measures of fat deposits (Arranz et al., 2004; Sengupta et al., 2008; Zhang et al., 2004). Furthermore, no substantial difference between drug-naive patients and control subjects in these various measures was found in the EUFEST study (Fleischhacker et al., 2013).

However, two recent meta-analyses conclude that there is evidence for impaired glucose tolerance and insulin resistance in first-episode schizophrenia (Perry et al., 2016; Pillinger et al., 2017). If this is due to an aetiological commonality between schizophrenia and diabetes, rather than being a consequence of certain symptoms or secondary behaviours, then any genetic risk factors identified in both disorders may be relevant. Impaired glucose tolerance has been reported in both drug-naive patients with schizophrenia and their relatives without psychotic symptoms (Spelman et al., 2007), indicating a predisposition to impaired glucose metabolism, which could be environmental or genetic and independent of the development of psychosis. However, a recent study, making use of risk genes derived from previous genome-wide association study (GWAS) data, has concluded that there is no significant increase in polygenic risk for type 2 diabetes in subjects with schizophrenia (Padmanabhan et al., 2016).

21.2.3 Tobacco Smoking

It has been recognized for over 50 years that people with schizophrenia have much higher rates of tobacco smoking than the general population (Kelly & McCreadie, 2000). Individuals in their first episode of illness are significantly more likely to be smokers than a population matched for age and sex (odds ratio 6.04, 95% CI 3.03 to 12.02; Myles et al., 2012). There is also evidence that nicotine has greater positive effects on some aspects of cognitive performance in people with schizophrenia (Barr et al., 2008) and that there is abnormal regulation of high-affinity nicotinic receptors compared with healthy people (Breese et al., 2000).

Smoking is an important risk factor for the development of coronary heart disease in the general population. Recent data from a primary care population in the UK confirm that smokers with severe mental illness acquire a similar level of risk from smoking as other smokers (Osborn et al., 2015). Smoking is also a risk factor for the development of diabetes (InterAct Consortium, 2014). There are probably a number of reasons for this, including some effect to increase blood glucose concentration and possible impairment of insulin sensitivity.

21.2.4 Misuse of Alcohol

Misuse of alcohol is a further risk factor for CVD and diabetes. A meta-analysis reported median current alcohol use disorder rates at 9.4% and median lifetime rates of 20.6% in people with schizophrenia (Koskinen et al., 2009). The *Adult Psychiatric Morbidity Survey: Mental Health and Wellbeing, England, 2014* suggests a figure of 3.1% for current alcohol use disorder in the general population in England (McManus et al., 2016). A register-based cohort study in Denmark reported that almost 31.7% of people with schizophrenia had a lifetime diagnosis of alcohol use disorder and that this was a significant factor in their increased mortality from cardiovascular-related disease (Hjorthoj et al., 2015).

General population studies show that heavy use of alcohol increases risk for CVD (coronary artery disease, stroke and peripheral arterial disease), hypertension, cardiomyopathy (and subsequent heart failure) and various cardiac rhythm disturbances (e.g. alcohol can prolong the QT interval). Controversy continues regarding whether light and moderate drinking may be protective for CVD for some individuals, but recent data suggest that any 'cardiovascular' benefits may be outweighed by other alcohol-related harms (Department of Health, 2016). The increased calorie intake from alcohol (60 Cals per unit) also increases the risk of overweight and obesity. Heavy drinking and binge drinking increase the risk of diabetes. (See Fernandez-Sola, 2015 for a review of these issues.)

21.3 Weight Gain and Metabolic Side Effects of Antipsychotic Drugs

21.3.1 Differential Effects of Antipsychotic Drugs

It is clear from the initial meta-analysis of RCT data by Allison et al. (1999) to the recent multiple treatments (network) meta-analysis from Leucht et al. (2013) that treatment with most antipsychotic drugs can lead to significant weight gain, and that antipsychotics vary in their liability to induce weight gain. The latter analysis employed data from 212 trials in people with schizophrenia, with a mean duration of illness of 12.4 years, and used data from the sixth week (or closest time-point to this) of each trial. (See Section 21.5.2 for more detailed discussion of the rationale for, and limitations of, this multiple-treatments meta-analysis.) It distinguishes three essentially discrete groups of drugs with respect to weight gain (Table 21.1). In a meta-analysis of 48 direct comparison RCTs, Rummel-Kluge et al. (2010) described three similar clusters and observed that the magnitude of changes in glucose and cholesterol fell broadly into the same clusters.

These differential risks for weight gain appear to be similar for younger people, who will make up the majority of those commencing antipsychotic treatment for the first time. There is some evidence that weight gain with antipsychotics may be disproportionately greater in young people compared with adults, though this may be an apparent effect because in clinical studies many older adults are starting from a higher baseline, often due to previous antipsychotic treatment. However, the risk of type 2 diabetes in children and young people taking antipsychotics is increased threefold compared with the risk in a healthy matched cohort (Bobo et al., 2013). Furthermore, in young people with diabetes, the decline in β-cell function is faster, and therapeutic failure rates are higher, than in adults.

21.3.2 Hormonal Mechanisms

Investigation of metabolic changes following initiation of antipsychotic drug treatment shows, in addition to the increases in cardiovascular and diabetes risk factors mentioned above, a substantial elevation in circulating leptin (Zhang et al., 2004), an anorexigenic hormone secreted by adipose tissue to influence hypothalamic control of food intake and body weight. Such changes in secreted leptin are expected in people with increasing fat mass, but in people gaining weight on antipsychotic drug treatment the effect of this hormone in diminishing food intake is lost. This has led to the suggestion that a major mechanism contributing to antipsychotic-induced weight gain is interference with the hormonal control of food intake and body weight (Reynolds & Kirk, 2010).

The effects of other hormones may also be disrupted by antipsychotic drug treatment. Adiponectin is an orexigenic hormone, also secreted by adipose tissue, with opposite effects to leptin on feeding behaviour. Its expression decreases with increases in adiposity, insulin resistance and type 2 diabetes. Treatment with olanzapine or clozapine, but not risperidone, is associated with decreases in adiponectin (Bartoli et al., 2015).

Ghrelin is a hormone secreted by the stomach, and like adiponectin, it opposes the effects of leptin in the hypothalamus. Ghrelin decreases with increases in adiposity but increases in starvation. However, reports of possible association between antipsychotic treatment and changes in serum ghrelin are inconsistent (reviewed by Jin et al., 2008).

Table 21.1 Rank order of liability for weight gain among oral antipsychotic drugs

	Risk of weight gain	Notes
Olanzapine	High	1
Clozapine	High	2
Chlorpromazine	High/Medium	3
Quetiapine	Medium	4, 5
Risperidone	Medium	4, 5
Paliperidone	Medium	4, 6
Asenapine	Low	7
Amisulpride	Low	7
Aripiprazole	Low	7
Lurasidone	Low	7, 8
Ziprasidone	Low	7, 8
Haloperidol	Low	8

Notes: (1) significantly greater than quetiapine; (2) not significantly greater than the 'medium' group due to the high reported variance of relative weight gain; (3) not significantly differentiated from either 'medium' or 'high' groups; (4) significantly lower than olanzapine; (5) significantly greater than asenapine; (6) significantly greater than amisulpride; (7) not significantly greater than haloperidol; (8) not significantly greater than placebo. Adapted from the multi-comparison meta-analysis by Leucht et al. (2013).

A recent study (Tagami et al., 2016) has suggested that olanzapine promotes appetite by enhancing ghrelin-receptor signalling, while long-term olanzapine administration inhibits post-prandial reduction of ghrelin in rats (Hegedűs et al., 2015).

21.3.3 Neurotransmitter Mechanisms

It is apparent that several antipsychotic drugs have relatively little effect on body weight. Aripiprazole, ziprasidone and lurasidone show little or no significant elevations over placebo in terms of mean weight change (Leucht et al., 2013). This may not be just due to the absence of a hyperphagic mechanism, these antipsychotics may offer protection from weight gain in people taking certain other antipsychotics. Thus, in rats, addition of aripiprazole or ziprasidone to olanzapine results in a significant decrease in food intake compared with olanzapine alone (Kirk et al., 2004; Snigdha et al., 2008). Recently, it has been found that lurasidone treatment can suppress both the increased food intake and short-term weight gain following olanzapine administration (Reynolds et al., 2019). Findings such as these suggest that pharmacological differences between antipsychotic medications may be relevant to their differential propensities for weight gain.

There have been attempts to identify receptor mechanisms behind weight gain by correlation between receptor affinities of drugs and their liability to induce weight gain in the clinic (Kroeze et al., 2003; Matsui-Sakata et al., 2005). However, such studies assume quantitative drug differences in a common pharmacological mechanism rather than allowing for multiple contributory, and possibly synergistic or protective, mechanisms (Reynolds & Kirk, 2010).

Histamine H_1 receptor: Both olanzapine and clozapine have high affinities at the H_1 receptor. Pharmacological support for the importance of histamine H_1 antagonism in antipsychotic-induced weight gain comes from a proposed relationship between the acute activation of AMP protein kinase mediated by H_1 receptor antagonism and food intake in mice (Kim et al., 2007). However, this conclusion assumes a qualitative difference between risperidone, described as non-orexigenic, and quetiapine, considered orexigenic and like clozapine and olanzapine, a distinction not seen in the clinic (Leucht et al., 2013).

This is not to say that histaminergic mechanisms are unimportant. Some recent studies have suggested that drugs that enhance histamine neurotransmission in the hypothalamus may be effective in ameliorating antipsychotic weight gain (e.g. Deng et al., 2012). It may also be that the H_1 antagonism contributes to the intermediate weight gain associated with drugs not demonstrating strong 5-HT_{2C} antagonism.

5-HT_{2C} receptor: Antagonism, or inverse agonism, at this receptor is a strong candidate for the particularly marked effects of olanzapine and clozapine on body weight. Serotonin (5-HT) has long been known to provide a hypothalamic satiety signal mediated by 5-HT_{2C} receptors. Antagonism or knockout of the 5-HT_{2C} receptor results in increased feeding and weight gain. A study in rats has indicated that effects at 5-HT_{2C}, rather than at H_1 receptors, can, in combination with dopamine D_2 antagonism, mimic olanzapine-induced food intake and weight gain (Kirk et al., 2009). It seems possible that the relatively weaker effects of quetiapine and risperidone at 5-HT_{2C} receptors differentiate them from olanzapine and clozapine in terms of weight gain.

Alpha$_1$-adrenergic receptors: Noradrenaline is known as a hypothalamic neurotransmitter involved in the control of food intake. For most antipsychotic drugs, α_{1A}-adrenoceptor antagonism is associated with weight gain, although the relative affinity, greatest for clozapine and quetiapine, does not closely reflect severity of weight gain. While there may be some synergistic effect of α_{1A}-adrenoceptor antagonism with other receptor activities in contributing to antipsychotic-induced weight gain (Reynolds & Kirk, 2010), there is little to suggest this is a primary mechanism.

Dopamine D_2 receptors: Dopamine D_2 receptor antagonism has long been known to influence feeding behaviour (e.g. Clifton et al., 1991). While hypothalamic dopamine may be involved in this process, it has been shown that the mesolimbic dopamine pathway, implicated in reward mechanisms, locomotor function and the antipsychotic response, can also mediate leptin's effects on food intake through leptin receptors on these dopaminergic neurons (Hommel et al., 2006). It seems likely that this may be disrupted by the dopamine D_2 antagonism of all antipsychotic drugs other than the partial agonism of aripiprazole, and may thereby interact with other, perhaps hypothalamic, receptor effects of these drugs.

Other effects of antagonism of D_2 receptors include elevations in prolactin secretion. While hyperprolactinaemia is associated with obesity, drugs with little effect on prolactin can induce high weight gain (e.g. olanzapine) while risperidone and amisulpride, associated with greater liability for prolactin elevation, have, respectively, intermediate or little effect on body weight.

Protective mechanisms: As described above, animal experiments have shown that several low weight gain antipsychotics can reduce olanzapine-induced food intake and weight gain. For aripiprazole this extrapolates to clinical experience: adjunctive aripiprazole can reduce the weight gain associated with olanzapine or clozapine. The underlying pharmacological mechanisms have yet to be identified. Actions at 5-HT receptors including 5-HT_{1A} and 5-HT_{1B} are possible candidates, while for aripiprazole the mechanism may also, or alternatively, include dopamine D_2 partial agonism.

21.3.4 Pharmacogenetic Mechanisms

While different drugs vary substantially in their effects on body weight, individual responses to the same drug vary considerably. Some people demonstrate rapid and substantial gains in weight on antipsychotic regimens that in others appear to have little or no effect (Bushe et al., 2012). While lifestyle and diet may contribute to this variation, it is apparent that genetic factors are also important. Common functional polymorphisms in many candidate genes implicated in the control of body weight, and various aspects of energy and lipid metabolism, have been investigated for association with weight gain in people receiving antipsychotic drug treatment and with metabolic pathology in chronic schizophrenia (Reynolds, 2012; Reynolds & McGowan, 2017).

The strongest and most replicated findings are the associations with promoter polymorphisms in the 5-HT_{2C} receptor and leptin genes. A recent meta-analysis (Zhang et al., 2016) identified effects on antipsychotic-induced weight gain from 13 polymorphisms of nine genes, including the genes for the 5-HT_{2C} receptor, α_{2A}-adrenoceptor (*ADRA2A*), dopamine D_2 receptor (*DRD2*) and for brain-derived neurotrophic factor (BDNF).

It is also apparent that genetic factors may influence the rate or extent of weight loss. Significant associations have been found for polymorphisms of *ADRA2A* and methylenetetrahydrofolate reductase (MTHFR) with weight loss in people who, having developed metabolic risk factors following antipsychotic drug treatment, were switched to treatment with an antipsychotic with low weight risk (Roffcei et al., 2014).

Difficulties in this area of research include ethnic differences, variations in weight gain relating to length of time on treatment and the possibility that some gene polymorphisms may relate to early weight gain (5-HT_{2C}) while others may be associated with persistence of obesity (e.g. fat mass and obesity-associated (FTO) gene). GWAS studies have so far not produced consistent results.

21.3.5 Effects on Lipids

An important characteristic of obesity is dyslipidaemia, which can include elevated levels of triglycerides, reduced levels of high-density lipoprotein (HDL) cholesterol and elevated levels of very low-density lipoprotein (VLDL), changes which are the main predictor for the development of CVD in those with obesity (Wang & Peng, 2011). Thus, the dyslipidaemia seen in many patients prescribed antipsychotic drugs is likely to be partly related to the development of obesity. However, there is evidence that the effect of antipsychotic drug treatment on lipids, which can occur rapidly, does not always parallel gain in body weight or, more precisely, fat mass (Correll et al., 2009).

There are differences between antipsychotic drugs in their propensity to dyslipidaemia relative to weight gain. Quetiapine, which is usually associated with less weight gain than olanzapine, can show equivalent increases in triglycerides and substantial effects on cholesterol (Meyer et al., 2008; Rummel-Kluge et al., 2010). On the other hand, risperidone, similar to quetiapine in its effect on body weight, has little effect on plasma lipids, with a lipid profile similar to that of the low weight gain drug ziprasidone (Daumit et al., 2008; Rummel-Kluge et al., 2010).

There have been several reports that elevations in blood lipids may correlate with improvement in psychotic symptoms. It is unclear whether this is a functional relationship or due to artefact (e.g. variations in drug availability or adherence). However, the Clinical Antipsychotic Trials of Intervention Effectiveness (CATIE) study, which to some extent controls for this factor and provides the biggest study of the relationship between metabolic factors and symptom change, does not demonstrate any relationship between lipid measures and treatment response (Hermes et al., 2011).

The effect of treatment with several antipsychotic drugs, including clozapine, olanzapine and quetiapine, is to elevate LDL with little if any compensatory elevation in HDL. Given the role increased LDL has in inducing atherosclerosis and CVD, using the current definition of metabolic syndrome which focuses solely on the HDL component of total cholesterol serves to underestimate cardiovascular risk in many patients receiving antipsychotic drugs.

21.3.6 Direct Effects on Glucose Control

While weight gain is a risk factor for the emergence of impaired glucose regulation and diabetes, there is evidence that treatment with some antipsychotic drugs, particularly clozapine and olanzapine, can directly affect pancreatic function, resulting in effects on glucose regulation independent of weight gain in people without diabetes (Newcomer et al., 2002). Insulin resistance has been demonstrated in non-obese individuals taking antipsychotic medications (Henderson et al., 2005), with the greatest effects on glucose elevation seen with olanzapine and clozapine (Newcomer, 2005; Rummel-Kluge et al., 2010). It appears that olanzapine may induce biphasic changes in insulin secretion in response to a hyperglycaemic challenge. This involves an immediate toxic effect on pancreatic β-cell function at the beginning of treatment, resulting in decrease of insulin secretion, possibly explaining why some patients develop diabetic ketoacidosis. This effect then diminishes over time, resulting in compensatory hyperinsulinaemia (Chiu et al., 2010; Henderson et al., 2006).

Acetylcholine acts to promote food intake via hypothalamic muscarinic M_3 receptors, thus it is unlikely that olanzapine and clozapine have their effects via their high-affinity antagonism at this receptor. However, parasympathetic (vagal) activation of insulin release acts through muscarinic M_3 receptors on pancreatic β-cells. In vitro studies suggest that M_3 antagonism may contribute to glucose dysregulation by inhibition of cholinergic-stimulated insulin secretion (Johnson et al., 2005).

21.4 Assessment of Physical Health Risk Factors

21.4.1 Guidelines

The NICE guideline CG178 *Psychosis and schizophrenia in adults: treatment and management* (NICE, 2014a) provides detailed guidance regarding the assessment of physical health (sections 1.1.3, 1.3.6.4, 1.3.6.5 and 1.5.3) and alcohol use (sections 1.3.3.1 and 1.3.6.7) – see Box 21.1. Similar guidance is provided for bipolar disorder (CG185; NICE, 2014c).

Box 21.1 CG178 guidelines for monitoring physical health in patients with psychosis

Parameter	Frequency	Notes
Weight	Weekly for first 6 weeks At 12 weeks At 1 year and then annually	Also need to calculate and record BMI. See note 1 below
Waist circumference	Annually and plotted on a chart	See notes 2 and 3 below
Pulse and blood pressure	At 12 weeks At 1 year and then annually	
Fasting plasma glucose (FPG), HbA_{1c} and lipids	At 12 weeks At 1 year and then annually	Early in treatment need FPG as HbA1c takes some weeks to show changes if glucose rises
Cigarette smoking	At all available opportunities	
Alcohol use	At all available opportunities	

Notes:

[1]BMI > 23 kg/m^2 is considered elevated for those of South Asian ethnicity.

[2]Assessment of waist circumference has some theoretical advantage over BMI in relation to prediction of cardiovascular morbidity. However, it is often measured incorrectly and loses validity above a BMI of 35 kg/m^2. The most recent NICE clinical guideline on obesity (CG189; NICE, 2014d) advises use of BMI, with waist circumference as a supplementary measure in certain circumstances (paragraphs 1.2.2 and 1.2.3) so CG178 is not entirely consistent with this. There is probably value in waist circumference for identifying changes early in the treatment of those in their first episode of psychosis, but weight and BMI are probably entirely adequate in the longer term.

[3]NHS Choices recommends measuring waist circumference as follows,

- find the bottom of your ribs (lower costal margin) and the top of your hips (ileac crest)
- wrap a tape measure around your waist, midway between these points
- breathe out naturally before taking the measurement.

21.4.2 Current Practice in the UK

Two national audit programmes have provided data on the extent to which NICE guidelines for the management of people with schizophrenia have been followed by Trusts. The Prescribing Observatory for Mental Health (POMH) is a national quality improvement programme within the Royal College of Psychiatrists' Centre for Quality Improvement, which examines discrete aspects of prescribing practice and in which all Mental Health Trusts in the UK are invited to take part. A POMH audit involving 48 Assertive Outreach clinical teams (n = 1966 service users from 21 Trusts) found no evidence that measures of obesity, blood pressure, blood glucose control and plasma lipids had been documented during the previous 12 months in 67%, 60%, 60% and 68% of patients, respectively (Barnes et al., 2007). In a questionnaire to clinical teams it emerged that around one-third of staff were uncertain whether responsibility for physical health screening lay with the mental health team or the primary care team, less than half were confident about interpretation of the results and there was a widespread lack of access to simple equipment for the task. Repeat audits, using samples from similar clinical teams, over the following six years have demonstrated substantial improvements in practice (Barnes et al., 2015).

The National Audit of Schizophrenia (NAS), renamed the National Clinical Audit of Psychosis (NCAP) for the third national report, has reported the results of an audit programme in which all 64 Mental Health Trusts in England and Wales participated (Royal College of Psychiatrists, 2012, 2014, 2018). Each Trust provided data on people with schizophrenia or schizoaffective disorder selected at random from among those managed in the community (100 cases per Trust for the first two audits and between 100 and 300 cases, depending on the size of population covered by each Trust, for the third audit). The third audit found some improvements in monitoring for cardio-metabolic risk factors, with 42% of patients having evidence that all five of the most important risk factors (smoking, BMI, blood glucose control, blood lipids and blood pressure) were monitored in the previous 12 months, compared to only 27% and 34%, respectively, in the 2012 and 2014 reports. In the third audit 65% had a record of BMI in the previous 12 months (compared to 48% and 52% in the previous audits), 59% a record of monitoring of glucose control (compared to 50% and 57%) and 66% a record of monitoring of blood pressure (compared to 57% and 62%). There was evidence of improvements in the frequency of offers of interventions for all risk factors: for example, in the third audit 75% had been offered an intervention for abnormal glucose control (compared to 26% and 34% in the previous audits) and 58% had been offered an intervention for elevated blood pressure (compared to 26% and 25% previously). However, the proportion of patients receiving adequate monitoring remains well below that recommended and though offers of interventions have improved this only applies to those cases identified through monitoring. (Note: selection criteria for patients included in these audits was changed for the third audit but data from the 2012 and 2014 reports were recalculated to allow proper comparison. Thus, some of the percentages provided here will differ from those in the original audit reports.)

In the second of these audits, data from a parallel service user questionnaire suggested that there were a significant number of instances where risk factors may have been assessed in primary care but that staff in the Trusts were unaware of the results. Further, data from the service user questionnaire suggested that potential adverse effects on physical health were often not adequately discussed in the process of deciding which medication to prescribe.

21.4.3 Risk Scores

If the results of monitoring show abnormalities it is then important to make some assessment of the level of risk, particularly cardiovascular risk, from these. A calculation of risk may be useful, for example, in persuading the person to adopt a change in lifestyle or in the decision to prescribe a statin. In primary care in the UK it is common practice to employ the QRISK2 CVD risk calculator (www.qrisk.org) to estimate the 10-year risk of a CVD event, such as stroke, transient ischaemic episode, myocardial infarction or angina.

Recently, a new version of QRISK has been launched, QRISK3 (Hippisley-Cox et al., 2017). This version includes 'severe mental illness' and prescription of 'atypical antipsychotic medications', as well as other additional factors not included in QRISK2. However, within 'severe mental illness' QRISK3 includes moderate/severe depression and the rationale for excluding all non-atypical antipsychotics, some of which can contribute to risk, and including all atypical antipsychotics, some of which carry low risk, is not clear. Thus, QRISK3 may not prove to have better validity for people with psychosis than QRISK2.

Existing 'risk scoring' systems, like QRISK, have been developed using data derived from samples of the general population. Osborn et al. (2015) have made the argument that such 'risk scores' may not properly reflect the risks faced by those with psychotic illness for whom there may be possible links to the illness itself, for whom physical inactivity can be a significant feature and for whom the effects of antipsychotic medications may play a part. A specific problem with QRISK is that it is only validated for people over the age of 30 years and thus may not adequately assess risk for younger people early in their illness.

Using data from the Health Improvement Network, collected as part of their PRIMROSE research programme (www.ucl.ac.uk\primrose), Osborn et al. (2015) have developed a CVD risk prediction model that predicts observed risk better in populations with severe mental illnesses than existing models derived from the general population. The variables employed are: gender, age, systolic blood pressure, weight, height, presence of diabetes, smoking history, prescription of antidepressants, presence of an alcohol problem, deprivation score, specific severe mental illness diagnosis and prescription of first- and/or second-generation antipsychotic medications. Work is in progress to develop this to a point where it could be used in the clinic.

Conventionally, in the UK, a high risk for CVD, with implications for treatment, was regarded as having a 20% or greater risk of such over the course of 10 years. More recent guidelines (NICE CG181) have proposed that a 10% risk should trigger consideration of treatment with statins (NICE, 2014b). Further work is essential to determine the optimal risk thresholds for people with psychotic illness and to explore the cost-effectiveness of such thresholds. In the meantime, the use of current risk prediction models remains appropriate and it is essential that people with psychosis receive timely screening for their risk of CVD and are considered for statins where their risk exceeds 10%. In this context it should be noted that in the recent NCAP audit only 4% of patients had evidence that a QRISK score had been calculated (Royal College of Psychiatrists, 2018).

Consideration should also be given to assessing the risk for development of diabetes using validated questionnaires or a web-based risk tool, e.g. http://riskscore.diabetes.org.uk/results on the Diabetes UK website. (See Section 21.6.3 for more detail.)

21.5 Interventions for Weight Gain and Obesity

Once individual risk factors have been identified it is important to intervene to attempt to reduce these. This section first reviews those interventions that merit definite consideration, depending on the clinical context, and then summarizes the situation regarding other interventions that have been subject to clinical studies but for which the evidence is either more limited or negative. Where appropriate, reference is made to the effectiveness of an intervention for obesity or risk of diabetes in the general population. In the context of evaluating the effectiveness of clinical trials of interventions for weight gain, widely accepted thresholds are that weight gain of ≥7% of body weight is regarded as clinically significant and weight loss of ≥5% of body weight is associated with a decrease in cardiovascular risk and mortality. It should also be remembered that this is an area of treatment where motivation and engagement is important and that this may be a factor in an individual's decision to enter a clinical trial. More detailed review of these interventions can be found in the British Association for Psychopharmacology (BAP) guidelines on the management of weight gain and metabolic disturbances and cardiovascular risk associated with psychosis and antipsychotic drug treatment (Cooper et al., 2016).

The clinical trial data come almost exclusively from studies in adult populations, usually over the age of 18 years. Lifestyle interventions have been studied in younger populations with largely similar results to those found in adults but for many of the interventions considered there is a lack of adequately powered RCT data in people under the age of 18 years. Thus, particularly in relation to pharmacological interventions, appropriate cautions and restrictions must be applied if these are being considered for children and young people.

21.5.1 Lifestyle Interventions

The NICE guideline on schizophrenia (CG178; NICE, 2014a, paragraph 1.1.3) and the NICE guideline on obesity in the general population (CG189; NICE, 2014d, paragraph 1.4) both recommend lifestyle interventions as the initial approach for people who have become overweight or obese. The NICE Public Health guidance on preventing type 2 diabetes (PH38; NICE, 2012) also recommends this approach as the first line for those in the general population at moderate or high risk of developing diabetes. Such lifestyle interventions involve strategies to: increase physical activity; improve eating behaviour; improve the quality of a person's diet; and reduce energy intake. These interventions are often termed 'behavioural lifestyle programmes' as they commonly include elements of counselling or cognitive approaches to understanding eating behaviours. Most involve group sessions to discuss diet and exercise programmes, but also offer individual sessions.

A systematic review of RCTs of lifestyle interventions for obesity, in adults in the general population, versus (for most studies) usual care or remaining on a waiting list, found 44 studies with data suitable for meta-analysis, with follow-up periods of between 3 and 12 months (Dombrowski et al., 2010). Studies that combined dietary and physical activity approaches, rather than providing either alone, were more successful with a mean difference in weight reduction from the control group of 2.9 kg (95% CI −4.3 to −1.5 kg) at 12 months, though managing diet appeared to be the more important factor.

Meta-analyses of RCTs in people receiving antipsychotic medication (the majority of whom had a diagnosis of schizophrenia) have demonstrated the effectiveness of similar lifestyle interventions for this population (Bruins et al., 2014; Caemmerer et al., 2012). However, there are large variations in study design and a paucity of studies with long-term (one year or more) follow-up. No clinical trial has directly compared the effectiveness of different types of lifestyle intervention programmes.

The largest meta-analysis included 25 RCTs (Bruins et al., 2014) with sample sizes varying from 14 to 291 patients and which, combined, included 1518 people with psychotic disorder (schizophrenia, schizoaffective disorder and bipolar disorder) treated with antipsychotics. Most studies combined physical activity and dietary restrictions. Some studies also included one or more of motivational interviewing, cognitive behavioural therapy or counselling. The various lifestyle interventions were aimed at either helping people to lose weight or prevention of weight gain from the outset of treatment.

In 14 studies, the duration of intervention was less than 3 months; in seven studies 3–6 months; and in only four studies did the interventions last for more than 12 months.

Data were reported in terms of standard mean differences and the overall effect size of lifestyle interventions on weight was −0.63 (95% CI −0.84 to −0.42; $p < 0.00001$), with effect sizes of −0.52 for weight loss interventions and −0.84 for weight gain prevention interventions. Comparison of individual trials did not show evidence for the superiority of any specific intervention. A combination of individual and group approaches appeared to be more effective than either alone, but this could not be tested statistically. These lifestyle interventions also demonstrated significant positive effects on waist circumference, triglycerides, fasting glucose and insulin. There were no significant effects on blood pressure or cholesterol. In the largest of these RCTs (Daumit et al., 2013; n = 291), 38% of the participants in the intervention group lost ≥5% of their initial weight versus 23% of the control group.

An earlier meta-analysis (Caemmerer et al., 2012) included 17 RCTs (15 of which were included in Bruins et al., 2014) which, combined, included 810 people with psychotic disorder. This meta-analysis reported data in terms of mean differences and found that intervention versus control treatment resulted in an overall mean reduction in weight of −3.12 kg (95% CI −4.03 to −2.21; $p < 0.0001$) and reduction in BMI of −0.94 kg/m^2 (95% CI −1.45 to −0.43; $p < 0.0003$). It also demonstrated that differences from control treatment were similar for weight gain prevention trials, in first-episode patients, and weight loss trials.

Two further large RCTs in established patients and two RCTs in first-episode patients have found similar results to those in these meta-analyses (data reviewed in Cooper et al., 2016). However, two of these studies have reported a narrowing of the difference between intervention and control groups with longer-term follow-up of six months or more.

However, since publication of the last relevant NICE guidelines (CG178; NICE, 2014a; and CG189; NICE, 2014d) and the BAP guidelines for the management of weight gain associated with psychosis and antipsychotics (Cooper et al., 2016), three studies have been published (one each from Denmark, USA and UK) which have not found a significant benefit for lifestyle interventions in patients with psychotic disorders (Druss et al., 2017; Holt et al., 2019; Speyer et al., 2016).

Thus, data from studies reported prior to 2016 suggest that 'behavioural lifestyle programmes', aimed at improving diet and increasing physical activity, can have a positive effect, compared with routine care, to help individuals reduce existing antipsychotic-induced weight gain or attenuate weight gain in those commencing treatment for their first episode of psychosis. Across these studies, mean reduction in weight, compared with control treatment, is around 3 kg and reduction in BMI, compared with control, is around 1 kg/m^2. A recent meta-analysis of studies focused mainly on nutrition interventions (Teasdale et al., 2017) described similar findings to the previous meta-analyses, with a mean weight loss of 2.7 kg, and found that the effect size was larger if the intervention began at the beginning of antipsychotic treatment. Nevertheless, attenuation of weight gain, compared with control treatment, in people experiencing a first episode of psychosis varies widely across studies from 2.8 kg to 6 kg.

However, the three negative studies, noted above, and not included in the Teasdale et al. (2017) analysis, and an apparent trend for the effect sizes from most studies published since 2011 to be lower than those from earlier studies, must suggest some caution regarding the effectiveness of lifestyle interventions for patients with psychosis in comparison to what appears to be more consistent evidence in the general population. Aspects that require clarification from future research include: whether such interventions are only useful for certain subgroups of patients (e.g. those commencing antipsychotics for the first time); are there benefits on parameters such as glucose control or blood pressure in the absence of significant weight loss; are there particular modes of delivery of intervention programmes that work better (e.g. patient narratives reported from some studies suggest that patients prefer to attend regimens designed specifically for them rather than generic regimens aimed at the general population, such as 'Weight Watchers')?

There is no clear evidence regarding the optimum length of engagement with such interventions. It is also clear that the trend in some studies is for benefits over routine care to diminish over time. This mirrors the findings for similar programmes in the general population (Aronne et al., 2009) and argues strongly for the need to make booster sessions available over the long term.

21.5.2 Antipsychotic Switching

Consideration of the potential role of the patient's existing antipsychotic medication is also important. Measurement of weight before starting treatment, and then following initiation of treatment, will provide a baseline and a trajectory of weight gain against which the effect of a first antipsychotic, or any subsequent change in medication, can be assessed. For most patients, low dosage or discontinuation of antipsychotic treatment is unlikely to be feasible without significant risk of clinical relapse. For certain dose-related adverse effects (e.g. sedation) a reduction in antipsychotic dose can be beneficial, where symptom control allows. However, for many adverse effects, including weight gain, there appears to be no clear relationship with antipsychotic dose (Simon et al., 2009). Switching to a different antipsychotic medication that may have a lower liability for weight gain is thus a treatment option that requires consideration.

Few clinical trials have directly examined the effect on weight and other metabolic measurements (e.g. plasma glucose or cholesterol) of specific switches of one antipsychotic medication to another. Thus, consideration of the likely benefits of switching antipsychotic medication must be approached mainly through consideration of the relative effects of different antipsychotics on these measures. The problem with such an approach is that the relative liability of individual antipsychotics to induce weight gain, and metabolic effects (Allison, 1999; Leucht et al., 2013; Taylor et al., 2012), is based on RCT data which have limitations. Firstly, most RCTs of antipsychotics are carried out to assess their effects on clinical symptoms and wider clinical outcomes – their effects on weight are not usually among the primary outcome measures. Secondly, many of the participants in these trials have had previous antipsychotic treatment and thus potentially already experienced some antipsychotic-induced weight gain. Thirdly, these problems are not always adequately reported in older antipsychotic trials. Fourthly, reports of side effects in antipsychotic RCTs may reflect a range of different assessment measures and criteria. Fifthly, the interpatient variation for these side effects may be greater than the differences in liability between individual drugs. The summary below refers primarily to differences in propensity for weight gain as fewer studies have provided comparable data for other metabolic variables.

The most comprehensive analysis of data from clinical trials of antipsychotic drugs is a multiple-treatments (network) meta-analysis of 212 short-term RCTs (Leucht et al.,

2013; summarized in Table 21.1). This type of analysis includes data from some direct comparisons of different antipsychotic drugs but also includes comparisons made between different drugs through their relative differences from placebo and/or other commonly used comparator drugs, mainly haloperidol, risperidone and olanzapine. Hence, this is sometimes referred to as an indirect or network meta-analysis.

The Leucht analysis suggested that all antipsychotics examined induced statistically significantly more weight gain than placebo, except for haloperidol, lurasidone and ziprasidone (not currently available in the UK). In this meta-analysis, the other antipsychotics examined were: aripiprazole, amisulpride, asenapine, paliperidone, risperidone, quetiapine, sertindole, chlorpromazine, iloperidone, clozapine, zotepine and olanzapine. (Note that this analysis did not include depot or long-acting injectable compounds.) As indicated in Table 21.1, antipsychotics could be divided into three essentially separate groups based on their influence on body weight, in which haloperidol, ziprasidone, lurasidone, aripiprazole, amisulpride and asenapine had the smallest effect. Most of the differences found were in the ranges of standard mean differences considered to be 'small' and 'medium'.

Direct meta-analysis can only compare those treatments for which specific comparative RCTs exist. Given the large number of possible direct comparisons between antipsychotics, it is not surprising that few of these have been subject to specific clinical trials. Hence, the value of the multiple treatments meta-analysis approach described above. Rummel-Kluge et al. (2010) identified 48 direct RCT comparisons, mainly comparing olanzapine or risperidone with another antipsychotic, in which there were usable data on weight, glucose or cholesterol. These trials included amisulpride, aripiprazole, clozapine, olanzapine, quetiapine, risperidone, sertindole and ziprasidone. The analysis suggested that the medications included would fall into the same three clusters identified by the much larger multiple treatments meta-analysis summarized in Table 21.1. The findings for changes in glucose and cholesterol fell broadly into these same clusters.

There are a small number of published clinical trials designed specifically to examine the effect on weight of switching from one antipsychotic to another. A Cochrane systematic review (Mukundan et al., 2010) identified four such studies (n = 636 participants) with adequate data. The conclusion was that switching from olanzapine to aripiprazole or quetiapine resulted in weight loss and decrease in fasting blood glucose. Only a switch to aripiprazole resulted in an improved lipid profile. There were no significant differences in clinical outcomes between switchers and those trial participants not switched.

The World Federation of Societies of Biological Psychiatry (WFSBP) has published a guideline on the long-term treatment of schizophrenia and management of antipsychotic-induced adverse effects (Hasan et al., 2013). Their conclusions in relation to effects on weight and metabolic measures were similar to those of the Cochrane review regarding a switch from olanzapine to aripiprazole or quetiapine. They also concluded that a switch from olanzapine or risperidone to ziprasidone, but not from first-generation antipsychotics to risperidone, was beneficial for both weight and metabolic measurements, though the data were derived from an open-label study (Weiden et al., 2008).

More recently, a pharmaceutical industry-sponsored trial of lurasidone demonstrated mean weight loss (observed cases analysis) of 1.9 kg over six months, with 29.0% showing >7% weight loss, when participants were switched to open-label lurasidone after six weeks of treatment with olanzapine (Stahl et al., 2013).

Thus, available data suggest three clusters of antipsychotic medications, with respect to liability for weight gain (Table 21.1). This provides a rationale for considering switching a patient from an antipsychotic with greater propensity for weight gain to one with a lower propensity, which in terms of medications available in the UK means to haloperidol, lurasidone, aripiprazole, amisulpride or (in bipolar mania) asenapine. The studies included in the Cochrane and WFSBP guidelines suggest that switching from olanzapine to aripiprazole may be worthwhile with more limited data supporting switches from quetiapine and risperidone to aripiprazole, olanzapine to quetiapine and olanzapine to lurasidone.

Any decision to switch antipsychotic must take into consideration the risk of reduced clinical efficacy in terms of psychotic symptom control and relapse prevention. It also requires discussion with the patient regarding the benefits and risks, including other potential adverse effects that may be more common with the alternative medication, and the possibility that the alternative antipsychotic medication may also cause weight gain in some individuals. Hence, though haloperidol is an available option, consideration must be given to the high risk of extrapyramidal side effects with this and the disincentive of these to good medication adherence, making it an unlikely choice.

In this context it is important to remember that other psychotropic medications being co-prescribed might also contribute to weight gain, e.g. sodium valproate or an antidepressant. Where appropriate, the possibility of switching, reducing the dose of or discontinuing such a co-prescribed drug should be considered. In a recent cohort study, in a UK population, mirtazapine was the antidepressant most implicated in weight gain (Gafoor et al., 2018). However, weight gain has been reported in some patients with all antidepressants, including all selective serotonin reuptake inhibitors (SSRIs), though it is much less common with SSRIs which may be the initial choice if a switch is feasible.

21.5.3 Adjunctive Aripiprazole

In patients who have gained considerable weight when prescribed clozapine it has become part of clinical practice in many clinics to consider adding aripiprazole as an adjunct to try to reduce weight. The initial rationale for this strategy was the observation that in many clinical trials, performed to assess efficacy for psychotic symptoms, patients on aripiprazole lost weight in comparison with those receiving the comparator treatment. For example, in a 26-week RCT of aripiprazole versus olanzapine ($n = 317$ patients), the aripiprazole group had a mean weight loss of 1.37 kg against weight gain of 4.23 kg in the olanzapine group ($p < 0.001$) (McQuade et al., 2004). An open-label trial of aripiprazole, 15–30 mg daily added to clozapine (mean dose 455 mg/day) for 6 weeks in 13 people with chronic schizophrenia (Henderson et al., 2006), then found a mean decrease in weight of 2.7 kg ($p < 0.003$).

A large multi-centre, double-blind RCT of aripiprazole versus placebo added to clozapine was carried out in 207 outpatients ($n = 190$ completers) with schizophrenia who had experienced weight gain of at least 2.5 kg on clozapine (Fleischhacker et al., 2010). The main, 16-week phase of the study was double-blind and was followed by a 12-week extension phase, on an open-label basis. At the end of week 16 the aripiprazole group had a greater mean decrease in body weight than the placebo group (mean difference −2.15 kg, 95% CI −3.17 to −1.12; $p < 0.001$). This difference was maintained in the open-label phase. Weight loss of ≥7% was achieved by 21% of the aripiprazole group and 13% of the placebo group. There were no changes in fasting glucose.

However, in a further double-blind placebo-controlled RCT of aripiprazole added to clozapine (n = 38), it was found that a measure of glucose metabolism (the primary outcome variable for this study) improved significantly in the aripiprazole group (Fan et al., 2013). There was a non-significant decrease in weight of −1.5 kg in the aripiprazole group and an increase of +0.3 kg in the placebo group.

Aripiprazole was examined as an adjunct to olanzapine in a 10-week placebo-controlled, double-blind, cross-over clinical trial in 15 overweight people with schizophrenia treated with a stable dose of olanzapine (Henderson et al., 2009). There was a significant decrease in weight with aripiprazole compared with placebo (−1.3 kg (SD 2.1) vs. +1.0 kg (SD 1.5); $p < 0.003$).

Meta-analysis combining the data from the two clozapine and single olanzapine double-blind studies (Mizuno et al., 2014) found a mean difference between aripiprazole and placebo of −2.13 kg (95% CI −2.87 to −1.39; $p < 0.00001$). There was evidence for reductions in total cholesterol and LDL cholesterol, but this is influenced by such changes in the single large study of Fleischhacker et al. (2010). There is no useful body of evidence regarding the use of adjunctive aripiprazole with other antipsychotics for control of weight.

The most commonly reported adverse effects of the combination treatment were nausea, headache, insomnia, anxiety and restlessness and it is important to remember that polypharmacy may result in an increase in adverse effects. The studies above did not find any significant changes in schizophrenia symptom scores. However, a 24-week double-blind RCT of adding aripiprazole in 40 patients receiving clozapine (31 completers), who were relatively unresponsive to treatment, found a significant improvement in total Scale for Assessment of Positive Symptoms score ($p < 0.0001$) for aripiprazole compared with placebo (Muscatello et al., 2011).

21.5.4 Adjunctive Metformin

Metformin hydrochloride is an oral glucose-lowering drug in the biguanide class. It is the first-line drug of choice for the treatment of type 2 diabetes in all national and international guidelines. Its main actions are to reduce hepatic glucose production and increase insulin sensitivity in muscle.

Many people in the general population are at increased risk of developing diabetes and some of these already show elevated fasting blood glucose though not to the extent it falls within a diabetic range; this latter group are sometimes referred to as having 'pre-diabetes'. NICE has published public health guidance relating to this situation: *Preventing type 2 diabetes: risk identification and interventions for individuals at high risk* (PH38; NICE, 2012). This guidance recommends risk assessment followed by lifestyle interventions for those at moderate or high risk of developing diabetes. However, for those in the general population at high risk of developing diabetes (fasting plasma glucose 5.5–6.9 mmol/L or HbA_{1c} 42–47 mmol/mol), and who continue to progress towards diabetes, and who are unable to comply with lifestyle interventions or who have failed to gain benefit from these, this NICE guidance recommends consideration of the prescription of metformin. There is evidence from large, long-term studies that, in the general population, metformin can reduce mortality and complications in those with diabetes, reduce the risk of progression to diabetes and reduce weight in overweight and obese individuals at risk of development of diabetes. The evidence for this is summarized in Cooper et al. (2016).

As discussed earlier, it appears that antipsychotic medications act to increase the risk of diabetes both through weight gain and direct effects on the pancreas, with both effects influencing insulin resistance. Many people with psychosis would meet the criteria for being at high risk of developing diabetes, as described in NICE PH38, and would also either have failed to gain benefit from lifestyle interventions or have failed to comply with these. Thus, they would meet criteria for consideration of prescription of metformin, as laid out for the general population, for whom it appears that metformin can be beneficial. While some of the factors important in weight gain and risk of diabetes may differ in patients with psychosis, nevertheless, there does not seem any clear reason not to consider application of the guidance in NICE PH38 for many of these patients.

A recent meta-analysis of studies where metformin was added to existing antipsychotic medication (most commonly clozapine, olanzapine or risperidone) identified 10 RCTs (Mizuno et al., 2014). The overall results of these studies favoured metformin over placebo with a mean difference of −3.17 kg (95% CI −4.44 to −1.90). There was evidence that metformin improved measures of glucose regulation and some aspects of lipid profile. The largest study (Jarskog et al., 2013) recruited 148 patients with schizophrenia or schizoaffective disorder who had a BMI ≥27 kg/m^2. At week 16 the mean weight change for the metformin group was −3.0 kg versus −1.0 kg for the placebo group ($p = 0.0065$). (All patients received a lifestyle programme.) The longest study, at a single site in China, recruited 84 female patients within their first year of commencing antipsychotic treatment (Wu et al., 2012). At 24 weeks the metformin group had lost −2.3 kg and the placebo group had gained +2.1 kg ($p < 0.01$). Doses of metformin in the RCTs were generally in the range 750 mg to 1000 mg per day.

While adverse effects in the studies above did not appear to differ between metformin- and placebo-treated participants it is important to remember that metformin can cause the serious effect of lactic acidosis, with a rate of around 9 cases per 100 000 person-years (often in the context of renal failure). For this reason, metformin is contraindicated in severe renal impairment (estimated glomerular filtration rate (eGFR) <30 ml/min), hepatic failure and heart failure. The risk may also be increased by alcohol consumption. Alcohol can also enhance the hypoglycaemic effect of metformin. Metformin can decrease absorption of vitamin B_{12} and 7% may develop deficiency of this over four years. The more common adverse effects are complaints of nausea, bloating, abdominal pain and diarrhoea in around 10–20% of patients, effects which often result in patients not being able to tolerate the drug. Thus, it is usually initiated at a low dose with gradual increase over two to three weeks.

Thus, metformin can reverse existing antipsychotic-induced weight gain, with a difference from placebo of approximately 3 kg and can help to attenuate weight gain in those commencing antipsychotics for the first time. However, many of the studies included some aspect of lifestyle management and most of the studies are of short duration and involve small numbers of patients.

21.5.5 Bariatric Surgery

Bariatric surgery has not been subject to any formal clinical trial in people with psychosis. There are reports of case series, extracted retrospectively from cohorts of all cases subject to bariatric surgery at specific surgical centres, but the numbers of people with a diagnosis of schizophrenia are usually less than 1% of such case series. Most of these case series also report people with a diagnosis of bipolar disorder, for whom such surgery appears to be performed more commonly. People referred for bariatric surgery in these centres generally have BMI >40 kg/m^2 and many have BMI >50 kg/m^2.

The general conclusion from these reports is that people with diagnoses of schizophrenia and bipolar disorder demonstrate the same post-surgical weight loss as others. Improvement is generally reported as percentage of excess weight loss (%EWL; i.e. % weight loss above ideal weight if BMI for their height was 25 kg/m^2). For example, at six months Hamoui et al. (2004) found %EWL was 39.5% (range 29.4% to 62.9%) in the schizophrenia group versus 46.9% (range 30.0% to 95.5%) in the control group (no statistically significant difference). There is no consistent evidence of post-surgical deterioration in mental state, but patients have presumably been carefully selected.

The available data are insufficient to be clear whether bariatric surgery will have the same persistence of effect in antipsychotic-treated patients, given that mechanisms other than increased food intake may be involved. There are no data regarding effects on absorption of antipsychotic medications. However, this is an approach which it may be appropriate to consider in cases of extreme weight gain, within the requirements of NICE guidelines for the management of obesity.

21.5.6 Other Interventions with Clinical Trials

Many other pharmacological approaches have been considered as possible adjunctive treatments for weight reduction in the context of antipsychotic-induced weight gain. Those for which clinical trial data exist are listed in Table 21.2, where these treatments are divided into four groups according to whether clinical trial evidence exists for their effects within antipsychotic-treated populations and/or within the general population and their availability in the UK.

The treatments listed in Group A (Table 21.2) are the only ones, aside from bariatric surgery (see above), that merit possible consideration for patients with intractable weight problems for whom other approaches have been either ineffective or impractical. It is not appropriate to recommend these drugs for routine consideration in the management of antipsychotic weight gain as currently available evidence for these is quite limited and/or the use of these drugs is limited by adverse effects. A more complete appraisal of these drugs can be found in a recent BAP guidelines document (Cooper et al., 2016). The evidence is summarized below.

Amantadine: Of six studies, four were open-label clinical trials or case series. None was longer than 16 weeks. Meta-analysis suggested a small mean difference from control treatment of 1.85 kg. Amantadine is a weak dopamine agonist and has been reported to induce psychotic symptoms as an adverse effect.

Melatonin: Melatonin has been shown to block olanzapine-induced weight gain and visceral adiposity in laboratory rats. Two double-blind RCTs have suggested difference from control treatment of 0.7 kg and 3.2 kg, respectively.

Table 21.2 Treatments as adjuncts to antipsychotic medication that have been studied for reduction of antipsychotic-related weight gain. (Listed in alphabetical order and not order of importance.)

Group	Evidence of efficacy for reducing weight gain and availability in the UK	Treatments given in alphabetical order within each group
A	Data available for these treatments from RCTs in antipsychotic-treated patients Treatments are available in the UK but only orlistat is licensed for the treatment of obesity	amantadine melatonin orlistat topiramate reboxetine zonisamide
B	These treatments have evidence of efficacy in the general population but noor very limited, trials in antipsychotic-treated patients The last two drugs are not currently available for use in the UK	bariatric surgery GLP-1 analogues (liraglutide & exenatide) lorcaserin phenteramine/topiramate combination
C	For most of these treatments only a single (negative) clinical trial has been carried out in antipsychotic-treated patients Treatments are available in the UK but are not licensed for the treatment of obesity	atomoxetine dextroamphetamine famotidine fluoxetine fluvoxamine nizatidine
D	Had limited or no evidence of effectiveness in antipsychotic-treated patients Treatments no longer available in the UK	d-fenfluramine phenylpropanolamine rimonabant rosiglitazone sibutramine

GLP-1, glucagon-like peptide-1.

Orlistat: Orlistat is an inhibitor of gastric and pancreatic lipase and prevents intestinal fat absorption. In the general population, it can reduce weight compared with control treatment with a mean difference of 2.9 kg. However, long-term adherence is only around 2%. In patients with schizophrenia, significant weight change, of similar magnitude, is only seen in males. If patients do not achieve weight loss in the first 16 weeks continuation does not appear to be beneficial.

Topiramate: Topiramate is a third-generation anticonvulsant introduced to the UK in 1995 and used as a first-line treatment for focal and generalized seizures. Weight loss has been reported in a proportion of people with epilepsy prescribed topiramate. A meta-analysis of studies of the effect of topiramate in overweight/obese people in the general population suggested a weight loss of 5.34 kg compared with placebo (Kramer et al., 2011). The proposed mechanism of action is a reduction in visceral fat associated with a decrease in plasma leptin concentrations. Meta-analysis of four double-blind, placebo-controlled RCTs, ranging from 8 to 12 weeks in length, concluded that augmentation of antipsychotic treatment with topiramate can prevent or reduce weight gain compared with control treatments, with a weighted mean difference of 2.83 kg.

However, adverse effects on cognition (the most common reason for discontinuation in one post-marketing surveillance study in epilepsy), in a population who already often suffer cognitive impairments, as well as the other known adverse effects (sedation, dizziness, paraesthesia and occasional psychosis) argue against consideration of topiramate as an adjunctive treatment for this clinical indication.

Reboxetine: There have been two studies examining the effect of the noradrenaline reuptake blocker reboxetine alone and one study of a combination of reboxetine and betahistine on olanzapine-related weight gain in people with schizophrenia. These studies are all from the same research group but do suggest a significant attenuation of weight gain by reboxetine, with a small weighted mean difference between reboxetine and placebo of 1.90 kg.

Zonisamide: Zonisamide is a sulphonamide anticonvulsant, unrelated to other anticonvulsants, approved in 2005 for use as an adjunctive therapy in adults with certain types of epilepsy. It has been found to cause weight loss in overweight people with epilepsy and in a one-year, double-blind, placebo-controlled RCT was shown to reduce weight in obese adults. One small, 10-week RCT in people with schizophrenia found significant reduction in weight gain compared with placebo.

21.5.7 Other Treatments

The treatments listed in Group B (Table 21.2) have RCT evidence of efficacy in inducing weight loss in the general population. Lorcaserin, a selective 5-HT_{2C} receptor agonist, and a phentermine/topiramate combination (Qsymia®) have been available in the USA since 2012 for the treatment of obesity in adults with BMI ≥30 kg/m^2 or those with BMI >27 kg/m^2 in the presence of one related co-morbidity. At the time of writing there were no trials of these two medications for antipsychotic-related weight gain and these medications were not approved for use in the UK.

The glucagon-like peptide-1 (GLP-1) receptor agonists are a class of injectable drugs that have been approved for the treatment of type 2 diabetes since 2006. Their use is associated with significant weight loss and this has led to clinical trials of their use in people with obesity. Liraglutide has been approved for the treatment of obesity in the USA, Europe and the UK (as Saxenda®). Although, in animal studies, liraglutide has been shown to reverse olanzapine-induced weight gain, it is less clear whether GLP-1 agonists have the same effect in humans. While a study of exenatide did not differ from placebo in its effects on obese antipsychotic-treated patients with schizophrenia (Ishøy et al., 2017), a larger study of liraglutide did show a significant reduction of clozapine- or olanzapine-induced overweight/obesity, as well as improvement in glucose tolerance (Larsen et al., 2017).

The treatments listed in Group C (Table 21.2) have been the subject of small numbers of clinical trials for antipsychotic-induced weight gain, all of which were negative. Phenylpropanolamine, rosiglitazone and rimonabant (Group D, Table 21.2) failed to show benefit for antipsychotic-induced weight gain and have been withdrawn for all indications because of safety concerns. There was limited evidence that D-fenfluramine and sibutramine could assist weight loss in patients with psychosis but both drugs were withdrawn from use for safety reasons. There was evidence that D-fenfluramine might exacerbate psychotic symptoms.

21.6 Other Relevant Interventions

While the effects of psychotropic drugs, and approaches to managing these effects, are the central focus of this chapter, it is important to remember that the development of weight gain, diabetes and elevated cardiovascular risk are usually multifactorial. Some of the interventions discussed above may be useful in reducing these problems whatever their cause, e.g. lifestyle interventions for weight gain. However, specific interventions may be necessary for some of the non-psychopharmacological risk factors (particularly smoking and misuse of alcohol) and general medical interventions (such as the prescription of statins) must also be considered where appropriate.

A useful resource to support clinical decision making in relation to cardiovascular risk factors is the Lester UK adaptation of the 'Positive Cardiometabolic Health Resource' (Shiers et al., 2014). This provides staff in mental health teams with a simple outline of which clinical measures should be monitored, what the appropriate values are for each measure and what interventions might be considered. (This resource is available at: www.rcpsych.ac.uk/docs/default-source/improving-care/ccqi/national-clinical-audits/ncap-library/ncap-e-version-nice-endorsed-lester-uk-adaptation.pdf?sfvrsn=39bab4_2.) Exercise may improve cardiovascular fitness even in the absence of weight loss.

The following sections provide a summary of relevant considerations in managing cardiovascular risk factors, other than weight gain, that are commonly encountered in people with schizophrenia and bipolar disorder.

21.6.1 Interventions for Tobacco Smoking

Smoking cessation rates for people with schizophrenia are poor – around half of those for the general population (Williams & Foulds, 2007). However, polycyclic aromatic hydrocarbons in cigarette smoke (not nicotine) induce the activity of cytochrome P450 1A2 and hence may reduce the plasma concentration of some psychotropic medications, particularly clozapine but also olanzapine, haloperidol and some antidepressants (Kroon, 2007). Thus, it is important that smoking is reduced in a controlled fashion with monitoring for indications of rising plasma drug concentrations (such as increased adverse effects) for all medications and monitoring of plasma drug concentrations for clozapine. Nicotine replacement therapy (NRT) does not affect P450 1A2 activity.

NICE public health guideline PH10 (NICE, 2008) recommends brief interventions as an initial approach to helping a person stop smoking with referral to a local smoking cessation service if appropriate. Pharmacological therapies, summarized below, are then available as a next step if required.

NRT is the most widely used treatment. Seven studies in people with chronic mental illnesses (summarized by Tidey & Miller, 2015) report abstinence rates between 9% and 23% at periods varying from 6 months to 12 months. These studies were all open-label as far as NRT was concerned but most provided some form of individual or group support, which was allocated at random. In general, the addition of such support improved abstinence rates.

There have been two small, uncontrolled studies of e-cigarettes in patients with psychosis. Both found considerable reductions in numbers of cigarettes smoked, accompanied by reductions in exhaled carbon monoxide (Minutolo et al., 2013 (n = 14 patients); Pratt et al., 2016 (n = 21 patients)). A recent uncontrolled pilot study, in the UK, recruited 50 patients (Hickling et al., 2018). These patients were offered free e-cigarettes for the first six weeks, encouraged to continue use of these, and were then followed up for 24 weeks. There was a statistically significant 50% reduction in the number of cigarettes smoked at six weeks, accompanied by reduction in exhaled carbon monoxide. The extent of these reductions diminished during the follow-up period. The patients in all of these studies found use of e-cigarettes to be acceptable and there did not appear to be relapses in psychosis related to their use.

Buproprion appears to assist initial smoking cessation in patients with schizophrenia but, as for most nicotine withdrawal treatments, relapse rates are high following discontinuation. Meta-analysis of six RCTs of buproprion, alone or combined with NRT, suggests a significant effect of buproprion (Tidey & Miller, 2015). Meta-analysis of three RCTs of the nicotinic partial agonist varenicline also suggests a significant effect (Tidey & Miller, 2015). For both buproprion and varenicline the individual studies are small and statistical significance is only seen when they are combined in a meta-analysis. There have been concerns that both buproprion and varenicline may cause adverse psychological effects (including suicidal ideation), but the evidence is conflicting.

Bennett et al. (2013) reviewed 11 studies which investigated psychosocial/behavioural approaches in people with schizophrenia and concluded there were reasonable short-term abstinence rates, but data were too variable to determine clear long-term effects. A recently reported UK pilot RCT of a bespoke smoking cessation programme for people with psychosis (SCIMITAR), compared with usual care, suggested that the bespoke programme resulted in greater effectiveness (Gilbody et al., 2015). This is being followed up with a full trial aiming to recruit 400 patients.

21.6.2 Interventions for Alcohol Misuse in Schizophrenia

There are limited data to guide clinicians in managing this situation (see Lingford-Hughes et al., 2012). A Cochrane systematic review of psychosocial interventions for co-morbid schizophrenia and substance use disorder found that none of the interventions showed clear superiority over 'treatment as usual' in reducing substance use, retention in treatment or improvement in mental state (Hunt et al., 2013). One small RCT of motivational interviewing for alcohol misuse showed some promise (Hunt et al., 2013) but many studies have focused largely on illicit drugs, such as cannabis, rather than on alcohol.

There is no consistent evidence that any individual antipsychotic drugs, whether first or second generation, are more likely than others to lead to reduction in misuse of alcohol or other substances (see Lingford-Hughes et al., 2012), but most studies in this area are either small or uncontrolled. Clozapine appears to have similar effectiveness for psychosis in patients with schizophrenia and substance abuse compared with those without substance abuse but there is no clear evidence about its effect on the substance abuse.

There are few studies examining the effects of treatments to prevent relapse of alcohol misuse in people with schizophrenia. For the general population with alcohol dependence, NICE guideline CG115 recommends that acamprosate or naltrexone be offered to all those with moderate to severe dependence, with disulfiram as second line (NICE, 2011, section 1.3.5). Acamprosate and naltrexone have been used safely in patients with schizophrenia and no specific considerations are required (Lingford-Hughes et al., 2012). Nalmefene is a newer licensed alternative to naltrexone that can also be considered when binge drinking is a problem.

Disulfiram has a propensity to increase psychosis as, probably through blockade of dopamine-beta-hydroxylase, it can increase dopamine levels. Its use in psychosis is listed as a contraindication, though there is a trial of disulfiram in psychotic patients (73% with bipolar disorder) demonstrating improved drinking outcomes, without adverse consequences (Petrakis et al., 2006). There are no studies of baclofen or topiramate for alcohol misuse in people with schizophrenia.

21.6.3 Interventions for Pre-Diabetes and Diabetes

The identification of a person's degree of risk for developing diabetes is an important step in determining the level of preventative measures required. The current NICE Public Health guidance (PH38) for the general population *Preventing type 2 diabetes: risk identification and interventions for individuals at high risk* (NICE, 2012) provides detail of how to approach this and is entirely consistent with the NICE guideline on schizophrenia (CG178; NICE, 2014a). Stage 1 of the NICE diabetes risk identification process recommends that clinicians and their patients should be encouraged to make use of validated questionnaires or web-based risk tools to assess the level of risk for an individual (e.g. http://riskscore.diabetes.org.uk/results on the Diabetes UK website).

For those at 'high risk', which includes people with psychosis and on antipsychotic medications, NICE recommends that a blood test should be offered at least once annually and more often if weight is increasing or symptoms of possible diabetes develop (polyuria, nocturia, polydipsia, tiredness, visual disturbance and candida infection). This can be a fasting plasma glucose or HbA_{1c}, the latter now being regarded as an appropriate alternative to fasting plasma glucose by the World Health Organization.

For the general population, NICE PH38 recommends a 'lifestyle' approach for those with increased risk of developing diabetes. However, as discussed earlier, it suggests that some individuals at high risk of developing diabetes may require to be considered for treatment with metformin. This guidance should be taken into consideration for people with psychosis.

Decisions regarding management of definite impairment of fasting glycaemia or glucose tolerance, or regarding the management of diabetes, should ideally be made by the patient's primary care physician or by a consultant physician. Initial risk assessment and investigation may be by the mental health team or primary care physician. Ideally medications that may contribute to weight gain should be avoided but this is often very difficult or impossible in the case of antipsychotic treatment. The NICE clinical guideline on the management of type 2 diabetes (*Type 2 diabetes in adults: management*, NG28; NICE, 2015) provides guidance on management and links to the relevant NICE pathway. It is important to remember to monitor patients for the many potentially serious consequences of diabetes.

21.6.4 Managing Dyslipidaemia and Hypertension

Patients with hypertension should be referred to their primary care physician for further investigation and management. Note that some antipsychotic medications may enhance the hypotensive effect of the commonly prescribed antihypertensive medications.

Dyslipidaemia in patients with psychosis may be associated with weight gain or the development of metabolic syndrome. The principal interventions described above for these problems (lifestyle change, antipsychotic switching, adjunctive aripiprazole, adjunctive metformin) have all been found to improve lipid profiles in most, though not all, clinical trials. Thus, if it has been feasible to employ one of these interventions, lipid profile should be reviewed after some weeks.

However, patients with persistent dyslipidaemia should be referred to their primary care physician. All people with dyslipidaemia should receive advice about diet, exercise, weight management and smoking cessation. After screening for the person's risk of CVD (usually with QRISK2 or QRISK3 in the UK), prescription of a statin should be considered for people who have a 10% or greater 10-year risk of developing CVD. Generally, people in these categories will be over 40 years of age. The cost-effectiveness and safety of prescribing statins before the age of 40 years is not clear, particularly for women of childbearing age. However, for people with diabetes aged 18 to 39 years who have one of: diabetic complications; poor blood glucose control; hypertension; features of the metabolic syndrome; or family history of premature CVD in a first-degree relative, at least one of which may often be present in a service user with psychosis, then some guidelines suggest commencing a statin (see Cooper et al., 2016 for further details).

Prescription of a statin requires monitoring of hepatic transaminase enzymes at baseline, 3 months and 12 months. Statins are contraindicated in pregnancy and ideally should be stopped 3 months before conception.

References

Alberti KGMM, Eckel RH, Grundy SM, et al. (2009). Harmonizing the metabolic syndrome. *Circulation*, 120, 1640–1645.

Allison DB, Mentore JL, Heo M, et al. (1999). Antipsychotic-induced weight gain: a comprehensive research synthesis. *Am J Psychiatry*, 156, 1686–1696.

Aronne LJ, Wadden T, Isoldi KK, et al. (2009). When prevention fails, obesity treatment strategies. *Am J Med*, 122(4 Suppl 1), S24–S32.

Arranz B, Rosel P, Ramirez N, et al. (2004). Insulin resistance and increased leptin concentrations in noncompliant schizophrenia patients but not in antipsychotic-naive first-episode schizophrenia patients. *J Clin Psychiatry*, 65, 1335–1342.

Barnes TRE, Mutsatsa SH, Hutton SB, et al. (2006). Comorbid substance use and age of onset in schizophrenia: the West London first episode study. *Br J Psychiatry*, 188, 237–242.

Barnes TRE, Paton C, Cavanagh M-R; UK Prescribing Observatory for Mental Health (2007). A UK audit of screening for the metabolic side effects of antipsychotics in community patients. *Schizophr Bull*, 33, 1397–1403.

Barnes TRE, Bhatti SF, Adroer R, et al. (2015). Screening for the metabolic side effects of antipsychotic medication: findings from a 6-year quality improvement programme in the UK. *BMJ Open*, 5, e007633.

Barr RS, Culhane MA, Jubelt LE, et al. (2008). The effects of transdermal nicotine on cognition in nonsmokers with schizophrenia and nonpsychiatric controls. *Neuropsychopharmacology*, 33, 480–490.

Bartoli F, Crocamo C, Clerici M, et al. (2015). Second-generation antipsychotics and adiponectin levels in schizophrenia: a comparative meta-analysis. *Eur Neuropsychopharmacol*, 25, 1767–1774.

Bennett ME, Wilson AL, Genderson M, et al. (2013). Smoking cessation in people with schizophrenia. *Curr Drug Abuse Rev*, 13, 180–190.

Bobo WV, Cooper WO, Stein M, et al. (2013). Antipsychotics and the risk of type 2 diabetes mellitus in children and youth. *JAMA Psychiatry*, 70, 1067–1075.

Breese CR, Lee MJ, Adams CE, et al. (2000). Abnormal regulation of high affinity nicotinic receptors in subjects with schizophrenia. *Neuropsychopharmacology*, 23, 351–364.

Brown S (1997). Excess mortality of schizophrenia. A meta-analysis. *Br J Psychiatry*, 171, 502–508.

Bruins J, Jorg F, Bruggeman R, et al. (2014). The effects of lifestyle interventions on (long-term) weight management, cardiometabolic risk and depressive symptoms in people with psychotic disorders, a meta-analysis. *PLoS One*, 9, e112276.

Bushe CJ, Slooff CJ, Haddad PM, Karagianis JL (2012). Weight change from 3-year observational data: findings from the worldwide schizophrenia outpatient health outcomes database. *J Clin Psychiatry*, 73(6), e749–e755.

Caemmerer J, Correll CU, Maayan L (2012). Acute and maintenance effects of non-pharmacologic interventions for antipsychotic associated weight gain and metabolic abnormalities: a meta-analytic comparison of randomized controlled trials. *Schizophr Res*, 140, 159–168.

Chiu C, Chen C, Chen B, et al. (2010). The time-dependent change of insulin secretion in schizophrenic patients treated with olanzapine. *Prog Neuropsychopharmacol Biol Psychiatry*, 34, 866–870.

Clifton PG, Rusk IN, Cooper SJ (1991). Effects of dopamine D1 and dopamine D2 antagonists on the free feeding and drinking patterns of rats. *Behav Neurosci*, 105, 272–281.

Connolly V, Unwin N, Sherriff P, et al. (2000). Diabetes prevalence and socioeconomic status, a population based study showing increased prevalence of type 2 diabetes mellitus in deprived areas. *J Epidemiol Community Health*, 54, 173–177.

Cooper SJ, Reynolds GP, Barnes TRE, et al. (2016). BAP guidelines on the management of weight gain and metabolic disturbances and cardiovascular risk associated with psychosis and antipsychotic drug treatment. *J Psychopharmacol*, 30, 717–748.

Correll CU, Manu P, Olshanskiy V, et al. (2009). Cardiometabolic risk of second-generation antipsychotic medications during first-time use in children and adolescents. *JAMA*, 302(16), 1765–1773.

Correll CU, Robinson DG, Schooler NR (2014). Cardiometabolic risk in patients with first-episode schizophrenia spectrum disorders. *JAMA Psychiatry*, 71, 1350–1363.

Daumit GL, Goldberg RW, Anthony C (2005). Physical activity patterns in adults with severe mental illness. *J Nerv Ment Dis*, 193, 641–646.

Daumit GL, Goff DC, Meyer JM, et al. (2008). Antipsychotic effects on estimated 10-year coronary heart disease risk in the CATIE schizophrenia study. *Schizophr Res*, 105, 175–187.

Daumit GL, Dickerson FB, Wang N, et al. (2013). A behavioral weight-loss intervention in persons with serious mental illness. *N Engl J Med*, 368, 1594–1602.

De Hert M, Dekker JM, Wood D, et al. (2009a). Cardiovascular disease and diabetes in people with severe mental illness position statement from the European Psychiatric Association (EPA), supported by the European Association for the Study of Diabetes (EASD) and the European Society of Cardiology (ESC). *Eur Psychiatry*, 24, 412–424.

De Hert M, Schreurs V, Vancampfort D, et al. (2009b). Metabolic syndrome in people with schizophrenia, a review. *World Psychiatry*, 8, 15–22.

De Hert M, Correll CU, Bobes J, et al. (2011). Physical illness in patients with severe mental disorders. I. Prevalence, impact of medications and disparities in health care. *World Psychiatry*, 10, 52–77.

Deng C, Lian J, Pai N, et al. (2012). Reducing olanzapine-induced weight gain side effect by using betahistine: a study in the rat model. *J Psychopharmacol*, 26, 1271–1279.

Department of Health (2016). *Alcohol Guidelines Review – report from the guidelines development group to the UK Chief Medical Officers*. London: Department of Health. Available at: www.gov.uk/government/consultations/health-risks-from-alcohol-new-guidelines (last accessed 16.8.19).

Dombrowsi SU, Avenell A, Sniehotta FF (2010). Behavioural interventions for obese adults with additional risk factors for morbidity: systematic review of effects on behaviour, weight and disease risk factors. *Obes Facts*, 3, 377–396.

Druss BG, Von Esenwein SA, Glick GE, et al. (2017). Randomized trial of an integrated behavioral health home: the Health Outcomes Management and Evaluation (HOME) study. *Am J Psychiatry*, 174(3), 246–255.

Fan X, Borba CPC, Copeland P, et al. (2013). Metabolic effects of adjunctive aripiprazole in clozapine-treated patients with schizophrenia. *Acta Psychiatr Scand*, 127, 217–226.

Faulkner G, Cohn T, Remington G, et al. (2007). Body mass index, waist circumference and quality of life in individuals with schizophrenia. *Schizophr Res*, 90, 174–178.

Fernandez-Sola J (2015). Cardiovascular risks and benefits of moderate and heavy alcohol consumption. *Nat Rev Cardiol*, 12, 576–587. doi:10.1038/nrcardio.2015.91.

Fleischhacker WW, Heikkinen ME, Olie J-P, et al. (2010). Effects of adjunctive treatment with aripiprazole on body weight and clinical efficacy in schizophrenia patients treated with clozapine, a randomized, double-blind, placebo-controlled trial. *Int J Psychopharmacol*, 13, 1115–1125.

Fleischhacker WW, Siu CO, Bodén R, et al.; EUFEST study group (2013). Metabolic risk factors in first-episode schizophrenia: baseline prevalence and course analysed from the European First-Episode Schizophrenia Trial. *Int J Psychopharmacol*, 16, 987–995.

Foley DL, Morley KI (2011). Systematic review of early cardiometabolic outcomes of the first treated episode of psychosis. *Arch Gen Psychiatry*, 68, 609–616.

Gafoor R, Booth P, Gulliford MC (2018). Antidepressant utilisation and incidence of weight gain during 10 years' follow-up: population based cohort study. *BMJ*, 361, k1951. http://dx.doi.org/10.1136/bmj.k1951.

Gilbody S, Peckham E, Man M-S, et al. (2015). Bespoke smoking cessation for people with severe mental ill health (SCIMITAR), a pilot randomised controlled trial. *Lancet Psychiatry*, 2, 395–402.

Hamoui N, Kingsbury S, Anthone GJ, et al. (2004). Surgical treatment of morbid obesity in schizophrenic patients. *Obes Surg*, 14, 349–352.

Hasan A, Falkai P, Wobrock T, et al. (2013). World Federation of Societies of Biological Psychiatry (WFSBP) guidelines for biological treatment of schizophrenia: part 2, update 2012 on the long-term treatment of schizophrenia and management of antipsychotic-induced side effects. *World J Biol Psychiatry*, 14, 2–44.

Hegedűs C, Kovacs D, Kiss R, et al. (2015). Effect of long-term olanzapine treatment on meal-induced insulin sensitization and on gastrointestinal peptides in female Sprague–Dawley rats. *J Psychopharmacol*, 29, 1271–1279.

Henderson DC, Cagliero E, Copeland PM, et al. (2005). Glucose metabolism in patients with schizophrenia treated with atypical antipsychotic agents. *Arch Gen Psychiatry*, 62, 19–28.

Henderson DC, Kunkel L, Nguyen DD, et al. (2006). An exploratory open-label trial of aripiprazole as an adjuvant to clozapine therapy in chronic schizophrenia. *Acta Psychiatr Scand*, 113, 142–147.

Henderson DC, Fan X, Copeland PM, et al. (2009). Aripiprazole added to overweight and obese olanzapine-treated schizophrenia patients. *J Clin Psychopharmacol*, 29, 165–169.

Hermes E, Nasrallah H, Davis V, et al. (2011). The association between weight change and symptom reduction in the CATIE schizophrenia trial. *Schizophr Res*, 128, 166–170.

Hickling LM, Perez-Iglesias R, McNeill A, et al. (2018). A pre-post pilot study of electronic cigarettes to reduce smoking in people with severe mental illness. *Psychol Med*, 49, 1033–1040. https://doi.org/10.1017/S0033291718001782.

Hippisley-Cox J, Coupland C, Brindle P (2017). Development and validation of QRISK3 risk prediction algorithms to estimate future risk of cardiovascular disease: prospective cohort study. *BMJ*, 357, j2099.

Hjorthoj C, Østergaard ML, Benros ME, et al. (2015). Association between alcohol and substance use disorders and all-cause and cause-specific mortality in schizophrenia, bipolar disorder, and unipolar depression: a nationwide, prospective, register-based study. *Lancet Psychiatry*, 2(9), 801–808.

Holt RI, Mitchell AJ. (2015). Diabetes mellitus and severe mental illness, mechanisms and clinical implications. *Nat Rev Endocrinol*, 11, 79–89.

Holt RI, Gossage-Worrall R, Hind D, et al. (2019). Structured lifestyle education for people with schizophrenia, schizoaffective disorder and first-episode psychosis (STEPWISE): randomised controlled trial. *Br J Psychiatry*, 214, 63–73.

Hommel JD, Trinko R, Sears RM, et al. (2006). Leptin receptor signaling in midbrain dopamine neurons regulates feeding. *Neuron*, 51, 801–810.

Hunt GE, Siegfried N, Morley K, et al. (2013). Psychosocial interventions for people with both severe mental illness and substance misuse. *Cochrane Database Syst Rev*, (10), CD001088. doi:10.1002/14651858.CD001088.pub3.

InterAct Consortium (2014). Smoking and long-term risk of type 2 diabetes, the EPIC-InterAct study in European populations. *Diabetes Care*, 37, 3164–3171.

Ishøy PL, Knop FK, Broberg BV, et al. (2017). Effect of GLP-1 receptor agonist treatment on body weight in obese antipsychotic-treated patients with schizophrenia: a randomized, placebo-controlled trial. *Diabetes Obes Metab*, 19, 162–171.

Jarskog LF, Hamer RM, Catellier DJ, et al.; METS Investigators (2013). Metformin for weight loss and metabolic control in overweight outpatients with schizophrenia and schizoaffective disorder. *Am J Psychiatry*, 170, 1032–1040.

Jin H, Meyer J, Mudaliar S, et al. (2008). Impact of atypical antipsychotic therapy on leptin, ghrelin, and adiponectin. *Schizophr Res*, 100, 70–85.

Johnson DE, Yamazaki H, Ward KM, et al. (2005). Inhibitory effects of antipsychotics on carbachol-enhanced insulin secretion from perfused rat islets: role of muscarinic antagonism in antipsychotic-induced diabetes and hyperglycemia. *Diabetes*, 54, 1552–1558.

Kahn RS, Fleischhacker WW, Boter H (2008). Effectiveness of antipsychotic drugs in first-episode schizophrenia and schizophreniform disorder, an open randomised clinical trial. *Lancet*, 371, 1085–1097.

Kelly C, McCreadie R (2000). Cigarette smoking and schizophrenia. *Adv Psychiatr Treat*, 6, 327–331.

Kim SF, Huang AS, Snowman AM, et al. (2007). From the cover: antipsychotic drug-induced weight gain mediated by histamine H1 receptor-linked activation of hypothalamic AMP-kinase. *Proc Natl Acad Sci U S A*, 104, 3456–3459.

Kinon BJ, Kaiser, CJ, Ahmed S (2005). Association between early and rapid weight gain and change in weight over one year of olanzapine therapy in patients with schizophrenia and related disorders. *J Clin Psychopharmacol*, 25, 255–258.

Kirk SL, Neill JC, Jones DN, et al. (2004). Ziprasidone suppresses olanzapine-induced increases in ingestive behaviour in the rat. *Eur J Pharmacol*, 505, 253–254.

Kirk SL, Glazebrook J, Grayson B, et al. (2009). Olanzapine-induced weight gain in the rat, role of 5-HT2C and histamine H1 receptors. *Psychopharmacology*, 207, 119–125.

Kodama S, Horikawa C, Fujihara K, et al. (2014). Quantitative relationship between body weight gain in adulthood and incident type 2 diabetes: a meta-analysis. *Obes Rev*, 15, 202–214.

Koskinen J, Löhönen J, Koponen H, et al. (2009). Prevalence of alcohol use disorders in schizophrenia – a systematic review and meta-analysis. *Acta Psychiatr Scand*, 120, 85–96.

Kramer CK, Leitao C, Pinto LC, et al. (2011). Efficacy and safety of topiramate on weight loss, a meta-analysis of randomized controlled trials. *Obes Rev*, 12, e338–e347. doi:10.1111/j.1467-789X.2010.00846.x.

Kroeze WK, Hufeisen SJ, Popadak BA, et al. (2003). H1-histamine receptor affinity predicts short-term weight gain for typical and atypical antipsychotic drugs. *Neuropsychopharmacology*, 28, 519–526.

Kroon LA (2007). Drug interactions with smoking. *Am J Health Syst Pharm*, 64(18), 1917–1921.

Larsen JR, Vedtofte L, Jakobsen MSL, et al. (2017). Effect of liraglutide treatment on prediabetes and overweight or obesity in clozapine- or olanzapine-treated patients with schizophrenia spectrum disorder a randomized clinical trial. *JAMA Psychiatry*, 74, 719–728.

Lawrence D, Hancock KJ, Kisely S (2013). The gap in life expectancy from preventable physical illness in psychiatric patients in Western Australia: retrospective analysis of population based registers. *BMJ*, 346, f2539.

Lester H, Marshall M, Jones P, et al. (2011). Views of young people in early intervention services for first-episode psychosis in England. *Psychiatr Serv*, 62, 882–887.

Leucht S, Cipriani A, Spineli L, et al. (2013). Comparative efficacy and tolerability of 15 antipsychotic drugs in schizophrenia: a multiple-treatments meta-analysis. *Lancet*, 382, 951–962.

Lingford-Hughes AR, Welch S, Peters L, et al. (2012). BAP updated guidelines: evidence-based guidelines for the pharmacological management of substance abuse, harmful use, addiction and comorbidity, recommendations from BAP. *J Psychopharmacol*, 26, 899–952.

Manu P, Dima L, Shulman M (2015). Weight gain and obesity in schizophrenia, epidemiology, pathobiology, and management. *Acta Psychiatr Scand*, 132, 97–108.

Matsui-Sakata A, Ohtani H, Sawada Y (2005). Receptor occupancy-based analysis of the contributions of various receptors to antipsychotics-induced weight gain and diabetes mellitus. *Drug Metab Pharmacokinet*, 20, 368–378.

McCreadie RG; Sottish Schizophrenia Lifestyle Group (2003). Diet, smoking and cardiovascular risk in people with schizophrenia. *Br J Psychiatry*, 183, 534–539.

McManus S, Bebbington P, Jenkins R, Brugha T (eds.) (2016). *Adult Psychiatric Morbidity Survey: Mental Health and Wellbeing, England, 2014*. Leeds: NHS Digital.

McQuade RD, Stock E, Marcus R, et al. (2004). A comparison of weight change during treatment with olanzapine or aripiprazole, results from a randomised, double-blind study. *J Clin Psychiatry*, 65, 47–56.

Meyer JM, Davis VG, McEvoy JP, et al. (2008). Impact of antipsychotic treatment on non-fasting triglycerides in the CATIE Schizophrenia Trial phase 1. *Schizophr Res*, 103, 104–109.

Minutolo G, Caponnetto P, Auditore R, et al. (2013). Management of smoking reduction and cessation in inpatients with schizophrenia: impact of electronic cigarettes. *Eur Neuropsychopharmacol*, 23(Suppl 2), S581–S582.

Mitchell AJ, Malone D, Doebbeling CC (2009). Quality of medical care for people with and without comorbid mental illness and substance misuse, systematic review of comparative studies. *Br J Psychiatry*, 194, 491–499.

Mitchell AJ, Vancampfort D, DeHerdt A, et al. (2013a). Is the prevalence of metabolic syndrome and metabolic abnormalities increased in early schizophrenia? A comparative meta-analysis of first episode, untreated and treated patients. *Schizophr Bull*, 39, 295–305.

Mitchell AJ, Vancampfort D, Sweers K, et al. (2013b). Prevalence of metabolic syndrome and metabolic abnormalities in schizophrenia and related disorders. A review and meta-analysis. *Schizophr Bull*, 39, 306–318.

Mizuno Y, Suzuki T, Nakagawa A, et al. (2014). Pharmacological strategies to counteract antipsychotic-induced weight gain and metabolic adverse effects in schizophrenia, a systematic review and meta-analysis. *Schizophr Bull*, 40, 1385–1403.

Mothi SS, Tandon N, Padmanabhan J, et al. (2015). Increased cardiometabolic dysfunction in first-degree relatives of patients with psychotic disorders. *Schizophr Res*, 165, 103–107.

Mukundan A, Faulkner G, Cohn T, et al. (2010). Antipsychotic switching for people with schizophrenia who have neuroleptic-induced weight or metabolic problems. *Cochrane Database Syst Rev*, (12), CD006629. doi:10.1002/14651858.CD006629.pub2.

Muscatello MRA, Bruno A, Pandolfo G, et al. (2011). Effect of aripiprazole augmentation of clozapine in schizophrenia, a double-blind, placebo-controlled study. *Schizophr Res*, 127, 93–99.

Myles N, Newall HD, Curtis J, et al. (2012). Tobacco use before, at, and after first-episode psychosis, a systematic meta-analysis. *J Clin Psychiatry*, 73, 468–475.

National Institute for Health and Care Excellence (NICE) (2008). *Stop smoking services*. Public health guideline [PH10]. London: National Institute for Health and Care Excellence.

National Institute for Health and Care Excellence (NICE) (2011). *Alcohol-use disorders, diagnosis, assessment and management of harmful drinking and alcohol dependence*. Clinical guideline [CG115]. London: National Institute for Health and Care Excellence.

National Institute for Health and Care Excellence (NICE) (2012). *Preventing type 2 diabetes: risk identification and interventions for individuals at high risk*. Public health guideline [PH38]. London: National Institute for Health and Care Excellence.

National Institute for Health and Care Excellence (NICE) (2014a). *Psychosis and schizophrenia in adults, prevention and management*. Clinical guideline [CG178]. London: National Institute for Health and Care Excellence.

National Institute for Health and Care Excellence (NICE) (2014b). *Cardiovascular disease: risk assessment and reduction*. Clinical guideline [CG181]. London: National Institute for Health and Care Excellence.

National Institute for Health and Care Excellence (NICE) (2014c). *Bipolar disorder, assessment and management*. Clinical guideline [CG185]. London: National Institute for Health and Care Excellence.

National Institute for Health and Care Excellence (NICE) (2014d). *Obesity, identification, assessment and management*. Clinical guideline [CG189]. London: National Institute for Health and Care Excellence.

National Institute for Health and Care Excellence (NICE) (2015). *Type 2 diabetes in adults: management*. NICE guideline [NG28]. London: National Institute for Health and Care Excellence.

Newcomer JW (2005). Second-generation (atypical) antipsychotics and metabolic effects: a comprehensive literature review. *CNS Drugs*, 19(Suppl 1), 1–93.

Newcomer JW, Haupt DW, Fucetola R, et al. (2002). Abnormalities in glucose regulation during antipsychotic treatment of schizophrenia. *Arch Gen Psychiatry*, 59, 337–345.

Olfson M, Gerhard T, Huang C (2015). Premature mortality among adults with schizophrenia in the United States. *JAMA Psychiatry*, 72, 1172–1181.

Osborn, DPJ, Levy G, Nazareth I, et al. (2007a). Relative risk of cardiovascular and cancer mortality in people with severe mental illness from the United Kingdom's general practice research database. *Arch Gen Psychiatry*, 64, 242–249.

Osborn DP, Nazareth I, King MB (2007b). Physical activity, dietary habits and coronary heart disease risk factor knowledge amongst people with severe mental illness, a cross sectional comparative study in primary care. *Soc Psychiatry Psychiatr Epidemiol*, 42, 787–793.

Osborn D, Hardoon S, Omar RZ, et al. (2015). Cardiovascular risk prediction models for people with severe mental illness. Results from the prediction and management of cardiovascular risk in people with severe mental illnesses (PRIMROSE) research program. *JAMA Psychiatry*, 72, 143–151.

Padmanabhan JL, Nanda P, Tandon N, et al. (2016). Polygenic risk for type 2 diabetes mellitus among individuals with psychosis and their relatives. *J Psychiatr Res*, 77, 52–58.

Perry BI, McIntosh G, Weich S, et al. (2016). The association between first-episode psychosis and abnormal glycaemic control, systematic review and meta-analysis. *Lancet Psychiatry*, 3, 1049–1058.

Petrakis IL, Nich C, Ralevski E (2006). Psychotic spectrum disorders and alcohol abuse, a review of pharmacotherapeutic strategies and a report on the effectiveness of naltrexone and disulfiram. *Schizophr Bull*, 32, 644–654.

Pillinger T, Beck K, Gobjila C, et al. (2017). Impaired glucose homeostasis in first-episode schizophrenia, a systematic review and meta-analysis. *JAMA Psychiatry*, 74, 261–269.

Pratt SI, Sargent J, Daniels L, et al. (2016). Appeal of electronic cigarettes in smokers with serious mental illness. *Addict Behav*, 59, 30–34.

Reynolds GP (2012). The pharmacogenetics of antipsychotic drug-induced weight gain – a critical review. *Clin Psychopharmacol Neurosci*, 10, 71–77.

Reynolds GP, Kirk SL (2010). Metabolic side effects of antipsychotic drug treatment – pharmacological mechanisms. *Pharmacol Ther*, 125, 169–179.

Reynolds GP, McGowan O (2017). Mechanisms underlying metabolic disturbances associated with psychosis and antipsychotic drug treatment. *J Psychopharmacol*, 31, 1430–1436. https//doi.org/10.1177/026988111772.

Reynolds GP, Dalton C, Watrimez W, et al. (2019). Adjunctive lurasidone suppresses food intake and weight gain associated with olanzapine administration in rats. *Clin Psychopharmacol Neurosci*, 17, 314–317.

Roffeei SN, Reynolds GP, Zainal NZ, et al. (2014). Association of ADR2A and MTHFR gene polymorphisms with weight loss following antipsychotic switching to aripiprazole and ziprasidone. *Hum Psychopharmacol*, 29, 38–45.

Royal College of Psychiatrists (2012). *Report of the National Audit of Schizophrenia (NAS) 2012*. London: Healthcare Quality Improvement Partnership.

Royal College of Psychiatrists (2014). *Report of the second round of the National Audit of Schizophrenia (NAS) 2014*. London: Healthcare Quality Improvement Partnership.

Royal College of Psychiatrists (2018). *National Clinical Audit of Psychosis – National report for the core audit 2018*. London: Healthcare Quality Improvement Partnership. Available at: www.rcpsych.ac.uk/docs/default-source/improving-care/ccqi/national-clinical-audits/ncap-library/ncap-national-report-for-core-audit-2018.pdf?sfvrsn=23c6a262_2 (last accessed 16.8.19).

Rummel-Kluge C, Komossa K, Schwarz S, et al. (2010). Head-to-head comparisons of metabolic side effects of second generation antipsychotics in the treatment of schizophrenia, a systematic review and meta-analysis. *Schizophr Res*, 123, 225–233.

Ryan MC, Collins P, Thakore JH (2003). Impaired fasting glucose tolerance in first-episode, drug-naive patients with schizophrenia. *Am J Psychiatry*, 160, 284–289.

Sengupta S, Parrilla-Escobar MA, Klink R, et al. (2008). Are metabolic indices different between drug-naive first-episode psychosis patients and healthy controls? *Schizophr Res*, 102, 329–336.

Shiers DE, Rafi I, Cooper SJ, Holt RIG (2014). *Positive Cardiometabolic Health Resource, an intervention framework for patients with psychosis and schizophrenia. 2014 update (with acknowledgement to the late Helen Lester for her contribution to the original 2012 version).* London: Royal College of Psychiatrists. Available at: www.rcpsych.ac.uk/workinpsychiatry/qualityimprovement/nationalclinicalaudits/nationalschizophreniaaudit/nasresources.aspx.

Simon V, van Winkel R, De Hert M (2009). Are weight gain and metabolic side effects of atypical antipsychotics dose dependent? A literature review. *J Clin Psychiatry*, 70, 1041–1050.

Snigdha S, Thumbi C, Reynolds GP, et al. (2008). Ziprasidone and aripiprazole attenuate olanzapine-induced hyperphagia in rats. *J Psychopharmacol*, 22, 567–571.

Spelman LM, Walsh PI, Sharifi N, et al. (2007). Impaired glucose tolerance in first-episode drug-naive patients with schizophrenia. *Diabetes Med*, 24, 481–485.

Speyer H, Christian Brix Nørgaard H, Birk M, et al. (2016). The CHANGE trial: no superiority of lifestyle coaching plus care coordination plus treatment as usual compared to treatment as usual alone in reducing risk of cardiovascular disease in adults with schizophrenia spectrum disorders and abdominal obesity. *World Psychiatry*, 15(2), 155–165.

Stahl SM, Cucchiaro J, Simonelli D, et al. (2013). Effectiveness of lurasidone for patients with schizophrenia following 6 weeks of acute treatment with lurasidone, olanzapine, or placebo: a 6-month, open-label, extension study. *J Clin Psychiatry*, 74, 507–515.

Stokes C, Peet M (2004). Dietary sugar and polyunsaturated fatty acid consumption as predictors of severity of schizophrenia symptoms. *Nutr Neurosci*, 7, 247–249.

Tagami K, Kashiwase Y, Yokoyama A, et al. (2016). The atypical antipsychotic, olanzapine, potentiates ghrelin-induced receptor signaling: an in vitro study with cells expressing cloned human growth hormone secretagogue receptor. *Neuropeptides*, 58, 93–101.

Taylor D, Paton C, Kapur S (2012). *The Maudsley Prescribing Guidelines in Psychiatry*, 11th ed. London: Wiley Blackwell.

Teasdale SB, Ward PB, Rosenbaum S, et al. (2017). Solving a weighty problem: systematic review and meta-analysis of nutrition interventions in sevmental illness. *Br J Psychiatry*, 210, 110–118.

Tidey JW, Miller ME (2015). Smoking cessation and reduction in people with chronic mental illness. *BMJ*, 351, h4065.

Tiihonen J, Lönnqvist J, Wahlbeck K, et al. (2009). 11-year follow-up of mortality in patients with schizophrenia, a population-based cohort study (FIN11 study). *Lancet*, 374, 620–627.

Toalson P, Ahmed S, Hardy T, et al. (2004). The metabolic syndrome in patients with severe mental illnesses. *Prim Care Companion J Clin Psychiatry*, 6, 152–158.

Vancampfort D, Wampers M, Mitchell AJ, et al. (2013). A meta-analysis of cardio-metabolic abnormalities in drug naive, first-episode and multi-episode patients with schizophrenia versus general population controls. *World Psychiatry*, 12, 240–250.

Vandenberghe F, Gholam-Rezaee M, Saigí-Morgui N (2015). Importance of early weight changes to predict long-term weight gain during psychotropic drug treatment. *J Clin Psychiatry*, 76, e1417–e1423.

Wang H, Peng D-Q (2011). New insights into the mechanism of low high-density lipoprotein cholesterol in obesity. *Lipids Health Dis*, 10, 176. https://doi.org/10.1186/1476-511X-10-176.

Weiden PJ, Mackell JA, McDonnell DD (2004). Obesity as a risk factor for antipsychotic noncompliance. *Schizophr Res*, 66, 51–57.

Weiden PJ, Newcomer JW, Loebel AD, et al. (2008). Long-term changes in weight and plasma lipids during maintenance treatment with ziprasidone. *Neuropsychopharmacology*, 33, 985–994.

Williams JM, Foulds J (2007). Successful tobacco dependence treatment in schizophrenia. *Am J Psychiatry*, 164, 222–227.

World Health Organization (2010). *Hidden cities: unmasking and overcoming health inequities in urban settings*. Geneva: WHO Press.

Wu RR, Jin H, Gao K, et al. (2012). Metformin for treatment of antipsychotic-induced amenorrhea and weight gain in women with first-episode schizophrenia, a double-blind, randomized, placebo-controlled study. *Am J Psychiatry*, 169, 813–821.

Yevtushenko OO, Cooper SJ, O'Neill R, et al. (2008). Influence of 5-HT2C receptor and leptin gene polymorphisms, smoking and drug treatment on metabolic disturbances in patients with schizophrenia. *Br J Psychiatry*, 192, 424–428.

Zhang JP, Lencz T, Zhang RX, et al. (2016). Pharmacogenetic associations of antipsychotic drug-related weight gain, a systematic review and meta-analysis. *Schizophr Bull*, 42, 1418–1437.

Zhang ZJ, Yao ZJ, Liu W, et al. (2004). Effects of antipsychotics on fat deposition and changes in leptin and insulin levels. Magnetic resonance imaging study of previously untreated people with schizophrenia. *Br J Psychiatry*, 184, 58–62.

Zhu Y, Krause M, Huhn M, et al. (2017). Antipsychotic drugs for the acute treatment of patients with a first episode of schizophrenia: a systematic review with pairwise and network meta-analyses. *Lancet Psychiatry*, 4(9), 694–705.

Index